Journal of Transcultural Nursing

Volume 21   Supplement 1   October 2010

Volume 21   Supplement I   October 2010

Journal of
Transcultural
Nursing

Core Curriculum for Transcultural Nursing and Health Care

Contents

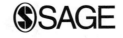

Los Angeles | London | New Delhi
Singapore | Washington DC

The **Journal of Transcultural Nursing** is the official journal of the Transcultural Nursing Society. The mission of the journal is to serve as a peer-reviewed forum for nurses, health care professionals, and practitioners in related disciplines to discuss issues related to the advancement of knowledge in the areas of culturally congruent health care delivery and to promote the dissemination of research findings concerning the relationship among culture, nursing and other related disciplines, and the delivery of health care.

Manuscripts: Visit http://mc.manuscriptcentral.com/tcn. For any difficulty with online submission, please contact Marjory Spraycar, editorial manager, at m.spraycar@verizon.net.

Journal of Transcultural Nursing (ISSN 1043-6596; ISBN: 1-4129-9249-4) (J381) is published quarterly—in January, April, July, and October—by SAGE Publications, Thousand Oaks, CA 91320. Send address changes to Journal of Transcultural Nursing, c/o SAGE Publications, 2455 Teller Road, Thousand Oaks, CA 91320.

Subscription Information: All subscription inquiries, orders, back issues, claims, and renewals should be addressed to SAGE Publications, 2455 Teller Road, Thousand Oaks, CA 91320; telephone: (800) 818-SAGE (7243) and (805) 499-0721; fax: (805) 375-1700; e-mail: journals@sagepub.com; http://www.sagepublications.com. **Current volume pricing:** Institutions: $621; Individuals: $136. For all customers outside the Americas, please visit http://www.sagepub.co.uk/customerCare.nav for information. **Claims:** Claims for undelivered copies must be made no later than six months following month of publication. The publisher will supply missing copies when losses have been sustained in transit and when the reserve stock will permit.

Member Information: Transcultural Nursing Society member inquiries, change of address, back issues, claims, and membership renewal requests should be addressed to Transcultural Nursing Society, Madonna University, College of Nursing and Health, 36600 Schoolcraft Road, Livonia, MI 48150-1173; telephone: (888) 432-5470; fax: (734) 432-5463; e-mail: staff@tcns.org; Web site: http://www.tcns.org/. The publisher will supply missing copies when losses have been sustained in transit and when the reserve stock will permit at the request of the Transcultural Nursing Society.

Abstracting and Indexing: Please visit http://tcn.sagepub.com and, under the "More about this journal" menu on the right-hand side, click on the Abstracting/Indexing link to view a full list of databases in which this journal is indexed.

Copyright Permission: Permission requests to photocopy or otherwise reproduce copyrighted material owned by SAGE Publications should be submitted to Copyright Clearance Center's Rightslink® service through the journal's Web site. Permission may also be requested by contacting the Copyright Clearance Center via their Web site at http://www.copyright.com, or via e-mail at info@copyright.com.

Advertising and Reprints: Current advertising rates and specifications may be obtained by contacting the advertising coordinator in the Thousand Oaks office at (805) 410-7772 or by sending an e-mail to advertising@sagepub.com. Acceptance of advertising in this journal in no way implies endorsement of the advertised product or service by SAGE, the journal's affliated society(ies), or the journal editor(s). No endorsement is intended or implied. SAGE reserves the right to reject any advertising it deems as inappropriate for this journal. To order reprints, please call (805) 410-7763 or e-mail reprint@sagepub.com.

Change of Address: Six weeks' advance notice must be given when notifying of change of address. Please send old address label along with the new address to ensure proper identification. Please specify name of journal.

Printed on acid-free paper

Preface

Journal of Transcultural Nursing
21(Supplement 1) 5S–6S
© The Author(s) 2010
Reprints and permission:
sagepub.com/journalsPermissions.nav
DOI: 10.1177/1043659610384464
http://tcn.sagepub.com
⑤SAGE

The development of this *Core Curriculum* has traveled a long and circuitous path. The field of transcultural nursing has its roots in the works of Madeleine Leininger, who in 1966, submitted her dissertation research on the Gadsup peoples of New Guinea (Leininger, 1966). Her subsequent publication in 1970, *Nursing and Anthropology: Two Worlds to Blend* (Leininger, 1970), ignited the flame that would inspire nurses and other health care professionals to explore the relationship between health and culture and its implications for the delivery of health care.

The field developed rapidly as numerous nurse researchers investigated culturally-based health care values, beliefs, caring practices and related phenomena of various ethnic and cultural groups. Ultimately, the need arose to define the distinct body of knowledge and practice that encompasses transcultural nursing (TCN). The first TCN certification examination was administered in 1987 under the auspices of the Transcultural Nursing Society (TCNS). The format of the early exams, however, limited the number of examinees while the demand grew.

In 2003, the Circle of Presidents, formed by then-President Dula Pacquiao, undertook as one of its major tasks to examine the structure and process of certification. As its initial work, a survey of members of the Transcultural Nursing Society (TCNS) was conducted; results indicated a need for more standardization of the exam, an independent credentialing body, and a request for a Core Curriculum that would outline the unique body of knowledge of transcultural nursing. The Certification Structure Task Force, chaired by Fran Wenger, was formed to develop a proposal that addressed these needs. In May, 2006, the Board of Trustees of the TCN Society approved the recommendations of the Task Force, which included the formation of the TCN Certification Commission and its accompanying by-laws, committee structure and business plan. Subsequently, in June 2007, the Board of Trustees of the TCN Society recommended that a comprehensive TCN Core Curriculum be developed, as per the report of the TCN Certification Task Force. The following text is a culmination of this work.

The *Core Curriculum* aims to establish a core base of knowledge that supports TCN practice. This body of knowledge is drawn from the breadth of substantive knowledge from the social and behavioral sciences, philosophy and nursing. This is reflected in the varied background of contributors and reviewers whose collective expertise facilitated the development of this *Core Curriculum*.

Transcultural nursing practice incorporates education, research, administration and direct care provision within the multilevel contexts of the individual, organization, community, society and the world as a whole. The goal of TCN practice is to promote health and well-being of individuals and populations by reducing health and care disparities through culturally congruent and competent approaches at the multilevel contexts of care.

The *Core Curriculum* is divided into four sections. Section I provides an overview of global health issues and a comparative examination of health care delivery systems in selected countries. Deeper awareness of health and care disparities is fostered by a comparative and global understanding of populations and health systems. Section II presents a comprehensive foundation of theories and concepts underlying TCN that are drawn from nursing and other relevant disciplines critical to the application of TCN in different practice roles and contexts. Cross-cultural communication transcends the various dimensions of TCN practices in the application of TCN knowledge. Section III focuses on TCN phenomena critical to direct care provision, explicating the universal and culture-specific aspects of care giving. Culturally congruent and competent care is built on an understanding of culturally-based health beliefs and caring practices and the process of cultural health assessment. Section IV focuses on TCN practice in education, administration and research. Sections III and IV provide a continuum of TCN practice from basic to advanced practice roles. The last chapter in this section focuses on the individual development of the professional role of a TCN, which links all the critical components to becoming a TCN nurse. The *Core Curriculum* is designed to facilitate the professional development of a TCN nurse capable of practicing in different roles and settings by demonstrating the application of TCN core knowledge.

Without the support and encouragement of numerous persons and agencies, this work would not have reached fruition. Dan Ruth, Acquisition Editor at Sage Publications, Inc., was the first and most steadfast in encouraging this work. Major funding was provided by The California Endowment, a private foundation dedicated to expanding access to affordable, quality health care for underserved individuals and communities. Additional funding was provided by the U.S. Health Resources and Services Administration *(HRSA)*, through a grant titled "Developing Cultural Competencies for Nurses: Evidence-based Best Practices," led by principal investigator Margaret Andrews.

This Core Curriculum is a compendium of the work of 53 authors, 37 reviewers and 4 Associate Editors, all with expertise in their particular aspects of transcultural nursing. The support staff, those indispensible members of the team who help meld the final product, included Maureen Thomas, TCN Production Manager, Lisa Dobson, Project Managing Consultant, and Michele Bitinis, Production Editor at Sage Publications, Inc. Graduate Assistant Beatriz Maria Yabur performed the unenviable task of checking the references for the entire text. The editors are deeply indebted to all of these persons and agencies for their support, diligence, persistence, and above all, for their efforts in producing a text of the highest quality. It is our hope and expectation that the reader will find this *Core Curriculum* a valuable and useful resource for the practice of transcultural nursing.

Marilyn "Marty" Douglas, DNSc, RN, FAAN
Editor, Journal of Transcultural Nursing
Dula F. Pacquiao, EdD, RN, CTN
Senior Editor, Journal of Transcultural Nursing

References

Leininger, M. (1966). *Convergence and divergence of human behavior: An ethnopsychological comparative study of two Gadsup villages in the Eastern Highlands of New Guinea.* Unpublished doctoral dissertation. University of Washington, Seattle. Accessed August 16, 2010, at http://depts.washington.edu/anthweb/programs/grad_phds.php

Leininger, M. (1970). *Nursing and Anthropology: Two World to Blend.* New York: John Wiley and Sons.

List of Contributors

Journal of Transcultural Nursing
21(Supplement 1) 7S–10S
© The Author(s) 2010
Reprints and permission:
sagepub.com/journalsPermissions.nav
DOI: 10.1177/1043659610385418
http://tcn.sagepub.com
⑤SAGE

Nancy L. R. Anderson, PhD, RN, FAAN
Professor Emerita, School of Nursing
University of California, Los Angeles
Los Angeles, California
Chapter 5: Explanatory Models of Health & Illness;
Adolescence: Rites of Passage
Chapter 7: Guidelines for Assessment of Persons from
Different Cultures; Interview Techniques; Community
Assessment

Margaret Andrews, PhD, RN, CTN, FAAN
Director and Professor of Nursing
School of Health Professions and Studies
University of Michigan-Flint
Flint, Michigan
Chapter 3: Transcultural Concepts in Nursing Care
Chapter 5: Child Care and Parenting Practices
Chapter 7: Andrews & Boyle Transcultural Nursing
Assessment Guide

Jeffrey R. Backstrand, PhD
Associate Professor, School of Nursing
Joint PhD in Urban Systems
University of Medicine and Dentistry of New Jersey
Newark New Jersey
Chapter 3: Archeology of Knowledge (Foucault);
Cultural Materialism (Harris); Ecosocial Model
(Krieger); Maintenance of Social Hierarchies
(Bourdieu); Symbolic Interactionism

Joyceen S. Boyle, PhD, RN, CTN, FAAN
Professor Emerita, College of Nursing
University of Arizona
Tucson, Arizona
Chapter 3: Transcultural Concepts in Nursing Care
Chapter 7: Andrews & Boyle Transcultural Nursing
Assessment Guide

Katherine N. Bent, PhD, RN, CNS
Chief, Healthcare Delivery and
Methodologies Integrated Review Group
National Institutes of Health
Bethesda, Maryland
Chapter 5: End-of Life Decisions and Practices

Josepha Campinha-Bacote, PhD, MAR, PMHCNS-BC,
CTN-A, FAAN
President
Transcultural C.A.R.E. Associates, Cincinnati, Ohio
Assistant Clinical Professor,
Case Western University, Cleveland, Ohio
Chapter 3: The Process of Cultural Competence in the
Delivery of Healthcare Services Model

Lauren Clark, PhD, RN, FAAN
Professor, College of Nursing
University of Utah
Sandy, Utah
Chapter 6: Complementary & Alternative
Therapies

Alison Colbert, PhD, APRN-BC
Assistant Professor, School of Nursing
Duquesne University
Pittsburgh, Pennsylvania
Chapter 6: Disaster Care: Care of Victims of Natural
Disasters

Ruth E. Davidhizar, DNSc, RN, APRN, BC, FAAN
  (deceased)
Former Dean and Professor, Division of Nursing
Bethel College
Mishawaka, Indiana
Chapter 3: The Giger and Davidhizar Transcultural
Assessment Model
Chapter 7: Cultural Health Assessment: Physical
Assessment

Marilyn K. Douglas, DNSc, RN, FAAN
Associate Clinical Professor, School of Nursing
University of California, San Francisco
San Francisco, California
Chapter 5: End-of-Life Decisions and Practices:
Organ Donation and Transplantation;
Chapter 10: Human Subjects Protection in Research

Dawn Doutrich, PhD, RN, CNS
Associate Professor, College of Nursing
Washington State University
Vancouver, Washington
Chapter 3: Worldviews; Essential Concepts
Related to Learning and Socialization;
Social Categories; Cultural Conflicts

Mercedes Echevarria, DNP, APN
Assistant Professor, School of Nursing
University of Medicine and Dentistry of
  New Jersey
Newark, New Jersey
Chapter 3: Cultural Safety

Cheryl V. Elhammoumi, MSN, RN, CCRN
Clinical Instructor, College of Nursing
East Carolina University,
Greenville, North Carolina
Chapter 5: Cultural Implications for Care of Patients
with Acute Illness & Trauma

Robin L. Eubanks, PhD
Associate Professor, School of Health Related
    Professions
Department of Interdisciplinary Studies
University of Medicine & Dentistry of New Jersey
Newark, New Jersey
Chapter 4: Health Literacy; Communicating with
    Established Family Hierarchy; Skills for Apologizing
    for Cross Cultural Errors

Jacquelyn H. Flaskerud, PhD, RN, FAAN
Professor Emerita, School of Nursing
University of California, Los Angeles
Chapter 6: Cultural Beliefs and Practices concerning
    Mental Health & Illness

Jody Glittenberg, PhD, RN, FAAN, TNS
Professor Emerita, Nursing, Anthropology, and Psychiatry
University of Arizona
Tucson, Arizona
Chapter 3: Project Genesis; Transdisciplinary/
    Transcultural Model for Health Care
Chapter 6: Intimate Partner Violence; Transcultural
    Nursing in War & Genocide

Joyce Newman Giger, EdD, APRN, BC, FAAN
Professor and Lulu Wolf Hassesnplug Endowed Chair in
    Nursing
School of Nursing
University of California, Los Angeles
Los Angeles California
Chapter 3: The Giger and Davidhizar Transcultural
    Assessment Model
Chapter 7: Cultural Health Assessment: Physical
    Assessment

Carol Holtz, PhD, RN
Professor, School of Nursing
Kennesaw State University
1000 Chastain Road
Kennesaw, Georgia 30144
Chapter 1: Global Health Issues
Chapter 2: Comparative Systems of Health Care Delivery
Chapter 3: Cultural Brokering

Marianne R. Jeffreys, EdD, RN
Professor, School of Nursing
City University of New York (CUNY)
Graduate College, New York, New York
College of Staten Island, Staten Island, New York
Chapter 3: Cultural Competence and Confidence Model
Chapter 8: Educational Issues for Students,
    Organizational Staff, Patients and Communities;
    Transcultural Self-Efficacy Tool (TSET) for students
    or staff

Ani Kalayjian, EdD, RN, DDL, BCETS
Professor, Psychology Department
Fordham University
New York, New York
Chapter 11: The Transcultural Nurse as an Advocate,
    Role Model, Entrepreneur, and in Policy Development

Janet R. Katz, PhD, RN
Associate Professor, College of Nursing
Washington State University
Spokane, Washington
Chapter 3: Worldviews; Essential Concepts Related to
    Learning and Socialization; Social Categories;
    Cultural Conflicts

Colleen Keenan, PhD, FNP-BC, WHNP-BC
Adjunct Associate Professor, School of Nursing
University of California, Los Angeles
Los Angeles, California
Chapter 5: Cultural Norms and Healthcare Disparities
    concerning Gender, Sexuality and Sexual Orientation

Jeanne K. Kemppainen, PhD, RN
Professor & Assistant Department Chair,
School of Nursing
University of North Carolina-Wilmington
Wilmington, North Carolina
Chapter 5: Cultural Factors in the Care of Patients with
    Sexually Transmitted Illnesses
Chapter 10. Critical Incident Analysis Research Method

Juliene G. Lipson, PhD, RN, FAAN
Professor Emerita, School of Nursing
University of California, San Francisco
San Francisco, California
Chapter 5: Living with Disabilities

Patti Ludwig-Beymer, PhD, RN, CTN, NEA-BC, FAAN
Chief Nursing Officer
Edward Hospital and Health Services
Naperville, Illinois
Chapter 6: Cultural Beliefs and Practices regarding Pain
    Management

Stephen R. Marrone, EdD, RN-BC, CTN-A
    Deputy Nursing Director
    Institute of Continuous Learning
State University of New York (SUNY)
Downstate Medical Center
    Brooklyn, New York
Chapter 9: Organizational Resources for Culturally
    Competent Care; Organizational Resources for Refugees
Chapter 11: Leadership Roles of the Transcultural Nurse:
    Collaboration, Scholarship, Evidence-based Practice,
    Credentialing and Certification; The Transcultural
    Nurse as an Educator and Researcher

Carolyn Thompson Martin, PhD, RN, CFNP
Assistant Professor, Department of Nursing
College of Human and Health Sciences
California State University, Stanislaus
Turlock, California
*Chapter 5: Cultural Influences on Aging and
    Older Adults*

Susan Mattson, PhD, RNC-OB, CTN, FAAN
Professor Emerita
College of Nursing & Healthcare Innovation
Arizona State University
Tempe, Arizona
*Chapter 5: Birth and Neonatal Care Practices;
    Reproduction, Pregnancy and Post-Partum Care
    Practices*

Marilyn R. McFarland, PhD, RN, FNP-BC, CTN-A
Associate Professor, Department of Nursing
School of Health Professions and Studies
University of Michigan-Flint
Flint, Michigan
*Chapter 3: Leininger's Theory of Cultural Care Diversity
    and Universality*
*Chapter 4: Leininger's Action Modes in Conflict
    Resolution; Case Study*
*Chapter 7: Leininger's Cultural Assessment Tools,
    Instruments and Guidelines*
Chapter 10: Ethnonursing Research Method

Gloria J. McNeal, PhD, MSN, ACNS-BC, FAAN
Dean, Mervyn M. Dymally School of Nursing
Charles Drew University of Medicine and Science
Los Angeles, California
*Chapter 3: Health Belief Model; Developing Mutually
    Beneficial Partnerships with Communities*

Sandra J. Mixer, PhD, RN
Assistant Professor, College of Nursing
The University of Tennessee
Knoxville, Tennessee
*Chapter 4: Leininger's Action Modes in Conflict
    Resolution; Case Study*

Cora Muñoz, PhD, RN
Professor, School of Natural Sciences, Nursing & Health
Capital University
Columbus, Ohio
*Chapter 4: Modes of Communication: Verbal and
    Non-Verbal Communication*

Sunita Mutha, MD, FACP
Associate Professor of Medicine
School of Medicine, Division of General
    Internal Medicine
University of California, San Francisco
San Francisco, California
*Chapter 9. Organizational Strategies to Address
    Discrimination; Workforce Diversity in Healthcare
    Organizations*

Akram Omeri, PhD, RN, CTN, FRCNA
Transcultural Nurse Consultant
University of Notre Dame
Sydney, New South Wales
Australia
Chapter 6: Care of Refugees and Asylees

Dula F. Pacquiao, EdD, RN, CTN
Associate Professor and Director
Stanley Bergen Center for Multicultural
Education, Research and Practice
School of Nursing
University of Medicine and Dentistry of NJ
Newark, New Jersey
*Chapter 3: Critical Pedagogy (Freire); Cultural Dimensions
    Model (Hofstede); Ecological Systems Theory
    (Bronfenbrenner); Organizational Culture (Schein);*
*Chapter 4: Nature of Cross-Cultural Communication;
    Cultural Context of Cross-Cultural Communication.*

Irena Papadopoulos, PhD, MA, RN, RM, FHEA
Professor of Transcultural Health and Nursing,
School of Health and Social Sciences,
Middlesex University,
London, England
*Chapter 3: Papadopoulos, Tilki & Taylor Model of
    Developing Cultural Competence*
*Chapter 7: Papadopoulos, Tilki & Lees Cultural
    Competence Assessment Tool (CCA Tool)*
Chapter 10: Participatory Action Research (PAR) Method

Larry Purnell PhD, RN, FAAN
Professor Emeritus, School of Nursing
University of Delaware
Newark, Delaware
Chapter 3: Purnell Model for Cultural Competence
*Chapter 7: Assessment of the Domains of the Purnell
    Model of Cultural Competence*

Marilyn A. Ray, PhD, MA, RN, CTN-A
Professor Emeritus
The Christine E. Lynn College of Nursing
Florida Atlantic University
Boca Raton, Florida
Chapter 3: Critical Theory, Transcultural Caring Dynamics
*Chapter 10: Phenomenology Research Method;
    Grounded Theory Research Method*

Janice M. Roper PhD, MS, RN
Assistant Dean of Evidence Based Practice & Research
American University of Health Sciences
Signal Hill, California
Chapter 10. Ethnography Research Method

Melissa Scollan-Koliopoulos, EdD, APRN, CDE
Assistant Professor
Department of Medicine, Division of Endocrinology,
University of Medicine and Dentistry of New Jersey
Newark, NJ, 07103
Chapter 10: Quantitative Research Methodologies

Jill Shapira, PhD, RN, FNP-C
Nurse Practitioner, Neurological Services Department
University of California Los Angeles Health Systems
Los Angeles, California
Chapter 10. Ethnography Research Method

Mary C. Sobralske, PhD, RN, CTN
Assistant Professor, College of Nursing
Washington State University
Spokane, Washington
Chapter 3: Worldviews; Essential Concepts Related to
*   Learning and Socialization; Social Categories;*
*   Cultural Conflicts*

Rachel Spector, PhD, RN, CTN-A, FAAN
Cultural Care Consultant
Needham, Massachusetts
Chapter 3: Cultural Diversity in Health and
*   Illness Model*
Chapter 7: The Heritage Assessment Tool

Aaron J. Strehlow, PhD, RN, FNP-BC, FNP-C, NPNP
Family and Neuropsychiatric Nurse Practitioner,
Administrator, UCLA School of Nursing
    Health Center
Assistant Clinical Professor
University of California, Los Angeles
Chapter 6: Ethnopharmacology and
*   Pharmocogenetics*

Kathryn Sucher, ScD, RD
Professor,
Dept of Nutrition, Food Science & Packaging
San Jose State University
San Jose, California
Chapter 6: Nutritional Practices: Diet & Culture

Gayle Tang, MSN, RN
Director, National Diversity
Kaiser Permanente
Oakland, California
Chapter 9: Language Services for Healthcare
*   Organizations*

Mary Tilki, PhD, MSc, RN
Principal Lecturer,
School of Health and Social Sciences,
Middlesex University,
London, England
Chapter 7: Papadopoulos, Tilki and Lees
*   Cultural Competence Assessment Tool*
*   (CCA Tool)*

Hsiu-Min Tsai, PhD, RN
Associate Professor and Dean of Academic Affairs
Department of Nursing
Chang Gung Institute of Technology
Taiwan
Chapter 10: Internet Research Method

Sheryl Tyson, PhD, RN, PMHCNS-BC
Professor, PhD Program, Director,
Psychiatric Mental Health Nurse Practitioner Program
Azusa Pacific University
Azusa, California
Chapter 6: Cultural Beliefs and Practices concerning
*   Mental Health & Illness*

Connie Vance, EdD, RN, FAAN
Professor, School of Nursing
College of New Rochelle
New Rochelle, New York
Chapter 11: The Mentoring Role of the Transcultural Nurse

Hiba Wehbe-Alamah, PhD, RN, FNP-BC, CTN-A
Assistant Professor, Department of Nursing
School of Health Professions and Studies
University of Michigan-Flint
Chapter 7: Leininger's Cultural Assessment Tools,
*   Instruments and Guidelines;*
Case Study: Assessment of a Traditional Lebanese
*   Muslim Patient*

Marian K. Yoder EdD, RN
Professor, School of Nursing
San Jose State University
San Jose, California
Chapter 3: Bridging Cultural Gaps

Anna Frances Z. Wenger, PhD, RN, CTN, FAAN
Professor and Director Emerita, Department of Nursing
Goshen College, Goshen, Indiana
Senior Scholar, Interfaith Health Program
Program Consultant, Rollins School of Public Health,
Ethiopia Public Health Training Initiative
Emory University, Atlanta, Georgia
Chapter 4: High and Low Context Communication;
*   Artifactual Cues in Non-Verbal Communication*

Rick Zoucha, PhD, PMHCNS-BC, CTN
Associate Professor, School of Nursing
Duquesne University
Pittsburgh, Pennsylvania
Chapter 3: Model for Multicultural Understanding (Locke)
Chapter 6: Disaster Care: Care of Victims of Natural Disasters

List of Reviewers

Journal of Transcultural Nursing
21(Supplement 1) 11S–12S
© The Author(s) 2010
Reprints and permission:
sagepub.com/journalsPermissions.nav
DOI: 10.1177/1043659610385419
http://tcn.sagepub.com
⑤SAGE

Nancy L. R. Anderson, PhD, RN, FAAN
Professor Emerita, School of Nursing
University of California, Los Angeles
Los, Angeles, California

Jeffrey R. Backstrand, PhD
Associate Professor, School of Nursing
University of Medicine and Dentistry of New Jersey
Newark, New Jersey

Joyceen S. Boyle, PhD, RN, CTN, FAAN
Professor Emerita, College of Nursing
University of Arizona
Tucson, Arizona

Karen Breda, PhD, RN
Associate Professor of Nursing
University of Hartford
Hartford, Connecticut

Sheila Bunting, PhD, RN
Professor, School of Nursing
Medical College of Nursing
Augusta, Georgia

Mary Lou de Leon Siantz, PhD, RN, FAAN
Assistant Dean of Diversity and Cultural Affairs
University of Pennsylvania School of Nursing
Philadelphia, Pennsylvania

Ruth De Souza, MA, RN
Senior Research Fellow
Centre for Asian and Migrant Health Research
Auckland University of technology
Aotearoa, New Zealand

Lydia DeSantis, PhD, RN, CTN, FAAN
Professor Emeritus
School of Nursing and Health Studies
University of Miami
Coral Gables, Florida

Marilyn K. Douglas, DNSc, RN, FAAN,
Associate Clinical Professor, School of Nursing
University of California, San Francisco
San Francisco, California

Marie Gates, PhD, RN
Professor Emerita, School of Nursing
Western Michigan University
Kalamazoo, Michigan

Guifang Guo, PhD, RN
Dean and Professor, School of Nursing
Peking University
Beijing, China

Karen Gylys, PhD, RN
Associate Professor,
School of Nursing
University of California, Los Angeles
Los Angeles, California

Jehad O. Halabi, PhD, RN
Assistant Dean for Development Affairs,
Faculty of Nursing
University of Jordan
Amman, Jordan

Carol Holtz, PhD, RN
Professor, School of Nursing
Kennesaw State University
Kennesaw, Georgia

Kathleen Huttlinger, PhD, RN
Professor, School of Nursing
New Mexico State University
Las Cruces, New Mexico

Margarita A. Kay, PhD, RN, FAAN
Professor Emerita, College of Nursing
University of Arizona
Tucson, Arizona

Jeanne K. Kemppainen, PhD, RN
Professor and Assistant Department Chair
School of Nursing
University of North Carolina
Wilmington, North Carolina

Anahid Kulwick, DNS, RN, FAAN
Associate Dean for Research
College of Nursing and Health Sciences
Florida Atlantic University
Miami, Florida

Teri Lindgren, PhD, MPH, RN
Assistant Adjunct Professor, School of Nursing
University of California, San Francisco
San Francisco, California

Juliene G. Lipson, PhD, RN, FAAN,
Professor Emerita, School of Nursing

University of California, San Francisco
San Francisco, California

Marlene Mackey, PhD, RN, FAAN
Associate Professor, College of Nursing
University of South Carolina
Columbia, South Carolina

Stephen R. Marrone, EdD, RN-BC, CTN-A
Deputy Nursing Director.
Institute of Continuous Learning
State University of New York (SUNY)
Downstate Medical Center
Brooklyn, New York

Carolyn Thompson Martin, PhD, RN, CFNP
Graduate Coordinator, Department of Nursing
California State University, Stanislaus
Turlock, California

Marilyn R. McFarland, PhD, RN, FNP-BC, CTN-A
Associate Professor of Nursing
University of Michigan-Flint
Flint, Michigan

Paula M. McGee, PhD, MA, RNT
Professor, Faculty of Nursing
Birmingham City University
Birminham, United Kingdom

Deanne K. Hilfinger Messias, PhD, RN, FAAN
Associate Professor, College of Nursing
University of South Carolina
Columbia, South Carolina

June Miller, PhD, RN
Adjunct Assistant Professor, School of Nursing
Johns Hopkins University
Baltimore, Maryland

Jan Nilsson, PhD, MSc, RNT
Senior Lecturer, College of Nursing
The Red Cross University
Stockholm, Sweden

Akram Omeri, PhD, RN, CTN, FRCNA
Adjunct Associate Professor, School of Nursing

University of Western Sydney
Penrith, NSW Australia

Huibrie Pieters, PhD, RN
Assistant Adjunct Professor
School of Nursing
University of California, Los Angeles

Dula F. Pacquiao, EdD, RN, CTN
Associate Professor and Director
Stanley S. Bergen Center for Multicultural
Education, Research & Practice
Univ. of Medicine and Dentistry of New Jersey
Newark, New Jersey

Larry Purnell, PhD, RN, FAAN
Emeritus Professor, College of Health Sciences
University of Delaware
Newark, Delaware

Antoinette Sabapathy, MSN, RN, SCM, WHNP, CNM
Assistant manager, School of Health Sciences
Nanyang Polytechnic
Singapore, Singapore

Donna Shambley-Ebron, PhD, MSN, RN
Assistant Professor, College of Nursing
University of Cincinnati.
Cincinnati, Ohio

Barbara Woodring, EdD, RN, CPN
Professor and Director
Byrdine F. Lewis School of Nursing
Georgia State University
Atlanta, Georgia

Fran Wenger, PhD, RN, CTN, FAAN
Senior Scholar, School of Public Health
Emory University
Program Consultant, Ethiopian Public Health Initiative
The Carter Center
Atlanta, Georgia

Karen Whitt, PhD, RN
Assistant Professor, Department of Nursing Education
George Washington University Medical Center
Washington, D.C.

Section I. Global Health and Health Care Issues

Associate Editor: Carol Holtz, PhD, RN

Chapter 1
Global Health Issues

Journal of Transcultural Nursing
21(Supplement 1) 14S–38S
© The Author(s) 2010
Reprints and permission:
sagepub.com/journalsPermissions.nav
DOI: 10.1177/1043659610368976
http://tcn.sagepub.com

⑤SAGE

Carol Holtz, PhD, RN[1]

I. INTRODUCTION

A. Health disparities are statistically significant difference in health indicators (burden of disease, morality and mortality rates) that persist over time, between groups (Centers for Disease Control and Prevention [CDC], 2008a), and which are associated with social inequalities.

B. Health care disparities are group differences in access to appropriate health care services that contribute to disparities in health status. In turn, poorer health status compromises the ability to obtain timely and appropriate health services.

C. Health and care disparities exist worldwide. Developing nations have a lower level of material well-being based on per capita income, life expectancy, and rate of literacy. These nations are also referred to as less economically developed, Third World, lower income nations, or resource-poor countries. Developed nations are also called industrialized societies, advanced economies, and higher income nations (UNDP, n.d.).

II. INDICES OF HEALTH DISPARITIES

A. Burden of Disease

1. Defined as the impact of a health problem in a given population measured by financial cost, mortality, morbidity, or other indicators, and often quantified in terms of *quality-adjusted life years* (*QALYs*).
2. This allows for comparison of disease burden due to various risk factors or diseases. It also makes it possible to predict the possible impact of health interventions.
3. The global burden of disease is shifting from infectious diseases to noncommunicable diseases, with chronic conditions such as heart disease and stroke now being the chief causes of death globally.

B. Mortality Rate

1. Defined as the number of deaths in a particular population, scaled to the size of that population, per unit of time.
2. Expressed in units of deaths per 1,000 individuals per year; thus, a mortality rate of 9.5 in a population of 100,000 would mean 950 deaths per year in that entire population.
3. The latest health trends indicate that the leading infectious diseases such as diarrhea, HIV, tuberculosis (TB), neonatal infections, and malaria will become less important causes of death globally over the next 20 years.

C. Infant Mortality Rate (IMR)

1. Defined as the number of deaths of infants (1 year of age or younger) per 1,000 live births.
2. Reported as number of live newborns dying under a year of age per 1,000 live births.
3. There are some discrepancies in calculating the IMR globally, making it difficult to compare rates in different countries of the world. The World Health Organization (WHO) defines a live birth as any born human being who demonstrates independent signs of life, including breathing, voluntary muscle movement, and/or heartbeat.
4. Infant mortality has significantly declined in the West because of improvements in basic health care, and advances in technology and medicine.

Funding: The California Endowment (grant number 20082226) and Health Resources and Services Administration (grant number D11 HPO9759).
[1]Kennesaw State University, Kennesaw, GA, USA

Corresponding Author: Carol Holtz, Email: choltz@kennesaw.edu

Suggested Citation: Douglas, M. K. & Pacquiao, D. F. (Eds.). (2010). Core curriculum in transcultural nursing and health care [Supplement]. *Journal of Transcultural Nursing, 21*(Suppl. 1).

5. IMR is a useful indicator of a country's level of health or development and a component of the physical quality of life index.
6. In the late 1990s, diarrhea was the most common cause of infant mortality worldwide. Successful dissemination of information on oral rehydration solution (a mixture of salts, sugar, and water) to mothers has decreased the rate of children dying from dehydration and electrolyte imbalance.
7. Currently, the most common cause of infant death is pneumonia.

D. Morbidity Rate
1. Defined as the number of individuals in poor health during a given time or the number who currently have that disease (*prevalence rate*), scaled to the size of the population.
2. The state of poor health; the degree or severity of a health condition; the total number of cases in a particular population at a particular point in time; the number of new cases in a particular population during a particular point in time irrespective of cause.

E. Life Expectancy
1. Defined as the average number of years of life remaining at a given age or the average life span; the average length of survival or expected age before death in a specified population based on the year of birth or other demographic variables.
2. *Healthy life expectancy (HALE)* is the average number of years that a person can expect to live in "full health" by taking into account years lived in less than full health due to disease and/or injury.
3. In countries with high IMRs, the life expectancy at birth is highly sensitive to the rate of death in the first few years of life. Hence, another measure such as life expectancy at age 5 is used to exclude the effects of infant mortality.
4. The estimated *global life expectancy at birth* between 2005 and 2010 was 67.2 years (65.0 years for males and 69.5 years for females; UN World Population Prospects 2006 Revision) compared with 2009 at 66.57 years (64.52 years for males and 68.76 years for females; Central Intelligence Agency [CIA] World Factbook, 2009).
5. Countries with the lowest life expectancies (Swaziland, Botswana, Lesotho, Zimbabwe, South Africa, Namibia, Zambia, Malawi, the Central African Republic, Mozambique, and Guinea-Bissau) have very high rates of HIV/AIDS infection, with adult prevalence rates between 10% and 38.8%.
6. In countries with high IMRs, the life expectancy at birth will be lower and may not reflect the life expectancy of a person who has survived infancy (CIA World Factbook, 2009).

F. Birth Rate
1. Defined as the number of childbirths per 1,000 people per year.
2. As of 2007 the average birth rate globally was 20.3 per year per 1,000 total population, which equals 134 million babies per year for a total population of 6.6 billion.

G. Total Fertility Rate
1. Defined as the average number of children born to each woman over the course of her life.
2. Fertility rates tend to be higher in developing countries and lower in more developed countries. *Global fertility rates* are declining in developed countries especially in Western Europe where populations are projected to decline over the next 50 years.
   a. Niger has the highest rate with 7.75 births per woman. Macaw and Hong Kong have the lowest, with 0.91 and 1.02 births per female, respectively.
   b. A rate of 2.33 children per woman is considered the stable replacement for a population.
   c. Rates above the replacement rate indicate populations growing in size with declining median age. Families may have difficulties to feed and educate their children and for women to enter the labor force.
   d. Rates below two children indicate decreasing size and aging of the population.
   e. In 1979, the government of China under Deng Xiaoping adopted a mandatory one-child-per-family policy to limit the population growth with some exceptions. The current leaders continue the policy through the 2006-2010 5-year planning period. Although designated as a "temporary measure," it has continued for a quarter century. The policy imposes fines, pressures couples to abort a pregnancy, and even forces sterilization (Population Reference Bureau, 2009).

H. Disability
1. Defined as the lack of ability relative to a personal or group standard or spectrum.
2. May involve physical, sensory, cognitive or intellectual impairment, or a mental disorder.
3. May occur during a person's lifetime or may be present from birth.

I. Nutritional Status
1. Influenced by diet, levels of nutrients in the body, and ability to maintain normal metabolic integrity.
2. Body fat may be estimated by measuring skin-fold thickness and muscle diameter.
3. For adults, general adequacy is assessed by measuring skin-fold thickness and muscle diameter.
4. For children, weight and height for age are compared with standards based on adequately nourished children. Increases in head circumference and bone development may also be measured.
5. Levels of vitamins and minerals are measured based on the serum levels, urine concentrations of nutrients and their metabolites, or by testing for specific metabolic responses.

III. GLOBAL HEALTH DISPARITIES
A. Mexico (Holtz, 2008b)
1. Health care system is challenged with malnutrition, infections, reproductive health problems, and injuries.
2. Approximately half of the population lacks adequate nutrition and access to health care.

B. China (Holtz, 2008b)
1. Has the most rapidly growing economy in the world in the past 3 years.
2. Income inequality has risen, with accompanying rural–urban income gap and the growing disparity between highly educated urban professionals and the urban working class.
3. Restrictions on rural–urban migration have limited opportunities for the relatively poor rural population.
4. Increasing inequalities are reflected in widening disparities in health and education outcomes.

C. Israel (Holtz, 2008a)
1. Life expectancy has increased to 76.69 for males and 80.4 years for females but extensive inequality continues to exist in health care delivery, health status, and health outcomes. Social inequalities in income, housing, education, and employment account for the bulk of health disparities. Many of the low-socioeconomic groups cannot afford to pay even the relatively low health care copayment required by law and unable to pay for medication or essential treatments.
2. In 2003, the total population of 6,600,000 consisted of two major groups, Jews and Arabs (19.3%). These groups differ in background, culture, and language. Low-socioeconomic Arab groups have poorer health indicators compared with the Jewish population (Israel Center for Disease Control, 2005). In 2002, life expectancy was about 3 years less for Arab Israelis than Jews (Israel Ministry of Health, 2003).
3. Although infant mortality is low in the general population, it is increasing among populations in the geographic periphery and large urban areas in the center of the country.

D. United Kingdom (Holtz, 2008a)
1. Disparities in health outcomes have been widening as the gap between the rich and poor increases.
2. The government is focusing on reducing class inequalities in health by 2010.

E. Japan (Tokyo Foundation, 2009)
1. Has one of the highest levels of health care in the world with very small disparities in health among its residents.
2. The first country in Asia to provide its citizens with comprehensive social insurance program. Universal health coverage was achieved through a mandate on all residents and all employers (with five or more employees) to contribute to their employees' health plan.

F. Canada (Holtz, 2008a)
1. Canadians are among the healthiest people in the world, but some major health disparities exist among specific populations influenced by gender, educational attainment, income, and other markers of disadvantages or unequal opportunities.
2. The universal single-payer health care system covers about 70% of expenditures, and the *Canada Health Act* requires that all persons be fully insured, without copayments or user fees, for all medically necessary hospital and physician care.
3. About 91% of hospital expenditures and 99% of total physician services are financed by the public sector.
4. Provides public coverage for private care delivery and is not a true system of socialized medicine.
5. A history of racism has resulted in poorer access and inadequate health care facilities for the Aborigines.

G. United States of America (CDC, 2004a: *National Healthcare Disparities Report*, 2004; Sridhar, 2005)
1. *African Americans* (Colen, Geronimus, Bound, & James, 2006).
   a. In 2000, 36.6 million (12.3%) people self-identified as African American and 35.4 million self-identified as non-Hispanic.

   b. Compared with White Americans, African Americans:
   1) Are twice as likely to have no health insurance.
   2) Bear a disproportionate burden of disease, injury, death, disability, risk factors, incidence and mor-bidity rates for diseases and injuries.
   3) Have 3 of the 10 leading causes of deaths (homicide, HIV, and septicemia) that are not among those listed in the 10 leading causes of deaths for whites
   c. Infant mortality and perinatal mortality, compared with White Americans, African Americans:
   1) Have an infant mortality rate average 13.9 per 1,000 live births as compared with 6.9 per 1,000 live births.
   2) An African American baby is 2.5 times more likely to die before reaching 1 year of age.
   3) Preterm birth is the leading cause of death
   4) Compared with White American women:
      a) African American women have higher pregnancy-related mortalities, including rates of pre-eclampsia, eclampsia, abruption placenta, placenta previa, and postpartum hemorrhage.
      b) Have a higher risk for having low and very low birth weight babies.
      c) Have lower number of females receiving prenatal care during the first trimester of pregnancy.
      d) Middle class African American women have access to fewer financial resources, more restricted opportunities for wealth accumulation, more likely to reside in racially segregated areas, and more affected by lifelong legacies of childhood poverty and psychological stress due to discrimination.
   d. Cancer
   1) Second leading cause of death for both non-Hispanic Whites and non-Hispanic African Americans. Compared with White Americans:
      a) African American females have substantially higher incidence of colon/rectal, pancreatic, and stomach cancers; have higher mortality rates from breast cancer.
      b) African Americans with rectal cancer are diagnosed at a younger age and with a more advanced disease stage.
      c) Had 25.4% higher adjusted death rate for cancer in 2001.
   2) Treatment disparities may contribute to differences in outcome among racial and ethnic groups. Health disparity may be partially explained by unequal access to screening, medical care, and "state of the art" surgical care.
   e. Other diseases—compared with White Americans, Non-Hispanic African Americans:
   1) Have higher rates of negative health indicators such as new cases of gonorrhea, deaths from homi-cide, and overweight or obesity.
   2) Had greater than twice the rate of diabetes in 2001
   3) Suffer from excess hypertension related health outcomes and blood pressures are often less con-trolled (Safford, Halanych, Lewis, Levine, & Howard, 2007).
   4) Have lower rates of vaccination against pneumococcal disease among those <65 years of age
   5) Had 18.2% lower adult influenza immunization rates in 2002
   6) Had twice the number of emergency room visits for chronic obstructive pulmonary disease (COPD) and were more likely to be hospitalized
   7) Had lower rates of <65-year-olds with health insurance resulting in poorer access to health care
2. *American Indians/Alaskan Natives* (CDC, 2008c).
   a. Represent 1.5% of the total U.S. population.
   b. More than 538,000 of American Indian/Alaskan Natives (one third of the total American Indian/Alaskan Native population) live on reservations or other trust lands with challenging climate, impassable roads, scarce transportation, and less accessible health care facilities (U.S. Census Bureau, 2007).
   1) Compared with the general population, health services and facilities are inadequate such as the insuf-ficient hospital beds available and ratios of doctors and nurses to patients in the Navajo areas.
   2) 60% rely on the Indian Health Service (IHS) for health care.
   3) The IHS goals include improving access to health care and providing comprehensive, culturally acceptable, personal and public health services to the population.
   c. Diabetes
   1) Diabetes and liver disease are greater than twice that of all other adults in the United States.

2) Greatest mortality rates are due to direct and indirect effects of type 2 diabetes. A special Diabetes Program for American Indians has provided funds for prevention and treatment of diabetes, yet rates remain higher than those of Whites.

3) Have higher levels of obesity, diabetes, and spend less time in physical activity than Whites.

d. Other health disparities

1) Leading causes of death are heart disease and cancer

2) Compared with Whites and other cultural groups, American Indians/Alaskan Natives:
   a) Have higher death rates of fetuses, infants, children, adolescents, and young adults
   b) Have higher preterm deaths, and fetal alcohol syndrome (FAS)
   c) Have lower rates of prenatal care.
   d) Have 1.7 times higher infant mortality rate
   e) Have twice the rate of sudden infant death syndrome
   f) Rates of sexually transmitted diseases (STDs) are 5.5 times higher for chlamydia, and 4 times higher for gonorrhea.
   g) Have higher levels of smoking and heart disease.
   h) Unintentional injuries are the third leading cause of death and the leading cause of death for the 1- to 44-year age group.
   i) Death rates for unintentional injuries and motor vehicle accidents are 1.7 to 2 times higher.
   j) Suicide rates are three times greater.
   k) Since the mid 1980s, mortality rates have been increasing

3. *Asian Americans* (CDC, 2008c)

a. In 2000, Asian Americans represented 4.2% of the U.S. population.

b. Have the lowest rates of fetal and infant very low birth weight births, preterm births, and cigarette smoking in pregnancy.

c. Have higher rates of breastfeeding in early and 6-month postpartum periods.

d. 21% lack health insurance as compared with 16% of the general population.

e. Rates for cervical cancer among Vietnamese women are 43 per 100,000, almost five times higher than non-Hispanic White women.

f. TB rates are higher than any other racial or ethnic group with 33 per 100,000 compared with 14 per 100,000 for African Americans; 12 per 100,000 for Hispanics; 11 per 100,000 for American Indians/Alaska Natives; and 2 per 100,000 for non-Hispanic Whites.

g. Rates for acute hepatitis B are twice the rate (2.95) of non-Hispanic Whites.

4. *Hispanic/Latino Americans* (Pew Hispanic Center, 2008)

a. Between 1990 and 2000, Latino population increased by 61%, becoming the largest minority group in the United States.

b. In 2004, there were 40.4 million Latinos, representing 14.2% of the population.

c. Latinos have multiple origins and cultures: Mexican (63.9%), Central American (10.2%), Puerto Rican (9.1%), South American (5.4%), Cuban (3.5%), other (8.5%).

d. Latinos have three times the rate for Whites of persons without health insurance.

e. Despite the fact that many Latinos have low income and educational levels and do not have health insurance, they have lower rate of low birth weight infants and infant mortality compared with other immigrant groups.

f. However, these low rates diminish with increased acculturation and assimilation to the dominant American culture as seen in increasing incidence of diabetes, mental illness, TB, and dental caries.

g. Language

1) Spanish is the primary language, although the vocabulary, accents, and idioms may vary among the subcultures depending on country of origin and level of education.

2) Among young children, it is common to mix English and Spanish; newer immigrants, especially women who are not working outside the home, tend to speak less English.

3) Use of interpreters is often necessary and ideally should be of the same gender; family and friends as well as children are much less ideal to interpret personal information to health care providers.

4) Latinos are four times more likely to misunderstand prescription labels than English-speaking patients. Many hospitals and outpatient facilities do not provide interpreter services, mainly because of cost.

5) Language differences and more limited access to health care contribute to patient safety problems.
6) Latinos living in rural areas are especially vulnerable to language and physical isolation limiting their access to treatment.

   h. Other disparities

1) HIV/AIDS is higher among Puerto Ricans than any other Latino group and six times the national average (5.4 per 100,000).
2) Mortality rates from diabetes is exceptionally high with 172 per 100,000 for Puerto Ricans, followed by Mexican Americans with 122 per 100,000, and Cuban Americans with 47 per 100,000.
3) Adult vaccination rates for pneumococcal diseases were 23.8% for Latinos as compared with 60.6% for Whites.
4) Asthma death rate for all Latino groups was more than twice the rate for Whites.

5. *Native and Other Pacific Islanders* (CDC, 2004a).

   a. According to the 2000 U.S. Census, Native and Other Pacific Islanders represent 0.3% of the population.
   b. 21% lack health insurance as compared with 16% of the general population.
   c. Have highest rates of TB (33 per 100,000) compared with African Americans (14), Latinos (12), American Indians/Native Alaskans (11), and non-Hispanic Whites (2).
   d. Diabetes rates are 2.5 times the rates for non-Hispanic Whites of similar ages.
   e. Hepatitis B rate of 3 per 100,000 is more than twice the rate for non-Hispanic Whites of 1.3 per 100,000.
   f. Asthma rate of 139.5 per 100,000 is twice the rate for all other groups in Hawaii.
   g. Higher cigarette smoking rate of 30.9% compared with 19.7% for other Hawaiian population groups.

IV. RELATIONSHP BETWEEN POVERTY AND HEALTH

A. Global Poverty

1. As of 2002, 1.5 billion people are exposed to poverty, particularly in the developing world. Nearly 3 billion people, half of the world's population, are considered poor.

   a. More than 100 million primary school–age children cannot go to school.
   b. More than 800 million go hungry each day.
   c. Those living in extreme poverty are 5 times more likely to die before the age of 5 years, and 2.5 times more likely to die between the ages of 15 and 59 years.
   d. More than 8 million people around the world die each year from lack of adequate finances to obtain clean, safe, and adequate food and water, and basic health care.

2. Funding for resources such as food, housing, and medical care programs greatly influence the health care of the poor in any society.

   a. Politics influences policies for funding health resources.
   b. The U.S. Census defines the *poor* as persons living in families whose household income falls below specific poverty thresholds, varying by family size and composition.
   c. Categories of poverty in the United States (U.S. Census Bureau, 2007):

1) *Extreme (absolute) poverty*: Households living with less than $1 a day and unable to afford the most basic needs to ensure survival. Eight million people a year die from absolute poverty.
2) *Moderate poverty*: Households living on about $1 to $2 a day and barely able to meet their basic needs, forgo many of the basic necessities such education and health care. The smallest misfortune (illness, job loss, etc.) threatens survival.
3) *Relative poverty*: Household income below the national average.

3. Those living in poverty are more prone to:

   a. Malnutrition
   b. Infectious and chronic diseases
   c. Inadequate housing conditions leading to diseases such as TB
   d. Higher morbidity and mortality rates due to decreased access to health services and quality care
   e. Inability to afford medications, treatments, and so on, needed for health maintenance
   f. Less access to preventive health education, treatments, and immunizations
   g. Food insecurity and poor nutrition (Pena & Bacallao, 2002)

1) *Food security* is having a steady access to sufficient, clean, safe, and nutritious foods for an active healthy life. They are able to acquire necessary foods without having to scavenge or steal.

2) *Food insecurity* exists when there is a limited or uncertain availability of safe and nutritious food. Food may not be easily acquired in safe and socially acceptable ways.

3) The long-term effects of food insecurity are ill health, reduction in physical and cognitive growth and development, disease vulnerability, and if untreated, eventual death.

4) The poor are more likely to become overweight or obese from energy-dense foods that cost less per calorie, low in fruits and vegetables, and contain more refined grain, sugars, and fats.

5) There is increasing concern worldwide that food and water supplies can become a weapon of bioterrorism and become vehicles for intentional spread of illness.

    a) Toxic substances such as radioactive particles, microorganisms (*Escherichia coli* 0517:H7, salmonella, shigella, or botulism toxin might be placed into the food and water supply.

    b) National policies and programs can promote food safety and improve assessment, monitoring, and control of food and water quality.

4. Poverty causes people to be exposed to environmental risks such as poor sanitation, unhealthy food, unsafe water, violence, and natural disasters.

5. The poor are less likely to be literate, educated, and prepared to cope with problems, increasing their risk for illness and disability.

6. Poor health can also lead to poverty.

7. Poverty varies by race and ethnicity in every country. For example, in the United States, in 2002, 24% of African Americans, 22% of Hispanics, 10% of Asians, and 10% of Whites were poor.

8. The poor often experience worse health and are more likely to die prematurely, mainly because of reduced access to high-quality care.

    a. *Access* is defined as the timely use of health services to achieve the best possible health outcome.

    b. In the United States, racial and ethnic minorities have consistently higher rates of uninsured persons than White Americans.

    c. Income-related differences in quality of care independent of having health insurance coverage have also been demonstrated.

    d. Community health centers (CHCs) are vital sources of health care for the poor.

    e. Those lacking access are less likely to have a regular source of care and more likely to receive lower quality care.

    f. Barriers that restrict Medicaid (government support for medical expenses for the indigent in the United States) patients, the uninsured and underinsured from accessing health care:

        1) Financial barriers: Health services for the poor are likely to diminish further as the cost of medical care continues to rise and public health services are being discontinued.

        2) Structural barriers: Low levels of reimbursement and complexity of the billing process discourage many physicians from participating in Medicaid.

        3) Personal barriers: Because of lack of knowledge of the medical system and low levels of education, many are not aware of their eligibility for Medicaid, or different levels of insurance.

B. Health Disparities in Vulnerable Populations (CDC, 2004a; *National Healthcare Disparities Report*, 2004; The Sullivan Commission, 2004)

  1. Definitions

    a. Groups in any society who have limited ability to control and make changes in their lives, because of physical, mental, material, and/or social factors.

    b. Because of multiple disadvantages, these groups are predisposed to cumulative health risks in their life course.

    c. Groups of people, whose options are severely limited, frequently subjected to coercion in their decision making, or who may be compromised in their ability to give informed consent.

    d. Includes groups of low socioeconomic status (poor, unemployed, lack education, lack health insurance and/or access to health care), marginalized and oppressed, those with limited capacity to choose the environment in which they live, and therefore at higher risk for poor health.

    e. Vulnerable groups are most affected by health disparities.

  2. The Elderly Poor

    a. Globally, the number of persons age 65 and older grows by 800,000 monthly (U.S. Census and the National Institute on Aging).

        1) More than one third of the world's oldest people (80 years and older) lived in three countries, China (11.5 million), the United States (9.2 million), and India (6.2 million).

    2) More than three quarters of the world's net gain of older people from 1999 to 2000 were in developing countries.

    3) There were more older women than older men in the majority of countries except India, Iran, and Bangladesh.

    4) In many countries, the fastest growing group is composed of persons 80 years and older.

b. Most elderly poor are women and very elderly women have higher poverty rates.

    1) Nearly one in five of single, divorced, or widowed women older the age of 65 years is poor; the risk of poverty for older women increases with age.

    2) Women aged 75 years and older are more than three times as likely to be living in poverty than their male counterparts.

c. Of the 227 countries or areas of the world with at least 5,000,000 people, 167 (74%) had some form of old-age disability or survivors' program in the late 1990s, compared with 33 in 1940.

d. Disability rates were declining in developed countries but were increasing in developing countries.

e. The elderly poor in the United States (65 years and older) and people of color experience poverty at higher rates than Whites.

    1) African Americans make up only about 9% of the elder population, yet they comprise 21% of elders living below the poverty line.

    2) Without *Social Security and Supplemental Security Income* benefits, about 44% of the elderly would be much poorer.

        a) 3.4 million live below the poverty line and millions more are just above poverty line who can barely make ends meet.

        b) In 2006, 9.4% had incomes below the poverty threshold of $9,669 for an individual and $12,186 for a couple.

        c) Nearly a quarter (22.4%) had family incomes below 150% of the poverty line.

    3) Those living in rural areas have higher rates of poverty.

    4) Higher health care expenditures stretch their limited budgets.

    5) 35% of households have incomes of less than $20,000 and experience the greatest energy burden, or percentage of income spent on energy costs.

    6) The U.S. Department of Agriculture (2006) estimates that almost 18% with incomes below 130% of the poverty line who live with others experience food insecurity compared with more than 12% of low-income seniors who live alone.

    7) Only one half of Americans 65 years or older have access to public transportation to meet their daily needs.

    8) The Federal Interagency Forum on Age-Related Statistics estimates that by 2030, there will be roughly 70 million Americans, age 65 years or older, which is more than double the number in 2000.

    9) In 25 years, the number of people aged 85 years or older is expected to double, whereas the number of people aged 100 years or older is expected to triple.

    10) One fourth of older adults have no supplemental health insurance, and 16% of Americans younger than 65 years have no health insurance.

    11) Preventive health screening rates are particularly low for minorities, low-income individuals, and older adults.

    12) Health care facilities are often not accessible or do not have the necessary equipment to serve elder people with disabilities.

    13) Older adults experience the effects of health care disparities more dramatically than any other population group and are particularly at risk because they are more likely than younger people to have chronic illnesses, make frequent visits to medical facilities, and live in poverty.

    14) Older adults are markedly underrepresented in clinical trials that have historically focused on relatively young participants. As a result, treatment decisions for older adults are based on knowledge gained from the younger population.

3. Infants and Children in Poverty (Aduddell, 2008; Global Health Council, 2006)

a. Most often the most vulnerable members of society, whose health serves as an index of the well-being of a society and its future potential.

b. 90% of global births are in Africa, Asia, and South America.

    1) Of the approximately 125 million infants born globally every year, 8 million die before reaching 1 year of life.

2) The greatest burden of infant mortality rate (IMR) is borne by the least developed countries.

3) A total of 20 children die every minute every day. Approximately 1,000 infants die every hour with 970 deaths occurring in developing countries; 300,000 children die each day from poverty in developing countries (Global Health Council, 2006).

4) In 2007, IMRs ranged from a low of 2.8 in Sweden to 184.4 per 1,000 live births in Angola.

5) The mortality rate of children 5 years and younger ranged between 8 in the United States to 86 deaths per 1,000, globally.

c. The major determinants of infant and childhood mortality globally are linked with poverty, lack of essential public health resources such as safe water and appropriate sanitation, absence of prenatal care, inadequate diet, exposure to insect vectors of disease, and lack of basic health and preventive services.

1) These conditions and situations put infants and children at a higher risk of death from numerous other conditions and diseases.

2) Malnutrition from inadequate diet contributes to approximately 53% of all child deaths.

4. **Childbearing Women in Poverty**

a. In the United States, improved perinatal care is considered one of the 10 medical achievements of the 20th century that dropped IMRs by 90% and maternal mortality rates by 99%. Similar trends have been noted in other developed countries.

1) Maternal mortality rates remain high in many developing countries.

2) Globally, 600,000 women die every year from pregnancy- and labor-related causes, equivalent to one death per minute.

3) The major causes of neonatal deaths (in descending order) include asphyxia, sepsis, pneumonia, and prematurity.

4) The major causes of maternal deaths include postpartum hemorrhage, sepsis, and complications of prolonged labor.

b. Reductions in maternal and neonatal mortality rates in the developing countries remain a major health challenge

1) Several programs have been initiated by major nongovernmental agencies (WHO, UNICEF, and World Bank) to improve the maternal and infant health indicators.

2) Women who start prenatal care in the third trimester or receive no prenatal care at all are at increased risk for poor pregnancy outcomes.

3) Low birth weight babies would be significantly reduced if women begin prenatal care in the first trimester of pregnancy.

5. **The Mentally Ill** (Camann, 2008)

a. There is often great difficulty in comparing rates or types of mental illness because of the great variations in the knowledge, recognition, acceptance and recording of cases among different countries or groups

b. In 2001, one in four people worldwide was affected by mental or neurological disorders at some point in their lives.

c. In developing countries, about 80% of serious cases go untreated compared with 35% to 50% in developed countries.

d. Approximately 26% of Americans have mental illness compared with 4% reported cases in Shanghai and 5% in Nigeria.

e. Between 1% and 5% of the world population has serious mental illness; 9% to 17% has had some episode of mental illness in the past year, whether serious or severe.

f. About 450 million people currently suffer from mental illness, placing mental disorders among the leading causes of illness and disability globally.

g. Mental illness is widespread and undertreated; wealthy people with mild illness receive more and better treatment than poor people with severe illness.

h. Mental illness causes so many lost days of work as any physical problem such as cancer, heart attack, or back pain

i. Even when treatments were available, nearly two thirds of people with a known mental disorder never sought help from health professionals.

j. Lack of understanding, stigma, discrimination, and neglect block individuals and groups from benefiting from known effective treatment.

k. Lack of resources and poor allocation of resources toward mental health care are significant barriers to addressing the problems of the mentally ill.

6. **Persons With Disabilities** (Human Rights of Persons with Disabilities, n.d.)
   a. According to the United Nations, more than half a billion persons globally are disabled as a result of one or more mental, physical or sensory impairments.
   b. Approximately 80% of the world's disabled population lives in developing countries.
   c. The disabled population often remains the most marginalized, discounted, invisible, and abused group of people within any society throughout the world.
   d. In spite of powerful international and national disability rights laws, persons with disabilities frequently live in deplorable conditions, facing barriers that prevent their integration and meaningful participation in mainstream society with protection of their basic human rights to freedom of movement, and access to education and health care.
   e. Health, especially mental health, of the disabled may further deteriorate because of added difficulties imposed by their disability, marginalization, invisibility and gross injustices from ignorance of their status.

7. **Persons With Illnesses That Are Socially Stigmatized** (Social Stigma, n.d.)
   a. Stigma, by definition, is a mark of disgrace or shame
   b. HIV/AIDS stigma
      1) Worldwide there are 31.1 million to 35.8 million people living with HIV/AIDS today. More than 25 million have died of AIDS since 1981 and in 2008 there were 2 million deaths from AIDS (HIV and AIDS Statistics, 2008).
      2) Prejudice and discrimination result in their rejection by their community, shunned, discriminated against, or even physically assaulted.
      3) HIV/AIDS stigma and discrimination occur globally, and is manifested differently across countries, communities, religious groups, and individuals.
      4) Possible consequences of HIV-related stigma include:
         a) Loss of income and livelihood
         b) Loss of marriage and childbearing opportunity
         c) Poor care within the health sector
         d) Withdrawal of care giving in the home
         e) Loss of hope and feelings of worth
         f) Loss of reputation
         g) Social isolation
   c. Mental health disorders and stigma ("Mental Health: Overcoming the Stigma," 2008)
      1) The term *mental illness* suggests that it is not the same as a medical or physical illness; *mental* may suggest that the illness is not a legitimate medical problem.
      2) Mental illnesses have very complex etiologies, consisting of a mix of genetics, biology, and life experiences, most of which are beyond one's control.
      3) The belief that a mentally ill person is dangerous is inflamed by media accounts of crime suspects as *mentally ill*.
      4) Stigma contributes to minimal reporting and denial of mental disorders with consequent delays in seeking treatment, lack of prevention, discrimination, and marginalization.
      5) Negative portrayals of people with mental illnesses fuel fear and mistrust and reinforce distorted perceptions that lead to even more stigma.
      6) Cultural behaviors also confound the diagnoses of mental illness.
      7) Harmful effects of stigma include:
         a) Rejection by family and friends
         b) Work problems or discrimination
         c) Difficulty finding housing
         d) Inadequate health insurance coverage for mental illnesses
         e) Social isolation
   d. Drug and alcohol addiction and stigma
      1) Alcohol and drug addiction are treatable diseases that can affect anyone.
      2) Stigma is similar to mental illnesses which affect one's social interactions, work, housing, and insurance coverage for adequate treatment.
      3) Consequences may result in incarceration, loss of custody of dependent children, loss of job, and/or abandonment by family/friends.
   e. Other addictions that are also stigmatized and of great societal concern include gambling, sex, and food

8. **Immigrants** (Avery, 2001)
   a. Immigrants and undocumented migrants in the United States (Kaiser Commission on Key Facts, 2003, 2007, 2008)
      1) In 2000, about 30 million persons in the United States were foreign born (Okie, 2007). Asians and Latinos are more likely to be foreign born.
      2) About 70% of Asians and 40% of Hispanics are foreign born compared with 6% of Whites and African Americans.
      3) An *immigrant* is a foreign-born person residing in the United States. Immigrants include naturalized citizens as well as non-citizens who belong under other immigrant categories.
         a) *Naturalized citizen* is a foreign-born person who has lawfully become a U.S. citizen, having all the rights of a citizen except to be president or vice-president of the United States.
         b) *Undocumented immigrant* is a foreign-born person residing in the United States who is not a legal resident.
         c) *Legal resident* or *permanent resident* is a person who is allowed to reside in the United States indefinitely despite not having citizenship. Permanent residents have the same rights as citizens *except* the right to vote, run for public office, apply for employment in public sector, and national security, have a U.S. passport and access consular protection.
         d) *Quasi-legal immigrants* are foreign-born persons who overstayed their visas, have temporary protective status with extended voluntary departure and those who have applied for asylum or waiting for green cards.
      4) Lack of health insurance coverage is a major issue facing immigrant populations. They have been identified as a vulnerable group.
      5) Vulnerability may vary within subgroups, including socioeconomic status, immigration status, English proficiency, access to publicly funded health care, residential location, stigma, and marginalization.
      6) Under current law, illegal immigrants are eligible for emergency medical services only through Medicaid. According to the *1996 Welfare Reform Law*, legal immigrants are not eligible for Medicaid (except emergency medical care) and *State Children's Health Insurance Program* (SCHIP) benefits for the first five years of residence in the United States (SCHIP, 2008).
      7) Exposure to traumatic circumstances may lead to mental health issues. Many immigrants experienced traumatic circumstances in their native country such as extreme poverty, human trafficking, exposure to war, and/or natural disasters.
      8) Some groups experience difficulty with acculturation to their new environments because of prejudice and discrimination.
      9) Paradox of acculturation and health of immigrants in some developed countries.
         a) The expectation is that new immigrants would have worse health problems as they arrive and better health as they assimilate, but the opposite is true.
         b) People who have not adopted mainstream attitudes and behaviors of the new culture tend to have some protection from adverse health outcomes.
         c) Low acculturation rates among U.S. Latinos have been linked to lower infant mortality rates, better immunization status, and lower mortality from cardiovascular disease and cancer, less cigarette smoking and drug use.
   b. Immigrant children in the United States
      1) Comprise 4% of the 78 million children.
      2) Undocumented immigrant children are not eligible for SCHIP or Medicaid regardless of how long they have been in the United States. Some states use other funds to cover health care for these children.
      3) Increased vulnerability to lead poisoning (Tehranifar et al., 2008).
         a) Despite a decline in lead poisoning in children, 1.6% of immigrant children aged 1 to 5 years have elevated blood lead levels and many may already have some cognitive impairments.
         b) The most common source is lead-based paint and exposure prior to immigration. Other sources of lead may be from old water pipes.
         c) Most immigrant families initially settle in urban neighborhoods with old, dilapidated buildings.
   c. Alien/asylee/refugees (Vergara, Miller, Martin, & Cookson, 2003)
      1) An *alien* is a person unable or unwilling to return to his or her country of nationality, or seek the protection of that country because of persecution or a well-founded fear of persecution. Fear of

persecution must be based on the alien's race, religion, nationality, membership in a particular social group, or political opinion.

2) *Refugees* and *asylees* are people seeking protection on the grounds that they fear persecution in their homeland. A refugee applies for protection while outside the country of destination.

3) An *asylee* differs from a refugee because the person first comes to the country of destination and once in the country, applies for protection.

   a) May be returned to their homelands when conditions change.

   b) Legally required to undergo a medical examination in their country of temporary asylum before obtaining admission to the United States.

   c) Presence of TB, Hansen's disease (leprosy), or a sexually transmitted disease (not including HIV as of August, 2008) prevents entry to the United States unless the disease is treated.

   d) May enter one of the eight ports of entry staffed by quarantine inspectors from the Centers for Disease Control and Prevention (CDC). New refugees are offered a health assessment on entry.

   e) Health risks include:

      (1) Malnutrition

      (2) Intestinal parasites

      (3) Hepatitis B, TB, malaria, STDs (syphilis, HIV)

      (4) Low immunization history

      (5) Dental caries

      (6) Long-term effects of rape, trauma, torture causing posttraumatic stress disorders

      (7) Mental health problems as a direct result of the refugee experience

      (8) Many often suffer from hunger, stress, grief, lack of cultural environment, change in climate, lack of clothing, dependency on others, and lack of local language skills.

   f) Relocation and acculturation issues of immigrants/refugees/asylees (Okie, 2007)

      (1) Housing

      (2) Health care access and treatment

      (3) New language and culture

      (4) Posttraumatic stress disorder

      (5) Legal issues

      (6) Societal prejudices

   g) Health insurance coverage (Kaiser Commission on Key Facts, 2007; Schwartz & Artiga, 2007).

      (1) Immigrants incur lower health care costs, because of lower utilization of health services.

      (2) Low-income non-citizens are more than twice as likely to be uninsured.

      (3) Medicaid, the nation's major health coverage for low-income people, assists children at higher income levels than adults.

      (4) Under the *Deficit Reduction Act of 2005*, most U.S. citizens and nationals applying for or renewing their Medicaid coverage for the first time must document their citizenship and identity.

      (5) Most legal immigrants are barred from Medicaid for the first 5 years in the United States; undocumented immigrants are eligible only for emergency Medicaid services.

      (6) Some groups are exempt, such as those receiving *SSI (Supplemental Social Security) and SSDI (Supplemental Social Security Disability Insurance)*.

      (7) All babies born in the United States are U.S. citizens.

      (8) Pregnant women, children and women are eligible for breast and cervical cancer screening; they can be granted presumptive eligibility for Medicaid without documenting their citizenship, but are required to file a regular application (Kaiser Commission on Key Facts, 2007).

      (9) Immigrants pay more of their own money for health care than native-born Americans.

     (10) Labor and delivery care costs for undocumented or uninsured immigrants are covered under the federal and state Emergency Medicaid Program, but most states do not cover prenatal care or family planning.

   h) Emergency room use by immigrants/refugees/asylees (Avery, 2001)

      (1) Visits to the emergency room are much higher than for native-born Americans.

      (2) Uninsured, low-income immigrants lack access to routine prevention and treatment; often wait until conditions are acute and receive more expensive treatment in hospital emergency rooms.

i) Infectious disease quarantines
   (1) CDC (2008d) guidelines for global migration and quarantine laws/regulations define *quarantine* as a restriction of activities of healthy persons or animals that have been exposed to a communicable disease.
   (2) The goal is to prevent transmission of disease from infected persons or animals to healthy persons during the disease incubation period.
   (3) Quarantine is an extreme form of isolation because it includes compulsory segregation of people from contacts with infectious cases. In 2007, Andrew Speaker was quarantined when he flew to Europe and returned to the United States with an extremely active case of drug resistant tuberculosis.
   (4) Often challenged for violating civil rights of individuals especially in cases of long confinement or segregation from society.
j) A medical examination is mandatory for all refugees coming to the United States and all applicants outside the US applying for an immigrant visa.
k) Treatments and immunizations for immigrants(Avery, 2001)
l) Immigrants with low income are immunized and often treated for malnutrition, intestinal parasites, hepatitis B, TB, dental caries, malaria, syphilis and other STDs, including HIV; children are often treated for rheumatic heart disease, high lead levels, and neonatal tetanus.
m) Mental health issues of anxiety and posttraumatic stress disorders associated with:
   (1) Long-term effects of loss, grief, rape, trauma, torture, mental health problems
   (2) Decreased sense of safety and security
   (3) History of imprisonment, witnessing violence or death of family and/or friends
   (4) Loss of homes and other possessions
   (5) Lack of resources and support system
   (6) Separation from family members and lack of awareness of the location or fate of loved ones
   (7) Problems associated with change in climate, inadequate food, clothing and shelter, role changes such as dependency on others, or unfamiliarity with new culture and local language.
n) *Immigration detention* is the policy of holding individuals suspected of visa violations, illegal entry or unauthorized arrival in detention until a decision is made by immigration authorities to grant a visa and release them into the community, or to repatriate them to their country of departure. *Mandatory detention* is the practice of compulsory detention or imprisonment of people seeking political asylum, or who are considered to be illegal immigrants or unauthorized arrivals in the country.
   (1) Detention centers for immigrants are often challenged with people who have numerous health care problems.
   (2) Immigrants often have no legal way to complain about care received.
o) Ethical and legal issues of immigrants (Yamin, 2005)
   (1) Legal due process
      (a) The *1990 Immigration Act (IMMACT)* limits the annual number of immigrants to 700,000 and emphasizes family reunification as the main immigration criterion, in addition to employment-related immigration.
      (b) The *Antiterrorism and Effective Death Penalty Act (AEDPA)* and *Illegal Immigration Reform and Immigrant Responsibility Act (IIRIRA)* describe many categories of criminal activity for which immigrants, including green card holders, can be deported.
      (c) Public funding of prenatal care for undocumented women has become a subject of intense public debate.
      (d) Undocumented immigrants who do not receive prenatal care are nearly four times as likely to have low birth weight infants and seven times as likely to have preterm births; their infants incur higher expenses for neonatal care.

9. **The Homeless** (National Coalition for the Homeless, 2007)
   a. The condition and social category of people who lack housing, because they cannot afford, or are otherwise unable to maintain, regular, safe, and adequate shelter.
   b. The term *homelessness* may also include people whose primary nighttime residence is in a homeless shelter, in an institution that provides a temporary residence for individuals intended to be institutionalized, or in a public or private place not designed for use as a regular sleeping accommodation.

   c. Major reasons for homelessness include:
   1) Lack of affordable housing
   2) Lack of employment opportunities
   3) Poverty, caused by many factors, including unemployment and underemployment
   4) Lack of affordable health care
   5) Substance abuse
   6) Lack of access to needed services
   7) Mental illness and lack of access to needed services
   8) Domestic violence
   9) Prison release and reentry into society
   10) Natural disaster

   d. Problems of homeless people
   1) Reduced access to health care
   2) Limited access to education
   3) Increased risk for violence and abuse
   4) Discrimination
   5) Not being seen as suitable for employment
   6) Lack of health care providers in homeless shelters
   7) Fear of imprisonment imposes isolation

   e. Assistance for the homeless
   1) Most countries provide a variety of services to assist with food, shelter and clothing that may be organized and run by community organizations (often with the help of volunteers) or by the government.
   2) These programs may be supported by government, charities, churches and individual donors.
   3) The United States has no national policy regarding the homeless, and their care and assistance fall on the state and local governments.

10. Groups in Inadequate Living Conditions (Probst, Moore, Glover, & Samuels, 2004)
   a. Residentially isolated (urban and rural areas)
   1) Two thirds of the estimated 1.8 billion people living in the rural areas of developing countries are at greater risk of being poor and living in poverty for a long time.
   2) Causes of isolation:
      a) Ecology: The soil quality, slope, rainfall quality and distribution, temperature, and vulnerability to natural hazards have a significant impact on a community's geographic isolation, amount of food produced, natural resources, such as clean water, fuel for heating and cooking, access to local markets, access to education and health care and overall poverty.
      b) Physical infrastructure: Poor roads, rail, or river connections often lead to high transport costs, which may cause a community to lack basic materials for construction, food, medical, and school supplies to maintain quality schools and health services
      c) Political parties: Weak political parties and networks are often linked to low level of government infrastructure and community resources, such as public services, food distribution, housing, and health care.
      d) Poverty: Low-income communities have inadequate tax revenues to support good infrastructure, trade, public education, health programs, housing, and food supply.
      e) Lack of transportation necessary to bring adequate goods and services to a community, for the people to get to and from their places of employment, trade with other communities, get to schools for education, and access health care services.

   b. Groups living in overcrowded and substandard housing (Myers, Baer, & Choi, 1996)
   1) A *substandard household* is overcrowded (has more than one person per room), lacks complete plumbing, does not have a private kitchen, lacks adequate heating, is physically deteriorated, or when the rent or mortgage payments cost more than 30% of the household income.
   2) The U.S. Census estimates that the national number of substandard households could be as high as one million.
   3) Worldwide, 1.6 billion people live in substandard housing and 100 million are homeless (Habitat for Humanity, 2009)

   4) The U.S. Department of Housing and Urban Development (HUD, 2008) acknowledges that conditions in many public housing developments are unacceptable due to poor management, poor maintenance, deterioration, and high crime rates.
   5) Unsafe environment is characterized by:
       a) High crime rate
       b) Overcrowded and substandard housing
       c) Unclean water supply
       d) High levels of nuclear and toxic wastes
   c. Groups with literacy and language difficulties include
       1) New immigrants/asylees/refugees
       2) Those with low education level or inadequate schooling
       3) Persons with learning disabilities
       4) Persons with mental retardation
       5) Persons with dementia
11. **Prisoners** (Prisoner Health Care, n.d.)
   a. The *US Marshals Service*
       1) Relies on state and local jails as well as the Bureau of Prisons detention facilities to provide medical care to inmates.
       2) Responsible for providing a secure escort and paying for medical care of prisoners in the local community.
       3) The U.S. Marshals Service faces an increasing number of prisoners and other challenges.
           a) Inmates suffer from extremely complex medical problems, such as cancer, terminal AIDS, and liver and kidney failure.
           b) Concerns with protecting staff, other prisoners and the general public from exposure to infectious diseases such as active tuberculosis.
           c) Has implement medical cost containment by establishing preferred provider medical networks, centralized medical bill review and pricing, locked hospital wards in local facilities, and interagency cooperative efforts with the U.S. Public Health Service and the Department of Veterans Affairs.
       4) The 1990 Resolution establishing *Basic Principles for the Treatment of Prisoners in the US* mandates that "Prisoners shall have access to the health services available in the country without discrimination on the groups of their legal situation."
       5) The *Standard Minimum Rules* give prisoners requiring specialized treatment the right to be transferred to special facilities or civilian hospitals.
       6) Preventive dental care is necessary for long-term dental health, but the U.S. Constitution does not give prisoners this right; except care related to treatment of dental pain and discomfort.
   b. There are more than 8.5 million prisoners held in penal institutions throughout the world, either as pre-trial detainees (*remand prisoners*) or having been convicted and sentenced.
       1) With a world population of 6.1 billion this represents an average incarceration rate of 140 prisoners per 100,000 of the population.
       2) Prison overcrowding leads to a multitude of other problems such as decreased living space, poor hygiene and sanitation.
       3) In some countries, there is insufficient bedding and clothing, food quality and quantity are compromised, health care is difficult to administer, and more tension and violence among prisoners as well as violence against staff occur.
   c. *Amnesty International* is a worldwide movement to campaign for internationally recognized human rights for all. Supporters are outraged by human rights abuses and inspired by hope for a better world. They work to improve human rights through campaigning and international solidarity, including prisoners.

V. GLOBAL DISPARITIES IN MORBIDITY AND MORTALITY FROM ACUTE AND CHRONIC DISEASES

A. Obesity
   1. Obesity prevalence is growing worldwide, in most developed and developing countries
       a. One third of the world's population aged 15 years or older is overweight or obese.

    b. In the United States, 66% of all adults are overweight (body mass index [BMI] equal to or greater than 25) or obese (BMI equal to or greater than 30).

    c. Within some ethnic groups (Latinos, American Indians, and African American women) obesity exceeds the overall U.S. estimates.

2. Factors contributing to increased obesity include:
    a. Modern technology and economic growth
    b. Shift toward highly refined foods, meat and dairy products containing high levels of saturated fats
    c. Reduction in energy expenditure and increased availability of food
    d. Greater inactivity

3. Obesity is a risk factor for a variety of health issues including diabetes, hypertension, cardiovascular disease, stroke, and certain cancers.

B. Malnutrition

1. A state of poor nutrition which can result from insufficient, excessive, or unbalanced diet, or from the inability to absorb foods.

2. Famine will continue due to political instability, repressive governments, internal conflicts, and natural disasters.
    a. Famine/starvation/malnutrition can result from political instability (Holtz, Plitnick, & Friedman, 2008)
    b. Starvation is used as a weapon in the Sudan's civil war.
    c. Malnutrition is widespread among Sudanese children living in Chad.

3. Considered to be the world's leading threat to life and health.
    a. Each day 24,000 people worldwide die from hunger and malnutrition, the majority of whom are young children.
    b. The WHO estimates that malnutrition is a contributing factor in at least 49% of deaths worldwide.
    c. Half of all malnourished children and a large proportion of malnourished adult women are in Bangladesh, India, and Pakistan.
    d. Nearly 33% of the world suffers from micronutrient malnutrition, resulting in the following:
        1) Decreased mental and physical development
        2) Poor pregnancy outcomes
        3) Decreased work capacity for adults
        4) Increased illness, disease susceptibility, and premature death
        5) Deficiencies in zinc, leading to immune deficiency, growth retardation, and diarrhea
        6) Bone loss
        7) Blindness

4. Key global future trends:
    a. Projected 20% increase in malnutrition in sub-Saharan Africa.
    b. Continuing growth of people affected by hunger worldwide; pattern of increase in the 1990s except in China.
    c. Iron deficiency and anemia will affect 3.5 billion people in the developing world.
    d. Food donations will decrease by one third.
    e. By 2015, worldwide nutritional issues will affect food distribution, access, and availability.

C. Diabetes Mellitus (Long, Rodriguez, & Holtz, 2008)

1. In the United States, more than 16 million people are affected, half of whom are unaware that they have the disease.
    a. Disproportionately affects older adults and ethnic minorities.
    b. The *health related quality of life (HRQOL)* of people with diabetes, a mainly self-managed disease, is related to glycemic control, duration of the disease, complications, and comorbidities.
    c. Elderly people living in rural communities have greater difficulty in self-managing diabetes because of limited access to medical specialists, places to exercise, special foods, and health education.

2. The International Diabetes Federation estimates that there are 246 million adults with diabetes.
    a. The Western Pacific region and Europe have the highest number of people with diabetes, approximately 67 and 53 million, respectively.
    b. The highest prevalence rates are found in North America (9.2%) and Europe (8.4%).
    c. The five countries with the largest numbers of people with diabetes are India, China, the United States, Russia, and Germany.

    d. The five countries with the highest prevalence rates are Nauru, United Arab Emirates, Saudi Arabia, Bahrain, and Kuwait.

    e. Developed countries have higher prevalence rates but developing countries are predicted to be hit the hardest by the epidemic.

    f. Increased urbanization, Westernization and economic development in developing countries have contributed to a substantial rise in diabetes.

    g. The number of people with diabetes is expected to increase to 380 million people globally in 2025. The number of people with diabetes is projected to rise from 171 million in 2000 to 366 million in 2030.

D. Tuberculosis (TB) (Akers, Blake, & Hansen, 2008)

    1. TB is a respiratory disease that spreads acid-fast bacilli through the air by means of infected, aerosolized droplets from people who cough, sneeze, or talk with vigor.

    2. TB has affected all nations and economic systems

        a. Approximately 8 million to 10 million new cases are reported globally each year, with almost 2 billion people, or one third of the world's population infected.

        b. TB is a preventable and curable but more than 1.7 million people die from TB annually, killing more people than any other infectious disease.

        c. The WHO estimates that Southeast Asia has the largest numbers of new TB cases, accounting for 33% of total cases globally.

    3. Drug-resistant TB is a major global problem often tied to HIV/AIDS.

E. Lead Poisoning (CDC, 2008a; Tehranifar et al., 2008)

    1. Almost half a million children in the United States have blood levels of lead that exceed 10 µg/dL of blood, a level at which adverse health effects are known to occur.

    2. Lead can be toxic when taken into the body through breathing, eating, or drinking; most dangerous to children, especially younger than 6 years of age.

        a. Lead poisoning can affect every body system and especially damaging to a child's kidneys, central nervous and reproductive systems.

        b. In young children, low levels of lead can be harmful and can result in decreased intelligence, impaired neurobehavioral development, decreased stature and growth, and impaired hearing.

        c. Because childhood lead poisoning often has no distinctive clinical symptoms, it can go unrecognized.

    3. The most significant sources of lead exposure for U.S. children are deteriorated lead-based paint and dust contaminated with lead. Lead-based paints were banned from housing in 1978, but about 85% of houses were built before the ban was instituted.

        a. Young children who live in older houses with deteriorating paint may eat paint chips that contain lead or ingest or breathe lead-contaminated dust from floors, carpeting, or toys.

        b. Because the exterior of houses may have been painted with lead-based paint, children may be exposed to lead in the soil when they play outdoors.

F. HIV/AIDS (Akers, Blake & Hansen, 2008)

    1. The WHO estimates that more than 65 million people have been infected with HIV; AIDS killed more than 25 million people.

        a. Almost 40 million people are living with HIV; most are unaware that they are infected (UNAIDS, 2006).

        b. Although HIV seems to be slowing down globally, there are regions and countries throughout the world that continue to see skyrocketing rates.

    2. The HIV virus is transmitted through blood, semen, vaginal fluids, and breast milk. The primary modes of transmission include unprotected sex and sharing of needles that contain infected blood.

    3. A mother can transmit HIV to her baby during pregnancy, childbirth, or breast-feeding (UNAIDS, 2006).

G. Malaria (Akers, Blake, & Hansen, 2008)

    1. The *World Malaria Report (2008)* describes the global distribution of cases and deaths, implementation of the WHO-recommended control strategies in countries where the disease is endemic, sources of funding for malaria control, and evidence that prevention and treatment can alleviate the burden of disease.

        a. Each year, there are approximately 515 million cases of malaria, killing between one and three million people, the majority of whom are young children in sub-Saharan Africa.

        b. Half of the world's population is at risk *for* malaria, and an estimated 247 million cases led to nearly 881,000 deaths in 2006.

2. A vector-borne infectious disease caused by a protozoan parasite, which is widespread in tropical and sub-tropical regions, including parts of the Americas, Asia, and Africa.
    a. In North America and Europe, *Anopheles* mosquitoes capable of transmitting malaria are still present, but the parasite has been eliminated.
    b. Socioeconomic improvements (e.g., houses with screened windows, air conditioning) combined with vector reduction efforts and effective treatment has led to the elimination of malaria without the complete elimination of the vectors.
    c. Vector control for the prevention of malaria includes insecticide, bed nets, indoor spraying, and larva control.
    d. No vaccine is available for malaria; preventive drugs must be taken continuously to reduce the risk of infection, but these prophylactic drug treatments are often too expensive for most people with malaria.

VI. EMERGING HEALTH THREATS
A. Natural Disasters
1. The public health infrastructure must be prepared to prevent illness and injury that would result from natural disasters such as hurricanes, fires, and tsunamis.
2. *The U.S. Model State Emergency Health Powers Act* or *Model Act* provides states with power to detect and contain bioterrorism, or a naturally occurring disease outbreak. This includes:
    a. Preparedness for a public health emergency
    b. Surveillance to detect and track public health emergencies
    c. Communication of clear and authoritative information to the public
    d. Management of property, ensuring adequate availability of vaccines, pharmaceuticals, and hospitals
    e. Protection of persons, vaccination, testing, treatment, isolation and quarantine when necessary

B. Bioterrorism (Gostin et al., 2002)
1. Early detection and control of biological or chemical attacks depends on a strong and flexible public health system at the local, state, and federal levels.
2. Biological or chemical terrorism ranging from anthrax spores to food product or water contamination; occurrence is impossible to predict.
3. The CDC's draft of a model law to assist states in responding to a bioterrorism event, gives state officials broad powers to close buildings, take over hospitals and order quarantines.

C. Nuclear Accidents (Gostin et al., 2002).
1. People are exposed to small amounts of radiation every day, both from naturally occurring sources (elements in the soil or cosmic rays from the sun), and human-made sources (electronic equipment, microwave ovens, and television sets), medical sources (x-rays, certain diagnostic tests and treatments), and fallout from nuclear weapons testing.
2. Amount of radiation to which people are exposed is usually small. A radiation emergency (nuclear power plant accident or a terrorist event) could expose people to small or large doses of radiation.
3. *Contamination* occurs when particles of radioactive material are deposited in places where they are not supposed to be (on object or a person's skin).
4. *Internal contamination* occurs when radioactive material is taken into the body through breathing, eating, or drinking.
5. *Exposure* occurs when radiation energy penetrates the body (when a person has an x-ray).
6. Radiation can affect the body in a number of ways and adverse effects of exposure may not be apparent for many years.
7. Nuclear warfare is an emerging threat especially when linked to terrorism that can potentially cause enormous radiation contamination leading to sickness and deaths.

VII. FACTORS CONTRIBUTING TO GLOBAL HEALTH DISPARITIES
A. Environmental/Ecological Causes of Health Disparities (Friedman, 2008)
1. *Pollution and toxins*
    a. Environmentally induced diseases can result from lack of knowledge about the adverse effects of radiation and toxic environmental chemicals.
    b. Epidemics have resulted from a failure to know and understand environmental risks from man-made and natural contaminants as well as those which resulted from societal, economic, or ethical decisions.

    2. ***Climate changes***
       a. Global warming create droughts, crop destruction, and starvation.
       b. Hurricanes, tornados, floods, and tsunamis create disasters causing destruction of human lives and properties.
       c. All the above increase mosquito breeding and mosquito-borne infections (malaria and dengue fever)

B. Socioeconomic and Gender Inequality (Holtz, 2008b)
    1. Global gender inequalities affecting health status are exemplified by:
       a. Female infanticide in countries such as China
       b. Inadequate feeding of female babies
       c. Female circumcision
       d. Domestic violence and homicide
       e. Childbirth without adequate family planning, health care, and nutrition
       f. Rape, incest, sexual slavery, and forced prostitution of women
       g. Male dominance and inadequate/unequal rights of women
       h. Slavery, sexual exploitation, child labor, and mass killings during wars

C. Political Instability and War (Ethnoviolence/Genocide) (Rummel, 1992)
    1. *Genocide* refers to violent crimes committed against groups with the intent to destroy the existence of these groups.
       a. World War II Asian Holocaust (Japanese killed 30 million people between 1937 and 1945; "the Rape of Nanjing")
       b. 1922-1945 genocide by German Nazis killed 15,200,000 people, including 6 million Jews in concentration camps.
       c. As of 1975, the Khmer Rouge regime killed about 3.5 million out of 7.1 million people in Cambodia through execution, starvation, and forced labor.
       d. 1945-1979 China's Cultural Revolution resulted in 70 million deaths.
       e. 16th century to 1900s, 20 million Americans were killed by Europeans
       f. 1971, Pakistani military atrocities against Bangladeshis and other ethnicities in East Pakistan caused 3 million deaths.
       g. Recent genocides of Iraqi Kurds, and the people of Bosnia-Herzegovina, Rwanda, and Darfur, Sudan.
    2. The *US Bill of Rights* and the *1948 UN Universal Declaration of Human Rights*, concern the rights of individuals and protection of all human lives.

D. Violence (Holtz, 2008d)
    1. *The World Report on Violence and Health* defines *violence* as the intentional use of physical force or power, threatened or actual, against oneself, another person, or against a group or community that either results in, or has a high likelihood of injury, death, psychological harm, maldevelopment, or deprivation.
    2. Violence includes: child abuse and neglect by caregivers; violence by youth (ages 10 to 29 years); intimate partner violence; sexual violence; elder abuse; self-inflicted violence; and collective violence, such as war or terrorism.
    3. Worldwide, an average of 4,500 people die a violent death every day.
       a. In 2000, there were 1.2 million violent deaths, one half from suicide, one third from homicide, and one fifth from war-related injuries.
       b. Intentional violence (homicide) is the greatest cause of death in many countries (approximately 120,000 deaths a year).
       c. Although the United States has lower rates of homicide and deaths related to firearms than developing countries, it has very high rates when compared with other developed countries.
       d. Homicide rates for Africa, Central America, and South America are three times the U.S. rate.

E. Accidents and Injuries (Holtz, 2008d)
    1. Injury is the ninth most common cause of premature death worldwide and the third most common cause of years lived with disability. Injuries cause about 10% of all deaths worldwide with traffic accidents, self-inflicted injuries, violence, and war, being the most common causes.
       a. The World Bank and the World Health Organization report that almost 12 million people die of traffic accidents injuries each year, and the number could increase by 65% in the next 20 years.
       b. The highest increase in deaths from injuries occurs in developing countries.
       c. Traffic accidents kill 1.2 million people (3,242 deaths per day) and injure or disable 20 to 50 million daily and injures more, globally.

   d. Most traffic-related deaths take place in developing countries, among young men 15 to 44 years old who are involved in 77% of all vehicular collisions and the riders of most motorized two-wheeled vehicles.
   e. In 2002, burns were responsible for nearly 322,000 deaths and more than 90% of fatal fire-related burns occur in developing countries.
   f. In 2002, an estimated 376,000 people drowned, making drowning the third leading global cause of death from unintentional injury after road traffic injuries and falls.
   g. In 2002, more than 390,000 deaths globally were caused by falls; adults older than 70 years of age, particularly women, have higher fall-related mortality/morbidity rates.
2. In the United States, the estimated cost of serious trauma care for each person is far greater than care for cancer and cardiovascular diseases.
   a. Advances in prehospital care with basic and advanced life support, helped decrease mortality rates from serious injuries.
   b. Advances in technology in hospital emergency rooms, operative care, and intensive care have significantly improved patients' chances of survival.
   c. In developing countries, many seriously injured patients may not have the benefit of advanced technology and care.
F. **Rape** (Waldsman, 2005)
   1. Women victims of rape face divorce, abandonment by family and community, or even death in cultures that prize female virginity and fidelity.
   2. Many women declare they would rather die than live to face the shame associated with being raped.
   3. Armies used rape to control the minds and bodies of the vanquished; rape demoralizes their prey, further asserting their power over the foreign "other."

VIII. HEALTH CARE DISPARITIES IN THE UNITED STATES
A. *Health care disparities* are gaps in health care across racial, ethnic, and socioeconomic groups.
B. Racial and ethnic minorities and low socioeconomic groups receive lower quality health care than whites, even when insurance status, income, age, and illness severity are comparable.
C. Causes of disparities
   1. Unequal and inadequate access to insurance coverage
      a. Health insurance directly affects access to health care regardless of race, ethnicity, or socioeconomic status.
      b. Without insurance, many people will go without medical care because they cannot afford to pay out-of-pocket for care.
      c. According to the U.S. Census Bureau (2007), 7% of non-Hispanic Whites were uninsured, compared with 20.1% of African Americans, 32.4% of Hispanics, and 18.4% of Asians.
   2. Lack of a regular source of health care
      a. Minority groups are less likely to have a regular source of health care.
      b. Those without a regular source of health care are less likely to access care.
   3. Lack of financial resources
      a. Those who have low income and are uninsured are particularly unlikely to access health care.
      b. Low-income immigrant minorities may be unable to obtain health insurance such as SCHIP.
   4. Physical barriers
      a. Inadequate or no transportation to health care services.
      b. Long waiting times for seeing a health care provider.
      c. Scarcity of health care providers and pharmacy services within inner city and isolated rural areas with higher concentrations of minorities.
   5. Language barriers
      a. Those with limited or no English speaking and understanding abilities are less likely to set up an appointment for medical care and will therefore rely on emergency rooms for care when vitally needed.
      b. Lack of English inhibits comprehension of health care advice.
   6. Lack of health literacy
      a. *Health literacy* is the ability to obtain, process, and understand basic health information to make appropriate health decisions.
      b. It is needed to access health care systems.
      c. A larger number of minority patients have challenges in health literacy.

7.   Lack of diversity in health care providers
   a. Minority patients, given a choice, are more likely to seek health care providers who are more like themselves and know their culture and language.
   b. Minority groups in the United States, together, represent 25% of the population, yet less than 9% of minority groups are nurses, 6% are physicians, and only 5% are dentists.
8.   Disparities in health care delivery (The Sullivan Commission, 2004)
   a. Racial and ethnic disparities in health care delivery are related to differences in treatment by health care providers.
   b. In 2002, the Institute of Medicine reported in *Unequal Treatment Confronting Racial and Ethnic Disparities in Health Care* that:
      1)   Minority groups are less likely than Whites to be given appropriate cardiac medicines or given cardiac bypass surgery when necessary.
      2)   Minority groups are less likely to receive renal dialysis or transplants than Whites.
      3)   Minorities are less likely to receive the best diagnostic tests or treatment for stroke or cancer than Whites.
      4)   Minorities are less likely to receive the best treatment for HIV/AIDS than Whites.
   c. Minorities often distrust health care providers, the majority of whom are White.
      1)   Less adequate health facilities and lower quality (education and experience) of health care providers are available to minorities.
      2)   African Americans are more likely than Whites to:
         a) Seek care from hospitals that have fewer resources and up-to-date technology.
         b) Have higher surgical mortality rates.
         c) Are more likely to receive care from physicians with less training.
         d) Have less access to specialists such as a cardiologist or neurosurgeon, as opposed to a family practitioner.

IX. "BRAIN DRAIN" AS A CAUSE OF GLOBAL HEALTH CARE DISPARITIES (Brush, 2008)
A. Health care providers migrate from developing to developed countries to seek better economic and working conditions, educational training, more stable political conditions, and hopes for a better future.
B. Large immigration of health care professionals creates acute shortages of skilled practitioners and educators in the home countries.
C. Developing societies make investments in the education of health care providers and lose their investments when these professionals leave.
D. Health care professionals who migrate from developing to developed countries may obtain more education and experience and bring back valuable expertise when they return to their native countries
E. The United States, Canada, New Zealand, and the United Kingdom have more than 20% foreign-born physicians and nurses. Although not all foreign health care practitioners are from impoverished countries, the majority are from developing countries.
F. Countries such as Jamaica, Haiti, Pakistan, India, Ghana, South Africa, and Uganda have lost more than 10% of their practicing physicians and nurses.
G. The United Kingdom, the United States, and Canada have hired large numbers of health care providers from the Philippines, India, Caribbean, and Africa.
H. In-country migration of health care workers from isolated rural areas to more populated and wealthier urban areas, and from public to private institutions) further limits care for low-income urban minorities.
I. Immigrant health care providers are generally placed in underserved inner cities and rural areas, and help address social justice issues in health care.

X. RECOMMENDATIONS FOR DECREASING HEALTH CARE DISPARITIES
A. Increase awareness of problem among providers, insurers, and policy makers.
B. Promote consistency and equity of care through evidence-based guidelines so treatment decisions are based on best available science.
C. Strengthen culturally competent health care delivery.
   1.   Culturally competent care has been identified in the United States as a moral obligation (Betancourt, Green, Carillo, & Park, 2005)
      a. *Cultural competence* in health care is the ability of systems to provide care to patients with diverse values, beliefs, and behaviors, including tailoring delivery to meet patients' social, cultural, and linguistic needs.

b. Cultural competency training has gained attention as a potential strategy to improve quality of care and eliminate racial and ethnic health disparities.

c. The goals are

1) Create a health care system and workforce that can deliver the highest quality of care to every patient, regardless of race, ethnicity, cultural background, or English proficiency.

2) Increase access and utilization of health care and mental health programs, and eliminate racial and ethnic health disparities.

3) Develop user-friendly and sustainable plan of care by assessing and incorporating the cultural needs of patients.

4) Negotiate with managed care and provider based on a comprehensive evaluation of the client's needs.

D. Increase diversity of the health care workforce to increase patients' choices of health care providers.

E. Measure health and health care quality

1. Clinical performance measures of how well health care providers deliver specific services, including communication with patients based on evaluations by patients, families, and communities.

2. Assessment by patients of how well providers meet their health care needs, such as whether providers communicate clearly with them.

3. Outcomes reflected in changes in morbidity, mortality, client utilization rates, and satisfaction with the system such as decreased death rates from cancers preventable by early screening.

F. Political activism to influence social and health policies

1. Grassroots organizations can encourage their members to write members of Congress, hold rallies, create websites, speak and write in public or private to address health care coverage and general health issues, such as clean air, water, decrease smoking in public facilities.

G. Use of mass media: Mass media information on health-related issues may cause changes in health service utilization through planned and unplanned coverage.

XI. GLOBAL AGENCIES/ORGANIZATIONS INVOLVED IN HEALTH PROMOTION AND REDUCING POVERTY

A. World Health Organization (WHO, 2008)

1. Direct and coordinate authority for health within the United Nations system
2. Provide leadership on global health
3. Shape the health research agenda
4. Set norms and standards or health care
5. Articulate evidence-based policy options
6. Provide technical support to countries
7. Monitor and assess health trends.

B. Organization for Economic Co-operation and Development (OECD, 2008)

1. Brings together governments of countries from around the world to support sustainable economic growth, boost employment, raise living standards, maintain financial stability, assist with economic development, and contribute toward growth in world trade.

C. The U.S. Agency for International Development (USAID, 2008)

1. Global health programs demonstrate the commitment and determination of the U.S. government to prevent suffering, save lives, and create a brighter future for families in the developing world.
2. Improvement of the quality, availability, and use of essential health services worldwide, including child, maternal, and reproductive health promotion, and reduction of disease prevalence, especially HIV/AIDs, malaria, and TB.

D. World Bank (World Bank, 2008)

1. Created in 1944 to rebuild a war-torn Europe after World War II.
   a. Began attempt to rebuild the infrastructure of Europe's former colonies.
   b. Focused largely on poverty alleviation, and later debt management.
      1) Provides loans to developing countries for programs, including reduction of poverty
      2) Current focus is the achievement of the Millennium Development Goals
      3) Financed through the sale of AAA-rated bonds in the world's financial markets, donations from forty donor countries that infuse money to the bank every 3 years, and from loan repayments.

E. The U.S. Centers for Disease Control and Prevention (CDC, 2008c)
1. Monitor local and global health
2. Detect and investigate health problems
3. Conduct research to enhance prevention
4. Develop and advocate for sound public health policies
5. Implement disease-prevention strategies
6. Foster safe and healthful environments
7. Provide leadership and training

F. The U.S. Department of Health and Human Services (USDHHS)
1. Has the following programs
    a. Health and social science research
    b. Disease prevention, including immunization services
    c. Assurance of food and drug safety
    d. Medicare (health insurance for elderly and disabled Americans) and Medicaid (health insurance for low-income people)
    e. Health information technology
    f. Financial assistance and services for low-income families
    g. Improvement of maternal and infant health
    h. Head Start (preschool education and services)
    i. Faith-based and community initiatives
    j. Prevention of child abuse and domestic violence
    k. Substance abuse treatment and prevention
    l. Services for older Americans, including home-delivered meals
    m. Comprehensive health services for Native Americans
    n. Medical preparedness for emergencies, including potential terrorism prevention
    o. Healthy People 2010 goals and objectives (CDC, 2008b)
        1) Goals include increasing years of healthy life and eliminate health disparities
        2) Purpose is to provide strategies to promote healthy behaviors, protect health, assure access to quality health care, and strengthen community prevention

G. U.S. Public Health Service
1. The principal agency for protecting the health of all Americans and providing essential human services, especially for those who are least able to help themselves.
2. The Office of Public Health and Science (OPHS) consists of 12 core public health offices and the Commissioned Corps, a uniformed service of more than 6,000 health professionals who serve at HHS and other federal agencies

H. U.S. Indian Health Service
1. A federal obligation to provide funding for health care services to American Indians and Alaska Natives
2. Designs health care programs, coordinates with other agencies, and obtains regulation waivers for selected Indian programs.

I. U.S. Veteran's Affairs (VA; http://www.va.gov/)
1. Medical benefits package for all enrolled veterans provides a full range of preventive outpatient, inpatient and long term care services within the VA health care system.
2. Has four goals:
    a. Restore the capability of veterans with disabilities to the greatest extent possible, and improve the quality of their lives and that of their families.
    b. Ensure a smooth transition for veterans from active military service to civilian life.
    c. Honor and serve veterans in life, and memorialize them in death for their sacrifices on behalf of the nation.
    d. Contribute to the public health, emergency management, socioeconomic well-being, and history of the nation.

XII. PUBLIC POLICY AND PROGRAMS TO REDUCE HEALTH AND HEALTH CARE DISPARITIES
A. Protection of Human Rights and Social Justice (de Chesnay & Anderson, 2008; Pacquiao, 2008)
   1. The World Health Organization goal of *Health for All* seeks highest attainable standard of health as a fundamental right of every human being. In the United States, 47 million people have no access to health care.

2. *Social justice* is the equitable balance between social benefits and burdens; movement toward a socially just world.

3. Human rights and equality principles require greater degree of economic egalitarianism through progressive taxation, income redistribution, and/or property redistribution.

4. Social justice implies access to needed health care is a right of citizenship.

5. Pacquiao (2008) proposed *cultural competence* as key to providing health care to vulnerable populations.
   a. Social justice means advocacy for elimination of health disparities by ensuring the basic human right to access quality health care.
   b. *Compassion* is critical to motivate people to act on behalf of others, and to identify those who are oppressed and/or disadvantaged.
   c. Collaborative partnerships with refugees and asylum seekers are needed to gain their respect and preserve their dignity and valued life ways.

6. Social justice gives moral privilege to the needs of the most vulnerable groups in an effort to promote justice within the society at large.

7. Within the context of social justice, all members of a society can demand and expect equal access to health care and the opportunity for good health.

8. Human rights principle imposes a moral duty on health care providers and society to give populations the right to access to health care.

9. Human rights reinforce the ethical principles of equity, the right to information and participation in decisions about one's health and care, beneficence and not doing harm.

10. Legal *right to health care*
    a. The *Universal Declaration of Human Rights*, adopted by the United Nations in 1948, proclaimed that "Everyone has the right to a standard of living adequate for the health and well-being of oneself and one's family, including food, clothing, housing, and medical care."
    b. The *US Bill of Rights* and the 1948 *UN Universal Declaration of Human Rights*, concerns the rights of individuals and is applicable to the protection of the lives of all humans in the world
    c. This statement was adopted at the urging of the US, and reflects the truth of the nation's founding documents, yet the government has achieved neither formal recognition nor practical realization of these rights.
    d. The *right to health care* under international law is a right not merely to health care but to the much broader concept of health.
    e. The initial right to health is found in the 1948 *Universal Declaration of Human Rights*, which was unanimously proclaimed by the UN General Assembly for all humanity. "The Declaration sets forth the right to a "standard of living adequate for the health and well-being of the [individual] and family including medical care and security in the event of sickness, disability" (WHO Constitution, Article 25; Yamin, 2005).

11. The U.S. government has undertaken not just a moral but a legal obligation to prohibit and to eliminate racial discrimination and to guarantee everyone without distinction as to race, color, or national origin, to equality before the law, which includes health care (Yamin, 2005).

12. Societal obligations
    a. Every woman, man, youth and child has the human right to the highest attainable standard of physical and mental health, without discrimination of any kind.
    b. Enjoyment of the human right to health is vital to all aspects of a person's life and well-being, and is crucial to the realization of many other fundamental human rights and freedoms.

13. Ethical issues
    a. Access to health care is a human right.
    b. Care of individuals is at the center of care delivery, and should be expanded to generate health for groups and populations.
    c. The responsibilities of the health care delivery system include the prevention of illness and the alleviation of disability.
    d. Collaboration with each other and those served is imperative for those working within the health care system.
    e. Violations human rights and social justice principles may be from unstable government/war, inadequate funding and other resources, inadequate health system and care providers, and geographic isolation.

14. Sources of injustices and lack of initiative to ensure health care to some groups may result from discrimination (racism, classism, ageism) or lack of support for vulnerable groups.

B. Initiatives to Promote Social Justice and Eliminate Health Disparities

 1. *Millennium Development Goals* (MDGs; Millennium Developmental Goals, 2008). The UN Millennium Summit (2000) set measurable goals and targets for combating poverty, hunger, disease, illiteracy, environmental threats, and discrimination against women.
 2. MDGs goals include:
    a. Reduce poverty and hunger by 50%; 1.2 billion people still live on less than $1 a day.
    b. Promote better education and achieve universal primary education. 113 million children globally, do not attend school.
    c. Reduce child mortality by three quarters.
    d. Improve maternal an reduce maternal mortality by 75%. In developing countries, the risk of dying in childbirth is 1 in 48.
    e. Reduce and someday eradicate HIV/AIDS, malaria, and other diseases.

XIII. SUMMARY

 A. Health disparities are a major challenge for health care agencies around the world. The burden of disease is growing disproportionately in regions of the world, which are commonly affected by poverty, isolation, marginalization, and acute manpower shortage.
 B. There is lack of an equal rights-based approach in the distribution of health care and resources.
 C. Advocacy for vulnerable populations should address equity in achieving quality of life and basic access to care that should emphasize improvement in basic life conditions, in general and health care, in particular.
 D. Knowledge of health disparities from local and global contexts is fundamental to understanding humanity as one and creating solutions that are informed by similarities and uniqueness of specific contexts.

NOTE: All references, additional resources, and important Internet sites relevant to this chapter can be found at the following website: http://tcn.sagepub.com/supplemental

Chapter 2
Comparative Systems of Health Care Delivery

Journal of Transcultural Nursing
21(Supplement 1) 39S–51S
© The Author(s) 2010
Reprints and permission:
sagepub.com/journalsPermissions.nav
DOI: 10.1177/1043659610368977
http://tcn.sagepub.com

Carol Holtz, PhD, RN[1]

I. INTRODUCTION

A. *Health care systems* are organized plans of health services that administer health care to a specified population. It includes a network of agencies, facilities, and health care providers. Funding is generally derived from public and private sources.

B. Nursing services are integral to all levels and patterns of care, and nurses form the largest number of providers in a health care system.

C. Comparison of health care systems requires understanding of the environmental, social, and cultural contexts that influence their establishment, resources, and service delivery.

D. Compared with Third World countries, developed nations have greater per capita health expenditures that can support higher quality of services, which are reflected in lower rates of infant, child, and maternal mortality, and greater longevity.

II. HEALTH STATUS

A. The current state of health, including status of wellness, fitness, and any underlying diseases or injuries.

B. Influenced by weight, nutrition, level of activity, smoking, alcohol and caffeine consumption, and compliance with prescribed medical regimen.

C. According to the World Health Organization (WHO), health is a state of complete physical, mental, and social well-being and not merely the absence of disease or infirmity.

III. DETERMINANTS OF HEALTH

A. The social, economic, and physical environment, and the person's individual characteristics and behaviors determine health.

   1. Income and social status—higher income and social status are linked to better health. The greater the gap between the richest and poorest people, the greater the differences in health.

   2. Education—low education levels are linked to poor health, more stress, and lower self-confidence.

   3. Physical environment—safe water and clean air, healthy workplaces, safe houses, communities, and roads contribute to good health.

   4. Employment and working conditions—employed people are healthier, particularly those who have more control over their work conditions.

   5. Social support networks—greater support from families, friends, and communities is linked to better health.

   6. Culture—customs, traditions, and beliefs of the family and community affect health.

   7. Genetics play a part in determining lifespan, health, and the likelihood of developing certain illnesses.

   8. Personal behavior and coping skills—eating habits, physical activity, smoking, drinking, and coping with life's stresses affect health.

   9. Health services—access and use of services that prevent and treat disease influences health.

   10. Gender—Men and women suffer from different types of diseases at different ages and rates.

Funding: The California Endowment (grant number 20082226) and Health Resources and Services Administration (grant number D11 HPO9759).
[1]Kennesaw State University, Kennesaw, GA, USA

Corresponding Author: Carol Holtz, Email: choltz@kennesaw.edu

Suggested Citation: Douglas, M. K. & Pacquiao, D. F. (Eds.). (2010). Core curriculum in transcultural nursing and health care [Supplement]. *Journal of Transcultural Nursing, 21*(Suppl. 1).

IV. FACTORS INFLUENCING HEALTH CARE SYSTEMS

A. Politics

1. Strongly influence health policy, legislation, and funding for health care.
2. Corrupt politicians may siphon off health care funds causing lack of or delays in new health care infrastructures.
3. Wars can cause violence, murder, rape, starvation, migration of populations, and inadequate food and health supplies resulting in significant morbidity and mortality within a nation.

B. Government

1. The dominant government philosophy such as socialist/communist or republic/democracy can guide the structure and function of the health care system in the country.
2. The degree of stability of the government can influence its ability to build an infrastructure and system of health care financing responsive to the needs and expectations of the population.
   a. Countries with unstable governments are unable to adequately fund a local health care system and develop enough well-prepared health care providers. As a result, they have little or no system of health care.
   b. Populations in unstable countries tend to use lay health care providers to meet their basic health care needs because of lack of accessible and affordable professional health providers.
   c. In stable societies, health care infrastructure is often better organized, better funded, and offers a higher level of health care with options for their residents.
3. Broad and equitable access to health care services is influenced by the political climate and commitment of governmental leaders.
   a. The governments of both developed and developing nations have limited resources for healthcare but should provide health care especially to vulnerable populations who cannot obtain it for themselves.
   b. Rationing may mean supplying services for those who are most likely to survive and cannot obtain services for themselves, for groups that are mandated by law or by ethical obligation, and in areas that can do the most good for the most people at the most reasonable cost.
4. The type of government influences the infrastructure of health care
   a. Dictatorship—has strict control over health care decisions such as types of treatment, birth control, abortions, access to health care, number of children allowed, and types of health care options.
   b. Democracy—offers more freedom to choose types of health care, refuse health interventions, and restrict dissemination of health information to others. Democratic nations may or may not have universal access to health care.
   c. Socialist or communist—often has a system with universal access depending on financial resources, and the type and stability of the government.
5. Laws and regulations influence health delivery systems. The *Patient Self-Determination Act* in the United States mandates that patients have a right to accurate and adequate information understandable to them regarding their care and treatment.

C. Health Policy (Toma, Zebich-Knos, Davis, & Paz, 2008)

1. Influences decision making, or organizational standards, which can facilitate or impede delivery of health care services, and the ability of providers to engage in practice that address health care needs.
2. Engagement in the process of policy development is central to creating a health care system that meets the needs of its constituents. Political activism and a commitment to policy development are central elements of professional nursing practice.
3. Influences multiple care delivery issues, including health disparities, cultural sensitivity, ethics, internationalization of health care concerns, access to care, quality of care, health care financing, and equity and social justice in the delivery of health care.

D. Style of Leadership ("Leadership Styles and Basis of Power," 2010)

1. The philosophy of leaders at the national and local levels directs the nature and function of a health care system. Leadership philosophy grounded in social justice ensures fairness in allocation of health care resources to all groups.
2. Leadership style affects the structure and processes of health care systems
   a. A bureaucratic leader is very structured and follows procedures as they have been established with minimal flexibility to explore new ways to solve problems; change is usually slow paced.
   b. An autocratic leader tends to make decisions alone and assumes total authority. Others in the group or society have no voice.
   c. A democratic leader listens to the team's ideas and studies them, but will make the final decision.

      d. A laissez-faire leader provides the least amount of direction or supervision; this style is suited for highly motivated and experienced employees.

E. The Nation's Economic and Financial Resources

    1. Adequate funding sources are needed to provide adequate quality health care to a population.

    2. The manner by which resources are allocated influence health outcomes. Equity in health outcomes stem from equitable allocation of resources.

    3. Health care expenditures are based on a nation's economic well-being. More developed countries with more established economies outspend developing countries.

    4. Health care facilities reflect the level of support allocated. Health systems in developed countries use more advanced technology in prevention, diagnosis and treatment, and patients have greater access to advanced and more costly medical procedures.

    5. The socioeconomic status of a population often affects the financial investment in health care services, including type and level of preparation of health care providers, and types of interventions available to the majority of the community.

    6. Health care financing may be drawn from direct out-of-pocket expenditures, general taxation, social health insurance, voluntary or private health insurance, and donations or community health insurance

    7. Funding for health care is drawn from public and private funds, including voluntary contributions from individuals and corporations.

    8. The U.S. government funding obligations for health care include Medicare, Medicaid, Indian Health Service, and the Veterans Administration Health Care System

F. Cultural Values, Beliefs, and Practices

    1. Caring rituals and practices are influenced by culture.

        a. Cultural and religious beliefs can influence support or prohibition of practices such as male circumcision, blood transfusion, fertility procedures, elective abortions, or organ transplants.

        b. Religion may dictate health care policies on euthanasia, birth control, sex education in schools, decisions about removal of life support, resuscitation of very low birth weight babies, infertility treatment options, and so on.

        c. Examples of culturally based practices in health care systems:

            1) Circumcision of males and/or females

            2) Roles of male or female caregivers

            3) Birthing rituals and caring practices

            4) Beliefs about use of blood products and blood removal

            5) Beliefs about the beginning of life

            6) Preferred healers and healing modalities

            7) Attitudes toward psych-mental health services

        d. Language, communication, and literacy levels of populations served by the health care system (National Network of Libraries of Medicine, 2008)

            1) Health literacy is important for general public health education, assessment and treatment, care management, and adherence to medical regime.

            2) Affect the methods and types of verbal and nonverbal communication

            3) Determine the different languages/dialects used in communication

    2. Ethical and moral assumptions of the society

        a. Ethics have strong implications for health policy regarding abortions, removal of life support, and universal access to health care.

        b. Nations that adopt ethical beliefs of social justice may create a health care environment that supports access to healthcare for all.

        c. Individuals or groups of people may not see the value in any or some health care practices and may not wish to financially support or participate in them.

        d. Societal belief that health care is a human right influences the health care delivery system.

            1) Care of individuals is at the center of health care delivery, but must be viewed and practiced within the overall context of doing the greatest possible health gains for groups and populations.

            2) Prevention and treatment of illnesses are inherent responsibilities of the health care delivery system.

            3) Requires cooperation among those working within the health system and those they serve.

            4) All individuals and groups involved in health care have the continuing responsibility to help improve its quality.

G. Geographic Location—Climate, Natural Resources

1. Countries and communities that are geographically isolated from sources of food, electricity, clean water, health care infrastructure and providers, and medicines have a tremendous limitation in providing adequate healthcare services for their population.
2. Climates suitable for large vector growth are confronted by infectious diseases such as malaria and dengue fever causing high rates of morbidity and mortality.
3. Lack of clean air and water can cause respiratory and gastrointestinal disorders.
4. Hurricanes, tornados, monsoons, floods, and droughts can cause contamination, inadequate food production, or overwhelm health care systems.
5. Natural resources, such as oil, natural gas, clean water, rich soil, and moderate climates can contribute to the economy and in establishing adequate health care delivery systems and food supply.

H. Ratio of Health Care Providers to Population (Millennium Developmental Goals, 2008)

1. The WHO requires a minimum of 20 doctors, 100, nurses and 228 total health care workers (professionals and nonprofessionals) for every 100,000 people.
2. Sub-Saharan Africa faces the greatest challenges.
   a. The shortage of health care workers is paralyzing the health systems in Lesotho, Malawi, Mozambique, and South Africa, and threatens the lives of millions, especially in rural areas.
   b. The vacancy rate for nurses in rural areas is 60%.
   c. Mozambique has only 2.6 doctors, 20 nurses, and 34 total health workers per 100,000 people.
3. Brain drain of health care providers
   a. Physicians and nurses from developing countries are recruited in large numbers by Western countries. The largest number of foreign doctors working in the United Kingdom, the United States, and Canada come from Nigeria and the Philippines.
   b. The shortage is complicating the fight against AIDS and other diseases in Africa. In Kenya, there is only one doctor for every 10,000 people. In many African countries, the scarcity is even greater.
   c. Although recipient nations and immigrating health care providers benefit from this migration, less developed countries lose important health capabilities because of loss of skilled health care providers.

I. Type of Health Care Financing

1. *Socialized medicine* is any system of medical care that is publicly financed, government administered, or both. The government operates health care facilities and employs health care professionals. Some countries differentiate tax-based universal insurance from social insurance (privately contributed by employees and employers).
   a. Examples of socialized medicine systems
      1) The British National Health Service (NHS) hospital trust
      2) Health care systems in most developed countries and Western European countries
      3) Health care system in Cuba.
      4) The United States has similar system for limited groups such as the Veteran's Affairs Health Care Systemand the Military Tricare program, Medicare (for the elderly and disabled persons) and Medicaid (for indigents).
      5) Countries with socialized health care may have open access to care with limitations for age and types of illnesses, and may also have long waiting times for appointments (Schwartz & Artiga, 2007).
   b. Health care can be financed through a *system of health insurance*, which is a type of protection that pays for medical expenses.
      1) Sometimes used more broadly to include insurance that covers disability, long-term nursing care, or medical needs.
      2) May be provided by a government-sponsored social insurance program or by private insurance companies, and may be purchased by a group or individual consumers.
      3) The covered groups or individuals pay premiums or taxes to help protect themselves from high or unexpected health care expenses.
      4) Similar benefits paying for medical expenses may also be provided through social welfare programs funded by the government.
      5) Health insurance works by estimating the overall risk of health care expenses and developing a routine finance structure (such as a monthly premium or annual tax) that will ensure that money is available to pay for health care benefits specified in the insurance agreement.
      6) Payments for medical services are administered by a central organization, most often by a government agency or a private or not-for-profit health plan.

7) A health insurance policy is a contract between an insurance company and an individual that is renewable annually or monthly. The contract specifies the type and amount of health care costs covered.

8) Individual policy holders' payment obligations may take several forms.

   a) Premium is the amount the policy holder pays to the health plan each month to purchase the health coverage.

   b) Deductible is the amount that the policy holder must pay out-of-pocket before the health plan pays.

   c) Copayment is the amount that the policy holder must pay out-of-pocket before the health plan pays for a particular visit or service.

   d) Co-insurance is the percentage of total costs that a policy holder must pay. A member may have to pay 20% of the cost of surgery, whereas the health plan pays the other 80%. There is no upper limit on co-insurance, the policy holder can end up owing very little, or a significant amount, based on cost of service used.

   e) Exclusions are services that are not covered by the insurance policy, which are paid by the policy holder.

   f) Coverage limits are the maximum amount that health plans will pay. The policy holder may be expected to pay any charges in excess of the health plan's maximum payment for a specific service. Some plans have annual or lifetime coverage maximums.

   g) Out-of-pocket maximums are similar to coverage limits, except that the members' payment obligation ends when they reach the out-of-pocket maximum, and the health plan pays for all further costs covered by the policy. Out-of-pocket maximums can be limited to a specific benefit category (such as prescription drugs) or can apply to all coverage provided during a specific period of time.

   h) Capitation is the amount paid by an insurer to health care provider, for which the provider agrees to treat all insured members.

   i) In-network providers are preselected health care providers by the insurer. The insurer offers discounted coinsurance or copayments, or additional benefits, to plan members who see them.

c. Private practice health care: Physicians and other health care providers provide legally sanctioned health care services, which are paid directly by the consumer, by an insurance company that collects premiums from consumers and/or by their employer, or by the government.

d. Managed care provider

   1) A health maintenance organization (HMO) is a type of managed health care system. HMOs and preferred provider organizations (PPOs) aim to reduce health care costs by focusing on preventive care and utilization management controls.

   2) Unlike many traditional insurers, HMOs provide both financing and care services. Doctors, hospitals, and insurers participate in HMOs.

   3) HMO members prepay a fixed monthly fee, regardless of how much medical care is needed in a given month to obtain a wide variety of medical services, from office visits to hospitalization and surgery.

   4) With a few exceptions, HMO members must receive their medical treatment from physicians and facilities within the HMO network.

V. TYPES OF HEALTH CARE PRACTITIONERS/PROVIDERS

A. Biomedical Health Care Professionals

1. Professional health care providers or practitioners undergo formal educational training and practice within the Western-based health care delivery system dominated by biomedicine. The length of education, types of degrees, and requirements for licensure and certification for advanced level of practice may differ worldwide. In each country, these are governed by governmental and sometimes nongovernmental agencies.

   a. Primary care providers (PCPs). First-line practitioners who are sought by patients for health maintenance and during illness. PCPs are general practitioners who refer patients to specialists and services for further treatment. In the United States, these can be doctors of medicine (MD) or osteopathic medicine (DO), nurse practitioners, dentists, or physician assistants in collaboration with a physician.

   b. Interdisciplinary professional providers consist of physicians, nurses, dentists, pharmacists, psychologists, and mental health practitioners, occupational therapists, physical therapists, speech therapists, nutritionists, medical technologist, etc. Each one has a specific specialized area of practice. Many undergo formal advanced training to qualify in a different specialty within their profession. For example, an MD may specialize in cardiology and a nurse can become a family nurse practitioner or nurse anesthetist.

   c. Professional support staff are formally trained in specific areas of practice within the discipline. For example, dental assistants or hygienists practice under the supervision of dentists, emergency medical technicians work under the supervision of MDs or DOs, and licensed professional nurses (LPNs) work in collaboration with registered nurses, and so on.

2. Nonprofessional support staff: Some healthcare systems provide on-the-job training for certain assistive personnel to assist professional staff and patients with their care.

   a. In the United States, *Unlicensed Assistive Personnel* consist of workers who are not licensed to perform nursing tasks; but were trained and certified to perform limited nursing tasks. These include certified nursing assistants, home health aides, and patient care technicians.

   b. In other countries, traditional birth attendants practice within the professional health system under the supervision and direction of licensed professionals such as nurses and medical doctors.

B. Practitioners of Integrative, Complementary, and Alternative Medicine (Johnson, 2008)

  1. *Practitioners of traditional Chinese medicine (TCM)*

   a. A complete medical system that has diagnosed, treated, and prevented illness for more than 2,500 years (as early as 1500-1000 BC) with books dating back to 221 BC.

   b. Korea, Japan, and Vietnam have developed their own unique versions of traditional medicine based on practices originating from China, using the ancient Chinese philosophy of yin and yang.

   c. Two polar principles in the body, *yin and yang*, are two opposing and complementary forces representing earth and heaven, winter and summer, night and day, inner and outer, cold and hot, wet and dry, body and mind.

   d. Balance between yin and yang regulates the flow of *qi* (or vital energy) throughout the body, which regulates a person's mental, physical, spiritual, and emotional states. Imbalances between yin and yang, disrupts the flow of *qi* and disease occurs.

   e. Diagnosis involves taking a history; inspecting facial complexion, body build, posture, and motion; examining the tongue and its coating; listening to the sound of voice, respiration, and cough; smelling the odor of the patient; and palpating the pulses.

   f. Treatments are directed at restoring harmony between yin and yang.

     1) Acupuncture

     2) *Tui na* (Chinese massage, a more powerful and stronger form of massage than those practiced in the United States)

     3) Herbal therapy

     4) Moxibustion (applying cones of herbal substances to the skin and igniting them to make smoke or holding a smoked-prepared strip of herbs close to certain parts of the body)

     5) Cupping (a small cup is attached to the skin of the patient creating a vacuum after the heated air inside the cup cools)

     6) Energetic exercises (*tai chi, qi gong*)

     7) Diet (adjusting the food based on its yin and yang properties).

   g. Examples of practitioners are acupuncturists, herbalists, and traditional Chinese medical doctors.

  2. Practitioners of chiropractic medicine

   a. Chiropractic medicine is a form of spinal manipulation, which is one of the oldest healing practices based on the belief that the nervous system is the most important determinant of health and most diseases are caused by spinal subluxations that respond to spinal manipulation.

   b. Manipulations or adjustment of the spine is the core procedure used that involves passive joint movement beyond the normal range of motion termed *adjustment.*

   c. Practitioners are called chiropractors or chiropractic doctors.

  3. *Massage therapists*

   a. Manipulate muscle and connective tissue to enhance their function, promote relaxation and well-being by increasing blood flow to the massaged areas, warm them, and decrease pain.

   b. First practiced thousands of years ago in ancient Greece, Rome, Japan, China, Egypt, and the Indian subcontinent. Massage therapy became popular in the mid-1800s in the United States and was promoted for a variety of health purposes. Interest in this therapy has increased since the 1970s.

    c. There are more than 80 types of massage therapy practices and techniques. In all of them, therapists press, rub, and/or manipulate the muscles and other soft tissues of the body, using varying pressure and movement through their hands, fingers, forearms, elbows, or feet.

4. ***Practitioners of energy medicine***
    a. Focus on *energy fields* (also called biofields) that are believed to surround and penetrate the human body. Therapies are based on the belief that human beings are permeated with a subtle form of energy, called *vital energy*.
    b. Therapies involve use of mechanical vibrations (sound) and electromagnetic forces, including visible light, magnetism, monochromatic radiation (such as laser beams), and rays from other parts of the electromagnetic spectrum. Specific, measurable wavelengths and frequencies are used to treat patients. Different degrees of heat produced by various heat lamps have been used in treating many disorders in China.
    c. Practitioners assert that they can work with subtle energy, see it with their bare eyes, and use it to cause changes in the physical body and influence health but have yet to be measured.

5. ***Reiki practitioners***
    a. Practice originated in Japan; *Reiki* means universal energy in Japanese.
    b. Based on the belief that a patient's spirit and physical body are healed when spiritual energy is channeled through a Reiki practitioner.
    c. It is not fully known how Reiki influences health.

6. ***Practitioners of therapeutic touch***
    a. Therapeutic touch is another form of energy therapy derived from the laying of hands.
    b. It is based on several ancient healing practices and the belief that each person has a unique energy field (sometimes visible as an aura) that is simultaneously inside and surrounding the person's physical body.
    c. A healthy person's energy field is flowing freely and in a state of balance. Therapeutic touch is used to balance or retain the free flow of life energy in an individual and restore health.

7. ***Practitioners of Ayurvedic medicine***
    a. *Ayurvedic medicine* (*ayurveda*) originated in India and practiced primarily in the Indian subcontinent for more than 5,000 years.
    b. It is based on the Hindu belief that everyone is born in a state of balance within themselves and in relation to the universe (interconnectedness).
    c. Good health is achieved when the person has effective and wholesome relationship with the immediate universe, and disease occurs when the person is out of harmony with the universe.

8. ***Practitioners of homeopathic medicine (homeopaths)***
    a. Also known as *homeopathy*, holds the *similia principle* or *like cures like*, *potentization*, and the belief that treatment should be selected based on a total picture of the patient, including physical symptoms, emotions, mental state, lifestyle, nutrition, and so forth.
    b. The principle of "like cures like" holds that symptoms are part of the body's attempt to heal itself and appropriately selected homeopathic remedy will support this self-healing process. The symptoms caused by a large dose of a substance can be alleviated by the extremely diluted small amount of the same substance.
    c. The concept of *potentization* holds that systematically diluting a substance, with vigorous shaking at each step of dilution, makes the remedy more effective by extracting the vital essence of the substance.
    d. *Homeopathy* believes that even when the substance is diluted to the point where no single molecule exists in the remedy, the remedy may still be effective because the substance's molecules have exerted their effects on the surrounding water molecules.

9. ***Practitioners of naturopathic medicine (naturopaths)***
    a. *Naturopathic medicine*, or *naturopathy*, is an eclectic system of health care originating in Europe.
    b. Many of its principles have been used for thousands of years in various healing traditions such as Chinese, Ayurvedic, Native American, and Hippocratic medicine.
    c. *Naturopathy* literally means "nature disease." Naturopaths treat illnesses by stimulating an individual's innate healing capacities through the use of organic, nontoxic therapies such as fresh air, pure water, bright sunlight, natural food, proper sleep, water therapies, homeopathic remedies, herbs, acupuncture, spinal and soft-tissue manipulation, hydrotherapy, lifestyle counseling, and psychotherapy.

10. ***Folk/generic healers***
    a. Healers are embedded in their communities and learn healing through observations, apprenticeship and handed down traditions of healing within a particular culture. Some examples of generic healers are:

   b. Curanderas/curanderos—traditional folk healers in Latino cultures.

   c. Parteras—female lay midwife in Latino cultures

   d. Voodoo/Santeria practitioners—traditional healers within the Afro-Caribbean religion. Magico-religious practice is often used as a strategy to resolve conflicts both within and between persons. Practiced within the bounds of nonmedical and psychic healing.

   e. Sobadores—within the Mexican American healing system, healers who specialize in the treatment of tense muscles and sprains.

   f. Shamans—intermediaries or messengers between the natural and spirit worlds; treat illness by mending the soul based on the belief that by alleviating traumas affecting the soul/spirit, the physical body achieves balance and wholeness. Shamans are capable of entering supernatural realms or dimensions to obtain answers to problems in their community.

VI. HEALTH SYSTEMS, AGENCIES, AND PROGRAMS

A. Global Health Care Service Programs

  1. World Health Organization (WHO, 2008)

    a. Goals

      1) Promote development and access to health promoting interventions

      2) Foster health security and protection from epidemic diseases

      3) Strengthen health systems to reduce poverty

      4) Provide worldwide guidance in the field of public health and set international standards

      5) Develop health research

      6) Enhance partnerships

      7) Improve performance

    b. Objectives

      1) Set global standards for health and provide technical assistance

      2) Strengthen national health programs

      3) Develop and transfer health information

      4) Promote improved standards of teaching and training in the health- and medical-related professions

      5) Establish and stimulate the establishment of international standards for biological, pharmaceutical and similar products, and standardize diagnostic procedures

      6) Foster activities in the field of mental health especially those activities affecting the harmony of human relations

    c. Policies

      1) Integrate health and human development into public policies

      2) Ensure equitable access to health care

      3) Promote and protect health

      4) Prevent and control specific health problems

    d. Constitutional mission

      1) Direct and coordinate authority on international health work

      2) Promote technical cooperation

      3) Assist governments, on request, in strengthening health services

      4) Furnish appropriate technical assistance and, in emergencies, necessary aid, on request or acceptance by governments

      5) Stimulate and advance work on the prevention and control of epidemic, endemic, and other diseases

      6) Promote, in cooperation with other specialized agencies, improvement of nutrition, housing, sanitation, recreation, economic or working conditions and other aspects of environmental hygiene

  2. USAID (USAID.gov)

    a. Global health programs represent the commitment of the U.S. government to assist families in the developing world. In 2007 its annual budget was nearly US$4.15 billion.

    b. Improve the quality, availability, and use of essential health services globally, including:

      1) Child, maternal, and reproductive health services

      2) Reduction of abortion and diseases (especially HIV/AIDS, malaria, and tuberculosis)

    c. USAID's Global Health Bureau supports field health programs, advances research and innovation in selected areas relevant to its overall objectives, and transfers new technologies to the field through its own staff, coordinates efforts with other donors, and offers a portfolio of grants.

3. **United Nations International Children's Emergency Fund** (UNICEF.org, n.d.)
   a. Supports global projects for child survival with evidence-based research interventions focusing on:
      1) Improving nutrition and environment
      2) Immunizations
      3) Emergency assistance in crisis situations
      4) HIV prevention among youth and adolescents
      5) Distribution of antiretroviral drugs to prevent maternal to fetus HIV transmission
      6) Prevention of child violence, exploitation, and abuse.
4. **Doctors Without Borders/Médecins Sans Frontières (MSF)**
   a. An international medical humanitarian organization created by doctors and journalists in France in 1971
   b. Provides aid in nearly 60 countries to people whose survival is threatened by violence, neglect, or catastrophe, primarily due to armed conflict, epidemics, malnutrition, exclusion from health care, or natural disasters.
   c. Operates independently of any political, military, or religious groups primarily through its sources of funding, which comes from private donors. The organization does not take sides in armed conflicts.
   d. Provides care on the basis of need and pushes for increased independent access to victims of conflicts as required by international humanitarian law.
   e. Teams comprise physicians and nurses who conduct health evaluations and provide care.
5. Cuban health care initiative
   a. The Cuban health care system has been producing a population that is as healthy as those of the world's wealthiest countries at a fraction of the cost.
   b. Has begun exporting its system to underserved communities around the world, including the United States.
   c. Everyone has access to doctors, nurses, specialists, and medications. There is a doctor and nurse team in every neighborhood and making house calls.
   d. Cuban doctors are trained in integrative, complementary and alternative healing.
   e. Cuba provides medical doctors to provide health care in other countries
6. **Centers for Disease Control and Prevention** (CDC, 2008a)
   a. Goals
      1) Promote population health
         a) *Populations* are aggregates or groups of individuals defined by a shared characteristic such as gender, diagnosis, or age.
         b) Traditionally physicians and nurse practitioners provide care to individuals and their families in a primary care practice and today it is essential that they practice with a broader perspective by noting health issue trends in the whole population.
         c) Focus the community, environmental/occupational, and cultural/socioeconomic dimensions of health.
      2) Prevent and control diseases in the United States and globally.
         a) Clinical prevention and health activities focus on the national goal of improving the health status of the populations. Unhealthy lifestyle behaviors account for more than 50% of preventable deaths in the United States.
         b) Worldwide programs include collection of epidemiological data and control of diseases. CDC works with partners to prevent and control infectious and chronic diseases; respond to international disasters; and build sustainable global public health capacity by training epidemiologists, laboratory scientists, and public health managers.
      3) Increase quality and years of life
         a) *Life expectancy* is a statistical measure of the average life span (average length of survival) of a specified population; often refers to expected age to be reached before death for a given population (by nation, by year of birth, or by other demographic variables).
         b) *Quality of life* is the degree of well-being felt by an individual or group of people. Quality of life has both physical and psychological components and includes a broad range of factors that impact on health such as diet, pain, stress, worry, emotional states, shelter, safety, as well as the freedoms and rights of the general population.
      4) Eliminate health disparities
         a) Also known as *healthcare inequality* in some countries, *health disparities* are gaps in the quality of health and health care across racial, ethnic, and socioeconomic groups. In the United States,

health disparities are well documented in minority populations such as African Americans, Native Americans, Asian Americans, and Hispanics. When compared with Whites, these minority groups have higher incidence of chronic diseases, higher mortality, and poorer health outcomes.

    b. The *Global Health Initiative* (GHI) will increases the U.S. government's investment to US$63 billion over 6 years to help partner countries improve health outcomes by strengthening health systems

        1) Particular focus on improving the health of women, newborns, and children through programs including infectious disease, nutrition, maternal and child health, and safe water.

    c. Global travel advisory

        1) CDC Traveler's Health Program gives advisory health information to more than 200 destinations, including recommendations for needed vaccinations, preparation for travel abroad, illness precautions, health references, and resources for travel destinations.

B. Global Food Programs

    1. Collaborative efforts among the Foreign Agricultural Service, the Agency for International Development, the World Food Program, the Five-A-Day Program, and the Office of the Global AIDS Coordinator

        a. Provide technical assistance and consultation to promote improved nutrition and food security in South Africa, Sierra Leone, Ethiopia, Hong Kong, Brazil, Tanzania, Swaziland, Mozambique, Uganda, Madagascar, Chile, United Kingdom, Argentina, Mexico, Israel, Italy, China, and Japan.

    2. China

        a. There is no official food stamp program in China.

        b. Unlike government subsidies in the West, the Chinese often manage on very little and do not desire beef as part of their diet.

        c. Rice, noodles, and basic vegetables are in great supply and are cheap. Even those who earn US$50 per month can have rice three times a day.

C. National Health Programs (this section is based on the United States)

    1. **U.S. Public Health Service** has national and local branches (USDHHS, 2008)

        a. Roles

            1) Environmental control

                a) Pollution control in food, air, water, or soil

                    (1) Pollution is the introduction of contaminants into an environment that causes instability, disorder, harm, or discomfort to the physical systems or living organism

                    (2) Pollution can come from chemicals, energy(noise, heat, or light), naturally occurring substances that occurs at such unnaturally high concentration, gaseous air pollutants, biological waste products, soil pollution, radioactive pollution, visual pollution (overhead power lines, motorway billboards, scarred landforms) or thermal (temperature change in natural water bodies).

            2) Coordinate climate preparedness and response

                a) Natural factors, such as volcanic eruptions, change in the earth's orbit and varying energy from the sun, have affected the earth's climate. Global warming, flooding, hurricanes, tornados, have caused such problems as dehydration, lack of water for growing food crops, drowning, mosquito infestations causing diseases, injuries, and mortalities.

                b) Vaccinations, mosquito spraying, temporary shelters, and treatment of related illnesses are sometimes needed.

            3) Disease prevention and treatment

                a) Facilitate access to health education, prevention, physical assessments, treatment, follow-up care, and immunizations.

                b) Historically, the leading causes of death were due to communicable diseases such as TB, polio, and measles, but with immunizations, the focus shifted from communicable diseases to chronic diseases such as heart disease, cancer, stroke, diabetes, hypertension, and injuries as leading causes of death.

                c) Conduct environmental health inspections of restaurants, public swimming pools, septic tanks, trailer parks, tourist accommodations, and air quality.

            4) Promote health of travelers. In conjunction with the CDC, health departments may have a special program for immunization and distribution of health literature for prophylactic medications, health education about a region and precautions/restrictions for safety and security.

    5) Promote emergency preparedness

       a) Provide in-depth information on specific hazards including what to do before, during, and after each type of hazard.

       b) Hazards covered include floods, tornadoes, hurricanes, thunderstorms, and lightning, household chemical emergencies, nuclear power plant accidents, and terrorism (including explosion, biological, chemical, nuclear, and radiological hazards).

    6) Conduct immunizations

       a) Developed ongoing programs to inform and educate providers and to promote appropriate immunization for all age groups.

       b) For children, the immunization program oversees the acquisition, distribution, and management of vaccines through the *Vaccines for Children (VFC) Program*, as well as vaccines acquired through state and other federal funding.

    7) Collect epidemiological data

       a) Health departments work with factors affecting the health and illness of populations

       b) Utilize evidenced-based interventions for public health and preventive medicine.

       c) Some of the programs include:

          (1) Assessing the health states and needs of a target population

          (2) Providing care for members using evidence-based practice derived from collected data from a population

          (3) Evaluating interventions designed to improve the health of the population

2. ***The National Institutes of Health*** (NIH) has several sections focusing on research (NIH, 2010)

  a. *The National Institute of Child Health Development* (NICHD) conducts and supports research training in reproduction, child health, and maternal health.

    1) Research includes studies on infant mortality, biometry, mathematics, statistical methodology and consultation, epidemiology, human fecundity and fertility, pregnancy complications and adverse outcomes, childhood injuries, teen driving, pediatric infectious diseases, birth defects, and behavioral research in health promotion and disease prevention.

    2) *The Epidemiology and Genetics Research Program* (EGRP) manages a comprehensive program of grant-supported, population-based research to increase understanding of cancer etiology and prevention. It is the largest grant funder for etiologic cancer epidemiology nationally and worldwide.

3. ***The U.S. Food and Drug Administration*** (FDA)

  a. Approves any prescription and over-the-counter drugs, before they can be sold; evaluates the safety of drugs.

  b. Promotes and protects public health by ensuring safe and effective products. Monitors products for continued safety.

  c. Does not regulate the safety or sale of herbs, food supplements, and other complementary and alternate medicine (CAM) medications.

  d. Provides guidelines and information for accrediting agencies for education of health professionals and health care organizations.

  e. Promotes timely availability of products in the market.

  f. Helps the public get the accurate, science-based information needed to improve health.

4. ***U.S. Environmental Protection Agency*** (EPA)

  a. The mission is to protect human health and environment; has been working for a cleaner, healthier environment since the 1970s.

  b. Leads the nation's environmental science, research, education, and assessment efforts

5. ***U.S. Department of Health and Human Services*** (USDHHS, 2008)

  a. Promotes health care access for undeserved people, including

    1) Organ and tissue donation and transplantation

    2) Blood cell (bone marrow and cord blood) donation and transplantation

    3) Injury compensation

    4) Emergency preparedness

    5) Poison control

    6) Construction of health care and other facilities

6. ***U.S. Department of Housing and Urban Development*** (HUD, 2008)
   a. Provides funding for supportive housing for very low income persons with disabilities who are at least 18 years of age.
   b. *Section 202—Supportive Housing for the Elderly Program* provides supportive housing for very low-income persons aged 62 years and older.
   c. *Section 8—Housing Choice Voucher Program* is the federal government's major program for assisting very low income families, elderly and disabled individuals to afford housing in the private market through various voucher options.
7. ***U.S. Department of Energy*** (DOE)
   a. The *Weatherization Assistance Program* enables low-income families reduce their energy bills by making their homes more energy efficient.
   b. During the past 30 years, the DOE's Weatherization Assistance Program has provided services to more than 5.6 million low-income families.
   c. Most of the population live in the countryside and grow their own food for personal consumption.

VII. COMPARATIVE HEALTH SYSTEMS WORLDWIDE

Table 2.1. Comparison of Health Care Systems of Selected Countries on Rank, Per Capita Health Expenditure, Life Expectancy, and Infant Mortality

Region/Country	Rank of Health System	Per Capita Expenditure on Health Care[a] ($)	Life Expectancy in Years (Healthy Life Expectancy)	Infant Mortality (Deaths Per 1,000 Live Births)
Western Europe				
United Kingdom	18	2,815	79.4 (71.7)	4.8
Spain	7	2,466	80.9 (72.8)	4.2
France	1	3,420	80.7 (73.1)	4.2
North America				
United States	37	6,719	78.3 (70.0)	6.3
Canada	30	3,673	80.7 (71)	4.8
Mexico	61	778	75.0 (65.0)	16.7
South America				
Brazil	125	674	72.4 (59.1)	23.6
Central America				
Nicaragua	71	235	72.9 (58.1)	21.5
Guatemala	78	267	70.3 (54.3)	27.8
Caribbean and Other Islands				
Puerto Rico	NA	NA	78.5 (68.0)	8.5
Cuba	39	674	78.3 (68.4)	5.1
Jamaica	53	307	73.5 (67.3)	15.2
Asia				
China	144	216	73.0 (62.3)	23.0
Japan	10	2,581	82.1 (74.5)	3.2
S. Korea	58	1,467	79.0 (65.1)	6.1
Philippines	60	120	71.1 (58.9)	23.1
Middle East				
Egypt	63	320	71.3 (58.5)	27.3
Saudi Arabia	26	720	72.8 (64.5)	18.8
Jordan	83	435	72.5 (60.0)	19.4
Sub-Saharan Africa				
Botswana	169	155	50.7 (32.3)	12.59
South Africa	175	715	44.0 (39.8)	44.42
Ghana	135	76	56.5 (45.5)	73.00

Note. NA = not available.
Source. The World Factbook (2009); WHO (2010a, 2010b).
a. Current U.S. dollars.

A. Table 2.1 compares the healthcare systems of selected countries in various regions worldwide using indices of total and per capita health expenditures, and two common indices of health outcomes, for example, life expectancy and infant mortality rates.

B. Comparison of health outcomes should be based on health expenditures and the region where these countries are located.

C. Among countries belonging to the Organization for Economic Cooperation and Development (OECD), increasing health expenditures do not translate to much better health outcomes. The United States is the only country in this group without universal access to care.

D. It should be noted that the statistics provided by both developed and developing countries, may differ from country to country based on data collection methods, actual year of data collection, publication of data, and the political agenda of a country.

E. Of particular note, is that some countries with greater health expenditures did not result in better infant mortality rates and life expectancy.

F. It is important to consider influences such as per capita income, number of new immigrants, geographic world region, heterogeneity of the cultures within the nation, numbers and level of education of health care providers, type of health infrastructure, type of health care system and access to the system, and funding for the system.

NOTE: All references, additional resources, and important Internet sites relevant to this chapter can be found at the following website: http://tcn.sagepub.com/supplemental

Section 11. Foundations of Transcultural Nursing and Health Care

Associate Editor: Gloria J. McNeal, PhD, MSN, ACNS-BC, FAAN

Chapter 3
Theoretical Basis for Transcultural Care

Journal of Transcultural Nursing
21(Supplement 1) 53S–136S
© The Author(s) 2010
Reprints and permission:
sagepub.com/journalsPermissions.nav
DOI: 10.1177/1043659610374321
http://tcn.sagepub.com
⑤SAGE

Margaret Andrews, PhD, RN, CTN, FAAN[1]
Jeffrey R. Backstrand, PhD[2]
Joyceen S. Boyle, PhD, RN, CTN, FAAN[3]
Josepha Campinha-Bacote, PhD, MAR, PMHCNS-BC, CTN-A, FAAN[4]
Ruth E. Davidhizar, DNSc, RN, APRN, BC, FAAN (deceased)[5]
Dawn Doutrich, PhD, RN, CNS[6]
Mercedes Echevarria, DNP, APN[7]
Joyce Newman Giger, EdD, APRN, BC, FAAN[8]
Jody Glittenberg, PhD, RN, FAAN, TNS[9]
Carol Holtz, PhD, RN[10]
Marianne R. Jeffreys, EdD, RN[11]
Janet R. Katz, PhD, RN[12]
Marilyn R. McFarland, PhD, RN, FNP-BC, CTN-A[13]
Gloria J. McNeal, PhD, MSN, ACNS-BC, FAAN[14]
Dula F. Pacquiao, EdD, RN, CTN[15]
Irena Papadopoulos, PhD, MA, RN, RM, FHEA[16]
Larry Purnell, PhD, RN, FAAN[17]
Marilyn A. Ray, PhD, MA, RN, CTN-A[18]
Mary C. Sobralske, PhD, RN, CTN[19]
Rachel Spector, PhD, RN, CTN-A, FAAN[20]
Marian K. Yoder, EdD, RN[21]
Rick Zoucha, PhD, PMHCNS-BC, CTN[22]

Funding: The California Endowment (grant number 20082226) and Health Resources and Services Administration (grant number D11 HPO9759).

[1]University of Michigan -Flint, Flint, MI, USA (Transcultural Concepts in Nursing Care)
[2]University of Medicine and Dentistry of New Jersey, Newark, NJ, USA (Foucault's Archeology of Knowledge; Harris' Cultural Materialism; Krieger's Ecosocial Model; Bourdieu's Maintenance of Social Hierarchies; Symbolic Interactionism)
[3]University of Arizona, Tucson, AZ, USA (Transcultural Concepts in Nursing Care)
[4]Transcultural C.A.R.E. Associates, Cincinnati, OH, USA (The Process of Cultural Competence in the Delivery of Healthcare Services Model)
[5]Bethel College, Mishawaka, IN, USA (The Giger and Davidhizar Transcultural Assessment Model)
[6]Washington State University, Vancouver, WA, USA (Worldviews; Essential Concepts Related to Learning and Socialization; Social Categories; Cultural Conflicts)
[7]University of Medicine and Dentistry of New Jersey, Newark, NJ, USA (Ramsden's Cultural Safety)
[8]University of California at Los Angeles, Los Angeles, CA, USA (The Giger and Davidhizar Transcultural Assessment Model)
[9]University of Arizona, Tucson, AZ, USA (Project Genesis; Transdisciplinary/Transcultural Model for Health Care)
[10]Kennesaw State University, Kennesaw, GA, USA (Cultural Brokering)
[11]Graduate College and College of Staten Island, CUNY, New York, NY, USA (Cultural Competence and Confidence Model)
[12]Washington State University, Spokane, WA, USA (Worldviews; Essential Concepts Related to Learning and Socialization; Social Categories; Cultural Conflicts)
[13]University of Michigan -Flint, Flint, MI, USA (Leininger's Theory of Cultural Care Diversity and Universality)
[14]Charles Drew University of Medicine and Science, Los Angeles, CA, USA (Health Belief Model; Developing Mutually Beneficial Partnerships with Communities)
[15]University of Medicine and Dentistry of New Jersey, Newark, NJ, USA (Freire's Critical Pedagogy; Hofstede's Cultural Dimensions Model; Bronfenbrenner's Ecological Systems Theory; Schein's Organizational Culture)
[16]Middlesex University, London, UK (Papadopoulos, Tilki & Taylor Model of Developing Cultural Competence)
[17]University of Delaware, Newark, DE, USA (Purnell Model for Cultural Competence)
[18]Florida Atlantic University, Boca Raton, FL, USA (Critical Theory, Transcultural Caring Dynamics)
[19]Washington State University, Spokane, WA, USA (Worldviews; Essential Concepts Related to Learning and Socialization; Social Categories; Cultural Conflicts)
[20]Cultural Care Consultant, Needham, MA, USA (Cultural Diversity in Health and Illness Model)
[21]San Jose State University, San Jose, CA, USA (Bridging Cultural Gaps)
[22]Duquesne University, Pittsburgh, PA, USA (Locke's Model for Multicultural Understanding)

Corresponding Author: Dula F. Pacquiao, Email: pacquidf@umdnj.edu or dulafp@yahoo.com

Suggested Citation: Douglas, M. K. & Pacquiao, D. F. (Eds.). (2010). Core curriculum in transcultural nursing and health care [Supplement]. *Journal of Transcultural Nursing, 21*(Suppl. 1).

I. INTRODUCTION

A. Increasing diversity in global and local populations intensified the realization that current models of health education and health care delivery are not adequately responsive to the changing needs of populations.

B. Widening health disparities across populations within countries and worldwide heightened the need for more comprehensive models and theories for care delivery that address social inequalities affecting population-based health outcomes.

C. This chapter provides a broad foundation for transcultural nursing and health care drawn from the social and behavioral sciences, philosophy and nursing to assist educators, practitioners and students to develop approaches to reduce differential outcomes of health care and education in populations.

II. CONCEPTS IN CULTURALLY COMPETENT CARE

A. The Concept of Culture

1. *Culture* is the complex whole, which includes knowledge, beliefs, art, morals, law, customs and any other capabilities and habits acquired by members of a society (Tylor, 1871).

2. Culture is an *ideational* system of shared ideas, concepts, rules and meanings that underlie and are manifested in the ways of life of human beings (Keesing & Strathern, 1998).

3. A set of explicit and *implicit guidelines* that individuals learn as members of a particular society, which guide how they view and affectively experience the world, and behave toward others, nature, supernatural forces, or gods (Helman, 2007)

4. Cultures are never homogeneous so one should avoid overgeneralizations or stereotyping about members of any group; differences between members of a particular group maybe just as distinct as differences across groups.

5. *Levels of culture* (Hall, 1984):

    a. Tertiary level—Explicit or manifest culture is the public facade that is visible to outsiders such as rituals, dress, cuisine, festivals.

    b. Secondary level—Underlying rules and assumptions known to members of the group but rarely shared with outsiders.

    c. Primary level—Deepest level of culture comprising implicit rules known and followed by members of the group but seldom stated.

6. Tertiary level is easily observed and manipulated but the deeper primary and secondary levels are most hidden, stable, and resistant to change.

B. Worldviews

1. *Worldview* is the perspective taken by an individual or group to explain the universe and life events, and understand and cope with the world around them and with life's experiences. It is often based on a strong sense of connection to a homeland.

2. Worldviews are illustrated by health belief systems (Andrews, 2008; Purnell & Paulanka, 2008).

    a. *Naturalistic paradigms* are based on the belief that health and illness are caused by the harmony, unity, and balance between humans and the universe. Examples are:

        1) Health and illness are influenced by the balance between opposing principles of *yin* and *yang*. Yin symbolizes feminine, winter and spring, cold, shady. Yang symbolizes masculine, summer and autumn, warm, sunny.

        2) Health and illness are influenced by the balance among the four body humors, began in ancient Greece.

          a) Excess of yellow bile is associated with anger and bad temper.

          b) Excess black bile is believed to cause melancholy or depression.

          c) Phlegm is associated with sluggishness, apathy, and evenness of temper.

          d) Blood is associated with cheerfulness and passion.

        3) *Ayurveda* originated in India and holds the belief that health and illness are influenced by the harmony between the five primary elements of ether (space), air, fire, water, and earth.

        4) A *moral paradigm* is based on a the worldview of goodness and rightness. Health is seen as a gift from God. Conversely, illness is believed to be a punishment or a special favor from God (Andrews, 2008). Illness and suffering may be viewed as enduring God's will.

        5) The *aesthetic paradigm* is based on a worldview of beauty and being in harmony with the environment, nature, and universe. An example is the Navajo Indian philosophy of *Blessing Way or Beauty Way*, that beauty surrounds the people and caring for nature contributes to health.

        6) The *magicoreligious paradigm* is dominated by the belief in supernatural forces as causes of health and illness. Examples are beliefs in voodoo, sorcery, witchcraft, and magic as causes of illness or can promote health among some Caribbean and African groups.

    7) The *social paradigm* holds that individual experiences, beliefs, and values are socially constructed and affect the way an individual perceives and responds to reality. Health and well-being are associated with freedom, peace, and tranquility; emphasizes importance of social relationships. Examples are.

      a) *Ubuntu* in African societies emphasizes harmony of difference and sameness.

      b) *Tanin* and *miuchi* (concepts of out and inner group) in Japanese society, emphasizes mutual interdependence with others (Doutrich, 2001).

C. Emic and Etic

1. Derived from linguistic anthropology (Pike, 1954), these terms are the two perspectives or worldviews used in studying cultural systems.
2. *Emic* refers to the perspective of the cultural insider (Takemura, 2005).
   a. The emic perspective focuses on the intrinsic cultural distinctions that are shared and meaningful to members of a given society (Pike, 1954).
   b. Emic worldview also refers to the lay, folk, or indigenous perspectives of a society about phenomena such as health and illness (Leininger, 2002).
3. *Etic* is the perspective of the cultural outsider that relies on extrinsic concepts and categories that have meaning for observers of a society (Pike, 1954).
   a. Etic is often the perspective of outsiders to the culture such as health care professionals and researchers.
   b. In research methods such as ethnography, study questions start from the etic perspective of the researcher (Spiers, 2000). The study attempts to draw the emic perspective of the phenomena by the research participants.

D. The Context of Culture

1. Individual or group values, beliefs, and behaviors are influenced by social and cultural contexts (Helman, 2007). Interpreting meanings of values, beliefs and behaviors should include understanding of contextual influences.
2. Individuals and groups will behave differently in different situations, thus, behaviors need to be contextualized and interpreted within particular contexts.
3. It is important to see culture within its particular context comprising historical, economic, social, political, and geographical elements that can influence individuals and groups at any particular point in time. It is impossible to isolate pure cultural beliefs and behavior from the socioeconomic context in which they occur.
   a. For example, individuals internalize discrimination by others and will respond differently in situations where discrimination is nonexistent.
   b. Sociocultural context consists of values, traditions, customs, and beliefs that are shaped by the history and experience of a group, including economic and political conditions.
   c. Individual factors such as age, gender, size, appearance, physical and emotional state, education, and occupation may pose differential influences on beliefs, values, and behaviors.

E. Dominant and Variant Cultural Patterns (Kluckhohn, 1976)

1. In any society there are certain groups whose lifeways are considered the norms for others and set the pathways to social acceptance, political and economic success. Dominant groups are sometimes referred to as *mainstream* groups in society.
2. Societies may have a predominant cultural ethos of individualism or collectivism.
3. Cultural clashes and misunderstandings are often seen between members of collectivistic and individualistic groups.
4. Some societies such as Japanese, Mexican, and African are predominately collectivistic (Doutrich, 2000; Maŕin, & Maŕin, 1991).
   a. They emphasize values of group belonging, unity, loyalty, harmony, maintenance of social relationships, mutual interdependence and empathy, self-sacrifice for the good of the group such as one's family (Purnell & Paulanka, 2008).
   b. They tend to be high context emphasizing maintenance of social relationships, status differences and social hierarchy in interactions with others.
   c. *Ubuntu* is a collectivistic worldview of most African societies that influences social conduct. It is a way of life that is fundamental to one's personhood, humanity, humanness, and morality (Broodryk, 1997).
      1) Integral to *ubuntu* is the idea of group solidarity and the survival of communities. An individual's existence is based on and expressed through relationships with others and caring for each other's well-being (Louw, 2005).
      2) Conformity, compassion, respect, human dignity, collective unity, and the spirit of mutual support are key to *ubuntu*.

    d. Individualistic cultures such as the United States consider self-identity as most important (Doutrich, 2000; Gudykunst & Ting-Toomey, 1988).

        1) They tend to be low context (Gudykunst & Ting-Toomey, 1988; Hall, 1976), emphasizing individualistic decisions and interactions.

        2) Emphasis is on personal autonomy, self-reliance, and self-responsibility and accountability.

F. Cultural Boundaries

    1. Differentiate one group from another and include practices and symbolic repertoires as modes of dressing, livelihood, language, cuisine, music, ritual, religious belief, and so on. Linked with ethnic identity versus identity piracy or pollution (Harrison, 1999).

    2. Linked with concepts of ownership, which differ culturally (Garmon, 2002). Different cultures may have legitimate positions on property rights that may conflict with the dominant Western ethos. For example, China had no copyright system until 1991.

    3. Globalization trends have shifted toward homogeneity, blurring some cultural boundaries (Friedman, 2005).

    4. Somerville (2007) defines *cultural boundary* within a context of nursing care. Nurses caring for patients and families from different cultures are "nursing across cultural boundaries." The principle of treating all patients the same was found to be inadequate because all people were not the same. Nurses treated all patients the same by "treating them differently." They were aware of the need to address differences within cultural groups as well as among different groups.

    5. Ramsden (2002) suggested that nurses "provide care *respective* rather than *irrespective* of all those factors which maintain [patients'] integrity as members of the human race" (p. 98).

    6. Nurses and other professionals are *edgewalkers* because they often practice across cultural boundaries (Boyd-Krebs, 1999).

    7. Individuals crossing cultural boundaries may be marginalized (Doutrich, 2000).

III. SOCIAL CATEGORIES

    A. Cultures have their own lens for categorizing their members that are arbitrary and unique. Cultures develop ways for moving people from one category to another such as the rites of passage.

    B. Most social scientists today agree that identity is a social construction, not "primordially given" (de Zwart, 2000, p. 15). The state (through its power to dominate discourse) is a key agent in the process of identity construction. For example, the government defines social categories using census—prescribed social categories may not be congruent with an individuals' self-identification.

    C. According to the Pew Research Center (2008), 4 out of 10 Blacks do not consider "Black" to be a single race. In the 2002 U.S. Census, 2.4% of the respondents self-identified with two or more racial categories (Pollock-Robinson, 2009, unpublished thesis).

    D. Farmer (2005) and Sherwin (1992) suggest the importance of understanding power balance in social categorization and identity development.

      1. Racial identity development in minority children is affected by how others categorize them (Tatum, 1997).

      2. Values revered by a culture are those that are embraced by the power elite (rich, White, and men in the United States). In contrast to Blacks, Whites enjoy racial privileges as having greater access to jobs and housing, able to shop without being followed, can buy hair products anywhere and negative behaviors are less likely labeled as racial attributes (McIntosh, 1990).

      3. People have multiple identities yet dominant culture is often assumed whereas minority is not (e.g., "gay," "lesbian" often included in list but "heterosexual" is assumed)

    E. Countries of Origin or Usual Residence—individuals may be categorized based on the country where they live, and have residency as established by the country's laws.

      1. *Nomads* are people who do not have a usual residence; they move from one site to another according to established patterns. Nomads may be considered stateless and may not be recognized as citizens by any of the countries through which they pass (Migration Policy Institute, 2008).

      2. People living outside their country of origin are

        a. *Refugees:* Persons fearing persecution because of race, religion, nationality, membership in a particular social group or political party, who are outside the country of their nationality (UN Migration Policy Institute, 1967).

        b. *Immigrants:* Persons who leave their country of origin to live in another country; may seek religious freedom or better economic status (Spector, 2009).

          1) Everyone in the United States is an immigrant except for the indigenous or American Indians and Native Alaskans.

2) Majority of immigrants in the United States today are from Mexico, India, Philippines, China, El Salvador, Dominican Republic, Vietnam, Columbia, Guatemala, and Russia (Migration Policy Institute, 2008).

3) Immigrants in Europe today come from Africa, China, and the Middle East.

3. ***Indigenous people*** are native, original inhabitants (United Nations, 2008). Indigenous people everywhere have undergone conflict over culture, land ownership, and industry due to colonization by nonindigenous people, for example, Spanish people colonizing parts of Central and South America; Dutch, French, English, and other Europeans colonizing South Pacific, North America, and Africa.

4. ***Nationality*** is a legal concept that refers to owning allegiance to a particular nation, regardless of race, ethnicity, culture, or religion. People within a nation usually have a shared history and political past. *Nationalism* is an idea, attitude, emotional response, and an opinion that focuses on the nation itself. The pursuit of nationalism has often led to conflict, war, and genocide (Connor, 1994).

5. ***Ethnicity*** is defined as the perception of oneself and a sense of belonging to a particular ethnic group, belonging to more than one group, or feeling of not belonging to any group because of multiethnicity.

   a. Ethnicity is integral to ethnic pride, identity, affiliation, and loyalty. An example is the concept of *on* in Japanese culture. *On* is a sense of obligation seen as a sacrifice of individual needs and personal goals for the sake of others (Doutrich & Colclough, 2008).

   b. Ethnicity is often determined by generation.

   c. Ethnicity is not equivalent to race. It is more than biological identification and includes commitment and involvement in cultural customs and rituals.

   d. Ethnohistory (Leininger & McFarland, 2006) influences ethnicity. Historical facts, events, personal demographics, and experiences of individuals and cultural groups over time help describe, explain, and interpret cultural patterns (Leininger & McFarland, 2006).

6. ***Race***

   a. In 2000, the Human Genome Project declared that there was no genetic basis for race (Hamilton, 2008).

   b. In total, 99.9% of all humans share the same genes; 0.1% genetic variations account for differences between humans.

   c. Race is a category used to place people in groups based on skin color, for example, non-White Hispanic or White Hispanic, or ethnic origins, for example, Jewish. It also includes geographical or country of origin, for example, Latin American or Spanish are Hispanic.

   d. Physical traits associated with race such as skin color, eye color, or hair tends to be related to common geographical location or origin.

   e. History of terminology (American Anthropology Association, 1998).

      1) The term *race* was used by colonizers to place a hierarchal value on people claimed to be determined by God. It was used to rationalize slavery and other unequal treatment that favored the colonizer.

      2) Physical traits were used to enforce this social construct, for example, dark skin was a characteristic of inferior people who could be enslaved because they were not like the enslavers.

      3) Early in the 19th century, some Europeans and Americans declared that White people were a separate and superior species. The Eugenics movement in America and the separation of Aboriginal children from their parents were based on the idea of having superior Whites reproduce more to increase the White race. In Australia, a reform movement sought to breed the blackness out of the Aboriginal people by mating their children with Whites.

      4) Race terminology was invented to assign low status to some and privilege, power, and wealth to others.

   f. According to the American Anthropology Association (1998), an individual's ability to succeed is not due to biological inheritance but to history, social, political, economic, and educational circumstance.

   g. Race is a recent human invention; it is about culture, not biology. Race and racism are embedded in institutions and everyday life (RACE, 2008).

   h. Race has an impact on health and health access and delivery.

   i. Race can affect culture and cultural identity.

      1) *Multiracial*—biological combination of two or more races; mixed race identity; unstable racial self-identification; possible sequelae include racial identity, confusion, and frustration over time (Tashiro, 2002).

      2) *Ascribed racial identity* emerges from how one's race is identified by others.

    j. Impact of governmental, legal, and national labeling and categories of mixed race
        1) Effects of policies on racialized tensions and interracial relations (Tashiro, 2002)
        2) Categories and labels of elements of race based on circumstances and context; for example, the U.S. Census (2000) first used *multiracial* as a category of more than one racial origin as a federally designated racial category.

7. **Religion**
    a. An organized system of beliefs or symbols concerning order and meaning of existence and nature; a belief in or worship of a god or gods (Andrews, 2007; Geertz, 1973).
    b. Concept of God or Deity, Supreme Being
    c. Religious beliefs dictate ideas, thinking, and behaviors
    d. Belief that religion and health are inseparable
        1) Spiritual health and illness
        2) Terms such as *holy*, *whole*, *heal*, and *hale*, are derived from same root word for health
        3) Integrated whole of mind–body–spirit such as the Native American tribal belief system, for example, Navajo spirituality
    e. World religions
        1) The three major religions are Judaism, Christianity, Islam
        2) Others include: Hinduism, Buddhism, Confucianism, Shintoism, Taoism, Animism
    f. *Atheism*—belief that there is no God or deity and may think that religion is harmful
    g. *Agnosticism*—doubts existence of God, spiritual world, or any ultimate reality
    h. *Maoism*—Belief that serving each other and all people as a whole transcends personal desires and ambitions
    i. *Spirituality* does not necessarily include religious beliefs. It can be based on the meaning a person gives to living, for example, meaning may be found in nature, relationships, or the arts. These manifestations of meaning provide a spiritual life. For example, balancing health or mind, body, and spirit may not involve religion.
    j. Religion and health—religious belief and traditions may be tied to behaviors, social interactions, explanations of environment and events. They affect health practices and reactions to illness, for example, praying to specific saints or deities based on the illness or problem; who to contact for help when ill, including type of healer consulted, and birth and death practices.
    k. Cultural background and religion may be connected and difficult to separate, but cannot assume persons of similar ethnic backgrounds have same religion (Spector, 2009).
    l. Religious beliefs can affect how people are treated within a society or community (Purnell & Paulanka, 2008).

8. **Gender**
    a. Culture dictates male or female gender behavioral characteristics and gender dictates roles and activities within a culture.
    b. Gender identity and the roles men and women play in society are determined by strong cultural norms and expectations.
    c. Family structures, gender roles, values, and beliefs differ across cultures and affect personality formation and developmental outcomes and manifestations of mental and physical illness (Hansen, Pepitone-Arreola-Rockwell, & Greene, 2000).
    d. This structure influences male–female relationships
        1) May clearly or generally define roles within the family structure
        2) Division of labor and authority in the family and in society
        3) Decision making, companionship, and family role in family communication are all affected.
    e. Examples: The traditional and historical belief that Chinese women are subordinate to men. In Japan, the woman or wife is typically the keeper of the household finances and doles out a daily or weekly allowance to her husband
    f. Hierarchical versus egalitarian family structure
        1) Typically, in high-context cultures there is hierarchical positioning and harmony is valued. For example, Hmong women make money doing sewing or other traditional crafts, whereas men may feel left out, thus increasing domestic discord within families.
        2) Legal ownership of land and property are often determined by gender.

    g. Models of women's health care do not always address integrating cultural values and lifeways that influence health and illness experiences (Meleis, 2003).

       1) Cultural models can inappropriately "stereotype women who share the same cultural heritage" (Meleis, 2003, p. 3).

       2) Individual experiences as well as culture will shape how women interpret and respond to health and illness.

    h. Gender roles in a culture vary and maybe manifested in

       1) Special traditions and rituals

       2) Sharing and reciprocity

       3) Household responsibilities

       4) Women may hold secondary status to men; wives may be submissive or obedient to husbands. Men may be considered the breadwinners and head of the household while women may be seen as the family caretaker. Men may have authority and power inside of the household.

       5) Family social hierarchy, for example, hierarchical versus egalitarian social structure.

       6) Collective versus individualistic social values can place differential roles and expectations on women. Collective societies emphasize harmony and conformity to traditional gender roles.

9. Education

    a. A social indicator that affects poverty and health status. People with more education have better health status, make better salaries, and are more likely to have children who become educated.

    b. Education in many countries affects economic status.

       1) In 2003, the typical full-time year-round worker in the United States with a 4-year college degree earned $49,900, or 62% more than a full-time year-round worker with only a high school diploma.

       2) Those with master's degrees earned almost twice as much, and those with professional degrees earned over three times as much per year as high school graduates (College Board, 2005).

    c. *Education for All* is the product of global efforts to improve levels of education for all children, youth and adults worldwide through six goals to be reached by 2015 (UNESCO, 2008).

       1) Goal 1: Expand early childhood care and education.

       2) Goal 2: Provide free and compulsory primary education for all.

       3) Goal 3: Promote learning and life skills for young people and adults.

       4) Goal 4: Increase adult literacy by 50%.

       5) Goal 5: Achieve gender parity by 2005, gender equality by 2015.

       6) Goal 6: Improve the quality of education.

    d. Educational attainment affects the status of a professional. In the United States, a physician's education is longer than that of a nurse, and physicians have higher status in general, than nurses (Purnell & Paulanka, 2008).

       1) Level of education is associated with a hierarchy model based on the years of education and degree earned. In the United States, entry to professional nursing education requires a high school diploma followed by an associate's degree or bachelor's degree. Nurses may then pursue a master's degree and possibly a doctoral degree, which is the highest or terminal degree.

       2) In health professions, the level of education required may be lower than the level preferred. For instance, a master's degree in nursing may be required in some countries to teach nursing while a bachelor's degree may be enough in other countries. A preferred level of education might be a PhD, or master's degree.

10. Occupation

    a. Patient's occupation, professional, and educational status are important to assess.

    b. Effects of immigration or migration on occupational status, access to health and emotional well being should be assessed. For example, a Russian engineer who moved to New York City and works as a cab driver may be due to the different requirements between the United States and Russia for professional eligibility.

    c. Consider workplace issues such as ethnic and racial tensions.

11. Sexual orientation

    a. Defined as the emotional and sexual attraction a person has toward others of a particular gender (Kaiser Permanente National Diversity Council, 2000).

    b. The term *sexual preference* is outdated and inappropriate because it "implies that sexual orientation is a behavioral choice rather than an intrinsic personal characteristic" (p. 2).

    c. *Homosexuality* is the attraction to another person or people of the same gender. *Lesbians* refer to females and *gays* refer to males.

    d. *Heterosexuality* is the attraction to another person or people of the opposite gender; considered the dominant norm in most societies.

    e. *Bisexuality* is the attraction to another person or people of both female and male gender.

12. ***Gender identity*** is a sense that one feels that he or she belongs to a particular gender (Sobralske, 2005). A strong and persistent *cross-gender identification* (Sobralske, 2008) occurs when one faces gender identity disorder and sexuality becomes confusing and sometimes distressing; a predominant sense of incongruity between birth gender and gender identity.

    a. Gender identity disorder has two components:

        1) Evidence of strong and persistent cross-gender identification that is not merely a desire for any perceived cultural advantage of being the other sex.

        2) Persistent discomfort with one's sex or sense of inappropriateness in the gender role of that sex (Sobralske, 2005). The degree of male or female characteristics of the sex of origin is not an indication of the degree of gender dysphoria (Kaiser Permanente National Diversity Council, 2000).

    b. *Transgendered* is the term used to include transsexuals, transvestites, and cross-dressers (Sobralske, 2008).

        1) Can represent one who has undergone hormone therapy or cosmetic surgery to live in the gender role of choice.

        2) The term does not include those who have undergone genital surgery.

        3) Some transgendered individuals have great difficulty accessing health and social services. Mental health care may be an ongoing need (Sobralske, 2005).

        4) *Transsexual* is someone who wishes to be of the opposite sex. The term is often applied to those seeking, undergoing, or completing a gender change.

        5) *Transvestite* is one who dresses in the clothing of the opposite gender. It is the clinical name for cross-dresser. *Cross-dressing* is wearing clothes, makeup, and other adornments assigned by society to the opposite sex. Generally, the body is not altered.

        6) *LGBT* is an acronym in Western societies for the lesbian, gay, bisexual, and transgendered population.

    c. *Heterosexism* is the belief that all people should be heterosexual and heterosexuality is normal, superior, or preeminent (Armstrong, 2003).

        1) Heterosexism can involve societal ignorance, irrational fears, stigmatizing, stereotyping and making false generalizations of the other.

        2) The extreme is "queer bashing," where homosexuals become targets of bullying and violence.

        3) In some countries, homosexuality or bisexuality is outlawed and discrimination is permitted.

13. ***Immigrants***

    a. People immigrate for a variety of reasons, including seeking religious and political freedom, economic and educational opportunities, and for a better way of life for themselves and their children or displacement caused by environmental disasters such as famine or forced relocation (Spector, 2009).

    b. May include wary refugees, sojourners, or those with personal ideologies that fit better in another nation (Purnell & Paulanka, 2008).

    c. There is emotional stress and drastic change involved in living within another culture and society (Schott & Henley, 1996). One experiences serious doubts, insecurity, need to compromise and make adjustments, and pressure to change.

    d. Immigration is driven by the supply and demand of human capital depending on the work force needs of the host country.

        1) Migration is dictated not only by immigrants wanting to immigrate but also by the desires of the host society, which values and needs their labor (Portes, 2007).

        2) Migration is big business. It is a complicated system, and in some cases, a highly organized migration industry exists worldwide.

    e. *Segmented-assimilation theory* identifies three distinct forms of adaptation: acculturation and integration into the middle class, acculturation into the "underclass" and downward assimilation, and selective acculturation into middle-class society through the preservation of culture (Piedra & Engstrom, 2009).

      1) Segmented acculturation is circular and continuous, occurring in segments (Portes, 2007). May result in upward economic mobility and greater health potential or downward mobility and worsening health (Yeh, Viladrich, Bruning, & Roye, 2009).

      2) *Downward assimilation* may affect the offspring of immigrant families when the family has immigrated illegally and are of low socioeconomic and class status in the new society. *Upward assimilation* is associated with human and social capital needed to support children in adapting to life in the host country. Families can provide economic resources, attention, and guidance for their children (Yeh et al., 2009).

  f. There are positive and negative effects of migration on health initially.

      1) Over time, the protective effect of migration on health may wane. Ongoing health effects may occur for years after immigration (Lassetter & Callister, 2009).

      2) Migration may involve transitional experience, poor access and barriers to health care, and vulnerability.

      3) Immigrants may behave in ways that the dominant population considers "odd or unique" (Meleis, 2003).

  g. Migration to the host country may impose changes in gender and family roles as immigrants meet new challenges with the values of the host culture (Spitzer, Neufold, Harrison, Hughes, & Stewart, 2003).

      1) Migration may create marginalization of female immigrants by being "set apart" and "at the periphery" in the host country because of their physical attributes, clothing, mannerism, accents, and language differences (Meleis, 2003).

      2) Women may be isolated from social networks, community resources, and health services. Appropriate assessment and interventions are needed to provide the care and attention for women embedded in new, strange, and intimidating situations.

  h. Large recruitment of professionals can cause a *brain drain* in their home countries. When institutions in developed countries recruit scarce professionals from developing countries, ethical questions arise. For example, a company in Florida engaged in recruiting scarce physicians from the Dominican Republic to retrain as Registered Nurse (RNs) in the United States in order to decrease the significant U.S. nursing shortage.

14. Vulnerable populations

  a. Traditionally defined as groups or individuals at risk for harm (Gueldner & Britton, 2005). As a general concept vulnerability means "susceptibility" (de Chesnay, 2008).

  b. Anyone can be vulnerable at a given point in time as a result of life circumstances (de Chesnay, 2008).

  c. Vulnerable populations are those with higher than average risk for developing health problems. This is a public health concept and rates populations vulnerable in relation to other populations.

  d. Reasons for vulnerability vary. Developmental, sociocultural, age, gender, or other characteristics may place a person more at risk to be a member of a vulnerable population. Typically, persons with physical and/or mental disabilities, drug dependent, elderly, indigent, homeless, illiterate, or poor are thought to be at higher risk for vulnerability (de Chesnay, 2008).

  e. People may be members of a vulnerable population yet not be vulnerable. Some people who are members of vulnerable populations identify as resilient rather than vulnerable (de Chesnay, 2008).

  f. The economic structure of a country is a powerful determinant of the health of the people.

      1) Wide economic disparities place populations at high vulnerability for health problems (Bezruchka, 2000, 2001; Wilkinson, 1997a, 1997b; Marmot, 2003).

      2) Economic, political, religious, and societal policies may increase or decrease population vulnerability (Hall, Stevens, & Meleis, 1994). Examples are the increased vulnerability to osteomalacia for *burqa*-wearing Afghan women; taxation policies that increase wealth disparities in the United States and decrease population health; laws that allow marginalization based on race/gender/ sexual orientation.

15. Disability

  a. Interpretation of disability varies across cultures and societies. What is considered disability in one culture may be highly regarded in another culture (e.g., homosexuality).

  b. Disability may be a spiritual rather than physical handicap. An example is the story of a Hmong child who was diagnosed with epilepsy by her American providers but interpreted as a spiritual condition in her culture (Fadiman, 1997).

16. **Variant or subcultures**
   a. A *subculture* is a small, distinct group of people whose experiences are different from those of the dominant society (Purnell & Paulanka, 2008).
   b. Variant experiences are associated with differences in socioeconomic status, ethnicity, place of residence, education, and philosophy. Examples of variant cultures include nurses, physicians, social workers, and skinheads.
   c. Social interactions and enculturation are unique among subcultures and may be viewed as positive and congruent or negative and variant by the dominant society.

17. **Marital status**
   a. Refers to the conjugal status of a person. In the United States, a committed relationship resulting in the legal bond of marriage usually occurs in young adulthood.
   b. The median age of marriage in the United States has increased over the past century with 21 years in the 1890s versus about 26 years of age in 2004.
   c. In Canada, *same sex marriage* has been legal since 2005 (Purnell & Paulanka, 2008).
   d. *Separated* refers to persons who are currently married, but who are no longer living with their spouse (for any reason other than illness or work) and have not obtained a divorce.
   e. *Divorced* persons have legally terminated their conjugal relationships from their spouses and have not remarried.
   f. *Widowed* persons have lost their spouse through death and have not remarried (Statistics Canada, 2008).

18. **Parental status**
   a. The typical U.S. family is *nuclear* with two parents, usually a man and woman and their children (Purnell & Paulanka, 2008).
   b. *Extended family* includes other relatives and is more common in countries outside the United States.
   c. *Alternative families* can include members not related through marriage or biologically related. Families consist of same sex parents or partners, and in states where it is legal, marriage can take place between two men or between two women.
   d. A parent may be a father or mother or a legal guardian.

19. **Residency location** (based on U.S. definitions)
   a. *Rural* locations are in counties of more than 10,000 residents with less than 50% living in towns of 2,500 or fewer people (Loue & Morgenstern, 2001).
   b. A *frontier* location has fewer than 6 people per square mile (Loue & Morgenstern, 2001).
   c. An *urban* location has a population density of 50,000 or more (Loue & Morgenstern, 2001).
   d. Location of residence affects health access and exposure to environmental health hazards.

IV. **CULTURE-BOUND PHENOMENA**
   A. Many anthropologists believe that all phenomena are embedded in particular sociocultural contexts, hence contextual interpretation of events and behaviors is extremely important.
   B. The dominant organizational cultures of schools, health care organizations, and government reflect the dominant societal ethos.
   C. Valued behaviors in one society maybe considered offensive or selfish in other contexts.
   D. Caring practices, professional socialization and ethics are examples of culture-bound phenomena.
   E. **Culture-Bound Syndromes**
      1. These are explicit health conditions recognized as particular, unique, and generally specific to a culture or geographic area (Giger & Davidhizar, 2008; Leininger, 1995).
      2. Culture-specific beliefs tend to produce a health/illness condition.
      3. Illness or impairment is created by personal, social, and cultural responses to dysfunctional biology and/or psychology (Andrews & Boyle, 2008).
      4. Understood only within a definite framework of meaning and social connection called *explanatory models* (Kleinman, 1980), which are the *emic* explanations of why an illness or symptom developed and how it should be treated. Explains the culturally based epidemiology of an illness. An example is physical pain without trauma experienced by some groups.
      5. *Conditions* are culture-related specific illness or afflictions. Often referred to as *folk illnesses* and have local names for conditions.
      6. *Disorders* are attributed to cultural rather than physiological factors, unique to one culture and may not be recognized by others.

7. There are no demonstrable scientific findings for the symptoms. Somatic symptoms reflect culturally specific patterns and tend to have psychological and/or religious overtones (Neff, 1999).
8. Treatment is usually culture based.
9. Some examples of culture-bound syndromes:
   a. *Ghost illness* in some Native American tribes and in north India where the individual experiences a sense of danger, terror, delirium (Andrews & Boyle, 2008)
   b. *Anorexia nervosa* seen in Western societies is characterized by an obsessive preoccupation with thinness and boy image distortion often leading to self-imposed starvation.
   c. *Empacho* seen in Latino cultures associated with the belief that a substance is stuck in the intestines or stomach and blocks digestion. Treatments include massaging with warm oil or stretching the skin over the abdomen or small of the back, imposing dietary restrictions, drinking herbal or laxative teas, instilling enemas, and using folk medicines.

F. **DSM-IV** (Diagnostic and Statistical Manual of Mental Disorders, Fourth Edition; American Psychiatric Association, 2004)
   1. Certain culture-bound syndromes are listed in the *DSM-IV* as meeting the criteria of psychiatric disorders. There is no one-to-one correspondence between a syndrome and a commonly recognized diagnosis in Western medicine.
   2. It is controversial whether culture-bound syndromes should be considered neurotic, psychotic, or personality disorders or if they are merely cultural variations of what is considered psychologically normal in Western societies.
   3. There is controversy on whether labeling and categorizing cultural responses to illness and impairment as psychiatric disorders or forms of ethnocentrism and cultural imposition by Western medicine.
   4. Examples of culture-bound syndromes labeled as psychiatric problems (*DSM-IV*):
      a. *Amok*—Withdrawal and explosive violence sometimes seen in Southeast Asia or in the Philippines
      b. *Mal de ojo* or *evil eye*—Fitful sleep, crying, and diarrhea usually seen in young female children (Andrews, 2008) that is believed to be caused by a stranger's attention to a vulnerable person, including health professionals.
      c. *Susto*—Loss of soul sometimes seen in Latin American cultures associated with fear, sudden fright, or witnessing a tragedy. Symptoms include anxiety, restlessness, and sometimes depression.
      d. *Rootwork*—Spells, sorcery, conjuring
      e. *Koro*—Imagination and fear of one's genitals shrinking or retracting, sometimes seen in Chinese and Hmong cultures (Garlipp, 2008).
      f. *Pasma*—Filipino folk illness caused by an imbalance between hot and cold. Common symptoms include facial paralysis, hand tremors, sweaty palms, numbness, and pain that can be relieved by massage.
      g. *Wendigo*—Belief among some Native American tribes of a malevolent creature that can transform or possess humans (Johnston, 1976).
      h *Hikikomori*—Acute extreme withdrawal from social interaction, resulting in self-imposed isolation and confinement from others.

V. **SOCIALIZATION**
   A. **Socialization** is the process by which members become part of a society by learning what is important and acceptable within a society such as how to live, work, and become an accepted member.
   B. **Socialization** to the norms of the middle and upper classes has significant impact on health status and access to health care in many countries.
   C. **Enculturation** is a conscious and an unconscious conditioning process (Hoebel, 1954). A natural process of learning accepted cultural norms, values, and roles in a society, and achieving competence in one's culture (Spradley, 1979). It is facilitated by growing up in a particular culture.
      1. *Informal enculturation* is similar to social learning that occurs by being with others and learning what behaviors are considered acceptable for that culture. An example is how competition may be viewed as positive or negative by different cultures.
      2. Education may be viewed as the acquisition of cultural knowledge and facilitating transmission of this knowledge to the next generation.
      3. Enculturation can be through formal education, apprenticeship, mentorship, role modeling, and so on.
      4. Valued teaching/learning methods and communication vary across cultures.

D. **Acculturation** involves changes when people from different cultures interact with each other over time. Changes occur in both directions although the sojourner or new comer will usually change more than the people in the established culture (Berry, 1980).

    1. Acculturation is not a linear process. Differences exist even among members of the same families. *Segmented assimilation* (Portes, 2007) is the term used to denote individual and group differences in acculturation that maybe influenced by specific networks and experiences of individuals within the new society.

        a. *Acculturative stress* refers to the disorganization or even disintegration of behavior that often accompanies social and cultural change (Berry, 1980).

            1) The individual experiencing acculturative stress may exhibit hostility, altered mental health especially confusion, anxiety, depression, feelings of marginality and alienation, a "heightened psychosomatic symptom level" and identity confusion.

            2) Berry (1990) suggests that symptoms are frequently present in acculturating individuals and represent the "negative side of acculturation" (p. 246).

        b. Successful adaptation to the new culture by learning the appropriate behavior of the host culture can take time. A positive outcome of acculturation is being recognized and accepted as a member of the new culture. Adaptation may be in the form of:

            1) *Bilingualism* is the ability to be fluent across two cultures. *Multilingualism* is the ability to be fluent across three or more cultures.

            2) *Biculturalism* is the ability to cope with all the demands of verbal and nonverbal behavior effectively.

        c. Acculturative style-continuum

            1) Traditional to identity explorer

            2) Identity acculturation: traditional, assimilated, marginal, bicultural behaviors of acculturation

E. **Assimilation** is a blending of *cultural heritage* and the new *host culture;* involves developing a new cultural identity and one takes on the worldview of the new culture over time.

    1. It is a more extreme process than acculturation is; to some degree it is preceded by acculturation and comes from the realization that one will never return to their society of origin (Clark & Hofsess, 1998).

    2. Assimilation is influenced by parental heritage and generational distance from the homeland.

    3. Language preference and physical similarities with the dominant groups are critical factors in the degree of assimilation.

F. **Transnational** migration is a global phenomenon reflecting the dynamic flow of people, their possessions, and commodities across national borders (Hilfinger Messias, 2002); a process that changes over time (Cano, 2005).

    1. Migrants maintain connection and linkage between the host and home countries.

    2. Health and health care are integral to transnationalism.

G. **Cultural relativism** refers to the notion that every culture is unique; therefore members of a particular culture should be evaluated according to their own values and standards (Haviland, Prins, Walrath, & McBride, 2007).

    1. Behavior is judged in relation to the cultural context.

    2. Patient interpretations of illness experiences are based on their own cultural belief systems. (e.g., allowing a deformed child to die because the culture believes the child cannot function in the society; Leininger, 1995).

    3. Many authors argue for awareness and understanding of cultural relativism and an avoidance of cultural imposition along with respecting differences in values, history, and sociopolitical ramifications unique to a culture.

    4. In part this counters ethnocentrism and embraces cultural difference.

        a. Farmer (2005) argues that it is important not to confuse cultural differences with poverty and structural violence. He argues against the tendency to view cultural relativism as a rationale for perpetuating inequalities between the First and Third World countries by equating inequalities with "otherness."

        b. Power differences need to be assessed in decision making before assuming a practice is endorsed by all people in a culture (Sherwin, 1992).Sherwin cites the example, when women perform and encourage clitorectomy, it may be in response to their oppressed position. She asserts that even considering cultural relativism, one cannot ethically encourage the practice.

  c. The issue has to do with ethics and what is useful and moral to support culturally.

  d. Ramsden (2002) argues that it is critical to understand not only the "cultural activities" of the patient but also analyze power structures. Although it is important to have respect and avoid cultural imposition it is critical to understand practices and beliefs within a power structure and historical and sociopolitical context.

H. Cultural Shock

  1. A normal response to a different culture that can be disabling due to strain in making adaptations, a sense of loss, feeling rejected or rejecting others, confusion with self identity, feeling powerless, feelings of disgust about the culture (Mumford, 1998).

  2. *Culture shock* is a term used to describe the anxiety and feelings (of surprise, disorientation, etc. felt when people have to operate within an entirely different cultural or social environment, such as a foreign country.

  3. Anxiety produced from the loss of familiar signs and symbols of social and cultural intercourse (Oberg, 1960), difficulty adjusting to a new country and culture that may be very different (Education USA).

  4. A period of time of unease or disorientation when placed within another culture and adapting to unfamiliar cultural practices (Akteos, 2008).

  5. Stage in the acculturation process. Being in a new place with a new language and different nonverbal cues leads to loss of power to communicate. This can disrupt self-identity (Haynes, 2008).

  6. Culture shock may be experienced by refugees and immigrants as well as travelers (Quartz Hill, 2008).

  7. *Culture Shock and Second Language* (Haynes, 2008)

    a. Symptoms of Second Language students and culture shock include emotional symptoms such as frustration, anger, sadness, homesickness, and loneliness, depression, sleeplessness, aggression, or withdrawal.

    b. Physical symptoms include stomachaches and headaches.

    c. Students may undergo a "silent period" characterized by unwillingness to speak in the second language that could last for one year. They should not be forced to speak until they are ready; Social support is important in alleviating culture shock problems (Pantelidou & Craig, 2006).

VI. CULTURAL CONFLICTS

 A. Cultural conflicts can result from injustices and lack of fairness, power struggles, lack of trust, presence of threats, unfulfilled promises, communication barriers, differences in styles of decision making, and so forth.

  1. *Cultural clash* and differences can play a central role in conflict between individuals and groups.

    a. The greater is the conflict of interest between the health care professional and the recipient of health care, the greater potential for ethnocentrism to exist (Leininger & McFarland, 2006).

    b. In conflicts, people tend to develop overly negative images of the other side. The opponent is expected to be aggressive, self-serving, and deceitful, whereas the other group view themselves in completely positive ways. If one side assumes the other side is deceitful and aggressive, the other side will tend to respond in a similar way.

    c. As communication is halted, conflicts heighten and there is increasing emotional tension. The resolution is to communicate and frame the conflict.

  2. *Cultural imposition and imperialism*

    a. *Cultural imposition* occurs when individuals or groups impose their beliefs, values, and behavioral attitudes on another culture (Leininger, 1995).

     1) Policies and practices of the dominant group are extended to other less powerful groups (Purnell & Paulanka, 2008).

     2) A belief that everyone should conform to the majority; for example, "we know what's best for you, if you don't like it you can go elsewhere." This may take the form of an active, formal policy or a general attitude (Wikipedia, 2008).

    b. *Cultural imperialism* is the practice of promoting, distinguishing, separating, or artificially injecting the culture or language of one culture into another. It is usually the case that the former belongs to a large, economically or militarily powerful nation and the latter belongs to a smaller, less important one.

    c. Cultural imposition and imperialism is more likely to take place in the socialization to professional education, which can result from an unconscious predilection for dominant cultural values or overt racism, classism, or prejudice (Doutrich, Wros, & Valdez, 2005; Hassouneh-Phillips & Beckett, 2003; Navarro, 1986; Terhune, 2008; Yu Xu, 2008).

d. Imbalance in the power relationships may manifest as cultural imposition, imperialism, *structural violence*, *institutional racism*, or *classism*.

  1) According to Farmer (2005), *structural violence* is difficult to grasp because groups have an ability to distance themselves from the suffering of "people not like them." There is difficulty in describing intense suffering adequately, and individual cases are unable to illustrate the extent of this suffering.

  2) While structural violence is often systematic and policy driven, it is seen through individuals' lived experience.

  3) According to Farmer, the rising tide of inequality breeds violence, and inequity constitutes and is constituted in structural violence. Thus, it is important not to confuse structural violence with cultural difference. For example,

    a) In the past 25 years, the United States pursued a drug policy based on prohibition and criminal sanctions for the use and sale of illicit drugs. Despite overall decline in prevalence of drug use since 1979, there is a 10-fold increase in imprisonment for drug charges. Although Black, Hispanic, and White Americans use illegal drugs at comparable rates, there are dramatic differences in the application of criminal penalties for drug offenses. African Americans are more than 20 times as likely as Whites to be incarcerated for drug offenses (Drucker, 1999).

    b) There are long-standing health disparities across population groups and between rich and poor countries. In the United States, there is a 41-year difference in the life expectancy of American Indian men on Indian reservations in South Dakota, and women of Asian descent in Bergen County, New Jersey (Murray, 1998). There is a difference of 48 years in life expectancy between Japan (developed country) and Zambia (developing country; United Nations, 2003).

3. **Ethnocentrism** is the tendency to comprehend and judge the world from the perspective of one's own culture; evaluate other cultures by the standards and practices of one's own cultural group; view one's own way of life as the only proper or moral way, resulting in a sense of personal and cultural superiority; confusing bias with truth (de Chesnay, 2008).

4. **Bias and prejudice** are prejudgments or a preconceived judgment or opinion usually based on limited information.

  a. Gadamer (1996) described prejudice as an unconscious understanding that influences all interpretation of meaning. Prejudice is rendered before all the elements that determine a situation have been fully examined.

  b. Individuals and people are constituted by their language and culture and they cannot always know or see our prejudices (Gadamer, 1996; Heidegger, 1927/1962). Hence, some prejudices are not recognized.

  c. Acknowledging that we all have biases affirms that we are human (de Chesnay, 2008). The more we can make transparent those blind prejudices/biases, and critically analyze our own values and beliefs in terms of how we see differences, the more enabling and less fearful we are with our biases and prejudices.

  d. *Self-reflection* and understanding one's culture is the process in becoming more familiar with one's biases (Heidegger, 1927/1962). This process of reflection on lived experiences should be fostered by educators and practicing nurses (Schön, 1983; Wepa, 2005; Ramsden, 2002; Spence, 2005).

  e. Some prejudices are *blind* whereas others are *enabling* (Spence, 2005).

    1) *Enabling prejudices* make ongoing development of understanding possible. In health care context, nurses may be willing to provide assistance, act on the belief in equal right to equal standards of care, engage with differences to extend understanding, question one's own beliefs and expectations, seek permission and being present with patients.

    2) *Blind or limiting prejudices* are seen in the nursing context as fearing and avoiding contact with differences, believing in the superiority of Western medicine, assuming understanding without checking its accuracy, being too busy to listen or expecting others to comply with one's beliefs and values.

5. ***Stereotyping***
   a. *Stereotyping* is the supposition that all people in a group are alike and share the same values and beliefs (Giger & Davidhizar, 2008).
   b. Having general and naïve impressions of a group of people based on physical appearance, history, characteristics, or unique aspects of a group.
   c. Having false associations between elements that are not interrelated or poorly connected.
   d. Stereotyping is often based on opinion and social convention. It is a form of social consensus often reinforced by the public media, health care systems, educational facilities, and societies at large.
   e. The danger of stereotyping is misunderstanding and closed mindedness. Stereotypes tend to be self-perpetuating.

6. ***Discrimination***
   a. *Discrimination* means unequal treatment in regard to law, health care, employment, housing, personal or social, political, institutional or organization.
   b. Discrimination can be based on any racial, ethnic, gender, nationality, religious, sexual orientation, socioeconomic differences, and so on, which may be manifested as:
      1) *Racism* can include unjust and unequal treatment based on skin color or physical features and characteristics, thus there are advantages based on race (Tatum, 1997).
         a) Discrimination stemming from a belief in the superiority of a particular race maybe manifested by overt expressions of racial superiority.
         b) Color is the strongest single factor central to racism (Rack, 1991).
         c) Cultural images and messages often affirm the assumed superiority of Whites and the assumed inferiority of people of color.
      2) *Sexism* is the oppression of one gender by another (Rothenberg, 2004) and associated with gender privilege of the oppressor. Most societies are patriarchal, male dominated, and male centered, which are often dictated and reinforced by religious beliefs.

VII. THEORIES, MODELS, CONCEPTUALIZATIONS FOR TRANSCULTURAL PRACTICE
A. Interdisciplinary Theories and Models
1. ***Cultural Materialism*** (Marvin Harris)
   a. Marvin Harris (1927-2001) was one of the most famous anthropologists of the latter half of the 20th century.
   b. He established the foundations of cultural materialism in his seminal book, *The Rise of Anthropological Theory* (Harris, 2000).
   c. Basic premises of *Cultural Materialism* (CM)
      1) Focus is on explaining the origins of the structure and content of culture.
      2) Views culture in an expansive way (in comparison to lay conceptions) that includes what people do, think, and create.
      3) CM views the origin and maintenance of culture and culture change as the outcome of probabilistic, not mechanistic, processes.
      4) Culture is seen as predominantly an outcome of human efforts to solve the basic biological problems of human existence, including issues such as food production, maintenance of health and safety, and the orderly reproduction of human society.
      5) Approach is *materialistic* in the sense that the primary influences on culture, in the long term, are assumed to be related to the material needs of humans.
      6) CM is *nomothetic* as it is focused on generating large-scale theory (*nomothetic theory*) that can be applied across human populations in space and time, and which will be generally true, but which may not be valid in all cases.
   d. Ideology and behavior
      1) Harris, like other cultural anthropologists, recognized that ideology and behavior are not synonymous. In fact, people often engage in behaviors that are apparently at odds with stated values, beliefs, and so on.
      2) As a result, anthropologists are presented with two types of data, observed phenomena and stated ideology.

e. The concepts of *emic* and *etic*

    1) *Emic* refers to the ideological and symbolic aspects of culture from the perspective of the individual who is embedded in that society (a native).

    2) *Etic* refers to the *observable* manifestations of culture (behaviors, social structure, etc.).

    3) Application of the concepts

        a) Harris (1989) considered the origin of Middle Eastern prohibitions against consumption of the "abominable" pig.

        b) From an *emic* perspective, the prohibition against pork is because the pig is considered unclean.

        c) From the *etic* perspective, pigs are poorly suited to the ecology of the Middle East and therefore are not worth the trouble of production, hence the cultural prohibition against the consumption (and production) of pigs.

f. The three basic components of culture

    1) *Infrastructure* is the technology and ideology by which a society engages with its environment. It is comprised of two components that can be known *reliably*:

        a) *Etic behavioral mode of production* is comprised of those behaviors that are used to satisfy human subsistence needs (e.g., modes of production such as hunting and gathering, or industrial production).

        b) *Etic behavioral mode of reproduction* is comprised of those practices or behaviors that maintain the population (e.g., medicine, contraception, child care)

    2) *Structure*

        a) *Domestic economy* consists of small-scale organization of human activities based on intimate human relations (family, friendship, etc.).

        b) *Political economy* refers to small or large scale organization of human activities based on impersonal relationships among people.

    3) *Superstructure* is the overarching structure of symbolic processes, which is composed of two components:

        a) Behavioral superstructure comprised of ritual, sport, art, folklore, and so on

        b) Mental superstructure comprised of beliefs, values, standards of behavior, and so on. These mental factors support the other three components of culture (structure, infrastructure).

g. Relationships between the three components of culture based on the principle of *Infrastructural Determinism*

    1) The *infrastructure* (modes of production and reproduction) will strongly influence structure (the political and domestic economy), which will in turn strongly influence the superstructure (beliefs, rituals, etc.).

    2) Although infrastructure is strongly influenced by the *infrastructure and structure*, the mental and behavioral *superstructures* are part of a cultural system. As a result, feedback from the infrastructure to the structure and superstructure occurs (but will be limited in the long run by the realities of providing for human needs).

    3) An example is North American slavery. A *materialist* would argue that the Jim Crow ideologies of 20th century America had their origins in the organization of agricultural production. In this view, Jim Crow was part of a complex system that maintained race-based agricultural production. So, instead of racism being the cause of slavery, it was the other way around (slavery was the cause of racist ideology).

h. Application of CM transcultural nursing and health care

    1) Emphasizes the infrastructural and social structural realities in shaping and reshaping values, beliefs, and practices of patients, communities, and practitioners.

    2) Shifts the focus of health care from a purely cognitive-oriented strategy in changing behaviors to include more holistic and structurally based approaches.

    3) Fosters understanding of human behaviors and health status as a product of life conditions that may be beyond the control of an individual patient/family.

    4) Analyzes the broader sociocultural, political and historical contexts to fully understand human motivation and health behaviors.

2. ***Symbolic Interactionism*** (SI)
   a. SI is an influential and enduring sociological paradigm that examines interactions among people. The term *symbolic interactionism* was coined in 1937 by the American sociologist, Herbert Blumer, a student of George H. Mead whose ideas are reflected in Blumer's theoretical construct.
   b. SI is associated with a number of sociological scholars and several different schools of thought and opinion. The approach has steadily evolved as new scholars modify and transform the basic paradigm.
   c. Prominent scholars associated to varying degrees with SI include George H. Mead, Herbert Blumer, Erving Goffman, Howard S. Becker, Norman K. Denzin, and Arlie Hochschild
   d. Scope of Symbolic Interactionism (Blumer, 1969)
       1) SI is concerned with the nature and structure of interactions that occur among humans.
       2) The theoretical scope is small scale (ideographic), and is largely restricted to the limited arena. of human interactions
       3) SI can also be considered to be largely fixed in the present and recent past (*synchronic*) with history being largely external to the analysis.
   e. Features of Symbolic Interactionism (Blumer, 1969)
       1) Humans act within frameworks of meanings (symbols).
       2) These symbols are used in active, creative ways and are continually shifting in meaning as individuals actively create and modify symbols to meet their needs (i.e., individuals have agency).
       3) Humans continually interact with each other and it is through these joint encounters that individuals in the process create their sense of self, the perception of themselves by others, and the larger social world.
       4) Humans actively monitor and interpret each other's actions.
       5) These interpretations (and the ensuing responses) are grounded in the meanings of words and behaviors (not the actual actions themselves). In other words, symbols mediate human interactions.
       6) Individuals are active, reflective and creative in forming responses to the actions of others.
       7) Meanings and symbols are derived from the community of social interactions.
   f. Methodology and Symbolic Interactionism
       1) The "bread and butter" of SI is participant observation.
       2) The approach is grounded in actual, observable behaviors.
       3) SI is essentially an inductive approach to sociological inquiry. The details of any particular subject matter are derived from the observations.
   g. Application in transcultural nursing and health care
       1) Critical to intercultural communication as it emphasizes clarifying and building common interpretation by patients/families of practitioner messages.
       2) Significance of observations and use of silence to validate meanings of intercultural encounters.
       3) Importance of meanings and reflection on them for effective cross cultural encounters.

3. ***Critical Theory***
   a. Philosophical underpinnings
       1) The philosophic forms of knowledge of *Critical Science/Theory* evolved from the philosophic traditions of Hegel, Marx, Kuhn, Popper, Parsons, Weber, Wittgenstein, Ricoeur, Gadamer, and Habermas.
       2) Habermas specified a comprehensive approach to the previously competing social paradigms of the *system* (structural functionalism) and the *lifeworld* (interpretive sociology/anthropology) by connecting them to formulate the *Theory of Rational Communicative Action*.
   b. Social paradigms in the treatment of modern society
       1) Structural-functionalist
       2) Lifeworld (phenomenology/hermeneutics)
       3) Communicative action

c. Constitution of knowledge and type of discourse—*Theory of Rational Communicative Action* is a systematic synthesis of three nonreducible cognitive interests related to the constitution of knowledge:

  1) *Technical* (functionalist) cognitive interest is established in the empirical-analytical sciences where the form of inquiry requires procedures which confirm or disconfirm empirical hypotheses or theories.

  2) *Practical* (interpretive) cognitive interest is highlighted in the phenomenologic-hermeneutic disciplines where the aim of inquiry is not knowledge gained from technical control and manipulation but knowledge that clarifies the condition for intersubjectivity and communication through reflective interpretation of meaning in the lifeworld.

  3) *Emancipatory* (assertoric) cognitive interest is the approach of critically oriented science that sets forth the claim that concepts related to control or concepts of meaning and understanding cannot make sense unless there is rational, moral evaluation with strong arguments made by community participants in communication with each other so that consensus can be reached.

d. The core of critical theory is the notion of emancipating people from oppressive social systems so as to co-create through negotiation and consensus improved conditions for individuals and communities. From this perspective, an adequate epistemology or foundation for knowledge in nursing is transcultural nursing as it takes into account the communicative caring relationship and reasoned moral action of diverse people in historical, political, and social contexts.

e. The core of Critical Theory

  1) *Emancipation (Assertoric)* knowledge to initiate freedom from oppression that comes about by rational communication and evaluation made by participants in community life

  2) *Communicative competence* (comprehensive theory of rationality) pertains to the meaning of language in the theory of communicative action (ideal speech situation, human agency, will, and choice)

  3) Responsible moral action (the meaning of ethical knowledge)

  4) Uncoerced negotiation through communicative action

  5) Reaching consensus through the better argument

f. Critique and changes of Habermas's Theory of Communicative Action resulted from several epistemologic developments:

  1) Transcultural knowledge, intersubjectivity, and skill

  2) Linguistic differences and understanding

  3) Ethics of caring, responsibility, and accountability

  4) Politics of identity (pan identity)

  5) Multiculturalism, interculturality, and transculturalism

  6) Politics of recognition, gender issues

  7) Relations between secular liberal state and religion

  8) New forms of power and new questions to manage them

g. Disciplinary origins and purpose of Critical Social Theory in Nursing

  1) Evaluation of empiric scientific approaches

  2) Evaluation of phenomenological–hermeneutic scientific approaches

  3) Embracing critical social science in nursing to gain in-depth understanding of the transcultural dynamics of the contemporary human conditions specifically in social and political contexts

  4) The social and cultural context of health and illness (*Journal of Transcultural Nursing*)

  5) Transcultural nursing knowledge (Leininger)

  6) Political, economic, and social vision of transcultural nursing (Ray)

  7) Caring, nursing, and caring in nursing (Roach, Sumner, Watson, Ray)

  8) The moral construct of caring and transcultural caring in nursing as Communicative Action (Ray, Sumner) is critical in nursing practice

    a) To enhance transcultural nursing knowledge and inquiry by understanding the nature of the social and cultural worlds

    b) To bring to consciousness the distinctive form of transcultural interaction as the dialectic between the ethical communicative caring life and the cultural world

    c) To understand the nature of empowerment and empowering relationships

        d) To illuminate the ways of communicating and reaching consensus for the purposes of emancipation (assertoric discourse) from oppressive conditions that fail to enhance the health, healing, and well-being of individuals, communities, and cultures

    9) Significance of the Theory of Communicative Action in Transcultural Nursing

        a) Effective organization of nursing theory, research, and practice using the Critical Theory of Communicative Action

        b) Political interaction and social justice

        c) Empowerment

        d) Transcultural political nursing interaction

        e) Policy development

        f) Human rights and interface with local, national, and international communities.

4. *Critical Pedagogy* (Paulo Freire)

  a. Freire was a Brazilian educator who dedicated his life to improve the lives of the poor.

  b. His philosophy of education published in his book, *Pedagogy of the Oppressed* (1970) has been widely influential worldwide.

  c. Born in a middle-class family, he experienced poverty and hunger when his family was severely affected by the Great Depression. This experience created the core of his philosophy linking social conditions with learning.

  d. Philosophy of *Critical Pedagogy* (Freire, 1970, 1976, 1987)

    1) *Critical Pedagogy* is a teaching approach grounded in critical theory to help students develop critical consciousness (*conscientization*) and question/challenge dominant beliefs and practices in society that create oppression.

    2) *Conscientization* uses education as a means of consciously shaping the person and society to allow maximum development of human potential.

        a) Critical thinking is making connections between individual problems and experiences in school and society.

        b) Education is not a neutral process but rather an instrument by which individuals deal critically with reality and discover how to participate in the transformation of their world.

    3) Education is not a mere transmission of facts to passive students (*banking education*), which perpetuates oppression and dehumanizes students and teachers.

        a) *Liberatory and dialogical pedagogy* raises individual consciousness of oppression and in turn transforms oppressive social structures through *praxis*.

        b) Many traditional and commonsense ways of education contribute to oppression in schools and society, and mask or exacerbate oppressive educational methods.

        c) Realizing one's consciousness (*conscientization*) is a needed first step of *praxis*, which is the power and know-how to take action against oppression through emancipatory or liberating education.

    4) *Praxis* is informed action derived from a balance between theory and action, which teaches people to be free from oppression.

        a) *Praxis* is the process by which a theory, lesson, or skill is enacted or practiced. It is practical and applied knowledge that has meaning in political, educational, and spiritual realms.

        b) Dichotomy between teachers and students should be replaced by a deep reciprocity where teachers learn and become learners who teach. Teachers should have a sense of humility to relearn that which they already think they know, through interaction with the learner.

        c) It is a continuous process of unlearning, learning and relearning, reflection, evaluation and the impact that these actions have on the students, particularly those who have been historically and continue to be disenfranchised by traditional schooling.

        d) *Praxis* involves the cycle of theory, application, evaluation, reflection, and then back to theory.

        e) Social transformation is the product of *praxis* at the collective level.

  e. Disciplinary Origins of Critical Pedagogy

    1) Freire's philosophy of education had origins from the classical approach of Plato, modern Marxist and anticolonialist thinkers, Rousseau's concept of the child as an active learner and John Dewey's democratic education.

2) Freire used Marxist class analysis in exploring the power relationships between the colonizer and the colonized and the powerful and the oppressed.

   f. Significance and application in transcultural nursing and health care

1) Relevant in analyzing issues related to lagging academic success of racial and ethnic minorities in a White-dominated educational system, which is reflected in decreased representation of these groups in health professions

2) Allows examination of the nature of relationships between teachers, and racial and ethnic minority students, and among multicultural peer groups in health professional schools

3) Exploration of power relationships between health care providers and patients, health disparities and unequal access to care

4) Understanding structural inequalities in social, health and organizational policies that impact on vulnerable populations

5) Importance in curriculum development, selection of clinical experiences for students, and evaluation of educational outcomes

6) Integration of social justice as an ethical framework of health care

5. **Archaeology of Knowledge** (Michel Foucault)

   a. Michel Foucault (1926-1984) was a French historian and philosopher whose work focused on understanding the nature of human knowledge. He was particularly interested in the rise of science and the resulting characterizations of human nature.

   b. Foucault argued that the apparently necessary and true aspects of the world are often on careful examination revealed as human creations.

   c. His work on the interrelations of power and knowledge has been very influential in contemporary humanities and social sciences.

   d. A selection of his books:

1) *The History of Madness in the Classical Age* (1961)

2) *The Birth of the Clinic: An Archaeology of Medical Perception* (1963).

3) *Discipline and Punish: The Birth of the Prison* (1975)

4) *The History of Sexuality, Volume One* (1976)

   e. Philosophical premises:

1) Foucault's research is rooted in philosophical inquiry about the nature of reason and knowledge (or the problem of objectivity).

2) The philosophical issue is how to reconcile the difference between the *objective* (the object itself) and the *subjective* (the human representation of the object).

3) Foucault's research centered on understanding and characterizing human knowledge without judging the *objectivity* of this knowledge, without imposing contemporary meaning upon the past, and without seeking to identify human universals (e.g., invariant biological or social determinants of knowledge).

4) Foucault engaged in small-scale "inquiry that was limited in place, time and subject matter." He forcefully rejected universalist inquiry as often misguided and potentially dangerous. For example, he rejected Marxist, socially determinant approaches.

   f. Major premises:

1) The relationship between knowledge/reason and "reality" cannot be known with clarity. However, the researcher can observe the representation of the object ("reality") by humans.

2) Thought (*epistemes* or discursive formations) is governed by rules that operate beyond the awareness of the individual.

   a) Words and actions are reflections of these underlying discursive formations.

   b) These *epistemes* set the boundaries of thought.

   c) Although researchers can identify *epistemes*, they cannot with certainty know the origins of these structures. However, they can use *Raw Data* to make tentative conclusions.

   d) Discursive formations are not the result of inevitable historical trends, but are often contingent on seemingly unimportant factors.

   g. Analytic Approach to History:

1) *Raw Data* are expressions of "truth" (*énoncés*) as accepted by both the speaker and at least some other individuals.

2) *Archaeology* is the analysis of the data with no consideration as to whether the statements are true or are even meaningful to the researcher.

    a)   Much like the archaeologist, the researcher uncovers artifacts that reveal the *episteme*.

    b)   The goal is to observe reflections of underlying, discursive systems of thought (*epistemes*) without imposing contemporary patterns of thought or theory on this structure.

3) *Genealogy*

    a)   Strict and exclusive use of the method of archaeology yields no insight into the origins of *epistemes* or provides no room for human agency.

    b)   *Genealogy* is Foucault's term for analysis that observes changes in *epistemes* over time.

    c)   He sought to scrupulously avoid any imposition of linear, historical, developmental or metaphysical or a sense of the "inevitability" of history on the text of history.

h.   Three *Theorizing Practices* (Foucault, 1988, 1989)

    1) *Refusal* to accept as self-evident the things that are proposed to us.

    2) *Curiosity* to analyze and to know, because we can accomplish nothing without reflection,

    3) *Innovation* is seeking out in our reflection those things that have never been thought and imagined.

i.   *Power* is relations among people. Power is not simply oppression or coercion or institutionalized power. It is the matrix of actions by individuals who influence or seek to influence others. For example, scolding of a friend is an application of power; guilt and shame can be manifestations of power.

    1) Power relations between individuals may occur in both direction, but becomes power when one has unequal effect on the other.

    2) Power operates within a field of practice that is defined by *epistemes* (discursive formations beyond the awareness of the individual).

    3) The relations of power are often "frozen" (institutionalized).

    4) Power relations are often "masked;" they are present, but not seen. For example, many power aspects of gender relations are masked.

    5) Crystallized power will ultimately become unfrozen as conditions change.

j.   Application in transcultural nursing and health care

    1) Understanding power imbalances and mechanisms by which these imbalances are created.

    2) Emphasizes the need for self-reflection on one's actions that can contribute to health and care inequities.

    3) Examination of practitioner interactions, decisions and actions that can result to objectification of patients and denial of their existential and subjective experiences.

    4) Critical examination of institutional policies and procedures that contribute to disempowerment and vulnerability of certain individuals and groups

6. *Maintenance of Social Hierarchies* (Pierre Bourdieu)

a.   Pierre Bourdieu (1930-2002) was a French architect and sociologist

b.   Bourdieu received his graduate training in philosophy

c.   After graduation, Bourdieu shifted his attention to sociology

d.   A selection of his books:

    1) *The Inheritors: French Students and Their Relations to Culture* (1964)

    2) *Reproduction in Education, Society and Culture* (1970)

    3) *Outline of a Theory of Practice* (1972)

    4) *Distinction: A Social Critique of the Judgment of Taste* (1979)

    5) *The Logic of Practice* (1980)

    6) *Language and Symbolic Power* (1982)

e.   The *Maintenance of Social Elites*

    1) Bourdieu's best-known work was focused on how social elites achieve and maintain power and high social status

    2) Bourdieu was interested in how individuals compete within social spheres for power, prestige, and economic resources.

f.   Philosophical premises:

    1) Much of Bourdieu's work is "critical first of inherited categories and accepted ways of thinking" (Wacquant, 2007).

2) Bourdieu challenges the sociologist to reflect on inherited conceptions of society, particularly those that conceive of society in terms of oppositional categories such as diachronic versus synchronic, macrolevel versus microlevel, subjective versus objective, and so forth.

3) In particular, Bourdieu sought to reconcile the "opposing" *structuralist* and *constructivist* perspectives.

    a) *Structuralist* perspectives tend to view social reality as a product of social structure (and which occurs largely beyond the consciousness of the individual actors).

    b) *Constructivist* perspectives tend to view social reality as an outcome of innumerable human actors who together actively *construct* society.

4) Bourdieu sought to create a theory of society in which individual actors both create society and are transformed themselves by that society

g. Society has three major components:

  1) *Capital* includes not only economic capital but also other types of resources that the individual can possess, including the social, cultural, and symbolic capital.

  2) *Field* represents a social space or sphere of life within which individuals learn and interact.

  3) *Habitus* "designates the system of durable and transposable dispositions through which we perceive, judge, and act in the world" (Wacquant, 2007)

h. *Capital*

  1) *Capital* is composed of those resources that the individual possesses that confer advantage in action within the field.

  2) The principal sources of capital are

    a) *Economic capital* is composed of the individual's economic, material, and financial resources.

    b) *Social capital* is the social advantage that is conferred by membership in a social network. For example, a young college student obtains a very desirable and well-paying summer internship via her wealthy uncle's contacts.

    c) *Cultural capital* is the socially valued knowledge or other characteristics that confer higher social status within the field. For example, knowledge of fine wines might confer social advantage within some social fields. Or, possession of a title that signifies nobility (Sir, Archduke, etc.) would be another form of cultural capital. The popular term *nouveau riche* has as its very definition the absence of cultural capital, despite the possession of economic capital.

    d) *Symbolic capital* is an individual advantage that accrues from social prestige. Because "prestige" is a group phenomenon, the presence or absence of symbolic capital derives from group definitions concerning worth. For example, the wealthy individual who donates large sums of money to charity can be said to possess both economic and symbolic capital.

      (1) *Symbolic violence* is the control over individuals by symbolic means generally, by the dominant society over a minority. For example, societal insistence on the superiority of "standard English" over "Black English" would constitute a form of symbolic violence.

      (2) Symbolic violence is a form of social control, and one that is often unreflectively taken to be "true."

  3) Capital in one form can be converted into capital of another form. For example, a wealthy individual might purchase symbolic capital in the form of expensive clothes or high-status social activities.

i. *Field*

  1) The field is a structured social "space" within which actors interact, compete, exchange information, make decisions, and so on.

  2) Examples of fields include the family, school, neighborhood, professional associations, court systems, and so on.

  3) In complex societies, an individual will be positioned within multiple fields

  4) Fields often fall within other fields (e.g., a school of nursing may be located within the larger field of the university).

  5) Each field has its own identity, rules, hierarchy, values, and so on.

        6) Fields are social locations at which political struggle occurs.

        7) Within each field, there will be individuals who struggle to support the field's *status quo* and others who will challenge this.

  j. *Habitus*

        1) *Habitus* is a system of enduring individual *dispositions* in thought and action.

        2) Bourdieu rejects mechanistic social formulations, such as the utilitarian Economic Man, who acts to maximize personal benefit. Instead, one can think of these dispositions as habits that manifest themselves in statistical, non-determinative manner.

        3) *Habitus* is learned by the individual via exposure to the world.

        4) Much of what constitutes *habitus* is learned early in life.

        5) *Habitus* is often comprised of elements that are self-evidently "true" (unquestioned by the individual).

        6) Because individuals are embedded within *fields*, learning is the means by which individuals incorporate social structure into their conception of the world.

        7) *Habitus* is comprised not only of ideals, values, modes of thinking and the like, but also includes learned modes of behavior and action.

  k. *Habitus*, the *Field*, and *Doxa*

        1) *Doxa* is a misrepresentation of reality that becomes established by consensus. Therefore, *Doxa* is a group phenomenon (a shared view of the world).

        2) *Doxa* is composed of generally accepted truths about the world. These may be so well ingrained in society that they are "taken for granted" and are not subject to examination except in the case of crisis.

        3) *Doxa* has its origins from the apparent coherence between *field* and *habitus*.

  l. Comparing *Habitus*, *Doxa*, and *Culture*

        1) *Culture* is defined variously even within the field of cultural anthropology. However, most cultural anthropologists would agree that culture is shared knowledge/information about the world, and passed down from one generation to the next.

        2) *Habitus* contains these same qualities, but also importantly shifts these conceptions.

        3) Habitus is shared *thought and action* that is learned through exposure to the world via human encounters that occur within multiple social fields.

        4) Therefore, an individual's *habitus* will include not only "ancient" knowledge (including *doxa*) that has been learned but also "new" information that has been accumulated over the course of a lifetime.

        5) *Doxa* shares many characteristics with the concept of culture, but has a focus on unexamined, "invisible" perspectives on the world.

  m. The Relationship of *Field* and *Habitus*

        1) Field and habitus can be viewed as reflections of each other

        2) Fields exist because of social actors each with habitus

        3) And, habitus exists via interaction with the field

  n. Application in transcultural nursing and health care

        1) Awareness of group differences between patients–providers, different groups and levels of providers, dominant organizational norms and those of patients/families and communities.

        2) Understanding sources of bias and prejudices from differential value premises of the powerful and influential that dominate organizational cultures in health care and education.

        3) Implications for capacity building for health in vulnerable communities and families

        4) Cultural sensitization and advocacy for diverse students to improve their academic success in health professions.

7. *Ecological Systems Theory of Human Development* (Urie Bronfenbrenner)

  a. Bronfenbrenner was a renowned Russian-born American psychologist known for his work in child development and advocacy for children and families.

  b. In 1979, his *Bioecological approach* led to a new direction in the study of human development across disciplines, emphasizing the linkage between the larger social structure across societies and the development of human potential.

   c.   His approach to the study of human beings and their environments led to new directions in basic research and influenced the design of programs and policies affecting the well-being of children and families both in the United States and abroad.

   d.   His work was the impetus for the creation of Head Start in 1965, the US federal child development program for low-income children and their families.

   e.   As the result of his groundbreaking concept of the ecology of human development, these environments from the family to economic and political structures were viewed as part of the life course.

   f.   Five propositions for child development (Bronfenbrenner, 1979; Seifert, 1999)

      1) The child must have ongoing, long-term mutual interaction with an adult(s) who have a stake in its development.

      2) Both the strong tie with adults and patterns of interpersonal interaction will help the child relate to the broader environment in later life.

      3) Attachments and interactions with other adults will help the child progress to more complex relationships.

      4) The relationships between the child and primary adults will progress only with repeated two-way interchanges and mutual compromise.

      5) The future relationships between the child and the adults require public support and affirmation of the importance of these roles.

   g.   *The Ecological Systems Theory* (Addison, 1992; Berk, 2000; Bronfenbrenner, 1979, 1992; Henderson, 1995)

      1) Views a child's development within the context of the system of relationships that forms its environment.

      2) Also known as the *bioecological systems theory*, it emphasizes that a child's own biology is a primary environment influencing its development. The interaction between factors in the child's maturing biology, its immediate family/community environment, and the societal landscape influences the child's development.

      3) Each of the complex *layers* of environment has an effect on a child's development. Each of these systems is characterized by roles, norms, and relationships.

        a)   The *microsystem* is the layer of structures in the immediate surrounding that interacts directly with the child. These structures include the family, school, neighborhood, or child-care environments.

        b)   The *mesosystem* is the layer that connects the structures of the child's microsystem such as the relationship between the child's teacher and the parents, the health providers and the parents, and so forth.

        c)   The *exosystem* is the layer of the larger social system external to the child's experience but affects his or her development by interacting with some structures in the child's microsystem. For example, the demands of the workplace on the parents or availability of child care services in the community where the family lives affect the interactions between parents and children.

        d)   The *macrosystem* is the outermost layer comprised of cultural values, customs, and laws that influence the interactions of all other layers. For example, a socialist philosophy provides universal access to health services, hence parents may readily seek professional health services for themselves and their children.

        e)   The *chronosystem* is the dimension of time and historical events in the child's environment such as timing of parental divorce, death of a parent, catastrophic illness of any family member, which can affect the life chances of the child.

      4) Changes or conflict in any one layer will affect other layers. When the relation between different microsystems is compatible, development progresses more positively. For example, when roles and expectations are consonant between home and school, children are likely to succeed.

      5) The interaction of structures within a layer and interactions of structures between layers, termed as *bidirectional influences*, is critical in all levels of the environment. At the microsystem level, bidirectional influences are strongest and have the greatest impact on the individual. For example, parental values and beliefs affect a child's behavior which also affects how parents and siblings interact with the child.

h. Bronfenbrenner argued against using the *deficit model* to determine the level of public support for struggling families who need to be declared deficient in order to get help, which fosters helplessness. In health care, this is evident in the eligibility requirements for Medicaid where families have to be evaluated as indigent before getting support.

i. Implications in transcultural nursing and health care
1) Conceptualization of health and illness as socially and culturally constructed
2) Understanding the complexity of health promotion within a multilevel systems/environment context
3) Emphasis on multidisciplinary and multisectoral collaboration in health promotion
4) Addressing health within the context of family, community, and society
5) Relevance in population-based health promotion
6) Significant in development, implementation, and evaluation of social, health, and organizational policies affecting health
7) Integration of historical and timing of events on the individual's life course
8) Shifting conceptualization of health from individual and biomedical to interactions between humans, society, and environment
9) Implications in education and health care of vulnerable individuals, families, and communities
10) Life course approach to health promotion
11) Importance of public support for families to ensure healthy children

8. ***Ecosocial Model (Social Epidemiology)*** (Nancy Krieger)
a. Krieger argues that health disparities are the result of complex, simultaneous interactions involving biological and social processes that are situated in space and time (Krieger, 2001, 2005, 2008).
b. She argues that prevailing theoretical approaches (both explicit and implicit) to the study of health disparities are too often restricted in scope, overly generic, and inadequately conceptualized. As a result, research has often been poorly positioned to reduce or eliminate health disparities.
c. She also argues that too often researchers have neglected the issues of agency and responsibility (i.e., who is responsible to fix the problem?).
d. Some limitations of two dominant theoretical perspectives according to Krieger (2001):
1) *Psychosocial theory*: Krieger argues that this perspective focuses on generic concepts of stress and coping at the individual level, and too little on the social, economic and political causes of stress.
2) *Social production of disease/political economy of health*: This perspective focuses on the social, economic, and political causes of disease, but generally provides little insight into the pathways by which ill health is influenced.
e. Krieger's model contains the following important features:
1) *Space and Time*: Health and disease are the outcome of processes that are uniquely rooted in space and time.
2) *Scale* is an important aspect of space and time. For example, the time effect may be acute or chronic, sustained or episodic. Spatial effects may be localized or widespread, densely organized or dispersed, and so on.
3) *Multilevel interactions*: Health and disease are the outcome of *simultaneous* interactions among levels that can range from the molecular to the sociopolitical.
4) *Uniqueness*: Each disease is the result of a unique process involving biological and social factors.
5) Example: the complex of biological and social factors that contribute to increased risk of conduct disorder will be different than those for anxiety disorders.
f. Five *ecosocial constructs* as identified by Krieger (2001):
1) *Embodiment*
a) *Embodiment* is the process by which the body is modified over time by exposure to the world (Krieger 2005).
b) An example of embodiment is *Death from suicide*: Suicides are the embodiment of many individual and societal factors, including the organization of health care, individual behaviors, and social, cultural, and biological factors.

2) *Pathways to embodiment*
   a) Embodiment is structured by the "constraints and possibilities of our biology" and social factors that influence these biological possibilities. Myocardial infarction might be a result of "biological susceptibility" to saturated fat intake, but also residence in a poor neighborhood with little access to exercise, fresh fruits and vegetables, and high-quality health care.
   b) *Cumulative interplay between exposure, susceptibility, and resistance:* Embodiment occurs across levels (molecular, physiological, social, political) and in multiple ecological domains (home, neighborhood, work).
   c) *Accountability and agency:* Researchers and practitioners should consider "who and what is responsible for social inequalities in health and for rectifying them" (Krieger 2008).
g. Application in transcultural nursing and health care
   1) Life course approach to health disparities.
   2) Consideration of social processes that create poor health and shorter life expectancy in populations.
   3) Moving way from victim blaming to more accurate approaches towards health problems in population groups.
   4) Forces biomedicine and disease-based models to include sociopolitical and environmental factors in addressing health problems.

9. ***Transcultural Caring Dynamics in Nursing and Health Care*** (Marilyn Ray)
   a. Assumptions guiding the framework
      1) Transcultural nursing focuses on the universality of human caring, and the comparative study and analysis of the diversity and dynamics of world cultures in relation to human caring values, beliefs, and behaviors (Leininger & McFarland, 2006; Ray, 1989, 1994, 2010).
      2) Transcultural caring illuminates the character of our moral lives by calling forth love as compassion and justice as right action within culturally dynamic communities.
      3) Transcultural caring organizes a systematic structure and process that elucidates the nature of the complexity of transcultural interaction, communication, and action in context.
      4) The systematic structure and process forms the foundation for competent/relevant transcultural nursing practice, and also for education, research, and administration within the discipline of transcultural nursing.
   b. Dimensions of the Framework
      1) *Essence of Caring* highlights the history of caring and its importance in human relationships and various disciplines, such as nursing, transcultural nursing, philosophy, anthropology, theology, ethics, science, and art.
         a) Caring is the essence of nursing. Although caring has many definitions, its focus in modern nursing relates to love and copresence in the context of complex systems (Morse, Bottorff, Anderson, O'Brien, & Solberg, 1992; Davidson & Ray, 1991).
         b) Roach (2002) defined the attributes of caring as the 6 Cs:
            (1) *Compassion* is an essential sensitivity to the suffering, pain, and brokenness of the other, and the quality of presence and right action when sharing in the life of the other.
            (2) *Confidence* is the basic responsibility to foster a trusting relationship with another.
            (3) *Conscience* is having an ethical sense of right and wrong in discerning what ought to be done in a particular situation.
            (4) *Competence* is defined as "the state of having the knowledge, judgment, skills, energy, experience, and motivation required to respond adequately to the demands of one's professional responsibilities (Roach, 2002, p. 54).
            (5) *Commitment* is a directed choice that the professional nurse has to make to intervene specifically in a nursing situation.
            (6) *Comportment* is the communicative interaction (knowledge, influence, demeanor, dress, language, or state of harmony) within the nurse–patient/family relationship.
         c) Transcultural caring is the quality of human caring communicative ethical activity within the dynamics of transcultural relationships and contexts.

2) *Transcultural Caring Ethics* is concerned with how we ought to live in complex dynamic cultures and society (Rachels, 2003).
   a) The pledge of transcultural nursing is to do good and do no harm for people of diverse cultures. Transcultural caring ethics helps us voice what is right, just or good for all people in any nursing situation.
   b) Thus, transcultural caring ethics is a set of principles, and code of conduct that facilitates understanding of the good and the potential for evil that can be perpetrated when conflict ensues within diverse cultures.
   c) The idea of good and evil is historical and traditional; they are cultural and religious and oriented to rules, principles, or ways of life.
   d) Understanding how sociocultural forms of ethical knowing and relating, how human ethical character and virtue are formed, co-created, changed and can be more understood is essential to all humans, and especially transcultural nursing interactions.
   e) Looking deeply into the lifeworld of the self and the other to become aware, to understand, and to seek the good illuminates the constructs of transcultural meaning, purpose, truth and beauty (Gadamer, 1986).
3) *Transcultural Context for Transcultural Nursing* identifies the centrality of the human-environment integral process, the unity of persons with the dynamic cultural contexts.
   a) Patterns of wholeness (integration of body, mind, spirit, and context) are essential to transcultural nursing.
   b) Transcultural context highlights the idea of culture from its earliest definitions to culture as dynamic, and continually unfolding as persons from diverse geographical and cultural communities interface within the world community.
   c) Transcultural context describes the person in the family, kinship system, community, society, and the globe.
   d) Transcultural context illuminates the complexity of ethnicity, identity and race within community, society, culture, and organizations.
   e) It examines changes in relationships due to globalization (transportation, economics, technology, computer technology, and cyberspace, and the space technology), and the potential for economic, geopolitical, and religious conflict.
   f) Thus, within the transcultural context, knowledge of concepts like racialized identity and panidentity, multiculturalism, the politics of recognition, interculturality, and transculturality emerge in the modern world.
   g) Transcultural context shows how transcultural nurses must be fully aware of changes in the world to deal with the difficulties and challenges of the unfolding meaning of diversity in culture to discover our common humanity and to provide culturally relevant care.
4) *Universal Sources* outline the importance of spirituality and/or religion in all transcultural nursing situations. From earliest records, there has been a belief in the Universal Mind, which has been described by a variety of names, among them, Logos, Jesus Christ, Brahman, the Absolute, Allah, Great Spirit, Holy Spirit, Weltgeist, or simply God (Margenau, 1984).
   a) Universal Sources identify many major religions and spiritual movements and how they become a part of the experience for choice making in health, healing, well-being or a peaceful death.
   b) Nursing is considered a sacred science and grounded in love and compassion and social justice (Ray, 1989; Watson, 2005).
   c) The integration of body, mind and spirit (holistic nursing) is the foundation to the choice for health and well-being.
   d) In this world, there is also a godless pursuit of happiness and health, and although not religiously grounded, appeals to the highest principle of ethics, doing good for diverse people in transcultural contexts.
   e) Transcultural nurses, thus, must be open to and integrate spirituality or ethics into their transcultural nursing practice to more fully recognize when patients are suffering with spiritual–cultural distress or when religious beliefs are or should be used in the decision-making caring process.

5) *Transcultural Caring Inquiry (Awareness, Understanding, Choice)* is the final dimension that highlights how transcultural nurses provided *transculturally* sensitive care.

    a) The final dimension offers a structure and process to synthesize and integrate all the dimensions as discussed to facilitate choices for health, healing, well-being, or a peaceful death.

    b) A number of assessment tools for inquiry and assessment (culturological assessment, culture-value conflict tool, and Ray's Transcultural Communicative Ethical CARING tool, and negotiation tools) have been co-created to facilitate growth and development in transcultural education, practice, administration and research.

    c) Ray's book also includes transcultural caring experiences/case studies/exemplars at the end of each chapter in the first section, and numerous transcultural nursing experiences of diverse and dynamics in the second section.

  c. A transcultural caring framework has been presented for the purposes of assessing and analyzing the complexity of transcultural nursing in a culturally diverse and dynamic world. The dynamic processes of the essence of caring, transcultural caring ethics, transcultural context for transcultural nursing, universal sources, and transcultural caring inquiry, awareness, understanding and choice, lay the foundation for interpretation, negotiation, reconciliation, and ultimately the development of competence of complex views of mutual caring in transcultural nursing situations.

10. *Model of Multicultural Understanding* (Locke, 1998)

  a. Purpose of the Model:

    1) Provides a comprehensive guide to gain knowledge and understanding of culturally diverse individuals and groups

    2) Provides a foundation to explore ethnic and cultural differences.

    3) Allows practitioners in the helping professions (teachers, counselors, etc.) to use this knowledge to engage in positive and meaningful relationships with culturally diverse individuals and groups

  b. Concepts underlying the model

    1) Sociological factors

      a) Family structure

      b) Child-rearing practices

      c) Self-determination within a cultural group

      d) Interest in political systems as important to advancement as a group

    2) Psychological and developmental (Sue & Sue, 1990)

      a) Awareness of knowing one's own bias, values, and interest

      b) Worldview is one's contemplation of the world

      c) Circumstantialist view of culture as socially constructed and reactive (Glazer & Moynihan, 1975)

    3) Multiculturalism

      a) Rights of individuals to be respected for their differences

      b) All cultures have values, beliefs, customs, language, knowledge, and worldview

    4) Culture as a socially transmitted system of shared ideas, that shapes behaviors, and provides names and categories for experiences (Locke, 1998)

  c. Disciplinary origins of the model

    1) Psychology

    2) Counseling

    3) Education

  d. Assumptions of the model (Locke, 1992, 1998)

    1) Self-awareness involves knowing one's biases and worldview.

    2) Awareness of cultural diversity is the understanding that not all cultures view the world in the same way.

    3) Cultural diversity creates a need for changes in research, theory and curriculum.

    4) Global events and influences may affect local and national views and events.

    5) Dominant culture is a backdrop for understanding cultural diversity.

    6) Cultural differences may stem from

    a) Acculturation

        (1) Members of a particular cultural group are not all alike

        (2) Different cultural groups immerse themselves differentially in the culture of the United States

        (3) Degrees of acculturation

            (a) Bicultural is the ability to function in the dominant and one's own culture

            (b) Traditional persons hold on to the majority of cultural traits from the culture of origin, while rejecting much of the dominant culture

            (c) Acculturated means that the individual has given up most of the cultural traits from the culture of origin and assumed the traits of the dominant culture

            (d) Marginal individuals are completely comfortable neither in the culture of origin nor in the dominant culture

    b) Poverty and economic capacity

        (1) Knowledge of historical reasons for poverty

        (2) Political and economic factors that influence poverty

        (3) Housing, employment, education, and life expectancy effect of poverty

    c) History of oppression—understanding the history as well as effects of historical and contemporary oppression

    d) Language and arts

        (1) Language is a transmitter of cultural values and viewed by the dominant culture as a reason for assimilation

        (2) Standard artistic forms may vary. In the United States, art form is linear versus circular in other cultures.

    e) Racism and prejudice

        (1) *Prejudice* is judging before fully examining the object of evaluation. *Racial prejudice* is judging based on racial/ethnic/cultural group membership before getting to know the person

        (2) *Personal prejudices* are beliefs about individuals as members of a particular cultural group.

        (3) *Institutional prejudices* are beliefs that have been incorporated into the structure of an institution

        (4) *Ethnocentrism* is a belief in the superiority of own cultural group over another

        (5) Racism (Locke & Hardaway, 1980) may be intentional or unintentional, covert or overt or a combination of the two types.

    f) Sociopolitical factors are the culturally unique factors that affect a particular culture

    g) Child-rearing practices are primary socializing agents to the culture

    h) Religious practices consist of the organized system of beliefs in god, gods or supernatural beings

    i) Family structure and dynamics are the basic unit of culture, responsible for the production and reproduction of culture

    j) Culture values and attitudes help emphasize what is known and how to interpret the world.

  e. Model strengths

    1) Comprehensive, easy to understand and use in practice

    2) Can be used as a conceptual framework for practice, education, and research

    3) Covers concepts beyond contemporary transcultural theories in health and nursing such as

        a) History of oppression

        b) Prejudice and racism

        c) History of poverty

    4) Offers a more comprehensive understanding of worldviews and environmental context of cultures

  f. Application in transcultural nursing and health care

    1) Should be used in conjunction with other nursing and health care theories and models

    2) No direct mention of implications to health care and nursing

3) Nurses and other health care providers must make the conceptual leap for the benefit of health care and nursing

4) The model is not predictive and there are no documented outcomes of the model.

11. *Cultural Safety Model* (Irihapeti Merenia Ramsden)

  a. Ramsden is best known in Aotearoa New Zealand and internationally for developing cultural safety as the main theme of her doctoral dissertation.

    1) She envisioned cultural safety as an educational framework for the analysis of power relationships between health professionals and those they serve.

    2) She consistently argued for the need to address the ongoing impact of historical, social, and political processes on Maori health disparities.

    3) Her ideas were both challenging and threatening to many *pakeha* (European) New Zealanders who were, and are, often ignorant of the country's history and fearful of difference.

  b. Philosophical underpinnings of the model

    1) Communication and recognition of diversity in worldviews

    2) Impact of colonization processes on minority groups

  c. Disciplinary origins

    1) Social/political policy

      a) *Treaty of Waitangi Act of 1975* is the formal agreement between Maoris and the Crown guaranteeing equity of health access and outcomes to the indigenous people of New Zealand.

      b) *A Model for Negotiated and Equal Partnership* was adopted to ensure that nursing education address health concerns of the Maoris using negotiation and partnership.

      c) *Kawa Whakaruruhau* was adopted by the Nursing Counsel of New Zealand in 1991 mandating the teaching of cultural safety in nursing and midwifery programs.

  d. Purpose of the model

    1) Improve the health status of all people in New Zealand based on the Treaty of Waitangi.

    2) Consideration of historically determined power relations between nurses and the indigenous people of New Zealand.

    3) Bridging differences that have evolved between nurses and the indigenous people of New Zealand.

  e. Concepts of Cultural Safety

    1) *Culture* incorporates many elements, such as a particular way of living in the world, attitudes, behaviors, links, and relationships with others (Nursing Counsel of New Zealand, 1992).

    2) *Cultural values* consist of morals, beliefs, attitudes and standards that derive from a particular cultural group (New Zealand Nurses Organisation, 1995).

    3) *Safety* involves actions by nurses and midwives nursing or midwifery to protect patient/client/ community from hazards to health and well-being. It includes regard for the physical, mental, social, spiritual, and cultural components of the patient/client and the environment (Nursing Counsel of New Zealand, 1992).

    4) *Unsafe nursing/midwifery practice* consists of any action or omission thtat endangers the well-being, demeans the person or disempowers the cultural identity of the patient/client (Nursing Counsel of New Zealand, 1992).

    5) *Cultural safety* is the outcome of nursing and midwifery education that enables safe service that is defined by those who receive the service (Nursing Counsel of New Zealand, 1996).

  f. Components of Cultural Safety

    1) Knowledge and understanding of the individual nurse or midwife

    2) Awareness of how own attitudes and assumptions affect others

    3) Concern with life chances of people rather than individual lifestyles

    4) Awareness of how differential social relations and the social/ political context affect life chances of people, including health

    5) Race relations addressed as a significant determinant of life chances in society

    6) Culture is not seen as ethnospecific but rather as a product of social/political realities and social inequalities

g. Principles of Cultural Safety
   1) Improving the health status of New Zealanders emphasizing health gains and positive outcomes, and acknowledgement of diverse beliefs and practices.
   2) Enhancing delivery of health and disability services by identifying power relationships, empowerment of the users of services and recognition of potential impact of diverse cultural reality on users of services.

h. Objectives of the model in education of nurses and midwives (Ramsden, 1996)
   1) Examine own "realities" and attitudes that have an impact on practice encounters.
   2) Be open minded and flexible in attitudes toward people who are different from oneself and to whom one offers or deliver service.
   3) Refrain from blaming victims of historical and social processes for their current plights
   4) Provide a workforce of well-educated, self-aware registered nurses and midwives who are culturally safe to practice.

i. Assumptions of the health care relationship between providers and care recipients (Ramsden, 1996)
   1) Each relationship is unique hence, differences among people must be recognized and care must be delivered regardful of these differences.
   2) Each relationship is power-laden; empowerment of recipients of care results in improvement of their health status as only the recipient of care determines if the care provided is safe.
   3) Each relationship is culturally dyadic, hence partnerships should be formulated so power is shared by providers and recipients of care.

j. Significance in transcultural nursing and health care
   1) Recognition of individual differences
   2) Provision of care respectful of individual differences
   3) Professional self-awareness of own attitudes and prejudices
   4) Understanding social and political influences in culture and power relations in health care
   5) Importance of empowerment in health status
   6) Active participation of care recipients in care decisions
   7) Focus on structural causes of poor health status minimizes stereotyping by not equating culture as ethnospecific.
   8) Recognition of subjectivity and power imbalance in health care interactions

k. Critique of the Model (Polaschek, 1998)
   1) Recognition of beliefs and assumptions and how one imposes these beliefs on others is of greater importance than self-attitude change
   2) Outcomes of indigenous people as key actors in their health development remain untested
   3) Definition of unsafe practice framed in terms of individuals while definition of safe practice refers to the Maoris collectively
   4) Relationship between individual Maori alienation and the social disadvantage of Maoris as a group not adequately explored

12. Cultural Dimensions Model (Geert Hofstede)
   a. Hofstede is a Dutch social scientist whose work originated from a large research project of workers in the multinational corporation, IBM in 64 countries.
   b. Subsequently, other groups (students, elites, pilots, consumers, and managers) in many different countries were also studied using his original work.
   c. Hofstede believes that in a globalized world intercultural understanding is essential to development of intercultural cooperation.
   d. Hofstede describes culture as the unwritten rules about how to be a good member of a group as it provides moral standards for group members. It inspires "symbols, heroes, rituals, laws, religions, taboo, and all kinds of practices but its core is hidden in unconscious values."
   e. Values are shared preferences with members of one's own collective that deal with what is good and bad, beautiful and ugly, normal and abnormal. Values are always collective within a group.
   f. Norms are rules we are supposed to respect, imposed by our environment (institutions/organizations), regardless of their compatibility with our own values. The government plays an important role in norm enforcement, but it has hardly any influence on our values, whatever some politicians may believe. One problem of norm enforcement is that it costs money, money that a

government can only spend once, and if you spend it on norm enforcement you cannot spend it on something else you also want.

g. Culture according to Hofstede (2001) can be a source of nuisance and conflict rather than synergy if not understood and dealt with properly

h. Independent dimensions of national culture differences (Hofstede & Hofstede, 2005)

1) Power distance is the extent to which the less powerful members of organizations and institutions (like the family) accept and expect that power is distributed unequally. Inequality is defined and endorsed by the followers as much as by the leaders. All societies are unequal, but some are more unequal than others.

2) Individualism versus collectivism is the degree to which individuals are integrated into groups. In individualist societies, social ties are loose and everyone is expected to look after himself or herself and his or her immediate family. Collectivist societies integrate members from birth to death into strong, cohesive in-groups, often extended families which provide them insecurity and expect loyalty.

3) Masculinity versus femininity is the distribution of roles between genders. Masculine values are associated with assertive and competitive behaviors, ambition, and accumulation of wealth whereas feminine values emphasize modesty, caring, and quality of life. Feminine values differ less among societies than masculine. Women in feminine countries have the same modesty, caring and quality of life values as men; in masculine countries they are somewhat assertive and competitive, but not as much as the men, so that these countries show a gap between men's values and women's values.

4) Uncertainty avoidance refers to a society's tolerance for uncertainty and ambiguity. Uncertainty avoiding cultures minimize uncertainty by strict laws and rules, safety and security measures, and by a philosophical belief in absolute truth. Uncertainty accepting cultures are more tolerant of opinions different from their own; have fewer rules and are relativist in their religion and philosophy. People within these cultures are more phlegmatic and contemplative, and less expressive of emotions.

5) Long-term orientation (LTO) versus short-term orientation (STO)—LTO is associated with values of thrift and perseverance whereas STO is associated with values such as respect for tradition, fulfilling social obligations, and protecting one's "face."

i. Findings of Hofstede's (1978) study

1) Power distance scores are high for Latin, Asian, and African countries and smaller for Germanic countries.

2) Individualism prevails in developed and Western countries, whereas collectivism prevails in less developed and Eastern countries; Japan takes a middle position on this dimension.

3) Masculinity is high in Japan, in some European countries like Germany, Austria, and Switzerland, and moderately high in Anglo countries; it is low in Nordic countries and in the Netherlands and moderately low in some Latin countries, like France and Spain, and Asian countries like Thailand.

4) Uncertainty avoidance scores are higher in Latin countries, in Japan, and in German speaking countries, lower in Anglo, Nordic, and Chinese culture countries.

5) LTO is mostly found in East Asian countries, in particular in China, Hong Kong, Taiwan, Japan, and South Korea.

j. Explanations for study findings

1) Hofstede relates these differences to historical roots of certain countries. For example, Latin countries such as Spain, Portugal, France, and Italy were ruled by the Roman Empire characterized by a central authority in Rome and a system of laws governing citizens everywhere. Centralization of authority fostered high power distance and a system of laws fostered strong uncertainty avoidance.

2) In contrast, the Chinese empire also knew centralization, but it lacked a fixed system of laws as it was governed by men rather than by laws, which fostered large power distance but medium to weak uncertainty avoidance.

3) The Germanic part of Europe, including Great Britain, never succeeded in establishing an enduring common central authority and countries which inherited its civilizations show smaller power distance.

4) Implications of findings

    a) Power distance is correlated with the use of violence in domestic politics and with income inequality in a country.

    b) Individualism is correlated with national wealth (per capita gross national product) and with mobility between social classes from one generation to the next.

    c) Masculinity is correlated negatively with the sharing of wealth by developed countries with the Third World.

    d) Uncertainty avoidance is associated with Roman Catholicism and with the legal obligation in developed countries for citizens to carry identity cards.

    e) LTO is correlated with national economic growth of the East Asian economies and its emphasis on future-oriented values of thrift and perseverance.

k. Application of model in transcultural nursing and health care

    1) Hofstede's model is applicable in intercultural communication, leadership, and management.

    2) Leadership and management are informed not only by workforce diversity in the organization but also by the dominant cultural ethos of the society in which organizations are situated.

    3) Applicable in dealing with diverse students in schools within specific sociocultural contexts.

    4) A significant criticism of the model is the idea of monolithic cultures especially in an era of global travel and more frequent cross-cultural exchanges.

13. *Organizational Culture* (Edgar Schein)

a. Schein is a social psychologist and professor emeritus of management at the Massachusetts Institute of Technology

b. Organizational culture is not the same as corporate culture as it involves broader and deeper concepts; it is what an organization "is" rather than what it "has" (Huczynski & Buchanan, 2007).

c. Organizations deal with two major problems: adapting to their external environment in order to survive and grow, and integrating internally in order to function and adapt. Organizational culture evolves to achieve stability, and patterning and integration.

d. Schein's views about organizational culture:

    1) Culture defines leadership. Good managers must work from a more anthropological model.

    2) Understanding the culture of the organization is critical to leadership success.

    3) Many of the problems confronting leaders can be traced to their inability to analyze and evaluate organizational cultures.

    4) Culture is the deeper level of basic assumptions and beliefs that are learned responses to the group's problems of survival in its external environment and its problems of internal integration, which are shared by members of an organization. Culture operates at the unconscious, and taken for granted level about itself and its environment (Schein, 1988).

    5) Culture is the most difficult organizational attribute to change, outlasting organizational products, services, founders and leadership and all other physical attributes of the organization.

    6) Schein's model examines organizational culture from the observer perspective.

    7) Strong culture exists when the staff response is aligned with organizational values. In such environments, organizations operate effectively. In a weak culture there is little alignment with organizational values, hence control must be exercised through extensive procedures and bureaucracy.

e. The three cognitive levels of organizational culture (Schein, 2005):

    1) Artifacts

        a) The first and most cursory level of organizational attributes that can be seen, felt, and heard by the uninitiated observer

        b) Include superficial, visible, tangible, and identifiable elements in an organization that are easily observed but difficult to decipher as they tend to be ambiguous

        c) Examples are the architecture, furniture, dress code, visible awards and recognition, the way members dress, how each person visibly interacts with each other and with organizational outsiders, company slogans, mission statements, and other operational creeds.

    2) Values or espoused values

        a) The professed culture of an organization is comprised of beliefs and ideas about what kinds of goals members should pursue and standards of behavior members should use to achieve these goals.

b) Desired cultural elements that are publicly advertised which originate from the founder, CEO or organizational leaders and are shared by the stakeholders. For example, the values of caring and professionalism are often part of leadership's values in health care organizations.

c) From organizational values develop organizational norms, guidelines, or expectations that prescribe appropriate kinds of behavior by employees in particular situations and control the behavior of organizational members toward one another (Hill & Jones, 2001).

3) Basic assumptions

a) The deepest level where the organization's tacit assumptions are found.

b) These are the actual values that the culture represents, not necessarily correlated to the espoused values. Often conflicts exist between espoused values and the day-to-day realities within organizations.

c) Well integrated in the organizational dynamic that they are hard to recognize from within. These may include elements of the culture that are often taboo inside the organization. Many of these "unspoken rules" exist without the conscious knowledge of the membership.

d) Elements of culture which are unseen and not cognitively identified in everyday interactions between organizational members.

e) These may evolve as solutions to repeated problems. The people eventually behave according to those assumptions in order to make their world stable and predictable.

f) Those with sufficient experience to understand this deepest level of organizational culture usually become acclimatized to its attributes over time, thus reinforcing the invisibility of their existence.

g) Culture at this level is the underlying and driving element and requires more in-depth means to draw its attributes.

h) Understanding the basic assumptions is critical to fostering change and identifying appropriate solutions to problems.

f. Application to transcultural nursing and health care

1) Critical in facilitating organizational climate for acculturation and enculturation of multicultural workforce in organizations.

2) Promotes understanding of paradoxical organizational behaviors and the difficulty in assimilating organizational culture by newcomers Explains why organizational change agents usually fail to achieve their goals.

3) Facilitate understanding of the relationship between the dynamics of interpersonal relationships and the dynamics of organizational culture in fostering change.

4) Instructive in the methodology of studying organizational cultures.

g. Critique of organizational cultural models have centered on the idea that many cultures exist in one organization. Emphasis on organizational culture alone neglects the structural components that have as much impact on the organization (Parker, 2000).

14. The Health Belief Model (HBM)

a. Disciplinary Origins

1) The HBM was first introduced in the 1950s by Hochbaum, Rosenstock, Kegeles, and Leventhal (Rosenstock, Strecher, & Becker, 1988).

2) The theory and development of the HBM was formulated from an interest among a group of social psychologists who were investigating the poor success rates of medical screening programs offered by the U.S. Public Health Service, particularly with regard to those screening programs designed to prevent the occurrence of tuberculosis (Rosenstock, 1974; Sharma & Romas, 2008).

3) The HBM is a psychosocial model that explains the correlation between an individual's health perceptions and the individual's health preventative behavior.

4) The HBM was heavily influenced by the theories of Kurt Lewin, which posits the existence of an individual's life space composed of regions having positive value (positive valence), negative value (negative valence), or regions that are relatively neutral. The presence of disease, represented as a negative valence, holds the potential to generate a force that can move the individual away from the negative region. In the Lewinian tradition, activities of daily living are conceptualized as processes pulled by positive forces and repelled by negative forces (Rosenstock, 1974).

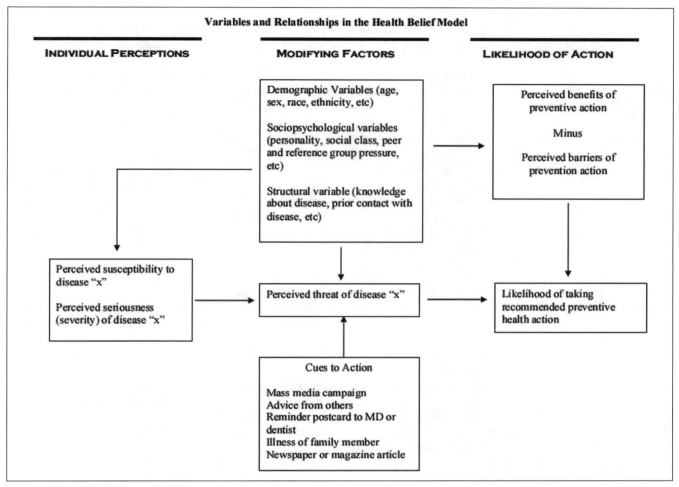

Figure 3.1. Health belief model
Adapted from Glanz, K., Rimer, B.K. & Lewis, F.M. (2002). *Health Behavior and Health Education. Theory, Research and Practice.* San Fransisco: Wiley & Sons. Reprinted with permission of John Wiley & Sons, Inc.

5) The HBM proposes that adherence to a preventive action is predicated on the individual's perception that the behavior needed to reverse a health threat will result in a perceived benefit. However, in order for the individual to change behavior to avoid disease, several psychological factors must be evident. The individual must believe that

   a) he or she is personally susceptible to the disease,
   b) the presence of disease would add a severity component to his or her life,
   c) a behavioral change would be beneficial in reducing susceptibility or severity, and
   d) the behavioral change would not result in perceived barriers to action, such as cost, inconvenience, pain, or embarrassment (Rosenstock, 1974).
   e) The construct has been used to examine health behavior adherence in weight management, exercise, vaccination, breast self-examination, and breast screening (Brewer et al., 2007; Daddario, 2007; Wood, 2008).

b. Theoretical Constructs (Figure 3.1)
   1) Perceived Seriousness
      a) Individuals vary widely in their understanding of the seriousness of a health problem.
      b) An individual's perception of the seriousness of an illness is influenced by his cultural beliefs, medical history, economic status, and other sociocultural and environmental factors (Rosenstock, 1974; Sharma & Romas, 2008).

c) The degree of seriousness is judged from both the impact of the illness on the personal well-being of the individual, as well as from the broader perspective of the effect of the disease on employment, family life, and social interactions (Rosenstock, 1974).

2) Perceived Susceptibility

   a) An individual's perception of risk is one of the more powerful motivating factors in the decision to change behavior. Studies have demonstrated that the perception of increased susceptibility to risk is directly related to an increased adoption of healthy behaviors and lifestyle changes (Mullens, McCaul, Erickson, & Sandgren, 2003; Turner, Hunt, DiBrezzo, & Jones, 2004).

   b) When both seriousness and susceptibility are perceived, there is an enhanced likelihood that the individual will perceive a greater threat to his well-being and will engage in preventive action (Sharma & Romas, 2008). Mullens et al. (2003) studied the behavior of colon cancer survivors and found that, due to the high incidence of recurrence, individuals previously diagnosed and treated for colon cancer were more likely to exhibit positive behavioral changes associated with diet, exercise, and weight management.

3) Perceived Benefit

   a) The perceived benefit associated with preventive action is based on the individual's belief that a change in a behavior will decrease the risk of developing a health problem.

   b) Perceived benefits are directly related to the enhanced adoption of secondary prevention behaviors. An increased number of health screenings conducted over a specified time period, for example, can be used to measure an enhanced adoption of secondary prevention when compared with a baseline database or national bench mark (Sharma & Romas, 2008)

4) Perceived barriers—refer to the individual's overall evaluation of the obstacles that prevent him or her from adopting a preventive action. For a change in behavior to occur the individual must believe that the change outweighs the negative consequences of continuing the old habit (Sharma & Romas, 2008). Costs, inconvenience, pain, and embarrassment are often cited barriers to change (Rosenstock, 1974).

5) Modifying variables—the four major constructs of perception are further influenced by three modifying variables

   a) Demographic variables (age, sex, race, ethnicity, etc.)

   b) Sociopsychological variables (personality, social class, peer and reference group pressure, etc.)

   c) Structural variables (knowledge about the disease, prior contact with the disease, etc.; (Sharma & Romas, 2008)

6) Cues to Action

   a) The HBM posits that in addition to perceptions and modifying variables, behavior is also affected by cues to action, such as, mass media campaigns, advice from others, reminder postcards, illness of a family member, newspaper or magazine article

   b) A cue to action may be an event, thing or person that drives an individual to adopt a preventive action. Media coverage of the widespread outbreak of a contagious disease, for example, can be a powerful influence on public action to prevent spread of infection. Similarly, an individual is more likely to change behavior when a close family member or friend contracts a preventable disease (Sharma & Romas, 2008).

7) Self-Efficacy—To achieve the desired outcome, the individual must believe in his own ability to perform a preventive action. If an individual perceives a behavioral change to be of benefit, but doubts his or her ability to perform the action, there is decreased likelihood that the behavior modification will occur (Bandura, 1977; Rosenstock, Strecher, & Becker, 1988; Sharma & Romas, 2008; Wood, 2008).

c. Application in transcultural nursing and health care

1) Fostering motivation for behavioral changes for health

2) Blends cultural and social cues in motivating individuals/groups to change behaviors

3) Weighs positive and negative forces for change in behaviors

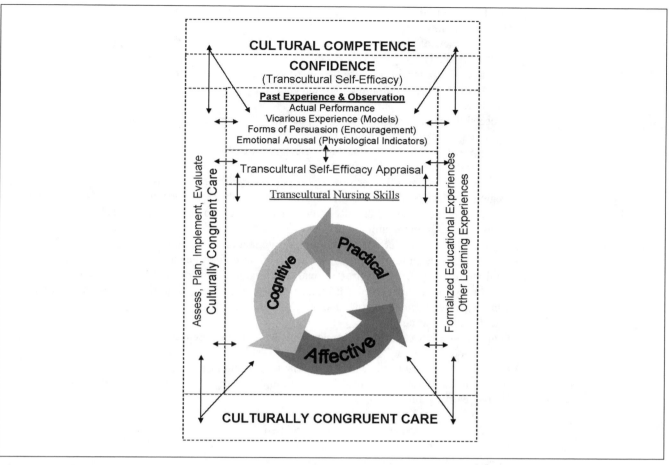

Figure 3.2. Jeffreys's cultural competence and confidence (CCC) model
Note: Please note that bidirectional arrows symbolize the ongoing, dynamic interaction between all components of the multidimensional learning process for cultural competence education.
Source: Reprinted with permission from Jeffreys, R. M. (2006). *Teaching cultural competence in nursing and health care: Inquiry, action, and innovation.* New York, NY: Springer.

15. *Jeffreys's Cultural Competence and Confidence (CCC) Model* (Marianne Jeffreys, 2006)
  a. Theoretical framework for teaching cultural competence; proposed as an organizing frame-work for examining the multidimensional factors involved in the process of learning cultural competence to
   1) identify at-risk individuals
   2) develop diagnostic-prescriptive strategies to facilitate learning
   3) guide innovations in teaching and educational research
   4) evaluate strategy effectiveness
  b. Interrelates concepts that explain, describe, influence, and/or predict the phenomenon of learning (developing) cultural competence and incorporates the construct of transcultural self-efficacy (confidence) as a major influencing factor (Figure 3.2).
  c. Based on the transcultural nursing literature, Bandura's self-efficacy theory psychology), Bloom's learning taxonomy (education), and results from numerous studies using the Transcultural Self-Efficacy Tool (TSET)—see Chapter 7 for questionnaire details and references.
  d. Cultural competence is defined as
   1) A multidimensional *learning process* (emphasizes that the cognitive, practical, and affective dimensions of transcultural self-efficacy can change over time as a result of formalized educa-tion and other learning experiences) that integrates

a) Transcultural skills in all three learning dimensions
   (1) Cognitive
   (2) Practical
   (3) Affective
b) Involves transcultural self-efficacy (confidence) as a major factor
c) Aims to achieve cultural congruent care

e. Transcultural skills
   1) Those skills necessary for assessing, planning, implementing, and evaluating culturally congruent care for diverse populations
   2) Incorporate cognitive, practical, and affective dimensions

f. Transcultural self-efficacy is defined as
   1) Perceived confidence for performing or learning transcultural skills
   2) Degree to which individuals perceive they have the ability to perform the specific transcultural nursing skills needed for culturally competent and congruent care despite obstacles and hardships

g. Cognitive learning dimension
   1) General: focuses on knowledge outcomes, intellectual abilities, and skills
   2) Specific to transcultural learning: knowledge and comprehension about ways in which cultural factors may influence professional care among clients of different cultural backgrounds and throughout the life cycle (different refers to clients representing various different racial, ethnic, gender, socioeconomic, and religious groups).

h. Practical learning dimension
   1) General: similar to psychomotor learning domain and focuses on motor skills or practical application of skills
   2) Specific to transcultural learning: refers to communication skills (verbal and nonverbal) needed to interview clients of different cultural backgrounds about their values and beliefs

i. Affective learning dimension
   1) General
      a) Concerned with attitudes, values, and beliefs
      b) Considered to be crucial for developing professional values and beliefs
   2) Specific to transcultural learning: Includes
      a) Self-awareness
      b) Awareness of cultural gap (differences)
      c) Acceptance
      d) Appreciation
      e) Recognition
      f) Advocacy

j. Cultural competence (CC) is influenced by
   1) Transcultural self-efficacy (TSE)
   2) The learning of transcultural skills (cognitive, practical, affective)
   3) Formalized educational experiences
   4) Other learning experiences

k. Transcultural Self-Efficacy Pathway
   1) Traces the proposed influences of TSE on a learner's actions, performance, and persistence for learning tasks associated with cultural competency development and culturally congruent care
   2) First step is self-efficacy appraisal, an individualized process influenced by four information sources: (Bandura, 1977, 1982, 1986, 1989, 1997)
      a) Actual performances
      b) Vicarious experiences (role models)
      c) Forms of persuasion (encouragement from others)
      d) Emotional arousal (physiological indices, such as sweating)
   3) Resilient individuals (realistically medium-high self-efficacy)
      a) Highly motivated and actively seek help to maximize their cultural competence and transcultural skill development
      b) Most likely to persist in cultural competence development

      c) Most likely to achieve cultural congruent care actions

      d) Following cultural competence educational interventions, changes in TSE noted

   4) Low self-efficacy (low confidence) individuals

      a) Poorly motivated and reluctant to actively seek help in cultural competence and transcultural skill development

      b) At risk for avoiding transcultural tasks

      c) Unlikely to persist in cultural competence tasks

      d) Unlikely to achieve cultural congruent care actions

      e) Most improvement noted in TSE gains following cultural competence educational interventions

   5) Supremely efficacious (overly confident) individuals

      a) May be totally unaware of their cultural incompetencies and weaknesses

      b) Likely to underestimate the transcultural task or its importance

      c) At risk for overestimating their abilities, overrating their strengths

      d) Unlikely to recognize the need for adequate preparation for cultural competence

      e) Unlikely to recognize the need to restructure priorities or time management to accommodate transcultural tasks

      f) Unlikely to achieve cultural congruent care actions

      g) Following cultural competence educational interventions, more likely to become more conservative (realistic) in TSE appraisals

l. Components of comprehensive cultural competence education

   1) Weave together cognitive, practical, and affective learning

   2) Encompass assessment, planning, implementation, and evaluation

   3) Integrate self-efficacy appraisals and diagnostic-prescriptive interventions

   4) Coordinated program planning and updates

m. Assumptions of CCC Model (Jeffreys, 2006, pp. 32-33)

   1) "Cultural competence is an ongoing, multidimensional learning process that integrates transcultural skills in all three dimensions (cognitive, affective, and practical), involves transcultural self-efficacy (confidence) as a major influencing factor, and aims to achieve cultural congruent care.

   2) Transcultural self-efficacy is a dynamic construct that changes over time and is influenced by formalized exposure to culture care concepts (transcultural nursing).*

   3) The learning of transcultural nursing skills is influenced by self-efficacy perceptions (confidence).

   4) The performance of transcultural nursing skill competencies is directly influenced by the adequate learning of such skills and by transcultural self-efficacy perceptions.

   5) The performance of culturally congruent nursing skills is influenced by self-efficacy perceptions and by formalized educational exposure to transcultural nursing care concepts and skills throughout the educational experience.

   6) All students and nurses (regardless of age, ethnicity, gender, sexual orientation, lifestyle, religion, socioeconomic status, geographic location, or race) require formalized educational experiences to meet culture care needs of diverse individuals.*

   7) The most comprehensive learning involves the integration of cognitive, practical, and affective dimensions.

   8) Learning in the cognitive, practical, and affective dimensions is paradoxically distinct yet interrelated.*

   9) Learners are most confident about their attitudes (affective dimension) and least confident about their transcultural nursing knowledge (cognitive dimension).*

   10) Novice learners will have lower self-efficacy perceptions than advanced learners.*

   11) Inefficacious individuals are at risk for decreased motivation, lack of commitment, and/or avoidance of cultural considerations when planning and implementing nursing care.

   12) Supremely efficacious (overly confident) individuals are at risk for inadequate preparation in learning the transcultural nursing skills necessary to provide culturally congruent care.

13) Early intervention with at-risk individuals will better prepare nurses to meet cultural competency.

14) The greatest change in transcultural self-efficacy perceptions will be detected in individuals with low self-efficacy (low confidence) initially, who have then been exposed to formalized transcultural nursing concepts and experiences.*"

B. **Transcultural Nursing Concepts, Models, and Theories**

1. *Theory of Culture Care Diversity and Universality* (Madeleine Leininger)

    a. Disciplinary Origins—based on Madeleine Leininger's work (McFarland in A. Tomey, 2008)

    1) Madeleine M. Leininger is the founder of transcultural nursing, a leader in transcultural nursing and human care theory and the first professional nurse with graduate preparation in nursing to hold a PhD in cultural and social anthropology.

    2) Born in Sutton, Nebraska, she completed her diploma from St. Anthony's School of Nursing in Denver, Colorado and joined the U.S. Army Nurse Corps while pursuing the basic nursing program.

    3) In 1950, she obtained a bachelor's degree in biological science from the Benedictine College in Atchison, Kansas with a minor in philosophy and humanistic studies in 1950.

    4) After graduation, she served as an instructor, staff nurse, and head nurse on a medical-surgical unit, and opened a new psychiatric unit as the director of the nursing service at St. Joseph's Hospital in Omaha, Nebraska.

    5) At the same time she took advanced study in nursing, nursing administration, teaching and curriculum in nursing, and tests and measurements at Creighton University in Omaha (Leininger, 1995c, 1996b).

    6) In 1954 Leininger obtained a master's degree in psychiatric nursing from the Catholic University of America in Washington, D.C.

    7) While employed at the College of Health at the University of Cincinnati, Ohio, she began the first master's level-clinical specialist program in child psychiatric nursing in the world; initiated and directed the first graduate nursing program in psychiatric nursing at the University of Cincinnati and the Therapeutic Psychiatric Nursing Center at the University Hospital (Cincinnati); coauthored one of the first basic psychiatric nursing texts, *Basic Psychiatric Concepts in Nursing* (Hofling & Leininger), which was published worldwide in 1960 in 11 languages

    8) While working at a child guidance home in the mid-1950s in Cincinnati, Leininger became concerned with the staff's lack of understanding of the cultural factors influencing the children's behavior.

        a) Children from diverse backgrounds responded differently to care and psychiatric treatments, and psychoanalytic theories and therapies were ineffective in reaching them.

        b) Leininger found few staff members who were interested or knowledgeable about cultural factors in the diagnosis and treatment of clients.

        c) When Margaret Mead became a visiting professor in the Department of Psychiatry at the University of Cincinnati, Leininger discussed the potential interrelationships between nursing and anthropology with Mead who provided her with no direct help, encouragement nor solutions.

    9) Leininger decided to pursue a doctoral study on cultural, social, and psychological anthropology at the University of Washington, Seattle. She studied many cultures and found anthropology to be an area that should be of interest to all nurses.

    10) She focused on the Gadsup people of the Eastern Highlands of New Guinea, where she lived alone with the indigenous people for nearly 2 years.

    11) She conducted an ethnographical and Ethnonursing study of two villages and observed the: unique features of the culture; and a number of marked differences between Western and non-Western cultures related to caring, health and well-being practices.

---

*Indicates assumptions with empirical support from research studies conducted using the CCC model's corresponding questionnaire, the Transcultural Self-Efficacy Tool (TSET)—see Chapter 7 for details.

12) From her study and firsthand experiences with the Gadsup, Leininger continued to develop her Culture Care Theory of Diversity and Universality (Culture Care Theory) and the enthnonursing method (Leininger, 1978, 1981, 1991, 1995c).

13) Her research and theory have helped nursing students understand cultural differences in human care, health, and illness.

14) She has been the major nurse leader to encourage many students and faculty to pursue graduate education and practice.

15) Her enthusiasm and deep interest in developing the field of transcultural nursing with a human care focus has sustained her for more than five decades.

16) During the 1950s and 1960s, Leininger (1970, 1978) identified several common areas of knowledge and theoretical research interests between nursing and anthropology (Leininger 1991, pp. 14, 18), formulating transcultural nursing concepts, theory, principles, and practices.

17) The book *Nursing* and *Anthropology: Two Worlds to Blend* (1970) laid the foundation for developing the field of transcultural nursing, Culture Care Theory and culturally-based health care.

18) Her next book, *Transcultural Nursing: Concepts, Theories, and Practice* (1978), identified major concepts, theoretical ideas, and practices in transcultural nursing, and became the first definitive publication on transcultural nursing (Leininger, 1991, p. 14; 1995, p. 81; 2002c, p. 72; 2006a, p. 4)

19) During the past 50 years, Leininger has established, explicated, and used the Culture Care Theory to study many cultures within the United States and worldwide.

20) She developed the enthnonursing qualitative research method to fit the theory and to discover the insider or emic view of cultures (Leininger, 1991b, 1995c), which was the first nursing research method developed for nurses to examine complex care and cultural phenomena.

21) During the past five decades, approximately 50 doctoral and many master's and baccalaureate students have been prepared in transcultural nursing and used Culture Care Theory (Leininger, 1990a, 1991; Leininger & McFarland, 2002; Leininger & Watson, 1990).

22) The first course offered in transcultural nursing was in 1966 at the University of Colorado, where Leininger became the first nurse to become a professor of nursing and anthropology in the nation.

23) In 1973, she initiated and served as the director of the first nurse scientist PhD program in the United States.

b. Philosophical Underpinnings (Leininger, 1991, pp. 14, 18)

1) The theory was drawn from Leininger's reflective and creative thinking about her past professional experiences in pediatric psychiatric nursing with children from diverse cultures (Appalachia, African, Anglo, Jewish, and German) and the interrelationships between *culture* and *nursing*.

2) She developed the theory concepts and constructs during and after further educational study and cultural experiences.

c. Care is the essence of nursing

1) There are different values, meanings, patterned expressions, and structured forms of care that are important to discover and establish transcultural and other comparative care knowledge, which predicted:

   a) These factors are influenced by worldview, social structure, ethnohistory, environment/ecology, and folk care/generic or lay practices screened through the lens of each culture's language and lifeways.

   b) Care beliefs and practices influence health, well-being, or illness expectations of people (Leininger, 2006c, p. 118).

2) Culture-specific care is essential to provide acceptable, effective, and satisfying care using the three modes of care action and decision.

3) Culturally congruent care is important for nursing care practices (Leininger, 2006c, p. 118).

4) Transcultural nursing is a substantive area of study and practice focused on comparative culture care (caring) values, beliefs, and practices of individuals or groups of similar or different

cultures, with the goal to provide culture specific and universal nursing care practices for the health and well-being of people or to help them face unfavorable human conditions (disabilities or death) Leininger, 2002b, p. 46)

d. Purpose of the theory
1) Discover, document, interpret, and explain the predicted and multiple factors influencing care from an emic and etic view as it relates to culturally based care (Leininger, 2002c, p. 76), and explaining care from a cultural holistic perspective (Leininger, 1997, p. 36).
2) Discover, document, know, and explain the interdependence of *care* and *culture* phenomena with differences and similarities between and among cultures to support the discipline of transcultural nursing and lead to therapeutic outcomes (Leininger, 2006a, p. 4).

e. Goal of the theory
1) Provide culturally congruent care that contributes to the health or well-being of people, or to help them face disabilities, dying or death using the three modes of nursing care actions and decisions (Leininger, 1997, p. 36; 2002, p. 76).
2) Use culture care research findings to provide specific and/or general care that would be culturally congruent, safe, and beneficial to people of diverse or similar cultures for their health, well-being and healing, and to help people face disabilities and death (Leininger, 2006a, p. 5).
3) Ethical and moral aspects related to transcultural nursing care will be identified and taken into consideration with the culture under study (Leininger, 1997, p. 36).

f. Significance in cultural competent care
1) Culturally congruent and competent care refers to the explicit use of sensitive, creative, and meaningful care practices to fit with the general values, beliefs, and lifeways and needs of clients (individuals or groups) for beneficial, satisfying, and meaningful health/care and well-being or to help them face illness, difficult life situations, disabilities, or death (Leininger, 2002a, pp. 12, 84).
2) Should become an integral part of a nurse's thinking and decisions for family and individual care practices.
3) Nurses need to reflect on the meanings of the definition to grasp its full and important dimensions.
    a) Definition incorporates the general purpose of transcultural nursing in discovering and using culturally based research care knowledge to promote healing and health or to deal with illnesses, life-threatening conditions, or death in beneficial ways with clients.
    b) Providing culturally competent, safe, and congruent care to people of diverse or similar cultures is the central and dominant goal of transcultural nursing and all health care providers worldwide.

g. Evolutionary Phases of Transcultural Nursing Knowledge and Use: All three phases help the nurse to assess how one is becoming a knowledgeable, competent, and confident transcultural nurse.
1) Phase I: Nurse is gaining cultural awareness and becoming sensitive to the needs of cultures.
    a) Sensitivity to another person, situation, or event is helpful but the nurse must go further and gain confirmed cultural knowledge and understanding.
    b) Superficial awareness or opinions can be dangerous and often lead to misunderstandings and problems.
2) Phase II: The nurse enters this phase to gain in-depth cultural knowledge and use transcultural nursing concepts and principles to guide his or her thinking and practices.
    a) The learner often needs a mentor in transcultural nursing to help see and reaffirm clients' beliefs and expressions.
    b) Newcomers to this field need a substantive course in transcultural nursing to discover differences and similarities, and for accurate assessments.
    c) Transcultural nursing holding or reflective culture care knowledge or concepts, principles, and theories are powerful guides to assess what one observes, hears, and experiences while in this phase of gaining in-depth knowledge and understanding.
    d) The Theory of Culture Care is an important guide to discover the largely unknown about individuals and groups of a culture; without the *theory*, one cannot discover and explain phenomena in a systematic way and arrive at credible ideas and decisions.

3) Phase III: The nurse uses observations, experiences, and knowledge documented with clients to provide culturally competent care.

a) This is the creative part of transcultural nursing in finding ways to use client and professional knowledge for beneficial outcomes.

b) The nurse documents and evaluates the outcomes when providing culturally based care; often done in conjunction with the observations of others working with the client.

c) The client's participation in the evaluation is very important and valued.

d) Discovers the importance of using theory-based knowledge along with transcultural nursing concepts, principles, and available research findings to provide meaningful, safe, and beneficial care.

e) The nurse assesses his or her competencies and areas that need to be strengthened or modified (Leininger, 2002a, p. 28; figure 1.3).

h. Scope of transcultural nursing (Leininger, 2002a, p. 20)

1) Local cultures

2) Regional/provincial cultures

3) National/societal cultures

4) Transnational cultures

5) Global human cultures

i. Concepts of the theory and orientational definitions (Leininger, 1991, p. 46; 1997, p. 38; 2002b, p. 83; 2006, p.12) [Sunrise Enabler Appendix A]

1) *Care*: The abstract and manifest phenomena or expressions related to assistive, supportive, enabling, and facilitating ways to help others with evident or anticipated needs in order to improve health, a human condition, a lifeway, or to face death.

2) *Culture:* The lifeways of an individual or group with reference to values, beliefs, norms, patterns, and practices that are learned, shared, and transmitted intergenerationally.

3) *Culture Care*: The culturally derived, assistive, supportive, or facilitative acts toward or for another individual or group with evident or anticipated needs which guides nursing decisions or actions, and held to be beneficial to the health or the well-being of people, or to face disabilities, death, or other human conditions.

4) *Culture Care Diversity*: The cultural variabilities or differences in care meanings, patterns, values, symbols, and lifeways within and among cultures.

5) *Worldview:* The way an individual or group looks out upon and understands their world to provide a value stance, picture, or perspective about their life and the world.

6) *Cultural and Social Structure Dimensions*: The dynamic, holistic, and interrelated patterns or features of culture (or subculture) related to religion or spirituality, kinship (social), political (and legal), economic, education, technology, cultural values, language, and ethnohistorical factors of different cultures.

7) *Environment Context*: The totality of an event, situation, or related life experiences that give meaning and order to guide human expressions and decisions within a particular environmental setting, situation, or geographic area.

8) *Ethnohistory*: The sequence of facts, events, or developments over time as known or witnessed by the people under study.

9) *Emic:* Refers to the local or insider's views and values about a phenomenon.

10) *Etic:* Refers to the outsider's views and values about a phenomenon.

11) *Health*: A state of well-being or restorative state that is culturally constituted, defined, valued, and practiced by individuals or groups that enables them to function in their daily lives.

12) *Nursing*: A learned humanistic and scientific profession and discipline that is focused on cultural care (caring), holistic knowledge and competencies to assist individuals or groups to maintain or regain their health or well-being or to deal with human life and death in meaningful and beneficial ways.

13) *Culture Care Preservation and/or Maintenance*: Assistive, supporting, facilitative, or enabling professional actions and decisions that help people of a particular culture to retain and/or preserve relevant care values so that they can maintain their well-being, recover from illness, or face handicaps and/or death.

14) *Culture Care Accommodation and/or Negotiations*: Assistive, supporting, facilitative, or enabling creative professional actions and decisions that help people of a designated culture or subculture to adapt to or to negotiate with others for a beneficial or satisfying health outcome with professional care providers.

15) *Culture Care Repatterning and/or Restructuring*: Assistive, supporting, facilitative, or enabling professional actions and decisions that help a client or clients to reorder, change, or greatly modify their lifeways for new, different, and beneficial healthcare patterns while respecting the client or clients' cultural values and beliefs and still providing beneficial or healthier lifeways than before the changes were co-established with the client(s).

16) *Culturally Competent Nursing Care*: [see above]

j. Theoretical Tenets and Hunches (Leininger, 2002a, pp. 17-18; 2002c, p. 78; 2006, p. 17)

1) Culture care expressions, meanings, patterns, and practices are diverse yet there are shared commonalities and some universal attributes.

2) Worldview, multiple, social structure factors, ethnohistory, environmental context, language, and generic and professional care factors are critical influencers of culture care patterns to predict health, well-being, illness, and ways people face disabilities and death.

3) Generic emic (folk or lay) and etic (professional) health factors in different environmental contexts greatly influence health and illness outcomes.

4) From the analysis of the above influences, three major care action and decision guides were predicted to provide ways to give *culturally congruent, safe, and meaningful health care to cultures*. These culturally based action and decision modes are

  a) Culture Care Preservation and/or Maintenance

  b) Culture Care Accommodations and/or Negotiation

  c) Culture Care Repatterning and/or Restructuring

5) Use of the Sunrise Enabler as a cognitive guide is important in the systematic discovery of the meaning and appropriateness of tailor making care actions and decisions (using the three modes) to fit with client needs in helping to prevent illness, disability, cultural pain, racism, and other problem care areas often neglected in traditional nursing practices. (Refer to #4 below)

k. Assumptive Premises of the Theory (Leininger, 1991, p. 44; 1997, p. 39-40; 2002c, p. 79; 2006, p. 18)

1) Care is the essence of nursing and a distinct, dominant, central, and unifying focus.

2) Care (caring) is essential for well-being, health, growth, survival, and to face handicaps or death.

3) Culturally based care is the broadest holistic means to know, explain, interpret, and predict nursing care phenomena and to guide nursing decisions and actions.

4) Nursing is a transcultural, humanistic, and scientific care discipline and profession with the central purpose of serving individuals, groups, communities, or institutions worldwide.

5) Care (caring) is essential to caring and healing, for there can be no caring without caring.

6) Culture care concepts, meanings, expressions, patterns, processes, and structural forms of care vary transculturally with diversities (differences) and some universalities (or commonalities).

7) Every human culture has generic (lay, folk, or indigenous) care knowledge and practices and usually some professional care knowledge and practices which vary transculturally.

8) Culture care values, beliefs, and practices are influenced by and tend to be embedded in the worldview, language, philosophy, religion (and spirituality), kinship, social, political, legal, educational, economic, technological, ethnohistorical, and environmental context of cultures.

9) Beneficial, healthy, and satisfying culturally based care influences the health and well-being of individuals, families, groups, and communities within their environmental contexts.

10) Culturally congruent or beneficial nursing care can only occur when individual, group, family, community, or institutional care values, expressions, or patterns are known and used explicitly in appropriate and meaningful ways.

11) Culture care differences and similarities between professionals and client participants exist in all human cultures worldwide.

12) Cultural conflicts, imposition practices, cultural stresses, and pain reflect the lack of professional care knowledge to provide culturally congruent, responsible, and sensitive care.

13) The ethnonursing qualitative research method provides an important means to discover and accurately interpret emic and etic embedded, complex, and diverse culture care factors.

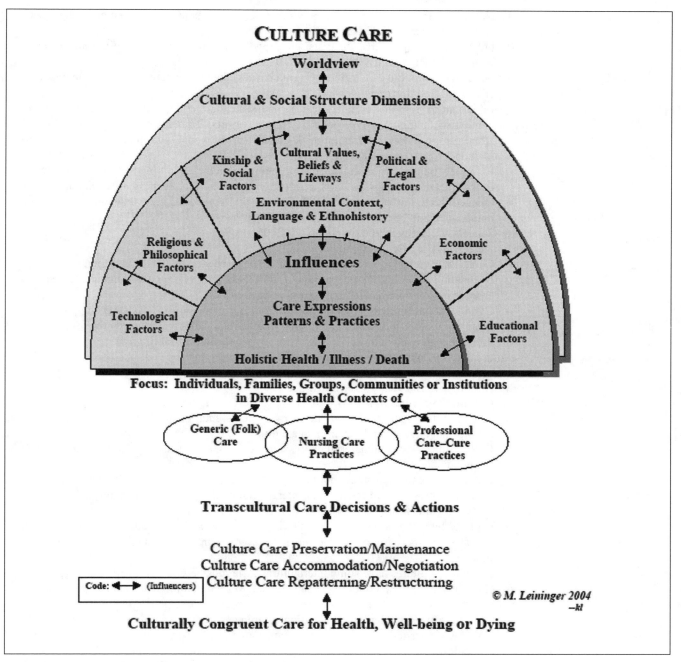

Figure 3.3. Leininger's Sunrise Enabler: Culture care theory
Reprinted with permission from M. Leininger.

1. Sunrise Enabler (Figure 3.3; Leininger, 1991, p. 49; 1997, p. 37 & 40; 2002c, p. 80-81; 2006, p. 25)
    1) *Let the sun rise* figuratively means to have nurses open their minds in order to discover many different factors influencing care and ultimately the health and well-being of clients.
    2) Developed as a conceptual holistic research guide and enabler to help researchers discover multiple dimensions related to the theoretical tenets.
    3) Enabler:
        a) Comprehensive and yet specific to depict different components that need to be studied systematically for the theory.
        b) Serves as a cognitive guide to tease out culture care phenomena from a holistic set of factors influencing care in cultures under study

    c) Not the theory per se but depicts areas that need to be examined in relation to the theory tenets and the specific domain of inquiry under study.

    d) Differs from other nurse theorists' concepts of models as it serves different purposes within the qualitative paradigm.

    e) Focuses on multiple care influencers (not causes) that can explain emic and etic phenomena in different historical contexts.

    f) Important to note that certain social structure factors gender, class, race, historical and contextual factors, kinship, politics, cultural norms, legal factors, religion/spirituality, ethnohistory, biophysical, emotional, genetic, professional, and generic health care are included.

    g) Extremely helpful in guiding nurses in thinking about these multiple factors and their influences on care meanings, patterns, symbols, and expression of care in different cultures.

    h) Opened the minds of nurses to look for new and embedded knowledge areas related to human care and health.

m. Major Concepts (Leininger, 2002b, pp. 46-47; 2006, pp. 3-5)

    1) Human care as the essence of nursing

      a) Care: (noun) refers to an abstract or concrete phenomenon related to assisting, supporting, or enabling experiences or behaviors, or for others with evidence for anticipated needs to ameliorate or improve a human condition or lifeway.

      b) Caring: (gerund) refers to actions and activities directed toward assisting, supporting, or enabling another individual or group with evident or anticipated needs to ease, heal, or improve a human condition or lifeway or to face death or disability.

    2) Culture and nursing, culture and subculture

    3) Other features of cultures (Leininger, 2002b, p. 48)

      a) Culture care is a synthesized construct

      b) Cultures have rules of behavior that are manifest or implicit

      c) Human cultures have material items or symbols such as artifacts, objects, dress, and actions that have special meaning in a culture.

      d) Cultures also have nonmaterial expressions, beliefs, and ideas to guide their members in unknown lands.

      e) Cultures have traditional ceremonial practices such as religious rituals, food feasts, and other activities that are transmitted intergenerationally and reaffirm family or group ties and caring ways.

      f) Cultures have their own local or emic (insider) views and knowledge about their culture that are extremely important for nurses to discover and understand for meaningful care practices

      g) All human cultures have some intercultural variations between and within cultures

        (1) Cultural variation is an important concept to keep in mind when studying individuals and different cultures, and observed in your response to people in your care.

        (2) There are slight and great variations within and between cultures.

        (3) One can usually find some common patterns of expressions and lifeways within cultures.

n. Associated Definitions (Leininger, 2002b, pp. 49-53)

    1) Ethnicity

    2) Cultural Values

    3) Western and non-Western values/modernism and progressivism

    4) Culture Shock

    5) Uniculturalism (monoculturalism)

    6) Multiculturalism

    7) Ethnocentricism

    8) Cultural Bias

    9) Cultural Relativism

    10) Cultural Imposition

    11) Cultural Blindness

           12) Cultural Pain

           13) Bioculturalism

           14) Culture-bound

    o. Other Related Concepts (Leininger, 2002b, pp. 53-55)

           1) Cultural Diversity

           2) Cultural Universals

           3) Racism

           4) Prejudice

           5) Cultural Backlash

           6) Cultural Overidentification

    p. Five Basic Interactional Phenomena (Leininger, 2002b, pp. 55-57)

           1) Culture encounter

           2) Enculturation

           3) Acculturation

           4) Socialization

           5) Assimilation

    q. Culture Care: A Central Construct With Related Concepts (Leininger 2002b, pp. 57-60). A *construct* has many ideas embedded in it (construction), whereas a *concept* is a single idea.

           1) *Culture Care* is the cognitively learned and transmitted professional and indigenous folk values, beliefs, and patterned lifeways that are used to assist, facilitate, or enable another individual or group to maintain their well-being or health or to improve a human condition or lifeway.

           2) *Culture-Specific Care/Caring* refers to very specific or particular ways to have care fit client's needs.

           3) *Generalized Culture Care* refers to commonly shared professional nursing care techniques, principles, and practices that are beneficial to several clients as a general and essential human care need, for example, respectful care.

           4) Culture Care Conflict/Clash

           5) Cultural Exports

           6) Cultural Imports

           7) Culture Time

           8) Social Time

           9) Cultural Space

           10) Body Touching

           11) Culture Context: high versus low

           12) Culture Care Therapy

    r. Generic and Professional Care/Caring (Leininger, 2002b, p.60)

           1) *Generic (lay or folk) Care*/Caring: Emic

           2) *Professional Care/Caring*: Etic

    s. Transcultural Nursing Care Principles (Leininger, 2002b, p. 61-62)

           1) Human caring with a transcultural focus is essential for health, healing, and well-being of individuals, families, groups, and institutions.

           2) Every culture has specific beliefs, values, and patterns of caring and healing that need to be discovered, understood, and used in the care of people of diverse or similar cultures.

           3) Transcultural nursing knowledge and competencies are imperative to provide meaningful, congruent, safe, and beneficial health care practices.

           4) It is a human right that cultures have their cultural care values, beliefs, and practices respected and thoughtfully incorporated into nursing and health services.

           5) Culturally based care and health beliefs and health practices vary in Western and non-Western cultures and can change over time.

           6) Comparative cultural care experiences, meanings, values, and patterns of culture care are fundamental sources of transcultural nursing knowledge to guide nursing decisions.

           7) Generic (emic, folk, lay) and professional (etic) care knowledge and practices often have different knowledge and experience bases that need to be assessed and understood before using the information in client care.

8) Holistic and comprehensive knowledge in transcultural nursing necessitates understanding *emic* and *etic* perspectives related to worldview, language, ethnohistory, kinship, religion (spirituality), technologies, economic, and political (legal) factors, and specific cultural values, beliefs, and practices bearing upon care, illness and well-being.

9) Different modes of learning, living, and transmitting, culture care and health through the life cycle across the lifespan are major foci of transcultural nursing education, research, and practice.

10) Transcultural nursing necessitates an understanding of one's self, culture, and ways of entering a different culture and helping others.

11) Transcultural nursing theory, research, and practice are interested in both universals (and commonalities) and differences to generate new knowledge and provide beneficial humanistic and scientific care practices.

12) Transcultural nursing actions or decisions are based largely on research care and health knowledge derived from in-depth study of cultures and the use of this knowledge in professional caring.

13) It is the culture care life cycle patterns, values, and practices of cultures that are valuable means to help sustain or maintain the health and well-being of people, or deal with other human conditions.

14) Transcultural nursing necessitates coparticipation of the client and the nurse for effective transcultural decisions, practices, and outcomes.

15) Transcultural nursing uses culture care theories to generate new knowledge and then to disseminate, use, and evaluate outcomes in practice.

16) Observations, participation, and reflection are essential modalities to discover and respond to clients of diverse and similar cultures with their care needs and expectations.

17) Verbal and nonverbal language with its meanings and symbols are important to know and understand to arrive at culturally congruent and therapeutic care outcomes.

18) Transcultural nurses respect human rights and are alert to unethical practices, cultural taboos, and illegal cultural actions or decisions.

19) Understanding the cultural context of the client is essential to assess and respond appropriately to clients and their holistic health care needs and concerns.

20) Culture care therapy may be needed for people who have been deeply hurt, insulted, or dehumanized because of cultural ignorance and noncaring modes. Specific application in cultural competent care (Leininger, 1997, p. 38; 2002c, pp. 78-79; 2006, p. 8).
  a) Culture Care Preservation and/or Maintenance: see previous definition
  b) Culture Care Accommodation and/or Negotiations: see previous definition
  c) Culture Care Repatterning and/or Restructuring: see previous definition

t. Strengths and Weaknesses of the Theory
1) Broad, holistic, comprehensive perspective of human groups, populations, and species.
2) Concepts and constructs related to social structure, environment, and language are extremely important to discover in order to obtain culturally based knowledge or knowledge grounded in the people's world.
3) Continues to generate many domains of inquiry for nurse researchers to pursue scientific and humanistic knowledge.
4) Challenges nurses to seek both universal and diverse culturally based care phenomena by diverse cultures, the culture of nursing, and the cultures of social unsteadiness worldwide.
5) Transcultural and global in scope; relevant to nurse researchers worldwide in conceptualizing the theory and research approaches and guide practice.
6) Both complex and practical and requires transcultural nursing knowledge and appropriate research methods to explicate the phenomena.
  a) Shows multiple interrelationships of concepts and diversity of key concepts and relationships, especially to social structure factors.
  b) It requires not only some basic anthropological knowledge but also considerable transcultural nursing knowledge, to be used in an accurate and scholarly fashion.

        c) Once fully conceptualized, Leininger's theory is practical, relevant, and useful for all levels of nursing research including undergraduate work.

        d) The Sunrise Enabler becomes imprinted as a way of knowing.

u. Applicability to the Discipline and Practice of Nursing

    1) Demonstrates the criterion of generality as a qualitatively oriented theory that is broad, comprehensive, and worldwide in scope.

    2) Addresses nursing care from a multicultural and worldview perspective.

    3) Useful and applicable to both groups and individuals with the goal of rendering culture-specific nursing care.

    4) Has broad or generic concepts that are well-organized and defined for study in specific cultures.

    5) Research led to a vast amount of expert knowledge largely unknown in the past.

    6) Enables many aspects of culture, care, and health to be identified, which have an impact on nursing. However, more research is needed for comparative purposes from both culture-specific data and some universal care knowledge, and for more world cultures. to be studied and compared to validate future caring constructs.

    7) Most helpful as a guide for the study of any culture and for the comparative study of several cultures.

        a) Findings from the theory are being used in client care in a variety of health and community settings worldwide to transform nursing education and services.

        b) Especially valued in developing a new and different approach to the traditional community nursing perspective.

    8) Transcultural nursing theory has important outcomes for nursing.

        a) Rendering culture-specific care is a necessary and essential new goal in nursing and places transcultural nursing theory center to the domain of nursing knowledge acquisition and use.

        b) The theory is highly useful, applicable, and essential to nursing practice, education, and research.

        c) The concept of care as the primary focus of nursing and the base of nursing knowledge and practice is long overdue and essential to advance nursing knowledge and practices.

        d) Although nursing has always made claims to the concept of care, rigorous research on care has been limited until the past five decades.

        e) This theory could be the means to establish a sound and defensible discipline and profession, guiding practice to meet a multicultural world.

2. *Glittenberg's Project GENESIS: Community-Based Action Research Model* (Jody Glittenberg)

a. Conceptual Differences Between Leininger and Glittenberg

    1) Leininger's conceptual foundation

        a) Based on doctoral studies at the University of Washington with prevailing theoretical foundations of ethnomethodology, ethnoscience, cultural particularism (Boas, Spradley), and psychological anthropology (Harris, 1968)

        b) Based on Leininger's inpatient psychiatric clinical experience

        c) Research threads include cultural competent individual nursing care, ethnonursing (Dreher, 2002) in multiple studies

        d) Founder and leader of the Transcultural Nursing Society model (forerunner of the Sunrise model) that emphasized cultural particularism.

    2) Glittenberg's conceptual foundation

        a) Based on doctoral studies at the University of Colorado 1970-1976 with prevailing theoretical foundations of cultural ecology, cultural materialism, applied anthropology, and biological anthropology

        b) Based on clinical experience in community health nursing

        c) Research threads include cultural ecological community studies

            (1) Longitudinal comparison (1977-1982) of 26 communities funded by the National Science Foundation

       (2) Quasi-experimental study of recovery from a national disaster, 1976 Guatemalan earthquake (Bates, Farrell, & Glittenberg, 1985)

       (3) Action research, empowerment philosophy, for example, Project GENESIS: Community Empowerment Partnership (CEPP) Project on violence (1997-2001) funded by NIDA (Glittenberg 2001a, 2008)

       (4) Primary health care, for example, building community capacity and sustainability (WHO Collaborating Center, University of Illinois, Western Pacific Region, WHO) (Glittenberg, 1986)

  b. Origin of Project GENESIS: A teaching and research model

    1) Model developed by Glittenberg for graduate studies in community health

    2) GENESIS, acronym stands for *G*eneral *E*thnography *N*ursing *E*valuation *i*n a *S*ystem or *S*tate funded for approximately $2,000 per community by AHEC (Area Health Education Center)

  c. Model Conceptual Framework (Glittenberg, 1981)

    1) Builds on a conceptual framework of holism and adaptation

    2) Community or system is composed of social institutions as family, religion, education, power/ politics, economics and health. Each system is studied individually and emically, and then combined into the whole.

    3) Simple or complex systems have the same organizational structure.

    4) Adaptation of communities or systems is a process that is always evolving and dynamic.

    5) Empowering *the people* through partnership with community/system people, and graduate student ethnographers (Glittenberg, 1982, 1992). Projects had students from nursing, anthropology, public health, public health administration and sociology (Glittenberg, 2008).

    6) Model is best described as *building a snowman* (partnership with participants in the system) *while studying snow in the middle of an avalanche* (doing an ethnography) (Glittenberg in Munhall, 2002).

    7) Model is still used at the University of Colorado and many community health nursing programs worldwide. It is often linked with primary health care programs in Australia, Israel, Philippines, and Papua New Guinea.

  d. Steps in doing a GENESIS:

    1) Invitation from a community or system (e.g., wide variety of small communities, retirement village, high school, slum in the Philippines, church-owned health care system, university-based health science, prison)

    2) Study a specific community or system's self-identified problem as high suicide rate, unsafe external environment, high alcohol consumption, gangs, rape in prison, and so on

    3) Contract made between students and community leaders for a partnership in completing the project

    4) Community/system leaders set up logistics of doing the ethnography, providing a diverse number of housing, eating, and other social activities for participant observation and full participation to "walk the talk"

    5) Students study the community/systems' sociocultural history, ecology, cultural context, and etic structure, and analyze vital statistics

    6) Collection of primary data through emic ethnographic interviews of a broad representative sample as identified by the community/system leaders

    7) Begin snowball sampling from the first level, self-identified representatives, inclusive of the total population and working toward saturation of data categories. Ask "do we know all we need to know?"

    8) Develop broad overview of the emic viewpoints of the identified problem by holding team meetings where the data are collapsed into themes of problems and identify local resources to solve or handle the problems.

    9) Students write a first level analysis and present findings to the community, at large. Based on community feedback, students revise findings and write a final evaluation that is presented to the community/system leaders

    10) Findings viewed as dynamic and changing with planned re-study at regular intervals

11) Build community capacity and sustainability through solving local problems using local resources

12) Evaluation of the method

   a) Done by students and outside groups (Glittenberg, 2008)

   b) Data-based interventions as empowerment, understanding of cultural ecology, importance of holism, and self-identified and inductively derived solutions, were found very positive (Glittenberg 2007)

3. Glittenberg's Transdiciplinary Model (Jody Glittenberg)

  a. Historical Influences

    1) Changing World: 1948-1968

      a) End of World War II, rebuilding of Europe, and colonialism in Africa and Asia shifted to infant nations. In the United States, events included civil unrests, the civil rights movements, women's liberation, legalization of interracial marriages, and population shifts and migrations (Glittenberg, 1988)

      b) Worldwide demographic changes

      c) Post–World War II GI Bill

      d) Publication of the Carnegie Corporation Report, *Nursing for the Future* by Esther Lucille Brown, a social anthropologist (Brown, 1948) which became the blueprint for initiating nursing education in universities

    2) 1956-1977

      a) Special pre-doctoral and the Nurse Scientist Graduate Training launched nurses into doctoral study in four fields: anthropology, sociology, psychology, and physiology (Bouregois, 1975; Leininger 1970; Schorr & Kennedy, 1999).

      b) Pioneer PhD nurse-anthropologists wrote theory and research methods linking anthropology and nursing (Aamodt,1982; Barbee, 1980; Bauwens, 1978; Brink, 1976; Clausen, 1973; DeSantis, 1988; Dougherty & Tripp-Reimer, 1985; Dreher, 1982; Evanesko & Kay, 1982; Kay, 1982; Glittenberg, 1974; Horn, 1978; Lipson 1980; Kayser-Jones, 1979; McKenna, 1984; Muecke, 1983; Osborne, 1969; Overfield, 1977, 1985; Leininger 1970, 1973, 1976, 2000, 2001;Tripp-Reimer, 1982, 1984).

        (1) These work centered primarily on cultural particularism using qualitative research methods (Benoliel 1974).

        (2) Later, nurses started publishing their work linking biology and culture (Glittenberg, 1980, 2002; Overfield, 1977, 1985; Tripp-Reimer, 1982).

      c) Professional societies established:

        (1) In 1968, *CONAA (Council on Nursing and Anthropology)*, a section of Medical Anthropology, American Anthropology Association was founded by Leininger.

        (2) In 1972, *Transcultural Nursing Society* was founded by Leininger who was instrumental in offering the first Certification as a Transcultural Nurse.

      d) Professional nursing journals were started

        (1) In 1978, Brink became the founding editor of the *Western Journal of Nursing Research*

        (2) In 1979, Leininger founded the *Journal of Transcultural Nursing*, which was originally the *Transcultural Nursing Annual Conference Proceedings* began in 1974.

        (3) In 1983, Janet Morse became the founding editor of the *Qualitative Health Research*.

      e) Graduates of PhDs in Transcultural Nursing published textbooks:

        (1) To assess various client cultural backgrounds and to develop culturally competent practice (Wenger, 1992). Examples include Andrews and Boyle's (2009) *Transcultural Concepts in Nursing Care* (6th ed.); Giger and Davidhizar's (1999) *Transcultural Nursing: Assessment and intervention* (3rd ed.); Purnell and Paulanka's (2003) *Transcultural Health Care: A Culturally Competent Approach* (2nd ed.); and Spector's (2000) *Cultural Diversity in Health and Illness* (5th ed.).

        (2) Provide the foundation for building further theories in transcultural nursing (Barbee, 1993; Clark, 1993; Ray, 1995).

    3) 2000 to Present: Transformation

      a) Focus on intervention and transdisciplinary

    b) Douglas (2000) argued for intervention studies in transcultural nursing.

    c) The Society was challenged to enter season of transition and evolutionary process (Ludwig-Beymer, 1996: Miller, Leininger, Leuning, Pacquiao, & Papadopoulos, 2008; Zoucha, 2001).

      (1) *Glittenberg's Transdisciplinary Transcultural Model for Health Care* presented at the 2002 TCN Conference as keynote speaker (Glittenberg 2004).

      (2) Action and intervention research (Glittenberg, 2001; McQuiston, Choi-Hevel, & Clawson, 2001).

  b. Origins of the Model

    1) Transdisciplinary Initiatives

      a) In 1840, William Whewell wrote about an inductive philosophy and "jumping together" of knowledge by linking facts across disciplines to develop a common explanation.

        (1) Developing a deeper understanding of human welfare by weaving together science and the humanities (Wilson, 1995) and synthesizing culture and genetics as bioengineering.

        (2) Wilber's (1995) *Sex, ecology, and spirituality* linked basic sciences and the humanities in understanding human evolution.

        (3) Holographic paradigm looks at discrete things as undivided and linked at a deeper foundational level (Wilber, 1995).

        (4) *Transdisciplinary* was first used by the physical anthropologist, Baker (1982) as the field of physical anthropology specific to human population biology and environmental ecology (Czech, 2002).

      b) Knowledge explosion, online teaching, computerized world, interdisciplinary knowledge.

      c) Ethnicity no longer discrete categories but rather as hyphenated and inclusive, for example, Mexican Americans, African Americans, Asian Americans, and so on; thus challenging cultural praticularism and difficulty in studying beliefs of one ethnic group (Dreher & MacNaughton, 2002).

    2) Transdisciplinary and Transcultural Initiatives

      a) 1970, Leininger was the first to combine nursing and anthropology

      b) 2004, Glittenberg developed the *Transdisciplinary, transcultural curriculum model for health care*

        (1) Differs from current interdisciplinary programs

        (2) Not additive but integrated new knowledge and theories

        (3) Transdisciplinary practices in university programs and partnerships (Grey & Connolly, 2008; Heitkemper et al., 2008; Knafl, & Grey, 2008; McDaniel, Champion, & Kroenke, 2008; Weaver, 2008).

      c) Examples of projects outside disciplinary boundaries

        (1) University of Washington (Heitkemper et al., 2008)

        (2) Indiana University (McDaniel, Champion, & Kroenke, 2008)

        (3) University of Arizona (Glittenberg, 2008)

        (4) Models of action, partnership research and practice (Glittenberg, 2001; McQuiston, Choi-Hevel, & Clawson, 2001).

      d) Challenges:

        (1) Out of safe, secure discipline boundaries

        (2) Questions about shared findings and shared indirect costs

        (3) Learning new, shared discipline language and new standards

        (4) Different promotion and tenure norms

      e) New opportunities

        (1) Geography has no boundaries; offers virtual reality centers

        (2) Contributors and students from multiple places

        (3) Linking to online courses

        (4) Creative partnerships

        (5) Need to do more research, publish, hold conferences, and organize new journal to illustrate new, emerging disciplines

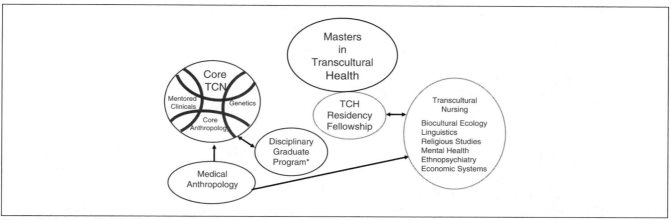

Figure 3.4. Glittenberg's transdisciplinary model
*MSN, MSW, MPH, PharmM, PharmD
Ref: Glittenberg, J. (2004). A transdisciplinary, transcultural model for health care. Journal of Transcultural Nursing. January, Vol. 14, Issue 1; pp.7-8. Reprinted with permission of Sage Publications, Inc.

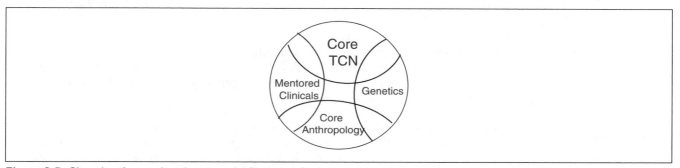

Figure 3.5. Glittenberg's transdisciplinary model: Basic certification
Ref: Glittenberg, J. (2004). A transdisciplinary, transcultural model for health care. Journal of Transcultural Nursing. January, Vol. 14, Issue 1; pp.7-8. Reprinted with permission of Sage Publications, Inc.

        (6) Funding streams from the National Institutes of Health (NIH) with its new agenda for translational research and interdisciplinary; some private foundations also need to be tapped for creative programs

    f) Basic model may lead to an advanced degree

        (1) Usually a master's level advanced model would lead to a PhD in Transcultural Health

        (2) Certificate may be either or both levels in place of or in addition to a degree indicating an accumulated, focused study

  c. The Model: Figure 3.4 describes two levels of preparation: the basic certification and the advanced.

    1) The Basic Level (Figure 3.5)

      a) Discipline specific

      b) Core of transcultural nursing studies using any of the textbooks, Leininger's Sunrise Model, ethnonursing and mixed methodology, genetics core anthropology originating in medical anthropology, mixed research methods.

      c) Each discipline mentored clinical practicum would be approved by specific State Boards (if needed)

      d) Transcultural nursing mentored clinical to practice application of principles of transcultural nursing in well-baby clinics in an underserved population, chronic illness clinic, geriatric center, a prison setting with mentally ill, healthy communities, and so on.

    2) The Advanced Level (Figure 3.6)

      a) Doctoral level with primary goal of research

        (1) Course work fieldwork in transcultural health in specific area of student research

        (2) Examples: transcultural nursing, ethics, biocultural disorders, human ecology, religious studies, linguistics, economic health care systems, international law, public policy, mental health/ethno psychiatry, and bioengineering

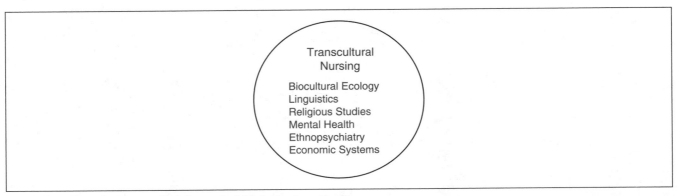

Figure 3.6. Glittenberg's transdisciplinary model: Advanced certification

Ref: Glittenberg, J. (2004). A transdisciplinary, transcultural model for health care. Journal of Transcultural Nursing. January, Vol. 14, Issue 1; pp. 7-8. Reprinted with permission of Sage Publications, Inc.

      (3) Research methods: mixed and action research

  b) Academic Minors

      (1) Individual learning needs of the graduate student accommodated through specific course work

      (2) Some online, others in classrooms

      (3) Possibilities are great for linguistics, religious studies, mental health, ethnopsychiatry, economics of the penal system, biocultural ecology, medical anthropology, psychopharmacology, forensics, criminology, energy medicine, and other courses with more depth

  c) Visionary Learning Environment

      (1) National or global virtual center could serve as a *reference point*

      (2) Centers of excellence for research projects carried out in many parts of the world

      (3) Many courses may be taught across disciplines and still retain a distinct discipline focus in the clinical application of the knowledge

      (4) Transcultural health residency, fellowship, and internships

      (5) Clinical settings, for example, prisons, industry, military, genetic laboratories, legal and correctional settings, health care settings of all types, integrative and alternative medicine, public health policy centers, religious orders, whole communities and systems

      (6) Transdisciplinary project partnerships maximize on the expertise of many people and many disciplines, either in classrooms or in virtual reality learning. This is important as cultural competence is mandated for all health care professionals.

      (7) Opportunities are endless!

4. ***Purnell Model for Cultural Competence*** (Larry D. Purnell)

  a. Philosophical underpinnings

    1) All health care professions need similar information about cultural diversity.

    2) All health care professions share the metaparadigm concepts of global society, family, person, and health.

    3) One culture is not better than another culture; they are just different.

    4) There are core similarities shared by all cultures.

    5) There are differences within, between, and among cultures.

    6) Cultures change slowly over time.

    7) The primary and secondary characteristics of culture determine the degree to which one varies from the dominant culture.

    8) If clients are co-participants in their care and have a choice in health-related goals, plans, and interventions, their compliance and health outcomes will be improved.

    9) Culture has a powerful influence on one's interpretation of and responses to health care.

    10) Individuals and families belong to several subcultures.

    11) Each individual has the right to be respected for his or her uniqueness and cultural heritage.

12) Caregivers need both cultural-general and cultural-specific information in order to provide culturally sensitive and culturally competent care.

13) Caregivers who can assess, plan, intervene, and evaluate in a culturally competent manner will improve the care of clients for whom they care.

14) Prejudices and biases can be minimized with cultural understanding.

15) To be effective, health care must reflect the unique understanding of the values, beliefs, attitudes, lifeways, and worldview of diverse populations and individual acculturation patterns.

16) Differences in race and culture often require adaptations to standard interventions.

17) Cultural awareness improves the caregiver's self-awareness.

18) Professions, organizations, and associations have their own culture, which can be analyzed using a grand theory of culture.

19) Every client encounter is a cultural encounter.

b. Disciplinary origins:

1) Conceptualized from biology, anthropology, sociology, economics, geography, history, ecology, physiology, psychology, political science, pharmacology, and nutrition.

2) Model builds on theories from communication, family development, and social support.

c. Purpose of the model

1) Provide a framework for all health care providers to learn concepts and characteristics of culture.

2) Define circumstances that affect a person's cultural worldview in the context of historical perspectives.

3) Provide a model that links the most central relationships of culture.

4) Interrelate characteristics of culture to promote congruence and to facilitate the delivery of consciously sensitive and competent health care.

5) Provide a framework that reflects human characteristics such as motivation, intentionality, and meaning.

6) Provide a structure for analyzing cultural data.

7) View the individual, family, or group within their unique ethnocultural environment.

d. Significance in cultural competent care

1) Includes *emic* and *etic* approaches to culture care and workforce issues

2) Used in research, practice, education, and research

3) Nonprescriptive approach that originated in practice

4) Overarching model covering all settings and disciplines

5) Used for practice, education, research, and management and administration

6) Applied in decreasing health disparities/inequities

7) Improves patient satisfaction and reduces health care cost

8) Focuses on patient-centered care and builds client trust

e. Concepts of the Model (Figure 3.7)

1) Metapardigm concepts: Global society, community, family, and person

2) General concepts

a) Overview, inhabited localities, and topography

b) Communication

c) Family roles and organization

d) Workforce issues

e) Biocultural ecology

f) High-risk behaviors

g) Nutrition

h) Pregnancy and childbearing practices

i) Death rituals

j) Spirituality

k) Health care practices

l) Health care practitioners

m) Specific applications in cultural competent care

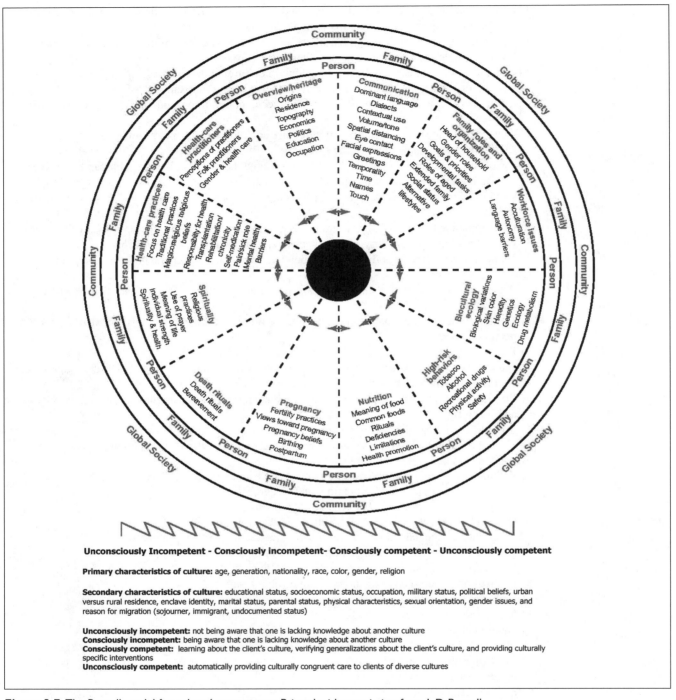

Figure 3.7. The Purnell model for cultural competence. Printed with permission from L.D. Purnell

f. Strengths of the model
    1) Holographic and complexity theory because it includes a model and organizing framework
    2) Can be used by all health care providers in various disciplines and settings
    3) Can be used in clinical practice, education, research, and the administration and management of health care services
    4) Can be used to analyze organizational culture

   5) Includes cultural workforce issues

   6) Comprehensiveness of cultural domains

  g. Weaknesses of the model

   1) Complexity of the model

   2) Can be interpreted by some as promoting stereotyping

  h. The model has been used extensively in research and publications. Studies and publications that used the Purnell model:

   1) Black, J., & Purnell, L. (2002). Cultural competence for the physical therapy professional. *Journal of Physical Therapy Education, 16*, 3-11.

   2) Black-Lattanzi, J., & Purnell, L. (2006). *Developing cultural competence in physical therapy practice*. Philadelphia, PA: F. A. Davis.

   3) Brathwaite, A. (2006). Selection of a conceptual model/framework for guiding research interventions. *Internet Journal of Advanced Nursing Practice*. Retrieved from http://www.ispub.com/ostia/index.php?xm1FilePath=journals/ijanp/vol6n1/research.xml

   4) Coakley, E., & Scoble, K. B. (2003). A reflective model for organizational assessment and interventions. *Journal of Nursing Administration, 33*, 660-669.

   5) Crandall, S. J., Geeta, G., Marion, G., & Davis, S. (2003). Applying theory to the design of cultural competency training for medical students: A care study. *Academic Medicine, 78*, 588-594.

   6) Eggenberger, S. K., Grassley, J., & Restrepo, E. (2006). Culturally competent nursing care for families: Listening to the voices of Mexican-American women. *Online Journal of Issues in Nursing, 11*(3). Retrieved from http://wee.nursingworld.org/MainMenuCategories/ANA-Marketkplace/ANAPeriodicals/OJIN/TableofContents/Volume112006/No3Sept06/ArticlePreviousTopics/CulturallyCompetentNursingCare.aspx.

   7) Hood, L., & Leddy, S. K. (2006). Multicultural issues in nursing practice. In L. Hood & S. K. Leddy (Eds.), *Multicultural issues in professional practice* (pp. 291-318). Philadelphia, PA: Lippincott, Williams & Wilkins.

   8) Nayar, S., & Tse, S. (2006). Cultural competence and models in mental health: Working with Asian service users. *International Journal of Psychosocial Rehabilitation, 10*, 79-87.

   9) Phelps, L. D., & Johnson, K.E. (2004). Developing local public health capacity in cultural competency: A case study with Haitians in a rural community. *Journal of Community Health Nursing, 21*, 203-215.

   10) Purden, M. (2005). Cultural considerations in interprofessional education and practice. *Journal of Interprofessional Care, 19*, 224-234.

   11) Purnell, L. (1999). Panamanians' practices for health promotion and the meaning of respect afforded them by healthcare providers. *Journal of Transcultural Nursing, 10*, 333-340.

   12) Purnell, L. (2000a). Guatemalans' practices for health promotion and wellness and the meaning of respect afforded them by healthcare providers. *Journal of Transcultural Nursing, 11*, 40-46.

   13) Purnell, L. (2000b). El Modelo de Purnell de competencia cultural: Una descripcion y el uso en practica, educación, investigación y de administracion. *Jornado de la Cultura y Antropología*, 46-55.

   14) Purnell, L. (2000c). A description of the Purnell Model for Cultural Competence. *Journal of Transcultural Nursing, 1*, 40-46.

   15) Purnell, L. (2002). The Purnell Model for cultural competence. *Journal of Transcultural Nursing, 13*, 193-197.

   16) Purnell, L. (2003, March-August). *Cultural diversity for older Americans. Cultural competence for the physical therapist working with clients with alternative lifestyles. A monograph*. Alexandria, VA: American Physical Therapy Association.

   17) Purnell, L. (2003). The Purnell Model for Cultural Competence: A model for all healthcare providers. *Medical Network, 1*, 8-17.

   18) Purnell, L. (2005). The Purnell Model for Cultural Competence. *Journal of Multicultural Nursing and Health, 11*(2), 7-15.

19) Purnell, L. (2007). Men in nursing: An international perspective. In C. E. O'Lynn & R. E. Tranbarger (Eds.), *Men in nursing* (pp. 219-241). New York, NY: Springer.

20) Purnell, L. (2009). *Guide to culturally competent care* (2nd ed.). Philadelphia, PA: F. A. Davis.

21) Purnell, L. & Foster, J. (2003a). Cultural aspects of alcohol use: Part I. *The Drug and Alcohol Professional, 3*(2), 17-23.

22) Purnell, L., & Foster, J. (2003b). Cultural aspects of alcohol use: Part II. *The Drug and Alcohol Professional, 3*(3), 3-8.

23) Purnell, L., & Paulanka, B. (2008). Transcultural health care: A culturally competent approach (3rd ed.). Philadelphia, PA: F. A. Davis.

24) Rosenberg, E., Kirmayer, L. J., Xenocostas, S., Dao, M. D., & Loignon, C. (2005). Impact of culture on the education of the geriatric patient. *Topics in Educational Intervention, 21,* 282-294.

25) Tortumuluogu, G. (2006). The implications of transcultural nursing models in the provision of culturally competent care. *Nursing Graduate* (25). ICUS Nursing Web: Turkey. Retrieved from http://www.nursing.gr/protectedarticles/trans.pdf

26) Voyer, P., Rail, G., Laberge, S., & Purnell, L. (2005). Cultural minority older women's attitudes medication and implications for adherence to a drug regimen. *Journal of Diversity in Health and Social Care, 2,* 47-61.

27) Williamson, G. (2007). Business and leadership: Providing leadership in a culturally diverse workplace. *American Association of Occupational Health Nurses Journal, 55,* 329-335.

28) Winn, J. M., & Riehl, G. K. (2001). Incoporating transcultural education in allied health curricula. *Journal of Allied Health, 30,* 122-125.

29) Yu, X., Shelton, D., Polifroni, E. C., & Anderson, E. (2006). Advances in conceptualization of cultural care and cultural competence in nursing: An initial assessment. *Home Health Care Management & Practice, 18,* 386-393.

5. ***The Giger and Davidhizar Transcultural Assessment Model*** (Joyce Newman Giger and Ruth Davidhizar)
   a. Origins of the Model
      1) The model was developed in 1988 in response to the need for nursing students in an undergraduate program to assess and provide care for patients that were culturally diverse.
      2) In 2007, the model was selected as Edge Runner for innovativeness by the American Academy of Nursing.
      3) Today, there is a fifth edition of *Transcultural Nursing: Assessment and Intervention* (Mosby, 1990, 1995, 2000, 2004, 2008).
      4) Supporting the textbook and the model is an online companion, which is titled "Evolve," which is available at http://www.evolve.elsevier.com/Giger complete with NCLEX questions and websites links for reference guidelines for the entire book and the supporting model.
      5) In 1998, Mosby Yearbook published a companion book that addresses Canadian ethnic groups (Davidhizar & Giger, 1998).
      6) A pocket guide was also published by Mosby that provides a quick user-friendly format to understand various cultural groups (Geissler, 1998).
      7) All the published books provide chapters on six cultural phenomena and chapters that address cultural groups, which have been authored by nurses who are experts in the culture or who are members of the cultural group.
   b. The Metaparadigm for the Giger and Davidhizar Model
      1) The model is premised on the fact that culture is a patterned behavioral response that develops over time as a result of imprinting the mind through social and religious structures and intellectual and artistic manifestations.
      2) Culture is also the result of acquired mechanisms that may have innate influences but are primarily affected by internal and external stimuli.
      3) Culture is shaped by values, beliefs, norms, and practices that are shared by members of the same cultural group.
      4) Culture guides our thinking, doing, and being and becomes patterned expressions of who we are.

5) These patterned expressions are passed down from one generation to the next.

6) Culture implies a dynamic, ever-changing, active, or passive process. Cultural values guide actions and decision making and facilitate self-worth and self-esteem.

7) Transcultural nursing: A culturally competent practice field that is client centered and research focused.

8) Culturally competent care: A dynamic, fluid, continuous process whereby an individual, system, or health care agency finds meaningful and useful care delivery strategies based on knowledge of the cultural heritage, beliefs, attitudes, and behaviors of those to whom they render care (Davidhizar & Giger, 1998; Giger & Davidhizar, 2008).

9) Cultural competence connotes a higher, more sophisticated level of refinement of cognitive skills and psychomotor skills, attitudes, and personal beliefs. To develop cultural competency, it is essential for the health care professional to use knowledge gained from conceptual and theoretical models of culturally appropriate care.

10) Achievement of cultural competence can help health care professionals in devising meaningful interventions to promote optimal health among individuals regardless of race, ethnicity, gender identity, sexual identity, or cultural heritage.

11) Culturally unique individuals: An individual is culturally unique and as such is a product of past experiences, cultural beliefs, and culturally norms.

12) Culturally sensitive environments: Culturally diverse health care can and should be rendered in a variety of clinical settings.

13) Health and health status: Health and health status are based on culturally specific illness and wellness behaviors. An individual's cultural beliefs, values, and attitudes all contribute to the overarching meaning of health for each individual.

c. The Model postulates that each individual is culturally unique and should be assessed according to six cultural phenomena:

1) *Communication*

a) Communication embraces the entire realm of human interaction, experience, and behavior.

b) Communication is the very means by which culture is actually transmitted and preserved.

c) Both verbal and nonverbal communication are actually learned in

2) *Space*

a) Space refers to the distance between individuals when they interact.

b) All communication occurs in the context of space.

c) There are four distinct zones of interpersonal space: intimate, personal, social and consultative, and public (Hall, 1966).

d) Rules concerning personal distance vary from culture to culture.

e) In terms of space, territoriality refers to feelings or an attitude toward one's personal area.

f) Each person has his or her own territorial behavior.

g) Feelings of territoriality or violation of the client's personal and intimate space can cause discomfort and may result in a client's refusing treatment or not returning for further care.

3) *Social organization*

a) Social organization refers to the manner in which a cultural group organizes itself around the family group but is also relative to clans, tribes, communes, and other such groups.

b) Family structure and organizations, religious values and beliefs, and role assignments may all relate to ethnicity and culture.

4) *Time* is an important aspect of interpersonal communication.

a) Cultural groups can be past, present, or future oriented.

b) Preventive health care requires some future time orientation because preventive actions are motivated by a future reward.

5) *Environmental control*

a) Environmental control refers to the ability of the person to control nature and to plan and direct factors in the environment that affect them.

b) Many Americans believe they control nature to meet their needs and thus are more likely to seek health care when needed.

    c) If persons come from a cultural group in which there is less belief in internal control and more in external control, there may be a fatalistic view in which seeking health care is viewed as tempting fate and encourage the unexpected to happen.

6) *Biological variations*

    a) Biological differences including genetic variations exist between individuals in different racial groups.

    b) It is a well-known fact that people differ culturally.

    c) Less understood and often less recognized are the biological differences that exist among people in various racial groups.

    d) Although there is as much diversity within cultural and racial groups as there is across and among cultural and racial groups, appropriate knowledge of general baseline data relative to a specific cultural group is an excellent starting point to provide culturally appropriate care and competent care.

    e) There is some evidence suggesting that different races metabolize drugs in different ways and at different rates (Echizen, Horari, & Ishizaki, 1989).

        (1) For example, Chinese people are thought to be more sensitive to the cardiovascular effects of certain drugs such as propranolol than are White people.

        (2) Many drugs are metabolized differently by race, for example, primaquine is metabolized by oxidation and is used in the treatment of malaria and yet when it is given to certain individuals who lack the enzymes necessary for glucose metabolism or the red blood cells, hemolysis of the red blood cells occurs.

        (3) It is postulated that approximately 100 million people in the world are affected by this particular enzyme deficiency and thus are unable to ingest primaquine.

        (4) Some 35% of African Americans have this particular enzyme deficiency.

        (5) Another category of drugs that are metabolized differently by race are antihypertensives.

        (6) For example, African Americans tend to need higher doses of beta-adrenergic blocking agents such as Inderal.

        (7) Chinese men tend to need only about half as much Inderal compared with White American males, and when angiotensin-converting enzyme inhibitors are given to African Americans they may cause coughing and may not produce the desired effect expected.

    f) One category of differences between racial groups is susceptibility to disease and the increased or decreased incidence may be genetically, environmentally, or gene–environmentally induced.

        (1) For example, American Indians have a tuberculosis incidence that is 7 to 15 times that of non-Indians, whereas African Americans have a tuberculosis incidence three times that of White Americans and urban American Jews have been the most resistant to tuberculosis.

        (2) Ethnic minorities now account for more than two thirds of all the reported cases of tuberculosis in the United States, partly as a result of the increased incidence of tuberculosis among ethnic minorities affected with HIV (Centers for Disease Control, 2007).

        (3) Whereas diabetes is quite rare among American Eskimos, it has a high incidence within certain American Indian tribes, including the Seminole, Pima, and Papago.

        (4) Non-insulin-dependent diabetes mellitus (NIDDM), or type 2 diabetes, is a major health problem for American Indians, occurring in American Indians as early as the teens or early twenties.

        (5) The age-specific death rates for diabetes appear to be 2.6 higher for Native Americans between 25 and 54 years of age, compared with the rest of the general population.

6. ***Spector's Model of Cultural Diversity in Health and Illness*** (Rachel Spector)

    a. Philosophical underpinnings of the model/theory—An in-depth knowledge and understanding of the traditional HEALTH/ILLNESS/HEALING beliefs and practices that vary between members of different communities both within the traditional community and within the larger society

        1) Health is the balance of the person, both within one's being, physical, mental, and spiritual—and in the outside world—natural, communal, and metaphysical.

        2) Illness is a state of imbalance among the body, mind, and spirit; a sense of disharmony both within the person and with the environment.

        3) Healing is a holistic or three-dimensional phenomenon that results in the restoration of balance, or harmony to the body, mind, and spirit; or between the person and the environment.

b. Disciplinary origins or emphasis (nursing, sociology, political, etc.).

        1) Nursing—Leininger, Boyle, and Andrews

        2) Sociology—Zola, Becker, Parsons, and Suchman

        3) Health Policy—National Standards for Culturally and Linguistically Appropriate Services in Health Care Title VI

        4) Theology

        5) Philosophy

c. Purpose of the model

        1) Assess degree to which patient/family/community identify with their *traditional* (ancient, ethnocultural–religious beliefs and practices that have been handed down through the generations) heritage

        2) Assess patient/family/community for personal knowledge and use of *traditional* HEALTH/ILLNESS/HEALING beliefs and practices

d. Significance in cultural competent care: Provision of culturally competent care rests in the knowledge the nurse has regarding the cultural heritage of the patient/family/community and their traditional HEALTH/ILLNESS/HEALING beliefs and practices.

e. Specific application in cultural competent care (specific populations, contexts)

        1) Universal—applicable to every patient/family/community

        2) Cultural Care needs predicated on the degree to which a given patient/family/community adheres to their ethnoreligious–cultural HEALTH/ILLNESS/HEALING perceived needs

f. Strengths and Weaknesses of the Model

        1) Strength—Greater knowledge gleaned to answer the question—"Who is this patient/family/community?"

        2) Weakness—Heritage assessment may lengthen the time necessary for patient admission interviews

g. Concepts of the Model

        1) Culturally competent care

        2) Culturally appropriate care

        3) Culturally sensitive care

h. *Heritage consistency*—(Spector, 2009, pp. 9-18)

        1 The degree to which a person's lifestyle reflects his or her traditional culture, whether American Indian, European, Asian, African, or Hispanic.

        2) The values indicating heritage consistency exist on a continuum, and a person can possess value characteristics of both a consistent heritage (traditional) and an inconsistent heritage (acculturated).

        3) The concept of heritage consistency includes a determination of one's cultural, ethnic, and religious background.

        4) Components of one's heritage to be assessed

            a) Culture

            b) Ethnicity

            c) Religion

        5) Determinants of heritage consistency

            a) The person's childhood development occurred in the person's country of origin or in an immigrant neighborhood of like ethnic group

            b) Extended family members encouraged participation in traditional religious or cultural activities

            c) Individual engages in frequent visits to country of origin or to the old neighborhood in the United States

            d) Family homes are within the ethnic community

Table 3.1. Spector's Health Traditions Model

	Physical	Mental	Spiritual
Maintain health	Proper clothing proper diet Exercise/rest	Concentration Social and family support systems Hobbies	Religious worship Prayer Meditation
Protect health	Special foods and food combinations Symbolic clothing	Avoid certain people who can cause illness Family activities	Religious customs Superstitions Wearing amulets and other symbolic objects to prevent the "evil eye" or defray other sources of harm
Restore health	Homeopathic remedies Liniments Special foods Massage Acupuncture/moxibustion	Relaxation Exorcism *Curanderos* and other traditional healers Nerve teas	Religious rituals—special prayers Meditation Traditional healings Exorcism

Source: Spector, R. E. (2009). *Cultural diversity in health and illness* (7th ed.). Upper Saddle River, NJ: Prentice Hall (pp. 78,79,365-367). Reprinted with permission from Pearson Education, Inc., Upper Saddle River, NJ.

      e) Individual participates in ethnic cultural events, such as religious festivals or national holidays, sometimes with singing, dancing, and costumes

      f) Individual was raised in an extended family setting

      g) Individual maintains regular contact with the extended family

      h) Individual's name has not been Americanized

      i) Individual was educated in a parochial (nonpublic) school with a religious or ethnic philosophy similar to the family's background

      j) Individual engages in social activities primarily with others of the same ethnic background

      k) Individual has knowledge of the culture and language of origin

      l) Individual possesses personal pride about heritage

6) Acculturation and assimilation

      a) Socialization

      b) Acculturation

      c) Assimilation

7) Ethnocultural life trajectories: Commingling variables

      a) Decade of birth

      b) Generations in the United States (Immigrant or native)

      c) Class

      d) Language (Native)

      e) Education

      f) Socioeconomic status

8) Cultural phenomena affecting health/HEALTH

      a) Environmental control

      b) Biological variations

      c) Social organization

      d) Communication

      e) Space

      f) Time orientation

i. *HEALTH Traditions Model*

1) Traditional HEALTH maintenance

      a) Physical—clothing/food activities

      b) Mental—concentration/support/hobbies

      c) Spiritual—religion/prayer/meditation

2) Traditional etiology

      a) Evil eye

      b) Envy

        c) Jealousy
        d) Hexes
        e) Soul loss
        f) Spells
     3) HEALTH protection
        a) Objects that protect HEALTH—amulets
        b) Substances that protect HEALTH
           (1) Foods—onions, garlic
           (2) Teas
        c) Spiritual—religious customs that protect HEALTH
     4) HEALTH restoration
        a) Herbal teas
        b) Massage
     5) Traditional healers
        a) Medicine man
        b) *Curandero/a*
        c) *Santero/a*
        d) *Partera*

j. Health/HEALTH care Philosophies
     1) Allopathic—dualistic—mind/body—modern
     2) Homeopathic—holistic—mind/body/spirit—traditional
        a) Folk medicine
        b) Natural
        c) Magicoreligious
        d) Health/HEALTH Care Choices
        e) Modern Health Care
     3) Public Health
     4) Primary Care
     5) Secondary care
     6) Tertiary Care
     7) Rehabilitation

k. Holistic HEALTH Care
     1) Homeopathic medicine
     2) Osteopathic medicine
     3) Chiropractic medicine
     4) Mesmerism
     5) Hypnotism
     6) Mind cure
     7) Christian Science

l. National Center for Complementary and Alternative Medicine
     1) Alternative or integrative care
     2) Traditional or ethnocultural care

m. HEALING
     1) Ancient forms of HEALING
     2) Religion and HEALING
        a) Old Testament
        b) New Testament
           (1) Saints
           (2) Spirituals journeys
           (3) HEALERS

n. HEALING and today's beliefs: Types of HEALING

o. Traditional rituals related to the life cycle
     1) Birth rituals
     2) Extensions of birth rituals to today's practices

3) Dying rituals

4) Death rituals

5) Extensions of death/dying rituals to today's practices

p. Target Community

1) Background

   a) Demographic Profile

   b) History

2) Traditional definitions of HEALTH

3) Traditional definitions of ILLNESS

4) Examples of traditional HEALTH beliefs and practices

5) Traditional HEALING beliefs and practices

6) Contemporary health problems—Disparities

7. ***Papadopoulos, Tilki, and Taylor Model of Developing Cultural Competence*** (Irina Papadopoulos)

a. Philosophical underpinnings of the model

1) Generic beliefs and values

   a) Human caring and the value of individuals

   b) Human rights, including the right to life, to dignity and to be treated with respect

   c) Socio-political systems, particularly society's constructions of power and disadvantage

   d) Culture, particularly intercultural relations and the belief in cultural diversities and similarities in health and illness

   e) Human ethics particularly transcultural ethics

   f) Anti-oppressive, anti-discriminatory practices

   g) Empowerment of clients to participate in health care decisions

   h) Promotion of equality

2) Specific beliefs and values related to nursing/healthcare professions

   a) The individual: All individuals have inherent worth within themselves as well as share the fundamental human values of love, freedom, justice, growth, life, health, and security.

   b) Culture: All human beings are cultural beings. Culture is the shared way of life of a group of people that includes beliefs, values, ideas, language, communication, norms and visibly expressed forms such as customs, art, music, clothing and etiquette. Culture influences individuals' lifestyles, personal identity and their relationship with others both within and outside their culture. Cultures are dynamic and ever changing as individuals are influenced by, and influence their culture, by different degrees.

   c) Structure: Societies, institutions, and family are structures of power that can be enabling or disabling to an individual.

   d) Health and illness: Health refers to a state of well-being that is culturally defined, valued, and practiced and which reflects the ability of individuals (or groups) to perform their daily role activities in culturally expressed, beneficial and patterned lifeways (Leininger, 1991).

   e) Illness refers to an unwanted condition that is culturally defined and culturally responded to.

   f) Caring: Caring is an activity that responds to the uniqueness of individuals in a culturally sensitive and compassionate way through the use of therapeutic communication.

   g) Nursing: Nursing is a learned activity aiming to provide care to individuals in a culturally competent way.

   h) Cultural competence: A process one goes through in order to continuously develop and refine one's capacity to provide effective healthcare, taking into consideration people's cultural beliefs, behaviors and needs, as well as the effects of societal and organizational structures which may help or hinder this process.

b. Disciplinary origins of the model

1) Community nursing

   a) Papadopoulos, a refugee to the United Kingdom, worked in the late 1970s to early 1980s in a deprived multicultural section of London as a community nurse.

       b) Her own experiences and those of her clients led her to believe that both the health care systems as well as those working in them were insensitive to patients' cultural needs.

   2) Nursing education

       a) Papadopoulos became a nurse educator in mid-1980s and realized that nursing students were not being prepared to provide effective and sensitive care to patients from different cultural backgrounds.

       b) Papadopoulos, with her colleagues Tilki, Taylor, and Alleyne set out to research and change the nursing curriculum.

       c) In 1998, to promote the inclusion of culture and cultural competence in the nursing curricula, Papadopoulos, Tilki, and Taylor published for the first time their model of cultural competence, which they had developed in 1994 following a research study into Transcultural nursing education (Papadopoulos, Alleyne, & Tilki, 1995).

  c. Purpose of the model

   1) To promote the development of culturally competent nurses and health care professionals because:

       a) The provision of cultural competent care for all is imperative.

       b) We are all cultural beings and culture matters to our health.

       c) Our culture is shaped by multiple influences such as ethnicity, socioeconomic status, gender, sexual orientation, religion, age, and so on.

       d) These factors impact on the ability of the health care systems to deal with this diversity.

       e) There are unacceptable national and global health inequalities.

       f) We have the right to access culturally competent health care that meets our fundamental health needs without discrimination or any form of oppression.

   2) To help staff develop the knowledge, skills, and attitudes necessary to plan and deliver services which

       a) promote equality

       b) value diversity

       c) challenge discrimination

       d) are appropriate to clients' needs

       e) are accessible to all clients

       f) are respectful to all clients

       g) are effective in every way, including the reduction of health inequalities.

  d. Significance in culturally competent care—cultural competence is both a process and an output, and results from the synthesis of knowledge and skills which we acquire during our personal and professional lives and to which we are constantly adding. To give this knowledge and skills some structure and to facilitate its learning, we proposed the following constructs and stages (see Figure 3.8)

  e. Key concepts of the model/theory

   1) Cultural awareness

       a) Cultural awareness is the degree of awareness we have about our own cultural background and cultural identity.

       b) This helps us to understand the importance of our cultural heritage and that of others, and makes us appreciate the dangers of ethnocentricity.

       c) It is the first step to developing cultural competence and must therefore be supplemented by cultural knowledge.

   2) Cultural knowledge

       a) This derives from a number of disciplines such as anthropology, sociology, psychology, biology, nursing, medicine, and the arts, and can be gained in a number of ways.

       b) Meaningful contact with people from different ethnic groups can enhance knowledge about their health beliefs and behaviors as well as raise understanding around the problems they face.

       c) Through, for example, sociological study we learn about power, such as professional power and control, or make links between personal position and structural inequalities.

   3) Cultural sensitivity

       a) This entails the crucial development of appropriate interpersonal relationships with clients through transcultural communication.

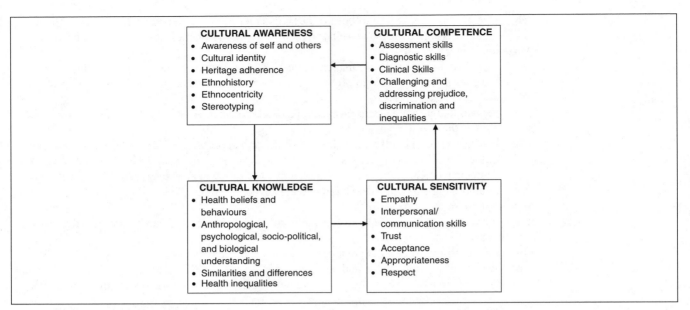

Figure 3.8. The Papadopoulos, Tilki, and Taylor model for developing cultural competence Source: Papadopoulos I (Ed) : (2006): Transcultural Health and Social Care : Development of Culturally Competent Practitioners. Edinburgh: Churchill Livingstone Elsevier. Permission from Elsevier Global Rights Department.

     b)   An important element in achieving cultural sensitivity is how professionals view people in their care.

     c)   Unless clients are considered as true partners, culturally sensitive care is not being achieved and we (nurses and other health care professionals) risk using our power in an oppressive way.

     d)   Equal partnerships involve trust, acceptance, and respect as well as facilitation and negotiation.

4) Cultural competence

     a)   Cultural competence is the capacity to provide effective health care taking into consideration people's cultural beliefs, behaviors, and needs.

     b)   Cultural competence is both a process and an output.

     c)   The achievement of cultural competence requires the synthesis of previously gained awareness, knowledge, and sensitivity, and its application in the assessment of clients' needs, clinical diagnosis and other caring skills.

     d)   A most important component of this stage is the ability to recognize and challenge racism and other forms of discrimination and oppressive practice.

     e)   This model combines both the multiculturalist and the antiracist perspectives and facilitates the development of a broader understanding around inequalities, human and citizenship rights, whilst promoting the development of skills needed to bring about change at the patient/client level.

f.   Applications of the model

  1) Nursing Education

     a)   Curriculum planning for undergraduate courses

     b)   Specific modules/courses for postgraduate courses

     c)   Development of cultural competence assessment tool

  2) Medical and paramedical professions

     a)   Recommended for use in medical education and in the education of clinical psychologist and physiotherapists.

     b)   Continues to be used in courses for professionals working in child and adolescent mental health services

  3) Research

     a)   Has been used in the development of a model of culturally competent research

           b) Is being used in doctoral studies

g. Strengths of the model

    1) Simplicity and user friendliness

    2) Focus on both culture and structure

    3) Transferability to different professions

h. Weaknesses of model

    1) Not as well known as other models

    2) Simplicity and user friendliness sometimes lead to its adoption without serious study

i. Studies and programs that used the model

    1) Knight Jackson A. E. (2007). *Cultural competence in community public health nurses: A case study* (Unpublished MPhil thesis). University of Birmingham, UK.

    2) Numerous master's projects from numerous universities, including Ben Gurion University, Israel)

    3) Masters in European Nursing collaboration between universities of Middlesex (U.K.), Tampere (Finland), Arcada (Finland), Athens (Greece), Malaga (Spain).

    4) Promoting Cultural Competence in Health and Social Care Practice (online course for the continuous development of health professionals—Middlesex University)

    5) National programme for CAMHS (Middlesex University).

    6) Undergraduate nursing programme. University of Adelaide (Australia)

    7) Web-based materials for nurses, Royal College of Nurses (UK)

    8) Papadopoulos, I., Tilki, M., & Lees, S. (2004). Promoting cultural competence in health care through a research based intervention. *Journal of Diversity in Health and Social Care, 1*, 107-115.

    9) Papadopoulos, I. (Ed.). (2006). *Transcultural health and social care: Development of culturally competent practitioners*. Edinburgh, Scotland: Churchill Livingstone Elsevier.

    10) Papadopoulos, I., Tilki, M., & Ayling, S. (2008). Cultural Competence in Action for CAMHS: The development of a cultural competence assessment tool and a short cultural competence training programme. *Advances in Contemporary Transcultural Nursing, 28*(1-2), 129-140.

8. *The Process of Cultural Competence in the Delivery of Health Care Services* (Josepha Campinha-Bacote)

a. Overview of Model

    1) The *Process of Cultural Competency in the Delivery of Health Care Services* is a practice model of cultural competence in health care delivery that defines cultural competence as the ongoing process in which the health care professional continuously strives to achieve the ability and availability to work effectively within the cultural context of the patient (individual, family, community).

    2) This model requires health care professionals to see themselves as *becoming* culturally competent rather than *being* culturally competent and involves the integration of cultural desire, cultural awareness, cultural knowledge, cultural skill, and cultural encounters.

    3) Cultural competence can be depicted as a volcano, which symbolically represents that it is cultural desire which stimulates the process of cultural competence (Figure 3.9).

    4) When cultural desire erupts, it gives forth the desire to enter into the process of becoming culturally competent by genuinely seeking cultural encounters, obtaining, cultural knowledge, conducting culturally sensitive assessments and being humble to the process of cultural awareness.

b. Philosophical Underpinnings of the Model

    1) The model is a complex whole, which includes knowledge, belief, art, moral, law, custom, and any other capabilities and habits acquired

    2) There is a direct relationship between culture and healthcare beliefs, values, and practices.

    3) Cultural groups are not limited to racial classification, ethnicity, or national origin; they are also based on factors such as

        a) geographical location

        b) gender

        c) sexual orientation

Journal of Transcultural Nursing 21(Supplement 1)

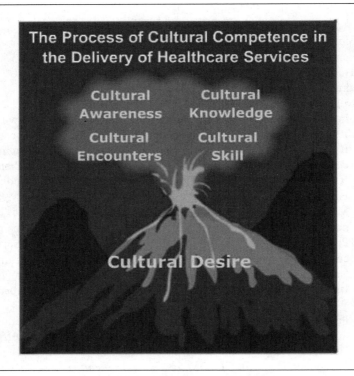

Figure 3.9. The process of cultural competence in the delivery of health care services
Copyrighted, Campinha-Bacote (2002).

       d) religious affiliation
       e) occupation
       f) disability—physical (e.g., blindness, deafness) or mental (e.g., mental retardation)
       g) socioeconomic status
       h) physical size
       i) age
       j) language
       k) political orientation
   4) Cultural competence is continuous and ongoing. It is a process, not an event; a journey, not a destination; dynamic, not static; a process of becoming, not a state of being; involves the paradox of knowing.
   5) Cultural competence requires healthcare professionals to continuously strive to achieve the ability and availability to work effectively within the cultural context of the patient (individual, family, community).
   6) The process of cultural competence consists of five interrelated constructs: cultural desire, cultural awareness, cultural knowledge, cultural skills, and cultural encounters.
   7) The spiritual and pivotal construct of cultural competence is cultural desire.
   8) There is variation within cultural groups as well as across cultural groups (intracultural variation).
   9) Cultural competence is an essential component in rendering effective and culturally responsive care to all clients.
   10) All encounters are cultural and sacred encounters.
 c. Disciplinary Origins
   1) Transcultural Nursing (Leininger, 1967, 1978, 1995, 2002, 2006)
   2) Nursing (Watson, 1979)
   3) Cultural Anthropology (Tylor, 1871)

      4) Transcultural Medicine (Kleinman, 1978, 1980)

      5) Cross-Cultural Psychology (Pederson, 1988)

      6) Pastoral Counseling (Law, 1993)

      7) Theology (Woods, 1998)

      8) Hospital Administration (Chapman, 2005)

      9) Medical Anthropology (Harwood, 1981)

      10) Philosophical Aspects of Cultural Differences (Nichols, 1987)

      11) Organizational Cultural Competence (Cross, Bazron, Dennis, & Isaacs, 1989)

d. Purpose of the Model

      1) Provide a framework for rendering culturally responsive health care services

      2) Provide a framework to teach health professionals cultural concepts

      3) Provide a framework for guiding culturally sensitive research

      4) Impact on eliminating health disparities

      5) Improve quality of health care delivery

      6) Add to the body of knowledge in transcultural nursing

      7) Respond to the current demographics of a culturally and ethnically diverse population

      8) Define the process of becoming a culturally competent health care professional

e. Significance in Cultural Competent Care

      1) Effective Organizing Framework for Health Professions Curricula

        a) Utilized as one of the two frameworks for proposed standards of practice for transcultural nursing (Leuning, Swiggum, Wiegert, & Mccullough-Zander, 2002)

        b) Physical therapy education (American Physical Therapy Association, 2008)

        c) Used in nursing programs (Kardong-Edgren & Campinha-Bacote, 2008)

        d) Used in pharmacy programs (Poirier et al., 2008)

      2) Effective for interdisciplinary training programs. Used as one of the training models to implement the Culturally and Linguistically Appropriate Standards (CLAS) in health care by these organizations:

        a) Department of Health and Human Services Office of Minority Health (USDHHS, OMH) in the development of the Cultural Competency Curricula Modules (CCCMs) for family physicians (USDHHS, OMH, 2007)

        b) USDHHS OMH in the development the Culturally Competent Nursing Modules (CCNMs) for healthcare professionals (USDHHS, OMH, 2007)

        c) National Minority AIDS Education and Training Center (NMAETC) as an organizing training framework. NMAETC's BESAFE Model is based on Campinha-Bacote's model of cultural competence (McNiel, 2003)

      3) Guides research studies, practice and educational programs (Cooper-Brathwaite, 2003). Constructs address all domains of learning: Cognitive (cultural knowledge), Affective (cultural desire and awareness) and Psychomotor (cultural encounter and skills)

      4) Instruments developed based on Model

        a) Inventory for Assessing the Process of Cultural Competence Among Health Care Professionals (Campinha-Bacote, 2002)

        b) Inventory for Assessing the Process of Cultural Competence Among Health Care Professionals (Campinha-Bacote, 2007)

        c) Cultural Diversity Questionnaire for Nurse Educators (Sealey, et al., 2006)

        d) Inventory for Assessing a Biblical Worldview of Cultural Competence Among Health Care Professionals (IABWCC) (Campinha-Bacote, 2005)

f. Concepts of the Model

      1) Cultural Desire—the motivation of the healthcare professional to "want to" engage in the process of becoming culturally competent, not because one "has to."

        a) The fuel necessary to draw us into a personal journey toward cultural competence

        b) Includes a genuine passion and commitment to be open and flexible with others

        c) Requires respect for differences, yet a commitment to build on similarities

        d) Willingness to learn from clients and others as cultural informants

        e) Caring and Love

(1) State in which something does matter; it is the source of human tenderness (May, 1975).

(2) Caring "comes from the heart; not from the mouth" (Campinha-Bacote, 1998).

(3) Caring is a virtue and should be seen as a practical comportment toward others, with the goal of enhancing the health-related existence of others (van Hooft, 1999).

(4) "Radical loving care, creating a continuous chain of caring light around each patient;" the passion to serve others; servant's heart that symbolizes love's greatest expression and assumes the full involvement of our best thought processes" (Chapman, 2005, p.10)

f) Sacrifice

(1) Willingness to sacrifice one's prejudice and biases towards culturally different clients.

(2) Sacrificing "proprietary assumptions of our own rightness and our unreflective grip on our own certainty" (Howard, 2003).

(3) Involves moral commitment to care for all clients, regardless of their cultural values, beliefs or practices.

g) Social justice

(1) Understanding of social inequalities and how they affect individuals and communities

(2) Direct correlation between inequality and negative health outcomes

(3) Achieve equality in health outcomes for all, regardless of race/ethnicity, language, gender, religion, or sexual orientation (Stacks, *Salgado, & Holmes*, 2004)

(4) Professional health care organizations' commitment to social justice

   (a) American Nurses Association's Position Statement on Ethics and Human Rights (1991)

   (b) Transcultural Nursing Society (Andrews, Bentley, Crawford, Pretlow, & Tingen, 2007)

(5) Socially just cultural competence requires entering into community partnerships.

h) Humility

(1) Cultural humility (Tervalon & Murray-Garcia, 1998)

   (a) Life-long commitment to self-evaluation and self-critique

   (b) Re-addressing power imbalances in the patient–health care professional relationship

   (c) Developing mutually beneficial partnerships with communities on behalf of individuals and defined populations

   (d) Seeing the greatness in others

(2) Realization of the dignity and worth of others

(3) Genuine desire to discover how your patients think and feel differently from you

(4) Humility is not thinking less of yourself, but thinking of yourself, less.

(5) Matthew 20:26-27 states, ". . . but whoever wishes to become great among you shall be your servant, and whoever wishes to be first among you shall be your slave" (New American Standard Bible, 2002)

(6) Directed toward serving our fellow human beings

(7) Paradox of possessing humility

(8) Theological ways to humble oneself (Ells, n.d.)

2) Cultural Awareness is the deliberate self-examination and in-depth exploration of our personal biases, stereotypes, prejudices and assumptions that we hold about individuals who are different from us as well as the acknowledgement of racism and other "isms" in health care delivery.

a) A health care professional's cultural and ethnic background can affect interpreting, assigning meaning to, and creating value judgments about their patients.

b) The process of gaining cultural awareness is an important first step in one's journey towards recognizing personal biases, prejudices, and discriminatory practices.

c) An affective or attitudinal construct.

      d) Involves "insight into personal cultural heritage, the disciplinary heritage into which one has been socialized as a healthcare provider, and the organizational culture within which services are delivered . . ." (Schim, Doorenbos, Benkert, & Miller, 2007, p. 107).

      e) Personal biases are ingrained in one's mind and not always directly available to our conscious thinking

      f) Serious barrier to culturally competent care is not a lack of knowledge of any given cultural group, but failure to develop self-awareness and a respectful attitude toward diverse points of view (Hunt, 2001)

      g) Avoid cultural imposition, which is the tendency to impose one's beliefs, values, and patterns of behavior on another culture (Leininger, 1978).

      h) Seek cultural openness, which is a " lifelong stance that promotes cultural self-awareness and continuing development of transcultural skills" (Wenger, 1998, p. 64).

      i) Techniques to stimulate cultural awareness:
          (1) Experiential exercises (role plays, role reversals, simulations)
          (2) Field trips
          (3) Guided self-study with a reading list
          (4) Critical incidents
          (5) Panel discussions
          (6) Audio-visual presentations
          (7) Interviews with consultants and experts
          (8) Bicultural observations
          (9) Cinematography

      j) Cultural competence continuum
          (1) Unconscious incompetence—being unaware that one is lacking cultural knowledge
              (a) Health care professionals not aware that cultural differences exist between themselves and the patient
              (b) Cultural blind spot syndrome—assume that there are no cultural differences (Buchwald et al., 1994)
          (2) Conscious incompetence—being aware one is lacking knowledge about other cultural groups
              (a) Possess the "know that" knowledge
              (b) Lacks the "know how" knowledge
          (3) Conscious competence—mindful act of learning about the patient's culture
              (a) Verify generalizations
              (b) Provide culturally relevant interventions
          (4) Unconscious competence—ability to spontaneously provide culturally responsive care to patients from a diverse culture

      k) Interacting styles (Bell & Evans, 1981)
          (1) Overt racism towards a particular group.
          (2) Covert racism - hiding or "covering up" one's true feelings is considered important to effective interactions
          (3) Culturally liberated- one does not fear cultural differences and interactions with specific cultural groups

      l) Lethal "isms": "ageism, sexism, ethnocentrism, classism, ableism, heterosexism, racism" (oppression and antiracist pedagogy; Hassouneh, 2006)

      m) Dominant culture privilege
          (1) White privilege (McIntosh, 1988)
          (2) Three principal presumptions of dominant culture privilege (Cullnan, 1999): presumption of innocence, presumption of worthiness, and presumption of competence

3) Cultural Knowledge: the process of seeking and obtaining a sound educational base about culturally diverse groups
      a) Intracultural variation—there are marked differences within cultural groups
      b) Stereotype versus archetype

    c) Focus on the integration of three specific issues: health-related beliefs practices and cultural values, disease incidence and prevalence, and treatment efficacy (Lavizzo-Mourey, 1996)

    d) The philosophical aspects of cultural differences (Nichols, 1987)

    (1) Axiology—what a culture values the highest

    (2) Epistemology—how a cultural group comes to know as truth or knowledge

    (3) Logic—cultural group's nature of reasoning

    (4) Process—cultural group's view of the nature of relationships in the world

    e) Disease incidence and prevalence

    (1) Common diseases and health conditions found among cultural/ethnic groups

    (2) Health disparities among cultural/ethnic groups

    f) Treatment efficacy; ethnic pharmacology

    (1) Environmental factors (e.g., diet, malnutrition)

    (2) Cultural factors (e.g., use of herbs)

    (3) Genetics

    (4) Generic substitution

    g) Diagnostic clarity: Culture-bound illnesses and misdiagnosis

    h) Interacting styles within cultural groups (Bell & Evans, 1981)

    (1) Acculturated—reject the values, beliefs, practices, and general behaviors associated with one's own cultural group

    (2) Culturally immersed—rejects all values, except those held by one's own cultural group

    (3) Traditional—neither rejects nor accepts one's cultural identity

    (4) Bicultural—demonstrates pride for one's history and cultural traditions, while still feeling connected and comfortable in the mainstream world.

4) Cultural Skill: the ability to collect relevant cultural data regarding the client's presentation problem, as well as accurately performing a culturally based, physical assessment in a culturally sensitive manner

    a) Cultural assessment

    (1) "Systematic appraisal or examination of individuals, groups, and communities as to their cultural beliefs, values and practices to determine explicit needs and intervention practices within the context of the people being served" (Leininger, 1978, pp. 85-86).

    (2) Goal is to obtain accurate information from the client that will allow you to diagnose the client's presenting problem and formulate a mutually acceptable and culturally relevant treatment plan.

    (3) Every client needs cultural assessment.

    b) Cultural assessment tools

    (1) 12 domains (Purnell, 2008)

    (2) Transcultural Assessment Model (Giger & Davidhizar, 2008)

    (3) Ethnocultural Assessment (Jacobsen, 1988)

    (4) Block's (1983) Assessment Guide for Ethnic/Cultural Variations

    (5) GREET (Chong, 2002)

    (6) CONFHER (Fong, 1985)

    (7) BATHE (Stuart & Lieberman, 1993)

    (8) ESFT (Carillo, Green, & Betancourt, 1999)

    (9) LEARN (Berlin & Fowkes, 1982)

    (10) ETHNIC (Levine, Like, & Gottlieb, 2000)

    (11) BELIEF (Dobbie, Medrano, Tysinger & Olney, 2003)

    (12) RISK (Kagawa-Singer & Kassim-Lakha, 2003)

    (13) ADHERE (Like, 2004)

    (14) SMARTS (Tang & Bozynski, 2000)

    c) Culturally sensitive medication assessment

    (1) Clinician's Inquiry Into the Meaning of Taking Psychotropic Medications (Gaw, 2001)

    (2) Assessment of Cultural Aspects of Disease Incidence and Medication Use (Kudzma, 2001)

    d) Campinha-Bacote's Integrated Model Approach to conducting a cultural assessment
        (1) Review several cultural assessment tools
        (2) Consider your discipline's and specialty's purpose in conducting an assessment
        (3) Consider your personal assets and liabilities as an interviewer
        (4) Integrate selected questions from a specific cultural assessment tool that will augment your existing patient assessment to yield culturally relevant data
        (5) Establish your own personal style of incorporating cultural content into your patient assessment

    e) Culturally based physical assessments
        (1) Melocentric versus a Eurocentric skin assessment (Salcido, 2002)
        (2) Skin Color Scale for Assessing Normal Skin Pigmentation in Asians (Parreno, 1977)
        (3) Biocultural Ecology (Bloch, 1983; Purnell, 2008)

    f) Skill acquisition
        (1) Eliciting cultural content in a sensitive manner
            (a) Remain nonjudgmental
            (b) Adopt less direct and more conversational approach
            (c) Attribute explanations to another person to help clients disclose health beliefs and practices that they may feel initially uncomfortable expressing
        (2) Levels of proficiency in skill acquisition (Dreyfus & Dreyfus, 1980)
            (a) novice
            (b) advanced beginner
            (c) competent
            (d) proficient
            (e) expert

5) Cultural Encounters: the act of directly interacting with clients from culturally diverse backgrounds
    a) Goals of cultural encounters (Sue et al., 1982)
        (1) Generate a wide variety of responses
        (2) Receive both verbal and non verbal communication accurately and appropriately in each culturally different context
    b) Culture is elastic—knowing the cultural norms of a given group does not predict the behavior of a member of that group (LeBaron, 2003)
    c) Every encounter is a cultural encounter
    d) Linguistic competence
        (1) "Capacity of an organization and its personnel to communicate effectively, and convey information in a manner that is easily understood by diverse audiences including persons of limited English proficiency, those who have low literacy skills or are not literate and individuals with disabilities" (Goode & Jones, 2004).
        (2) Resources to support linguistic competence (Goode & Jones, 2006):
            (a) Bilingual/bicultural or multilingual/multicultural staff
            (b) Cultural brokers
            (c) Cross-cultural communication approaches
            (d) Sign language interpretation services
            (e) Printed material in easy to read, low literary, picture and symbol formats
            (f) Foreign language interpretation
            (g) Materials in alternative formats (e.g., audiotape, Braille, enlarged print)
            (h) TTY and other assistive devices
            (i) Materials tested for specific cultural ethnic and linguistic group
            (j) Computer-assisted real-time translation (CART) or viable real-time transcriptions (VRT)
        (3) Health literacy
        (4) Models for cultural encounters
            (a) PEARLS (Clark, Hewson, & Fry, 1996)
            (b) RESPECT (Bigby, 2003)

    (c) LIVE & LEARN (Carballeria, 1996)

    (d) CRASH (Satcher, Ninan, & Masand, 2005)

    (e) TRANSLATE (Like, 2000) model for working with interpreters

  e) Conflict and compassion (Gallaher, 2007)

   (1) Culture is always a factor in conflict

   (2) Cultivating compassion requires that we understand from the other's point of view

   (3) Cultivating compassion requires that we engage in self-reflection of how our actions are affecting the other person

  f) Sacred encounters (Chapman, 2005, p. 58)

   (1) Occurs whenever we meet another's deep need with a loving response

   (2) Making a connection

   (3) Attentive listening—listen responsively resulting in the following outcomes (Ting-Toomey, 1999):

    (a) Feeling of being understood

    (b) Feeling of being respected

    (c) Feeling of being supported

  g) Non-face-to-face encounters

   (1) Telephonic communication

   (2) Electronic communication (e.g., email)

 g. Specific Application in Cultural Competent Care

  1) Clinical/Practice Examples

   a) Home care (Campinha-Bacote & Narayan, 2000)

   b) Rehabilitation (Campinha-Bacote, 2001)

   c) Case management (Campinha-Bacote & Munoz, 2001)

   d) Spiritual care (Campinha-Bacote, 1995, 2003, 2005)

   e) Psychiatric care (Campinha-Bacote, 1994, 1995, 2002, 2003)

   f) Mental health care (Campinha-Bacote 1991)

   g) Pediatric care (Campinha-Bacote & Ferguson, 1991)

   h) Care to special population—Examples

    (1) HIV/AIDS (McNeil, Campinha-Bacote, & Vample, 2002)

    (2) Lesbians (Dinkel, 2005)

  2) Education examples

   a) Continuing education (Campinha-Bacote, Yale, & Langerkamp, 1996)

   b) Health Professions' Curricula (Campinha-Bacote, 2006, 2008; Campinha-Bacote et al., 2005; Kardong-Edgren & Campinha-Bacote, 2008; Nash et al., 2006)

   c) Mentoring Minority Nursing Students (Rivera-Goba & Campinha-Bacote, 2008)

   d) Transcultural Nursing courses (Anderson, 2004; Cooper-Brathwaite, 2005; Marcinkiw, 2003)

  3) Research examples

   a) Organizing framework (Campinha-Bacote & Padgett, 1995)

   b) Tool development (Fitzpatrick, Cronin, & Campinha-Bacote, under review)

  4) Administration Examples

   a) Managed care organizations (Campinha-Bacote & Campinha-Bacote, 1999)

   b) Nursing management (Campinha-Bacote, 1996)

  5) Health Policy Examples

   a) Child health policy (Campinha-Bacote & Ferguson, 1997)

   b) Health law (Campinha-Bacote & Campinha-Bacote, under review)

  6) Nursing Assessment and Intervention Examples

   a) Assessment (Campinha-Bacote, 1988)

   b) Ethnic pharmacology (Campinha-Bacote, 1995, 1997, 2008)

   c) Ethno music Therapy (Campinha-Bacote, 1993; Campinha-Bacote & Allbright, 1992)

   d) Ethno humor therapy (Campinha-Bacote, 1995, 1997)

  7) Technology—Serves as a template for web pages (Darling-Fisher, 2000)

 h. Strengths (Cooper-Brathwaite, 2006; Tortumluoglu, 2006)

  1) Comprehensive

2) Conceptual clarity, logical congruence
3) Clinical utility, useful for all patients, practice-oriented, patient-centered
4) Advocates the experiential–phenomenological perspective of culture
5) Explicit, parsimonious
6) Provides direction for empirical research
7) Contributes to development of cultural competence by providing concrete guide for clinical, research, organizational, and educational use
8) Multidisciplinary use and application: medicine, nursing, physical therapy (American Physical Therapy Association, 2008), social work, occupational therapy, dentistry, theology, psychology, allied health professions
9) Pictorial representation (see Figure 3.9)
10) Mnemonic representation—ASKED Model: awareness, skill, knowledge, encounters, desire
11) Constructs can be measured
    a) Inventory for Assessing the Process of Cultural Competence among health care professionals—revised (IAPCC-R; Campinha-Bacote, 2002)
    b) Inventory for Assessing the Process of Cultural Competence among health care professionals—student version (IAPCC-SV; Campinha-Bacote, 2007)

  i. Weaknesses of the Model (Campesino, 2008; Duffy, 2001)
1) Lacks theoretical level of development (e.g., does not have a set of interrelated statements about the constructs)
2) Constructs not operationalized
3) Lack of significant attention to inequitable historical and social conditions
4) Limited attention to environmental factors (e.g., structural systems of power)
5) Lack of clarity between culture, race, and ethnicity
6) Limited attention to globalization issues

  j. Studies Demonstrating Outcomes of Model Application
1) Clinical Examples
    a) Ethnographic study of patients with cervical cancer in Iquitos, Peru (Hunter, 2008)
    b) Population-based nursing care to the Hutterites (Fahrenwald, Boysen, Fischer, & Maurer, 2001)
2) Education Examples
    a) Faculty development (Sealey, 2003)
    b) Curricula framework for undergraduate students (Kardong-Edgren & Campinha-Bacote, 2008)
    c) Framework for integrative simulation (Rutledge et al., 2008)
    d) Framework for health professions' courses
      (1) Pharmacy (Poirier et al., 2008)
      (2) Nursing (Brathwaite, 2005, 2006; Hunter, 2008; Sargent, Sedlak, & Martsolf, 2005)
      (3) Study abroad (Koskinen & Tossavainen, 2003)
3) Research Examples: Measuring cultural competence in nursing (Seright, 2007) and among osteopathic medical students (Anderson-Warts, 2005)

9. *Transcultural Concepts Guiding Nursing* Care (Margaret Andrews and Joyceen Boyle; Figure 3.10)
  a. Developing cultural competence
1) *Cultural competence* is a process that involves a complex integration of knowledge, attitudes, beliefs, and skills. Health care professionals become *culturally competent* to provide *culturally congruent care* to persons from different cultures.
    a) Individual cultural competence
    b) Linguistic competence
2) Cultural self-assessment is awareness of your own cultural values, attitudes, beliefs, and practices. These insights enable you to overcome your own ethnocentric tendencies and cultural stereotypes.
3) Skills needed for cultural competence include both psychomotor and behavioral skills. They include assessment skills that focus on communication, hygiene, activities of daily living, and religion or spirituality.
  b. Transcultural Concepts that guide nursing practice

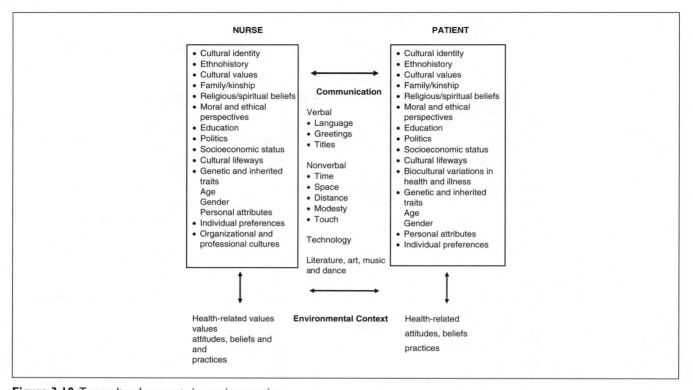

Figure 3.10. Transcultural concepts in nursing practice
Source: Adapted from Andrews, M. M., & Boyle, J. S. (2008). *Transcultural concepts in nursing care.* Philadelphia, PA: Lippincott Williams & Wilkins. Reprinted with permission.

1) Cross-cultural communication
   a)   An exchange of messages and the creation of meaning.
   b)   Effective communication brings about a mutual understanding of the meaning attached to the message.
   c)   Consider the ways in which people from various cultural backgrounds communicate with one another.
   d)   In addition to oral and written communication, messages are conveyed nonverbally through gestures, body movements, posture, tone of voice, and facial expressions.
   e)   Be aware of how the environmental context can influence communication with clients from a different culture.
   f)   Avoid technical jargon, slang, colloquial expressions, abbreviations, and excessive use of medical terminology.
2) Communication patterns with family members and significant others
   a)   Identify who is responsible for decision making that affects the client's health care
   b)   Ascertain the value, decision-making patterns, and overall pattern of communication within the client's household
   c)   Familism (often seen in Hispanic cultures) emphasizes
      (1) interdependence over independence
      (2) affiliation over confrontation
      (3) cooperation over competition
   d)   Assess how kinship terms and relationships vary among cultures
   e)   Individual values orientation in North America often leads to decision making about health and illness becoming an individual matter
3) Cultural perspectives on intimacy
   a)   Interactions between the nurse and the client may vary from very formal interactions to close personal relationships

(1) Some clients of Asian origin expect health care professionals to be authoritarian, directive, and detached. They may appear to be reserved and place an emphasis on social harmony

(2) Appalachian clients often have interaction patterns that lead them to expect close personal relationships with health care providers

(3) Hispanic cultures, such as Mexican Americans and Cuban Americans may emphasize values and behaviors related to *simpatico* and *personalismo*

   b) Ensure a mutually respectful relationship by introducing yourself and indicate to the client and family how you prefer to be addressed. Elicit the same information from the client and family members

4) Nonverbal communication patterns vary widely among cultures.

   a) Periods of silence

   b) Silence among some Native Americans may indicate understanding and respect. It may indicate thoughtful consideration

   c) In traditional Japanese and Chinese culture, silence may mean that the speaker wishes the listener to consider the content of what has been said before continuing the conversation

   d) Silence may be interpreted by Russians persons as a sign of agreement. However, in some African Americans, silence is used in response to a question perceived as inappropriate

5) Eye contact

   a) Eye contact is most likely the most culturally variable nonverbal behavior

   b) Direct eye contact may be considered an affront or impolite or aggressive by Asian, Native American, Indochinese, Arab, and Appalachian clients

   c) Direct eye contact may be related to modesty in Arab, Latino, and African American groups

6) Touch

   a) Physical contact with clients conveys various meanings cross-culturally

   b) Arab and Hispanic cultures may culturally prohibit male health care providers from touching or examining part or all of the female body

   c) Some cultures have strict norms related to touching children. Touching a child on the head should only be done with parental permission

7) Space and distance

   a) Space and distance "comfort levels" can cause uncomfortable feelings and reactions when interacting with persons from another culture

   b) Individuals from Middle Eastern origins, Hispanic, or even East Indian are generally more comfortable with close physical proximity

   c) Nurses frequently interact with clients in the intimate or personal distance zones

8) Sex and gender

   a) Violation of norms related to gender may be a serious transgression

   b) Males from Middle Eastern cultures may avoid being alone with members of the opposite sex. Men and women do not touch each other outside the marital relationship

   c) Same sex relationships also vary culturally. What may be culturally acceptable expressions of friendship and affection may be misinterpreted

9) Language

   a) Nearly 1 in 5 persons, age 5 years or older, speak a language other than English at home

   b) Use of interpreters in health care encounters

   c) Recommendations for institutions who hire interpreters

   d) What to do when there is no interpreter

10) Sick role behaviors are those socialized and culturally acceptable ways of behaving when one is ill.

VIII. STRATEGIES FOR REDUCING BIAS AND PREJUDICE

   A. Cultural Brokering (Jezewski, 1990)

      1. Cultural brokering on behalf of clients is the act of bridging, linking or mediating between groups or persons of differing cultural backgrounds for the purpose of reducing conflict or producing change.

      2. The culture broker acts as a go-between, one who advocates or intervenes on behalf of another individual or group.

3. Culture brokering gives professionals the tools to assess cultural factors so they can work more productively with clients from diverse backgrounds.

4. A systematic way to analyze the role culture plays in an individual's or family's experiences with disability services.

5. Important strategy as communities become increasingly multicultural and health care providers work with more and more clients from diverse cultural and linguistic backgrounds.

6. With the current immigration trends, it is critical for service providers and educators to work across cultures to support people with disabilities and for families to access services and resources.

7. Jezewski's (1990) Culture Brokering Model
   a. A conflict resolution and problem-solving model
   b. Recognizes that there is a problem or potential problem in the consumer's encounter with the health care system
   c. The culture broker looks at the problem from a cultural perspective. Potential problems are anticipated, prevented, or minimized.
   d. A breakdown in communication between providers and consumers and differences in beliefs about appropriate services are examples of problems that can be resolved by using the culture-brokering model as a guide.
   e. In the intervention phase, mediating and negotiating strategies are put into practice in order to resolve the identified problem or problems.
   f. Advocating is another strategy used to promote the rights or change the system on behalf of an individual or group.
   g. Involves activities that are aimed at the redistribution of power and resources to the individual or group that has demonstrated a need.
   h. Networking is another culture brokering strategy by which the health care provider establishes links with other professionals who can provide services to consumers.
   i. The broker evaluates the degree to which the problem has been resolved. If resolution does not take place or the problem is not resolved satisfactorily, the culture broker reverts back to reassessing the problem or using additional strategies.

B. Bridging Cultural Gaps

1. The strategies for reducing bias and prejudice by *bridging cultural gaps* were identified in a qualitative study on the processes by which nurse educators teach ethnically diverse nursing students (Yoder, 1996, 1997, 2001).

2. Data were obtained from in-depth interviews with 26 nurse educators and 17 nurses representing Asian Americans, African Americans, and Mexican Americans.

3. Of the five patterns of teaching that emerged, the *Bridging pattern* provides useful strategies applicable for nurse educators working with nursing students, staff or client learners.
   a. *Bridging educators* encouraged learners to maintain their ethnic identity, and modified teaching–learning strategies to meet the cultural needs of learners.
   b. Educators managed teaching by an interactive process with three components:
      1) Sending cues
      2) Interpreting cues
      3) Acting/interacting based on cues

4. *Cultural awareness* of the educator significantly influenced bridging.
   a. Broad structural issues, as well as conditions influencing the individual, bear upon cultural awareness.
   b. Individual level cultural awareness was influenced by educators' lived experience, participation in sensitivity sessions, experience interacting with diverse students, and level of commitment to equity.
   c. Differing levels of cultural awareness resulted in varying levels of responding in culturally sensitive ways. Educators' responses ranged from no accommodation for the needs of ethnically diverse students to a high adjustment of teaching strategies to meet the needs of students as illustrated by the Bridging educators.
   d. Teaching approaches resulted in different consequences for the nurse educators and the ethnic students, but consequences of the *Bridging pattern* were positive for students.

5. Unique characteristics of *Bridging educators*
    a. Bridging educators were all ethnic minority persons who demonstrated a high level of cultural awareness.
    b. Level of awareness significantly influenced by experience as ethnic minority, identification with students' experiences, extent of valuing diversity, and formal educational preparation.
    c. Retained strong ethnic identification that affected their responses to students, and capacity to identify with the experiences and feelings of ethnically diverse learners.
    d. Life experiences provided informal education for interpreting lerner cues.
    e. Valued diversity, appreciated unique backgrounds of students, and viewed working in a diverse setting as rewarding experience. Value of diversity was communicated to learners and used to enhance the learning environment.
    f. Identified with students' experiences because of their own experiences with same issues in personal and professional life.
    g. Clinical experience with diverse clients helped prepare them in working with diverse students.

6. Interactions of *Bridging educators* with diverse learners
    a. Interaction process involved assessing cues students sent, distinguishing cultural problems, and recognizing barriers students face.
    b. Bridging educators analyzed students' cultural frames of reference and effect of students' cultural views on their understanding of nursing concepts.
    c. Explored differences in perceptions and built teaching strategies relevant to learners.
    d. Identified differences in students' cultural frames of reference based on assessment of cultural cues from students.
    e) Major cultural conflict issues that emerged were differing definitions of health, alternative views of appropriate relationships with teachers, and varied ideas about suitable learning approaches.
        1) Ethnic students' assumptions about basic nursing concepts differed from those of majority students as nursing concepts are culturally based.
        2) Students' cultural values influenced their perceptions of teacher role and apprehensions about approaching teachers.
        3) Students' approaches to learning were grounded in their cultural system leading to conflicting values about learning approaches. In the dominant cultural system that values individualism and independence, educators stress the importance of independent learning and competition.
        4) An independent learning approach present problems for some ethnic students who were enculturated in family systems that encourage interdependence.

7. In contrast to other educators, *Bridging faculty* identified cultural barriers that learners faced:
    a. Majority believed that prejudice, discrimination, and racism presented major problems for ethnic learners in school and clinical agencies.
    b. Students faced social and interpersonal barriers as unfavorable faculty attitudes, lack of faculty awareness of racial/ethnic issues, negative stereotyping, and unfavorable peer group attitudes.
    c. Students were expected to adopt the professional nursing system grounded in the norms and values of America's dominant society although they often held different health beliefs, assumptions, and theories. Consequently, ethnic students have difficulty relating with these concepts.
    d. Although majority of faculty assumed that students' clinical problems resulted from lack of competence, *Bridgers* believed that problems often arose from resistance within agencies.
    e. *Bridgers* differed from other educators in their perceptions of the amount of prejudice students encountered and the number of barriers they faced.

8. Effective strategies of *Bridging educators*
    a. Recognized subtle needs and feelings of ethnic students, and identified many of the same needs that students' expressed.
    b. Respected cultural differences of students, and developed actions that were culturally adaptive using four major strategies.
        1) Incorporating *Student's Cultural Knowledge* validated students' valuable contribution.
            a) Goal was not to encourage students to adopt majority cultural views but rather to enrich the knowledge system.
            b) Related course content to cultural views of ethnic and majority students.

    c) Careful assessment of student's conceptualization of a situation, allowed discovery of how students' values affected their clinical performance.

    d) Clarified cultural expectations of the dominant group, without conferring inferior status to students' own values.

    e) Accommodated different worldviews in managing conflicts based on own repertoire of experiential knowledge.

2) Preserving student's ethnic identity

    a) Enhancing student's ethnic self-concept, providing successful role models, and encouraging students to function biculturally

    b) Selecting experiences to provide a comfortable environment for students to develop positive ethnic identities

    c) Using anecdotes and illustrations from their own diverse ethnic backgrounds, to create safe environment for students to share their own ethnic beliefs

    d) Advocating for students to retain their own cultural beliefs and behaviors as they developed proficiency to function in the dominant culture.

    e) Providing successful ethnic role models to foster positive ethnic identity by

        (1) linking students with ethnic role models in the clinical settings

        (2) developing mentor programs with Black, Hispanic, and Asian nurses in the community

        (3) encouraging ethnic support groups for students

        (4) connecting students with ethnic professional nursing organizations

        (5) developing mentoring relationships between the teacher and students.

3) Facilitating Student Negotiation With Barriers

    a) Considered prejudice, discrimination, and racism as realities of ethnic students' experiences, and assisted them to cope with them

    b) Permitted student expression of problems related to prejudice or discrimination, and validated their experience as reality

    c) Engaged in collaborative problem solving with students and role modeled how to handle cultural conflicts

    d) Drew from own experience with barriers, commitment to social change, and investment of energy to assist students in dealing with racism and prejudice.

4) Advocating for System Change

    a) Advocated for structural and policy changes

    b) Assisted students to form ethnic student support groups to identify and advocate needed policy changes

    c) Developed liaisons with ethnic community groups and professional associations to support students.

    d) Realized difficult process of advocating for commitment and change supportive of diversity

9. Consequences of the bridging pattern; resulted in many positive consequences for both faculty and students.

a. Faculty

    1) Believed that large numbers of ethnic students enhanced their teaching and provided positive reinforcement

    2) Faculty "learned from students," which increased teaching effectiveness.

    3) Structured teaching to incorporate cultural knowledge of ethnic students

    4) Incorporating aspects of students' worldviews allowed expression of a broader range of viewpoints in the classroom and increased all students' awareness

    5) Enhanced ethnic identity and self esteem of students

b. Consequences of bridging pattern for students

    1) When barriers were acknowledged, students' perceptions were validated, which assisted them to address racial issues.

    2) Comfortable learning environment reinforced students' cultural perspectives.

    3) Environment enhanced students' self-confidence and identity as ethnic nurses.

    4) Students' cultural perspectives were reinforced and cultural differences were viewed as an asset rather than a liability or deficiency.

        5) When clinical experiences were organized to use students' strengths, their self-esteem was raised and the students' contributions were validated.

        6) Students' unique strengths were recognized and their contributions were valued.

        7) Students' input was not suppressed but rather drawn upon to provide valuable content for all students.

        8) Students felt they were welcomed in the educational environment and valued for the contributions to the profession.

C. Developing Mutually Beneficial Partnerships With Communities

    1. *Effect of Social Environment on Health and Illness* (CDC/ATSDR, 1997)

        a. Studies have demonstrated that the social environment in which individuals live can significantly affect the incidence of illness within a population (Institute of Medicine, 1988).

        b. Researchers stress the importance of engaging the community in the development of health promotion and disease prevention efforts using community-based participatory methodologies (Andrews et al., 2007; Di Bari et al., 2007; Dale, Shipman, Lacock, & Davies, 1996; Fawcett et al., 1995; Israel, Schulz, Parker, & Becker, 2001; Krueger & King, 1997; McNeal, 1996; McNeal, Doherty, O'Donnell, & Mallory, 1997; Murray & Graham, 1995; Murray et al, 1994).

        c. The process of community engagement is achieved through collaborative initiatives that involve groups of individuals affiliated by geographic region, special interests or common situations, who seek to address issues impacting the health and well being of their respective neighborhoods

        d. Supportive community collaboration effort leads to the creation of positive environments, which promote the establishment of long term partnerships that inform population-based interventional strategies aimed at disease prevention.

    2. *Definition of Community Systems* (CDC/ATSDR, 1997)

        a. Communities are systems composed of individuals and sectors that have an array of distinct characteristics.

        b. Membership of each sector consists of individuals who represent specific functions or interests within the community system.

        c. Overall operation of each sector is oriented toward meeting the needs of its members.

        d. Functionality of a community system is determined by the interrelationships of its various sectors. For example, the focus of the educational sector is on student education; the economic sector, on enterprise and employment; the faith-based sector, on spirituality; the healthcare sector, on health promotion and disease prevention, etc.

        e. Individuals may belong to one or more community systems.

        f. Communities can also be defined from the broader sociological perspective of those social and political networks, which form linkages between and among individuals, community organizations and leaders

    3. *Organizing Concepts to Guide Approaches to Effective Community Engagement* (CDC/ATSDR, 1997)

        a. Social Ecology

            1) Social ecological theories seek to describe the community as a dynamic interplay between individuals and the environment in which they live (Stokols, 1996).

            2) Interventions designed to change individual health behaviors must be grounded within the social and cultural context of the lived experience (Spector, 2000).

            3) Motivation and attitudes of individuals within a designated community are heavily influenced by community norms and the structure of community services (Goodman, et al., 1996)

        b. Cultural Influences

            1) Health behaviors are significantly influenced by the cultural orientation of community members.

            2) Culture influences one's health beliefs and practices, including perceptions of health and illness, disease prevention methods, treatments for illness, and utilization of healthcare services (Spector, 2000)

            3) Community based interventional strategies must consider the cultural orientation of the community and its members

        c. Community Participation

            1) Key element in community engagement is the participation of those most closely affected by the effort, which includes individuals, community-based organizations and institutions.

    2) Community participation leads to neighborhood improvement and a stronger social fabric that can serve as a catalyst for change, especially as it relates to community health decision making and action.

  d. Community Empowerment

    1) Process by which communities are mobilized to act at the grass roots level to take action and influence decisions on critical issues

    2) Requires collaboration of individuals and institutions working together to effect mutually agreed upon outcomes

  e. Capacity Building

    1) Process by which individuals and organizations are assisted to acquire resources, knowledge, and skills needed to gain control and influence decision making and action (Fawcett et al., 1995)

    2) Additional training in the acquisition of resources may be required prior to initiating a community-based intervention

  f. Coalitions

    1) Rooted in political science; involves development of formal alliances among organizations, groups and agencies united for a common purpose (Florin, Mitchell, & Stevenson, 1993)

    2) Long-term partnerships formed by diverse groups of entities that plan, coordinate, and advocate for the needs of communities served (Butterfoss, Goodman, & Wandersman, 1993)

  g. Community Organization Approach (Minkler, 1990)

    1) Provides a path to engagement that facilitates identification of common problems, mobilization of resources, and development and implementation of strategies to reach mutually established goals

    2) Brings about change at the community level based on principles of empowerment, participation and capacity building

4. *Methods Used to Assess Community Assets*

  a. Asset Mapping (Parks & Straker, 1996)

    1) The boundaries of a community can be mapped to identify its primary, secondary and potential building blocks (CDC/ASTDR, 1997)

      a) Primary building block refers to those community assets and capacities located within the neighborhood and under its control.

      b) Secondary building block refers to community assets that are within the neighborhood but are largely controlled by outsiders.

      c) Potential building blocks refer to resources that originate inside of the neighborhood but are controlled by outsiders.

  b. Steps in the asset mapping process (CDC/ATSDR, 1997)

    1) Emphasis on problems and needs of communities highlights community weaknesses and dependence on outside solutions (Parks & Straker, 1996).

    2) Community capacity perspective capitalizes on resources and strengths available in the community as well as service gaps

    3) Stresses positive aspects of community, local definition and control, and relationships among community institutions (Parks & Straker, 1996)

    4) Develops inventories of local community institutions and agencies

    5) Includes identification of available medical resources (hospitals, primary care providers, local health centers, specialists, health education classes, etc.)

    6) Identifies health providers, elements of routine health assessment, health promotion, counseling and guidance, and provider barriers to care

    7) Process includes contact with clinical and administrative personnel to establish a link and working relationship between a community health project and area health care providers.

  c. Rapid Participatory Appraisal (Dale, Shipman, Lacock, & Davies, 1996; Murray, 1999; Murray, Tapson, Turnbull, McCallum, & Little, 1994)

    1) Successfully used to assess community level health service needs and develop meaningful interventions fully embraced by the community (Murray & Graham, 1995; Wilkinson & Murray, 1998)

    2) Process of discovery and engagement, ensuring locally relevant programs and evaluation measures as well as community commitment

3) Designed to maximize efficiency for data collection, analysis and reporting back to community in a very short time period

4) Focused on collection of action-oriented information to be used for planning and management

5) Multidisciplinary data collectors and different sources of data used to triangulate on problems and solutions; emphasizes community involvement in both data collection and analysis.

6) Pyramid conceptual structure of inquiry is based on community composition, organization and capacity to act at its base. The next level is made up of socioecological factors that influence health. The third level comprises existing social, health, and educational services. The top level is health policy.

7) Flexibility of model permits modification to local circumstance and opportunity to direct the inquiry to specific problems, such as minority health disparities.

8) Involves intensive semistructured interviews with key informants from the community, supplemental data from outside sources, analysis of major themes, presentation of themes to community informants for validation and formulation of action plans (Murray, 1999)

5. *Key factors to Success of Community Engagement* (CDC/ATSDR, 1997)
   a. Environmental
      1) History of collaboration or cooperation in the community
      2) Collaborating group and agencies seen as leader in community
      3) Favorable political and social climate
   b. Membership
      1) Mutual respect, understanding, and trust
      2) Appropriate cross-section of members
      3) Members see engagement benefits their self-interest and offset costs
      4) Ability to compromise
   c. Process/Structure
      1) Members feel ownership and share stake in both process and outcome
      2) Every level of collaborating groups participates in decision-making
      3) Flexibility of collaborating group
      4) Clarity of roles and guidelines
      5) Ability to sustain itself in the midst of changing conditions
   d. Communication
      1) Open and frequent interaction, information, and discussion
      2) Informal and formal channels of communications

6. *Purpose*
   a. Goals clear and realistic to all partners
   b. Shared vision
   c. Unique to the effort (i.e., different at least in part from mission, goals or approach of member organizations)

7. *Resources*
   a. Sufficient funds
   b. Skilled convener

8. *Nine Principles of Community Engagement* (CDC/ATSDR, 1997)
   a. Be clear about the purposes and goals of engagement effort and population to be served
   b. Become knowledgeable about the community's economic conditions, political structures, norms and values, demographic trends, history and experience with and perception of engagement efforts
   c. Go into community, establish relationships, build trust, work with formal and informal leadership, and seek commitment from community organizations and leaders to create processes for mobilizing community
   d. Accept that community self determination is the responsibility and the right of all people who comprise the community. No external entity should assume it can bestow on a community the power to act in its own self-interest.
   e. Partnering with the community is necessary to create change and improve health.
   f. All aspects of engagement recognize and respect community diversity. Awareness of various cultures and other factors of diversity needed in designing and implementing approaches

g. Only sustained by identifying and mobilizing community assets, and by developing capacities and resources for community decisions and action

h. Engaging organization or individual change agent must be prepared to release control of actions or interventions to community, and be flexible to meet changing needs of community.

i. Requires long-term commitment by engaging organization and its partners.

9. *Strategies to Building a Mutually Beneficial Partnership*

a. Develop partnerships with key community stakeholders

b. Conduct a community needs assessment

c. Identify disease/condition for the interventional project

d. Plan the intervention methodology with the community.

IX. SUMMARY

A. The chapter gave an overview of major thoughts drawn from selected disciplines and seminal examples of approaches supported by empirical and theoretical literature.

B. Health achievement is multidimensional requiring a broad foundation beyond nursing and individual-focused care to population-based care.

C. This chapter established the foundation for the remaining sections and is anticipated to assist health educators and practitioners to conceptualize innovative approaches to health care and education.

NOTE: All references, additional resources, and important Internet sites relevant to this chapter can be found at the following website: http://tcn.sagepub.com/supplemental

Chapter 4
Cross-Cultural Communication

Journal of Transcultural Nursing
21(Supplement 1) 137S–150S
© The Author(s) 2010
Reprints and permission:
sagepub.com/journalsPermissions.nav
DOI: 10.1177/1043659610374322
http://tcn.sagepub.com
SAGE

Robin L. Eubanks, PhD[1]
Marilyn R. McFarland, PhD, RN, FNP-BC, CTN-A[2]
Sandra J. Mixer, PhD, RN[3]
Cora Muñoz, PhD, RN[4]
Dula F. Pacquiao, EdD, RN, CTN[5]
Anna Frances Z. Wenger, PhD, RN, CTN, FAAN[6]

I. INTRODUCTION
    A. This chapter presents cultural concepts and principles essential to effective cross-cultural communication.
    B. It focuses on building cross-cultural communication skills, critical in transcultural nursing and health care.
    C. A case study is presented at the end of the chapter to enhance application of cultural knowledge and communication.

II. NATURE OF CROSS-CULTURAL COMMUNICATION
    A. Cross-cultural communication skills are critical in a global society where encounters with diverse groups are part of everyday life. All interactions are cross-cultural, as human beings tend to be bounded by a set of *symbols* and *meanings* that have been culturally imprinted in time (Samovar, Porter & McDaniel, 2004).
    B. Communication is a process that occurs whenever meaning is attributed to behavior or the residue of behavior.
        1. Cross-cultural or intercultural communication is between individuals and groups whose perceptions and symbol systems are distinct enough to alter the communication event (Samovar & Porter, 1995). Differences can occur across and within the same groups.
        2. Communication is symbolic, as it uses verbal, nonverbal, and visual representations to create shared meanings.
        3. Culture and communication are intricately bound; one cannot understand communication without understanding its social and cultural context.
        4. Communication is a complex process; language is at best an approximation of reality.
        5. In communication, one can only infer about the other; hence, seeking and giving feedback, facilitating comfort in the exchange, listening and observing, and using other resources, such as interpreters, are critical.
    C. Elements of Cross-Cultural Communication
        1. Perception (Singer, 1987)
            a. Process by which an individual selects, evaluates, and organizes stimuli from the external world.
            b. Based on beliefs, values, and attitude systems
        2. Verbal processes—how we talk to each other and think
        3. Nonverbal processes—use of actions to communicate

III. CULTURAL CONTEXT OF CROSS-CULTURAL COMMUNICATION
    A. Cultural values and beliefs
        1. Influence perceptions of the other's credibility, trustworthiness, and acceptance
        2. For example, belief in a person's capacity to bear pain as a sign of moral strength is likely to be associated with intolerance of patients overtly complaining of pain.

Funding: The California Endowment (grant number 20082226) and Health Resources and Services Administration (grant number D11 HPO9759).
[1]University of Medicine and Dentistry of New Jersey, Newark, NJ, USA (Health Literacy; Communicating with Established Family Hierarchy; Skills for Apologizing for Cross Cultural Errors)
[2]University of Michigan-Flint ,Bay City, MI, USA (Leininger's Action Modes in Conflict Resolution; Case Study)
[3]University of Tennessee -Knoxville, Knoxville, TN, USA (Leininger's Action Modes in Conflict Resolution; Case Study)
[4]Capital University, Columbus, OH, USA (Modes of Communication: Verbal and Non-Verbal Communication)
[5]University of Medicine and Dentistry of New Jersey, Newark, NJ, USA (Nature and Cultural Context of Cross-Cultural Communication)
[6]Goshen College, Goshen, IN, USA (High and Low Context Communication; Artifactual Cues in Non-Verbal Communication)

Corresponding Author: Dula F. Pacquiao, Email: pacquidf@umdnj.edu or dulafp@yahoo.com

Suggested Citation: Douglas, M. K. & Pacquiao, D. F. (Eds.). (2010). Core curriculum in transcultural nursing and health care [Supplement]. *Journal of Transcultural Nursing*, 21(Suppl. 1).

3. The value attached to cleanliness and absence of body odor in the dominant American culture creates bias against those who appear unkempt and those with strong body odor.

4. Cultural Dimensions affecting interactions (Hofstede, 1980)
   a. Collectivism vs. individualism
      1) Members of collectivist groups tend to value cooperation, harmony, and agreement with the group.
      2) Communication is less likely to be individualistic, competitive, or assertive.
      3) Face saving, conflict avoidance, and euphemistic communication prevails.
   b. Uncertainty avoidance—degree to which a culture feels threatened by ambiguous situations.
      1) Countries such as Germany and Japan tend to have high uncertainty avoidance.
      2) Trust takes longer to establish with different and new groups.
      3) Detailed communication and planning are needed.
      4) Long-term relationship is important.
   c. Power Distance—degree to which subordinate members accept power differences.
      1) The dominant culture in America values egalitarian relationship.
      2) Communication between superiors and subordinates is less formal.
      3) Use of first and nicknames in conversation is common.
   d. Masculinity and femininity—degree to which masculine or feminine traits are valued
      1) In feminine cultures, caring and nurturing behaviors are valued.
      2) Interdependence, supportive, and sympathetic interactions are preferred.
      3) Masculine cultures value success, materialism, competitiveness, and individual control of the situation that are reflected in assertive communication.

5. Cultural patterning of worldview (Kluckhohn & Strodtbeck, 1960)
   a. Belief in human nature
      1) The puritanical belief that man is essentially evil but perfectible is dominant in American culture.
      2) An individual is valued and trusted based on his/her good deeds and achievement.
      3) Reason and self-discipline are valued, minimizing emotionality in interactions.
   b. Relationship between humans and nature
      1) Cultures that subscribe to the belief that humans are subject to nature and gods may be prone to fatalistic beliefs.
      2) Fatalism is reflected in acceptance of status quo and risk avoidance.
      3) Individuals are less likely to take preventive actions and challenge authority believing that they cannot change fate.
   c. Time orientation
      1) Cultures place different emphasis on past, present, and future dimensions.
      2) Present time orientation is a characteristic of cultures that value present events and relationships.
      3) Present time–oriented communication is likely to be circuitous and indirect, emphasizing relationship rather than task completion.
      4) Present time–oriented individuals could pose challenge to future-oriented individuals, who care more about tasks than relationships and whose communication tends to be direct, businesslike, and cold.
      5) Edward T. Hall (1976) differentiated polychronic from monochromic cultures.
         a) *Monochronic* time-oriented individuals tend to focus at one task at a time and hate interruptions or distractions.
         b) In contrast, *polychromic*-oriented individuals focus on many aspects at the same time and may be more concerned by the character of the communication than completion of the task at hand.
   d. Activity orientation
      1) Cultures may value activity as *being* (spontaneous), *being-in becoming* (spiritual rather than material), or *doing* (accomplishments are measurable and observable).
      2) Latin cultures, for example, value spontaneous (being) activities. Interactions are personalistic and friendly and emphasize social acceptance.
      3) In contrast, the dominant American culture values achievement (doing), and members tend to be impatient with small talk, long-winded conversations, and prolonged greetings.
   e. Relational orientation
      1) Cultures prescribe the manner by which individuals and groups relate with each other.
      2) Authoritarian societies emphasize hierarchical and linear communication from the top down to those in the lower levels of hierarchy.

3) Negotiations are not encouraged between different levels of hierarchy.

4) Patients from these cultures may not question physicians, who are perceived to be in positions of higher authority.

6. High- and low-context communication

a. *High and low context* refers to the degree of context used in communication. Edward T. Hall (1976) first described a high-low context continuum.

b. Role of context in communication (Hall, 1976, pp. 85-86)

1) Culture as a selective screen

2) Code, context, and meaning as different aspects of a single event

3) High and low ends of the continuum

4) High-context communication has most of the information in the surrounding context and/or internalized by the actors within the culture or event.

5) Low-context communication has most of the information within the communication code itself.

7. Context and meaning

a. Context refers to the situation in which an event occurs (American Heritage Dictionary, 1991).

b. Spiro (1965) was one of the first anthropologists to study the role of context in determining meaning.

c. Hall (1976, 2000) argued that the meaning of a communication should be understood within its context.

d. Cultural context refers to the entirety of the life experiences and shared meanings of a particular group of people (Leininger, 1970; Leininger, 1995, p. 78).

8. High- and low-context cultures

a. All cultures have degrees of high- and low-context communication.

b. Specific cultures have characteristics that tend to be higher or lower in context and therefore can be known as high- or low-context cultures (Hall, 1976).

c. Major characteristics contrasting high- and low-context cultures (Wenger, 1991a & 1991b)

9. High- and low-context communication

a. Comparison of characteristics (Hall & Hall, 1990; Samovar, Porter, & McDaniel, 2004)

b. Emic and etic approaches (Gudykunst, Ting-Toomey, & Nishida, 1996)

c. Research studies

d. Phenomenon of care in a high-context culture (Wenger, 1988, 1991a)

e. Culture context and health care decision making (Wenger, 1995)

f. "Here-there" theme in a comparative study of two high-context refugee communities within a low-context dominant culture (Wenger, 2006)

g. High- versus low-context comparison of three cultures (Kim, Pan, & Park, 1998).

B. Environmental Context includes temporal, spatial, and social contexts.

1. Spatial environment refers to the location of communication

a. Conversations in hospital corridors are not conducive to elicit confidential information or build comfort of participants.

b. Private space is best for in-depth assessment.

2. Temporal factors affect the level of comfort and type of interactions.

a. Busy time schedules or end-of-shift times are not ideal in eliciting in-depth information.

b. An individual who is rushed is not likely to take time to interact.

3. Social environment refers to the people present, the relationships, level of trust, and acceptance among participants.

a. Gender, race, ethnicity and age differences can influence the nature and level of comfort of participants.

b. Class, economic, and educational differences can influence power and control by individuals of the interaction.

IV. MODES OF COMMUNICATION

A. Nonverbal Communication

1. Artifactual cues

a. *Artifacts* are objects produced or shaped by human workmanship that may be of archeological or historical interest (American Heritage Dictionary, 1991).

b. Tangible elements of culture consisting of physically existing objects that have meaning within the culture (Langness, 1980, p. 157)

   c. *Artifactual cues* refers to the relationships of artifacts to the cultural context that may assist one to understand the emic and etic meanings.
   d. Material culture as artifact
      1) Marvin Harris (1968) considered overt observable behavioral patterns as artifactual cues (Langness, 1980, p. 84)
      2) Cultural idealism views culture in mental and symbolic ways thus symbols and ways of thinking can be viewed as artifactual cues also (Langness, 1980, p. 84)
   e. Artifacts and Context (Malinowski, 1935, in Langness, 1980, p. 78)
      1) Danger of studying cultural objects in isolation
      2) Potential for changing the artifact into something it is not
   f. *Artifactual communication* refers to nonverbal ways that objects within the culture communicate preferences, ideas, tastes, values, and so on (Wood, 2004). Example of artifactual communication related to gender and nonverbal communication (http://www.saintmarys.edu/~berdayes/vincehome/courses/comm200/notes/nonverbalf02.htm)
   g. Importance of learning the *emic* meanings of artifactual cues before subjecting these to *etic* categorization and/or comparisons
2. **Eye contact**—degree of eye contact differs from culture to culture.
   a. Those with Eurocentric perspective perceive direct eye contact as positive and necessary in any communication.
   b. Others may interpret direct eye contact as rude, disrespectful, or even aggressive since the significance of eye contact is viewed differently in various cultures.
   c. Health care providers in Eurocentric society tend to view negatively patients who do not have direct eye contact during communication and interactions.
3. **Gestures and expression of emotion**—the White middle-class culture values open and direct expression of emotions.
   a. However, they differ in the amount of expressiveness of emotions, tone, pitch, and volume of voice compared to other groups.
   b. For example, African Americans express emotions in more dramatic way with a louder tone, pitch, and volume of voice.
   c. Asians tend to be more quiet, withdrawn, and private in their expression of emotions.
   d. Amount, types, and meanings of gestures used by individuals are also influenced by their culture.
4. **Use and meaning of silence**
   a. Silence is a therapeutic communication technique that is appropriate when allowing time for patient to reflect and then respond or when patients prefer not to disclose information.
   b. Use of silence and touch in communication are culturally influenced.
   c. Giger and Davidhizar (2003) identified the following techniques for responding to patients' silence:
      1) Avoid interrupting silence
      2) Analyze the meaning of silence considering patients' nonverbal behavior
      3) Have an accepting demeanor and attitude
      4) Provide support based on emotional behavior of the patient
      5) Encourage patient to break the silence and initiate conversation
5. **Use and meaning of touch**
   a. *Touch* is appropriate only when it is acceptable to the patient.
   b. Cultures differ radically as to what kind of touch is permitted and when.
   c. In general, it is more acceptable to touch a child or an elderly person in a comforting manner than an adult.
   d. Muñoz and Luckmann (2005) identified the following examples to minimize potential problems with regard to touch:
      1) Touching the head of a Southeast Asian child is unacceptable since the head has traditionally been considered the site of the soul in these cultures.
      2) Many Hispanic patients are accustomed to supportive touch or a gentle embrace.
      3) It is usually acceptable to touch a Hispanic patient when paying a compliment, because touch is generally viewed as a gesture of sincerity in this culture.

4) When talking with a Hispanic child, praise and smile while gently touching the head or the hand of the child or the baby.

5) Tapping the shoulder or touching the hand is generally considered appropriate for Asian and Hispanic adolescents.

6. **Spatial distancing**

a. Each cultural group defines its own rules for personal, social, and public space.

b. Use of personal space between individuals who are interacting is culturally influenced.

c. For some cultures, it is acceptable to stand closer while talking, have closer face-to-face interactions, and even touch more frequently.

d. Individuals from other cultures may tend to stand farther apart from each other and may have less touching.

e. Distance between people are respected and maintained as a wider space around individuals is established.

7. **Translation** (Martin & Nakayama, 2004)

a. *Translation* generally refers to the process of producing a written text that refers to something said or written in another language.

b. The original language text of a translation is called the *source text* and the text into which it is translated is the *target text*.

c. Translation studies traditionally emphasize issues of *equivalency*; however, intercultural communication process emphasizes more on the meaning and accuracy from one language to another.

d. Some languages have tremendous flexibility in expression; others have limited range of words.

8. **TRANSLATE Model** (Like, 2000): Considerations for translation

a. **Trust**

1) How will trust be developed in the triadic relationship between patient, interpreter, and health care provider?

2) How will trust be developed with patient's family and other health care providers?

b. **Role**

1) Identify role of the interpreter.

2) What is the role of the interpreter in the clinical encounter process?

3) Would it be a language translator, culture broker, interpreter of biomedical culture, patient advocate?

c. **Advocacy**

1) Advocacy for patient and family

2) How will advocacy and support for patient- and family-centered care occur?

3) How will power and loyalty issues be handled?

d. **Nonjudgmental attitude**

1) How can fair and nonjudgmental attitude be maintained during health care encounters?

2) How will personal beliefs, values, opinions, biases, and stereotypes be dealt with?

e. **Setting**

1) Where and how will medical interpretation occur during health care encounters?

2) Will salaried interpreters, contract interpreters, volunteers, or AT&T Language Line be used?

f. **Language**

1) Communication styles and methods

2) What methods of communication will be employed?

3) How will linguistic appropriateness and cultural competence be assessed?

g. **Accuracy**

1) Information is complete, thorough and factual.

2) How will knowledge and information be exchanged?

h. **Time**

1) How will time be monitored during the encounter?

2) How will time be appropriately managed during health care encounters?

i. **Ethical issues**

1) Privacy and confidentiality of information

2) How will potential ethical conflicts be handled during health care encounters?

3) How will confidentiality of clinical information be maintained?

C. Verbal Communication

   1. ***Interpretation***

   a. Interpretation is the process of verbally expressing what is said or written in another language.

   b. Interpretation can be either *simultaneous*, with the interpreter speaking at the same time as the original speaker, or *consecutive*, with the interpreter speaking only during the breaks provided by the original speaker.

   c. *CLAS standards*

   1) CLAS—Culturally and Linguistically Appropriate Services (CLAS)

   2) The first national standards for cultural competence in health care was developed in 2000 by the Department of Health and Human Services. (See Figure 1.)

   3) The 14 standards are organized in the following themes:

   a) *Culturally Competent Care*—health care organizations need to ensure that all their patients and consumers of services receive care that is sensitive and respectful of their cultural beliefs and practices and in their *preferred language.*

   b) *Language Access Services*

   (1) Health care organizations must provide language assistance to all patients and consumers of services with *limited English proficiency* at no cost to the patients/consumers and at all *points of contact* in the health care system.

   (2) Easily understood patient information and signage in the languages of the groups represented in the service area must be available.

   c) Organizational Supports

   (1) Health care organizations must develop and implement a strategic plan that includes clear goals and policies to provide culturally and linguistically appropriate services.

   (2) Organizational self-assessment and data collection must be integrated and periodically updated in the organization's management information system.

   (3) Collaborative partnerships with communities need to be developed.

   d. *Medical Interpreter Code of Ethics* (Muñoz & Luckmann 2005)

   1) *Confidentiality*—treat all information shared by the patient as confidential and will not be disclosed unless the patient provides consent.

   2) *Accuracy*—the spirit of the message must be conveyed thoroughly with no omissions or additions and ensure that the patient understands the questions and other information.

   3) *Completeness*—all information must be interpreted fully *except* when the information is offensive or insulting; in this case, the interpreter needs to discuss it with the health care provider before interpreting is done.

   4) *Conveying cultural frameworks*—since some words may not be interpreted directly or literally, the interpreter must explain relevant cultural practices to the health care provider.

   5) *Nonjudgmental attitude*—interpreters must not screen out any information that is disagreeable; rather, all information need to be interpreted and no judgments must be placed on the patients' comments and responses.

   6) *Client self-determination*

   a) The interpreter needs to provide opportunities for the patient to make a decision based on the information provided.

   b) The interpreter must refrain from any actions or words that may influence the patient's decision.

   7) *Attitude toward clients*—the interpreter must treat patients with dignity and respect and maintain a trusting relationship.

   8) *Acceptance of assignments*—interpreters need to recognize their own limitations and accept only assignments that suit their level of expertise and experience.

   9) *Compensation*—interpreters must accept only the fee that has been agreed upon; no other money, services, or favors can be accepted in their contractual obligation as interpreters.

   10) *Self-evaluation*—interpreters are responsible for necessary training, certifications, or continuing education to maintain professional status as interpreter.

   11) *Ethical violations*—interpreters need to adhere to the Code of Ethics and must withdraw from assignments that may be perceived as violations of ethical principles and practices.

   12) *Professionalism*—professionalism must be maintained at all times during the interaction including being punctual, respectful, and professional in appearance.

e. Role of interpreter
1) Adhere to Code of Ethics—interpreters must abide by the Code of Ethics and maintain ethical principles during interpretation.
2) Recognize own limitations—interpreters must not accept any assignment that requires skill and knowledge that they do not possess. Continuing education and further training may be needed to accomplish this task.
3) Be transparent—interpreter must have an open attitude and receptive demeanor during encounters.

f. Rationale for using interpreters
1) Quality of Care—use of interpreters leads to better outcomes in terms of health care services since communication of important information, instructions, and planning of care is facilitated.
2) Legal Mandate—the Civil Rights Act requires using interpreters for patients with limited language proficiency.
3) Cost-Effective
   a) When communication/linguistic barriers are addressed, patient-provider interaction is promoted.
   b) When patient and provider do not speak the same language, the provider tends to prescribe more diagnostics, which increase cost of health care.
4) Social Justice—every individual has the right to obtain quality health care from the providers, including the right to obtain understandable information on health care services.

g. Interpreter Competencies
1) Proficiency
   a) Level of skill and expertise in interpretation must be evaluated.
   b) This includes use of interpreters who are proficient in the language through formal training or certification or credentialed.
   c) Use of family members, friends, or hospital personnel who may be proficient in the language but do not have the qualifications mentioned should not be used as interpreters in a health care setting.
2) Linguistic parallels
   a) Knowledgeable about cultural beliefs, practices, and cultural framework to convey the spirit of the message when word to word interpretation is not possible.
   b) Convey the relevant concept in a manner that is culturally respectful and appropriate.

h. *National Standards of Practice for interpreters in Health Care* (National Council on Interpreting in Health Care, 2005; http://www.ncihc.org).
1) Statements of expectations and skills of trained/professional interpreters in health care to maintain consistent provision of quality services.
2) Standards are used for selecting and hiring interpreters as well as in training and monitoring their performance.
   a) Accuracy
      (1) Render all messages accurately
      (2) Replicate style and tone of speaker
      (3) Explain the interpreting process
      (4) Manage the flow of communication
      (5) Correct mistakes as soon as possible
      (6) Maintain transparency
      (7) Take into consideration the cultural context of the conversation in recognizing that there may not be a precise equivalent of the words in another language.
   b) Confidentiality
      (1) Does not disclose information other than with the team or with client's permission or if required by law
      (2) Maintains confidentiality of all written information
      (3) Maintains trust and honors private and personal nature of the interaction
   c) Impartiality
      (1) Remains objective
      (2) Discloses potential conflict of interest and withdraws from assignments if necessary
      (3) Refrains from counseling, advising, or projecting personal biases or beliefs

    d) Respect
       (1) Recognizes the inherent dignity of patients
       (2) Conveys respect in a professional and culturally appropriate manner
       (3) Promotes direct communication and patient autonomy
    e) Cultural Awareness
       (1) Develops awareness of the cultures encountered in the performance of interpreting duties
       (2) Alerts all parties to any significant cultural misunderstandings
    f) Role Boundaries
       (1) Maintains professional role boundaries
       (2) Limits personal involvement
       (3) Limits professional activity to interpreting within an encounter
       (4) Adheres to standards of practice while interpreting
    g) Professionalism
       (1) Honest and ethical
       (2) Prepared for all assignments
       (3) Discloses skill limitation
       (4) Avoids sight translation especially of complex or critical documents such as a consent form
       (5) Accountable
       (6) Advocates for working condition that support quality interpreting
       (7) Shows respect for other professionals
       (8) Behaves in a professional manner appropriate to the setting
    h) Professional Development
       (1) Furthers own knowledge and skills through independent study, continuing education, and actual interpreting practice
       (2) Seeks feedback to improve interpreting performance
       (3) Supports professional development of other interpreters
       (4) Participates in organization and activities that contribute to the development of the profession of interpreters
    i) Advocacy
       (1) Speaks out to protect an individual from serious harm
       (2) Advocates for a party or group to correct mistreatment or abuse
       (3) Advocates when the patient's health, well-being, or dignity is at risk

  i. INTERPRET MODEL (Medrano, 2002)
    1) **I**—Introduction; introduce and identify all participants.
    2) **N**—Negotiation; negotiate clear role for interpreter; agree on mode of interpretation (simultaneous or interval); clarify need for interpreter as culture broker.
    3) **T**—Trust; establish atmosphere of mutual trust.
    4) **E**—Engagement; speak directly to patient; use short, simple sentences; allow for patient to speak and interpreter to interpret before proceeding.
    5) **R**—Room-set-up; place interpreter's chair slightly behind patient.
    6) **P**—Patient centered; make an effort to ensure the history is complete and accurate; establish and address patient' agenda; ensure patient agreement and understanding of treatment plan and follow-up.
    7) **R**—Respect for cultural beliefs; elicit and acknowledge patient's cultural beliefs without necessarily agreeing with them.
    8) **E**—Ethical considerations; address ethical issues, such as confidentiality, gender issues, use of children as interpreters.
    9) **T**—Time management; manage the interview efficiently.

V. HEALTH LITERACY (Baker et al., 2002; Baker, Parker, Williams & Clark, 1997)

  A. *Illiteracy* has become an increasingly important problem, especially as it relates to health care. More than 90 million people in the United States have difficulty reading (Stedman & Kastle, 1991).
    1. According to the National Assessment of Adult Literacy, only 12% of adults score "proficient" on health literacy.
    2. Nearly 9 out of 10 adults may lack the skills needed to manage their health and prevent disease.

3. Fourteen percent of adults (30 million people) have "below basic" health literacy.
4. These adults were more likely to report their health as poor (42%) and are more likely to lack health insurance (28%) than adults with proficient health literacy.

B. Implications of poor health literacy (Andrus & Roth, 2002; Like, 2007; U.S. Department of Health and Human Services[USDHHS], 2008)
    1. Patients
        a. Poor health status, needless suffering
        b. Poor understanding and use of appropriate services
        c. Lack of knowledge of medical conditions
        d. Poorer compliance rates
        e. Increase health care cost; more experience with preventable hospital visits
        f. Higher rates of hospitalization
        g. Underutilization of preventive services (e.g., mammograms, pap smears, flu shots)
        h. Increased needless suffering and higher care dissatisfaction
    2. Increased provider frustration

C. ***Health literacy*** (Rudd, 2007; Shohet, 2002)
    1. According to *Healthy People 2010, health literacy* is the degree to which individuals have the capacity to process and understand basic health information and services needed to make good health decisions.
    2. *Health literacy* is the ability to act on health information.
    3. A functional type of literacy that allows adults to obtain, interpret, understand, and use information to promote and maintain health (Greenberg, 2001; Shohet, 2002).
    4. Health literacy goes beyond the ability to read health information; it includes the ability to describe symptoms, request information, advocate for one's rights, and take medication safely.
    5. It is dependent on both systemic and individual factors (Like, 2009), including:
        a. Demands of the health care and public health systems and situational context (USDHHS, 2008)
        b. Individual oral communication and comprehension skills, cultural background, and understanding of specific contexts (health topic, physician's everyday language) (Davis, Williams, Marin, Parker & Glass, 2002)

D. Health literacy includes numeracy skills
    1. Calculating cholesterol
    2. Blood sugar levels (McConnell-Imbriotos, 2001)
    3. Measuring medications (Estrada, Martin-Hryniewicz, Peek, Collins, & Byrd, 2004)
    4. Nutritional labels (Boehl, 2007)
    5. Calculating premiums and copays

E. Challenges to health literacy (Rudd, 2009)
    1. Medical and legal jargon (Castro, Wilson, Wang & Schillinger, 2007)
    2. Words with dual meanings
    3. Conceptual understanding of risks and benefits
    4. Comfort in asking questions

F. Importance of health literacy (Baker, 2006)
    1. Assists individuals in navigating the system
    2. Enables individuals to engage in self-care and chronic disease management
    3. Enables individuals to respond appropriately to health-related news

G. Misconceptions about people with low health literacy (Doak, Doak, and Root, 1996)
    1. People of low literacy are more likely to be intellectually impaired or slow learners.
    2. Majority of people with low literacy are poor, immigrants, and minorities.
    3. People with low literacy will tell you if they cannot read.

H. Components of basic health literacy
    1. Capacity to read and understand the "structure" of the text (e.g., prescription label)
    2. Familiarity with various text features (e.g., font, layout, or design)
    3. Visual, computer, and information literacy

I. Culture and health literacy
    1. Culture impacts interpretations, understanding, and implementation of diverse aspects of health literacy.
    2. Health care professionals have their own "culture" and language, which can affect how they communicate with the public.

3. A cultural group's ideas about authority, hierarchy, and communication style will impact the degree to which a person will obtain and process basic health-related information.

4. For example, reading skills in a second language may take 6 to 12 years to develop, and a patient's cultural background may express verbal and not written communication style.

5. Patients' perspectives on culturally and linguistically appropriate services provide important data and create opportunities for health care providers to improve the quality of care provided (Ngo-Metzger et al., 2006).

6. Culture affects communication styles (Viswanath & Kreuter, 2007), views of health and sickness (Spector, 2008), healers and caregivers, and responses to treatment and recommendations.

7. Culture affects appropriateness of cultural competency tools.

8. There are differences between lay/generic medicine and Western medicine (Spector, 2008).

9. Culture impacts on food practices, gender roles, body language, and so on

J. Vulnerable population groups at risk for poor health literacy

   1. Elderly (Kutner, Greenberg, Jin & Paulsen, 2006).

   2. Minority groups

   3. Immigrants

   4. Low-income groups

   5. People with chronic mental and/or physical health conditions

K. Negative psychological effects of Low Health Literacy

   1. Stigma and shame (Parikh, Parker, Nurss, Baker & Williams, 1996).

   2. Tendency to hide reading difficulties to maintain dignity (Baker et al., 1996)

   3. May develop ineffective strategies to compensate for difficulty

L. Practical signs of low health literacy

   1. Patient returning forms without completion

   2. Consistently arriving late for appointment

   3. Require several calls between appointment for clarity of instructions

   4. Patient's comments (e.g., "I forgot my glasses" or "My eyes are tired")

M. Assessment of Adult Literacy in the Health Context

   1. Individual Literacy

      a. REALM—Rapid Estimate of Adult Literacy in Medicine (Davis et al., 1993)

      b. TOFHLA—The Test of Functional Health Literacy in Adults (Parker, Baker, Williams & Nurss, 1995).

      c. SAHLSA—Short Assessment of Health Literacy for Spanish Speaking Adults (Shoou-Yih, Bender, Ruiz, & Cho, 2006).

   2. Issues regarding measures:

      a. Limited range of health literacy skills assessed

      b. No accounting of cultural differences in approaches of health.

N. Challenges in achieving health literacy

   1. Limited training and education of health providers (Nielsen-Bohlman, 2004)

   2. Long-term nature of educational programs

   3. Health information materials exceed reading ability of population being served

   4. Skills of navigation and negotiation of health care system not included in most training (Cegala, 2003).

O. Practical Strategies for Improving Health Literacy

   1. Identify population using the information (National Cancer Institute, 2008)

      a. Do materials reflect the population?

      b. Assess communication capacity of intended users.

      c. Utilize community's input in formatting and designing brochures and applicable forms.

      d. Utilize posttest to assess effectiveness of information.

   2. Health literacy screening questions (Wallace et al., 2007)

      a. How often do you have someone help you read hospital materials?

      b. How confident are you in filling out medical forms by yourself?

      c. How often do you have problems learning about your medical condition because of difficulty understanding written information?

   3. "Ask Me 3" Format (Partnership for Clear Health Communication/Ask Me 3, 2002)

      a. What is my main problem? (Diagnosis)

      b. What do I need to do? (Treatment)

      c. Why is it important for me to do this? (Context)

4. Use medically trained interpreters if necessary
5. Check for understanding—"check-back" method (Schillinger et al., 2003)
6. Establish a patient navigator program (National Literacy Act, 1991)
7. Revise forms to improve clarity and simplicity
8. Supplement instructions with visuals (Doak et al., 1996)
9. Plain Language Initiative (http://execsec.od.nih.gov/plainlang/)

P. Health Literacy and Reduction of Health Disparities
1. Address the challenges of informed consent forms (Paasche-Orlow, 2005).
2. Promote effective diffusion of health information at the community level (Nielsen-Bohlman, 2004).
3. Promote collaboration between health professionals, health and educational organizations, and communities.

VI. PRINCIPLES OF CROSS-CULTURAL COMMUNICATION IN SELECTED SITUATIONS

A. Negotiating with differences in status hierarchy
1. Identify members accorded higher status and authority in the family or group
2. Criteria used to define status and authority may differ from those used by health care professionals and mainstream society
3. Seek input from group members and observe their interactions with different members of their family or group
4. Observe cultural rules in addressing persons in authority
   a. Adapt degree of eye contact
      1) Use variable distance
      2) Direct questioning may be perceived as too intrusive
      3) Close may be perceived as rude
      4) Caution regarding use of touch; ask permission before touching
      5) Observe cultural norms in negotiating with gender and age differences
      6) Use honorific terms (mister, sir, ma'am); be formal unless corrected
      7) Use respectful tone of voice
      8) Consult/suggest rather than be directive with persons in authority

B. Apologizing for cultural mistakes
1. Do not hesitate to apologize.
2. Demonstrate congruent verbal and nonverbal behaviors when apologizing.
3. Admit own ignorance/limitations and state willingness to learn from the other.
4. Demonstrate how you can correct mistakes if possible; inform other staff about correct norms.
5. Avoid sounding defensive.
6. Open the interaction by admitting own cultural ignorance and seek cultural knowledge from others actively.
7. Seek feedback regarding behavior from the cultural context of the other.
8. Show appreciation for learning gained.
9. When in doubt, seek validation from the other about what you plan to do.

VII. USE OF LEININGER'S ACTION MODES IN CONFLICT RESOLUTION

A. Leininger's culture care theory uses three modes for transcultural nursing care decisions and actions:
1. Culture care preservation and/or maintenance refers to those assistive, supportive, facilitative, or enabling professional actions or decisions that help people of a particular culture to retain, preserve, or maintain beneficial care beliefs and values or face handicaps and death.
2. Culture care accommodation and/or negotiation refers to those assistive, accommodating, facilitative, or enabling creative provider care actions or decisions that help people from a culture (or subculture) adapt to or negotiate with others for culturally congruent, safe, and effective care for their health or well-being or to deal with illness or dying; achieve a beneficial/satisfying health outcome with professional care providers.
3. Culture care repatterning and/or restructuring refers to those assistive, supportive, facilitative, or enabling professional actions and mutual decision that would help people to reorder, change, modify, or restructure their lifeways and institutions for better (or beneficial) health care patterns, practices, or outcomes (Leininger, 1991, pp. 48-49; Leininger, 2002, p. 84; Leininger, 2006, p. 8).

B. Transcultural care decisions and action modes are used in contrast to nursing interventions. Nursing interventions are viewed by people in some cultures as "too controlling or all knowing" (Leininger, 2006, p. 9).

1. Leininger's actions and decision modes are essential for caring. Nurses use research data about cultural caring to apply to patient caring

    a. "Holding knowledge" guides nurses' actions and decisions.

    b. "Holding knowledge" is integrated with cultural assessment data to provide culturally congruent care specific to the person/family.

2. Modes incorporate patient/family "insider" knowledge with nursing "outsider" or professional knowledge.

3. Goal of the modes is meaningful care for patient/family satisfaction, recovery, and healing (includes death) (Leininger, 2002).

4. Once the nurse has completed a cultural assessment, the nurse uses the modes to facilitate creative and flexible ways to be sensitive to and meet the culture care needs of patients and families.

5. Since patients and families have strong desire for their cultural values, beliefs, and lifeways to be honored and respected, the nurse works with person(s) to determine what to preserve and maintain.

6. The nurse and patient/family discuss what can be accommodated and what may need to be negotiated.

7. As one proceeds toward restructuring/repatterning, the nurse treads lightly. Actions and decisions should reflect the patient and family health and well-being needs rather than the nurse's cultural bias, ethnocentrism, or cultural imposition (Leininger, 1991).

8. Thus, Leininger's transcultural nursing action and decision modes provide a concrete and practical way to provide culturally congruent care.

C. The following examples of research findings with application of Leininger's transcultural care decisions and action modes are useful for nurses in applying the culture care theory in their practice. These efforts build relationships among patients, families, and nurses, which contribute to effective cross-cultural communication and the provision of culturally congruent care.

    1. In a study of Mexican Americans receiving professional nursing care, Zoucha (1997) identified the following culture care modes necessary to provide culturally congruent nursing care:

        a. Mexican Americans identified the need for family and friend presence during health care delivery to promote a sense of security and connectedness.

            1) ***Preserve*** this care practice by allowing family members or friends to stay with the client in the health care delivery area (Zoucha, 1997, p. 39). Include family and friends in nursing and health care decisions and actions.

            2) Many Mexican Americans speak Spanish only and view a nurse who attempts to speak Spanish as caring.

        b. ***Accommodate*** by attempting a few Spanish phrases. Use an interpreter for accurate assessment data and communication.

            1) Other care needs of Mexican Americans are a context of friendlike relationship with the nurse to build understanding of one another. They also desire confidence in the nurse. Confidence in the nurse must be earned and is built through this relationship.

            2) ***Negotiate*** to spend more time with Mexican American clients to build this relationship and ***Accommodate*** the need for a personal and attentive relationship.

            3) To provide culturally congruent care, nurses must combine Mexican American generic care values within professional care practices.

        c. ***Restructuring*** and ***Repatterning*** of institutional and clinic contexts is required. Restructure work hours and provide financial support for nurses to learn Spanish. Employ nurses prepared in transcultural nursing with expertise in the Mexican American culture to teach colleagues and facilitate these restructuring and repatterning efforts (Zoucha, 1997).

            1) A study of chronically mentally ill persons living in the community provides another example of application of Leininger's action modes to provide culturally congruent care. George (2000) identified chronically mentally ill persons as a subculture. They desire normalcy while fearing rejection from the dominant culture.

            2) Nurses are encouraged to ***Preserve*** strengths exhibited by clients as they work toward increased independence in home and work settings. Positive lifeways can be supported through encouragement and praise.

            3) As nurses support clients' participation in the dominant culture, ***Accommodation*** and ***Negotiation*** are useful. For example, in planning a trip to attend the symphony, nurses negotiated with clients to dress properly. Clients were accommodated when nurses arranged to have a few of the musicians visit the mental health activity center to meet clients before the concert.

4) ***Restructuring*** was suggested for clients with survival care needs. For example, sleeping in a packing box was viewed as a potentially harmful lifeway. Nurses are encouraged to assist clients in restructuring to locate and accept temporary shelter and eventually find more permanent living quarters.

VIII. SUMMARY

A. Cross-cultural communication is a key instrument in the provision of cultural competent care that can impact on reducing health disparities.

B. Understanding and negotiating with social and cultural contextual variables of communication are significant in cross-cultural interactions.

C. Health care is primarily interactive, and cross-cultural communication skill bridges differences between professionals and laypeople and between diverse values, beliefs, and attitudes.

Case Study

Objectives: The learner will:

1. Describe the importance of cross-cultural communication in assessing cultural values, beliefs, and practices of patients to provide culturally congruent care.
2. Discuss strategies to address cross-cultural communication using Leininger's modes for transcultural nursing care decisions and actions.

As part of a transcultural nursing course, a student conducted an interview with a person from another culture to learn about providing culturally competent nursing care. The nursing student, Abasi (pseudonym), was born and raised in Nigeria and has been living in the United States for 9 years. She is married and the mother of two sons, one born in Nigeria and one born at a local urban medical center.

Abasi chose to interview a mother who is Haitian to learn about culture, values, beliefs, and practices surrounding her postpartum care. The mother described that in an effort to avoid postpartum complications, Haitian women eat hot spicy soup three times a day for a least 1 month. The soup, which consists of seaweeds, rice, beans, and other ingredients, is believed to "help clean the blood, provide calcium, and improve the breast milk supply." Mothers are not allowed to drink cold fluids, as they are believed to be harmful to their bodies, causing headaches, arthritis, or digestive dysfunction.

The mother described the care she received at an area medical center during the postpartum phase of having her last child. She stated that she tried to tell the nurse she could have only hot spicy soup or hot water; however, the nurse insisted she drink ice water and apply cold compresses to her wounds. The mother, whose cultural values, beliefs, and practices involve respecting persons in authority and avoiding conflict, "at last had to obey the American culture and drink cold water instead of hot fluid." The mother reported that her wounds healed; however, she had diarrhea and was worried she would develop chronic diseases. She stated that despite this incident happening 5 years ago, it is still just as vivid today.

Abasi, the nursing student reflected:

From this experience, as a foreigner and mother, I can understand her painful feelings because cultural misunderstandings always happen to people on the other side of the culture. Most of the time, foreigners have to comply with the American culture and abandon their own culture, leading to feelings of extreme sorrow. Through my paper, I hope that the new generation of nurses would understand patients' feelings and learn to negotiate and/or accommodate their needs. As an illustration, in this case, if the hot spicy soup has no implications for the treatment of the new Haitian mother, I think the nurses should have accommodated her desire to eat the soup and negotiate with her to also drink ice water since that is the norm in the United States (R. Omitaomu, Personal Communication, December 5, 2008).

<u>Critical Thinking Questions:</u>

1. Neither the nurse nor the patient ever came to a common understanding of one another or the pathophysiological or cultural concerns underlying this conversation. After learning about Leininger's modes for nursing actions and decisions, how would you handle this situation if you were the nurse?
2. How might you encourage a fellow nurse to address a similar situation in the future?
3. What central constructs and theoretical tenets described by Leininger and expressed in her culture care theory would be useful to apply in this scenario?

Discussion:

1. Integrating cultural values, beliefs and practices into pregnancy and postpartal care:
   a. Nurses struggle to provide culturally congruent postpartal care
      1) Complicated by limited postpartal time in the acute care setting.
      2) "The first step toward cultural competence . . . is to acknowledge overtly the value and respect of the women to be served" (Mayberry, Affonso, Shibuya, Clemmens, 1998, p. 19).
      3) Nurses need to be open-minded, be creative, and have a presence with patients.
      4) Daily lifeways, such as diet, are essential for a woman's adaptation, recovery, and the health of her child (Mayberry et al., 1998).
2. Hispanic women's perceptions of patient centeredness:
   a. Identified the need for emphasis on warm, interpersonal relationships; relaxed atmosphere and sense of time; and interpreters for effective communication
      1) Hispanic mothers felt less respected by doctors and nurses than non-Hispanic mothers.
      2) Due to language barriers, many Hispanic mothers did not understand information shared by doctors and nurses.
   b. Findings suggest these issues may be contributing to Hispanic mothers' underutilization of services (Tandon, Parillo, & Keefer, 2005).
3. Health seeking behaviors of Haitian families:
   a. Haitian families generally reported satisfaction with health care providers; may be due to local physician commitment to serving families in their communities and many staff were Haitian.
   b. Importance of culturally diverse workforce.
      1) Families reported using a combination of biomedical health care services and folk/traditional practices
      2) Drinking tea was widely reported and reflective of Haitian belief that illness is a disequilibrium between hot and cold factors (Schantz, Charron, & Folden, 2003, p. 67).
      3) Overall use of home remedies was less than expected. Researchers are concerned that participants may have been reluctant to admit folk remedy use, or the findings could reflect assimilation into American culture (Schantz, Charron, & Folden, 2003).

NOTE: All references, additional resources, and important Internet sites relevant to this chapter can be found at the following website: http://tcn.sagepub.com/supplemental

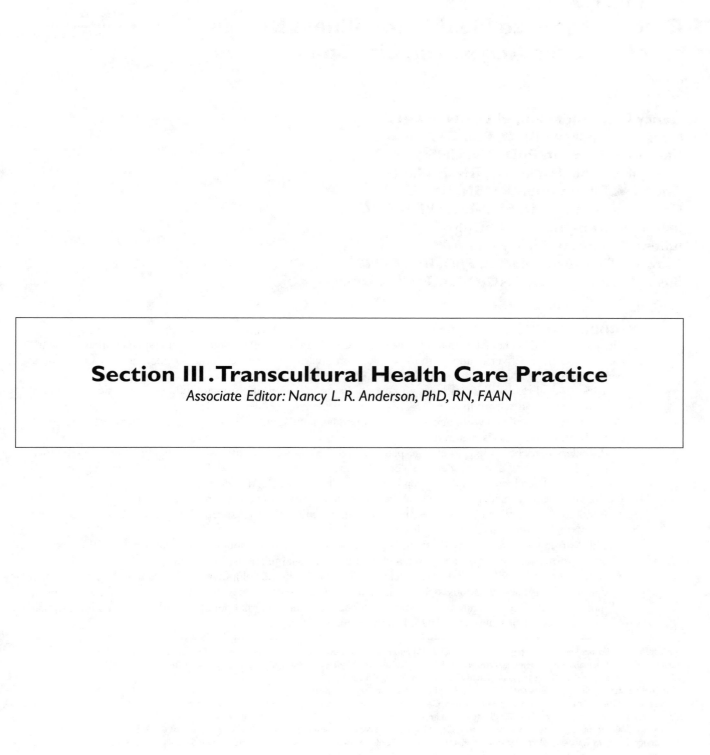

Section III. Transcultural Health Care Practice

Associate Editor: Nancy L. R. Anderson, PhD, RN, FAAN

Chapter 5
Culturally Based Health and Illness Beliefs and Practices Across the Life Span

Journal of Transcultural Nursing
21(Supplement 1) 152S–235S
© The Author(s) 2010
Reprints and permission:
sagepub.com/journalsPermissions.nav
DOI: 10.1177/1043659610381094
http://tcn.sagepub.com
⑤SAGE

Nancy L. R. Anderson, PhD, RN, FAAN[1]
Margaret Andrews, PhD, RN, CTN, FAAN[2]
Katherine N. Bent, PhD, RN, CNS[3]
Marilyn K. Douglas, DNSc, RN, FAAN[4]
Cheryl V. Elhammoumi, MSN, RN, CCRN[5]
Colleen Keenan, PhD, FNP-BC, WHNP-BC[1]
Jeanne K. Kemppainen, PhD, RN[6]
Juliene G. Lipson, PhD, RN, FAAN[4]
Carolyn Thompson Martin, PhD, RN, CFNP[7]
Susan Mattson, PhD, RNC-OB, CTN, FAAN[8]

I.   INTRODUCTION

A.   The purpose of this chapter is to anchor health care within the context of the ethical responsibilities of health care providers to deliver quality care to people from diverse personal, cultural, social, and global contextual backgrounds.

   1.   These ethical responsibilities must go beyond the assimilation of cross-cultural and linguistic knowledge, competence, and sensitivity.

   2.   An appreciation of and willingness to learn individual, family, cultural, and social group perspectives regarding health and illness is required.

   3.   Providers must be willing to engage patients and their families in assessment, dialogue, and negotiations regarding patients' and providers' explanatory models (Ems; Helman, 2000; Kleinman, Eisenberg, & Good, 1978, 2006) and health and illness representations (Farmer & Good, 1991).

B.   Health beliefs are formed and health practices are enacted within the context of everyday life.

   1.   Beginning at the time of birth, people learn and assimilate their perspectives regarding health and illness within their cultural and social worlds.

   2.   This learning becomes internalized and is gradually modified throughout their lives as a result of their experiences, formal and informal education, and their interpersonal relationships.

   3.   Bronfenbrenner (1995) describes this as a gradually evolving developmental process based on a culturally defined age, role expectations, opportunities, and the timing of the person's life course. Within this context, individuals engage in a mutual accommodation between their internal beliefs and an ever changing external environment (Bronfenbrenner, 1995; Bronfenbrenner & Ceci, 1994).

Funding: The California Endowment (grant number 20082226) and Health Resources and Services Administration (grant number D11 HPO9759).

[1]University of California at Los Angeles, Los Angeles, CA USA (Explanatory Models of Health & Illness; Adolescence: Rites of Passage)
[2]University of Michigan -Flint, Flint, MI, USA (Child Care and Parenting Practices)
[3]National Institutes of Health, Bethesda, MD, USA (End-of-Life Decisions and Practices)
[4]University of California at San Francisco, San Francisco, CA, USA (End-of-Life Decisions; Organ Donation & Transplantation)
[5]East Carolina University, Greenville, NC, USA (Cultural Implications for Care of Patients with Acute Illness)
[6]University of California at Los Angeles, Los Angeles, CA USA (Cultural Norms related to Gender, Sexuality and Sexual Orientation)
[7]University of North Carolina -Wilmington, Wilmington, NC, USA (Cultural Factors in the Care of Patients with Sexually-Transmitted Illnesses)
[8]University of California at San Francisco, San Francisco, CA, USA (Living with Disabilities)
[9]California State University Stanislaus, Turlock, CA, USA (Cultural Influences on Ageing and Older Adults)
[10]Arizona State University, Tempe, AZ, USA (Birth and Neonatal Care Practices; Reproduction, Pregnancy and Post Partum Care Practices)

Corresponding Author: Marilyn K. Douglas, Email: martydoug@comcast.net

Suggested Citation: Douglas, M. K. & Pacquiao, D. F. (Eds.). (2010). Core curriculum in transcultural nursing and health care [Supplement]. Journal of Transcultural Nursing, 21(Suppl. 1).

C. Discussion of *theories of disease causation* and the *meaning of symptoms* and symptom management provides a basis for the exploration of ethical issues in health promotion, prevention and treatment across the lifespan.

   1. Clinicians need to learn how to partner with socioculturally and economically diverse patients in assessing how they manage health and illness in the context of their gender identity, religious and spiritual beliefs and practices, and *culturally ascribed sick roles.*

   2. This requires commitment from clinicians to determine patients' perceptions of their health or illness, and to negotiate and/or partner with them to achieve the best approaches to health promotion and disease treatment.

II. CULTURAL EXPLANATORY MODELS OF HEALTH AND ILLNESS

A. Cultural Definitions of Health

   1. Health is often defined by people from many cultural groups as the *absence of illness* and is based on
      a. Personal perceptions of well-being and personal health
      b. Family and cultural health beliefs and practices
      c. Sociocultural systems of beliefs and practices in dynamic interaction within the context of the environment (Foster, 1976; Foster & Anderson 1978)
      d. Beliefs about the structure and functions of the body (Helman. 2000).
         (1) Optimal body shape
         (2) Body boundaries
         (3) Inner structure
         (4) Body function

   2. The meaning of health derives from its relationship to social and cultural roles and the ability to carry out responsibilities for
      a. Family
         (1) Care and protection of children and elders
         (2) Economic support
         (3) Education and enculturation to family and cultural values
      b. Work
      c. Community

B. Cultural Definitions of Illness: Cultural Beliefs and Theories of Disease Causation

   1. *Background*
      a. "Understandings of disease causation, its dynamics, and treatment are elements of the culture of an individual" (Fabrega & Manning, 1979, p. 41).
      b. Even highly acculturated people from diverse and mixed ethnic and cultural backgrounds retain perceptions about illness from their culture of origin and family folklore.
      c. Social science and clinical research, field studies, and clinical experiences contribute to our understanding of theories of disease causation and illness experiences of diverse cultures.

   2. *Health and Illness Belief Systems*
      a. Personalistic systems based on the belief that illness is caused by ". . . active, purposeful intervention of a *sensate* agent . . ." (Foster & Anderson, 1978, p. 53)
         (1) Supernatural being (a deity, god)
         (2) Nonhuman being (ghost, evil spirit)
         (3) Human being (witch, sorcerer)
         (4) Examples of personalistic causes of illness
            (a) Evil eye (Aguirre Beltran, 1963; Dundes, 1992; R. Spector, 2000, 2008; see Table 5.1 on selected folk illnesses)
            (b) Witchcraft
      b. Naturalistic systems based on the belief that illness results from imbalance of *insensate* elements or humors in the body (e.g., heat and cold, yin and yang).
         (1) Rooted in the early Greek characterization of the four elements (earth, water, air, and fire), the bodily humors included (Foster & Anderson, 1978, p. 56)
            (a) Blood (hot, moist)
            (b) Phlegm (cold, moist)
            (c) Black bile (cold, dry—melancholy)
            (d) Yellow bile (hot, dry—choler/anger)

Table 5.1. Selected Folk Illnesses

Folk Illness	Groups	Symptoms	Emic Etiology	Folk Treatment	Healer	Citations
Falling-out (fainting, indisposition)	African Americans, Bahamians, Haitians	Collapse without warning; no convulsions or epileptic signs	Blood rises to head and brain in times of extreme anger, fear, uncertainty; spirits, God, omens may be seen as cause	Prayer and spiritual healing	Orthodox, spiritualist, or sorcerer	Weidman (1979)
Empacho	Latino/Hispanic	Diarrhea, bloating, indigestion, vomiting, lethargy	Food believed to form a ball that clings to the stomach resulting in cramps and pain; linked to gastroenteritis in infants and children	Massage of the abdomen, teas, and in some cases lead-based remedies	Home treatment by mothers and folk healers	Andrews and Boyle (1999), Spector (2000), Weller et al. (1993), Baer et al. (1998)
Pibloktoq (Arctic hysteria)	Polar Eskimos	May be preceded by irritability; speaking meaningless words, phrases, running away, taking off clothing, imitative behaviors, acting in a bizarre manner	Considered to be a physical illness like a cold—seen in humans and dogs	Patient does not respond to others, often sleeps after the episode and wakes up feeling normal		McElroy and Townsend (1989)
Koro	Chinese	Intense fear, nausea, dysuria, diarrhea, anxiety	Pathological fear that penis will retract into abdomen followed by death		Traditional healer, or orthodox care	Bartholomew (1994), Kleinman (1980)
Susto	Latino/Hispanic	Anxiety, trembling, phobias, listlessness, anorexia, loss of strength, depression	Sudden fright, emotional stress, soul loss	Massage, encourage to relax, rites to coax the soul back to the body	Curandero or Curandera	Rubel, O'Nell, and Collado-Ardon (1985), Spector (2000, 2008)
Evil eye	Greek, Central American, Iranian, Islamic peoples, Southeast Asians, Hindus (dates back to ancient times, continues today in some form among some members of all groups and socioeconomic levels)	Varies based on the specific illness following perception that the patient was the object of envy	Staring at or praising the person or person's possessions (often a child); perceived by the offended family that the offending person is motivated by envy	Rituals; wearing an amulet (such as a blue bead, medal, string, or visible or invisible mark on the face or body)	Protection against evil eye is practiced in many families; most protective strategies are employed by the person or the family	Aguirre Beltran (1963), Dundes (1992), Kaya et al. (2009), Spiro (2005)

Table 5.2. Hot and Cold Illnesses and Respective Treatment Examples

Illness Category and Designation	Cultural Group(s)	Folk Remedies and Designation	Sources
Arthritis (cold)	Puerto Ricans, Guatemalans	Hot (such as chili peppers, corn meal, kidney beans)	Harwood (1971), Helman (2000)
Diabetes mellitus (hot)	Hispanics	Cold [Nopal (cactus), aloe vera juice]	Ortiz et al. (2007)
Asthma (cold)	Hispanics	Hot (oregano, onion/garlic, lemon, honey)	Bearison et al. (2002), Ortiz et al. (2007)
Nausea in Pregnancy (too much yin—a cold condition)	Chinese	Yang—hot (soup, broth, and hot herbal remedies)	Lipson and Dibble (2005), Yeh et al. (2009)

Notes: Hot/cold therapies and herbal remedies are most commonly used in conjunction with Western and/or traditional therapies as complementary or alternative medicine (CAM). Although many of the folk remedies are safe, others are not (See Table 6.9 (Chapter 6) describing safety of CAM remedies in Complementary and Alternative Therapies below). The methods used to obtain emic data regarding hot/cold treatments may have overemphasized and perpetuated the concept of hot/cold dichotomous folk remedies (Tedlock, 1987).

(2) Dual forces of yin and yang considered to maintain harmony in all aspects of life and health (Chinese medicine)

(3) Maintaining body equilibrium of the humors often requires the proper balance (see also Complimentary and Alternative Therapies below):

    (a) Foods designated as "hot" or "cold" (Andrews & Boyle, 2008; Bearison, Minian, & Granowetter, 2002; Foster & Anderson, 1978; Harwood, 1971; Helman, 2000; Ortiz, Shields, Clauson, & Clay, 2007; Yeh et al., 2009) in:

        i. India (Ayurvedic medicine)

        ii. China, and some other Asian countries

        iii. Some Arab and north African countries (and among some Moslems and Jewish people)

        iv. Some Hispanic countries

    (b) Prescriptions and proscriptions of hot and cold foods are based on the humoral concept rather than temperature or spiciness of the foods.

    (c) The goal is to create a balance in the body when exposed to or experiencing an illness (see Table 5.2 on hot and cold illness remedies)

        i. Illnesses considered to be hot are treated with cool or cold foods

        ii. Illnesses considered to be cold are treated with hot foods

    (d) Tedlock (1987) cautions care in the conduct and interpretation of research regarding the hot–cold dichotomy. She blended depth interviewing in highland Guatemala, examination of curing texts, with formal healing training and found that healers did not include hot–cold categories in their explanatory models of illness etiology.

c. Helman (2000) characterizes lay beliefs about causation as emerging from four areas in a model of four concentric circles, one inside the other beginning with the inner circle and proceeding to the outside:

    (1) The individual

    (2) The natural world

    (3) The social world

    (4) The supernatural world

3. *Explanatory Models (EMs)*

a. Definition

    (1) An EM serves as a definition of the etiology and experience of sickness. Based on their varied background knowledge and experience patients and health care providers often define sickness in different ways creating a potential for misunderstanding and health disparities (Kleinman et al., 1978, 2006).

    (2) People make sense of their own and family members' illnesses by trying to figure out the cause and the meaning of the illness experience in their everyday lives.

    (3) Western health care providers focus primarily on the physical aspects of disease.

b. Kleinman (1988) identified two primary EM categories or causal models:

    (1) Beliefs originating in the experience of *illness* (patients'/families' perspectives)

    (2) Beliefs originating in biomedical and physical concepts of *disease* (clinicians' perspectives)

(3) These different ways of viewing sickness may lead to confusion between patients and providers resulting in undesired health outcomes.

c. The etiology of perceived sickness rarely resides in only one causation and treatment arena

d. Rather a combination of explanations often occurs:

(1) Patients may accept some aspect of clinicians' explanations based on the Western medical EM, and

(2) at the same time retain naturalistic or personalistic components in their EM

(3) Rarely communicated to clinicians. For example, Farmer and Good (1991) describe a case of a Haitian man who, while accepting the biomedical cause of HIV/AIDS as a virus, continues to express concern about "who sent the virus" thus simultaneously maintaining the biomedical explanation and a personalisitc belief that some being sent the virus to sicken him.

4. *Assessment of Explanatory Models* (see Table 5.3 for studies evaluating EM examples)

a. To avoid miscommunication between patients' *illness* perceptions and clinician's biomedical *disease* perceptions, health providers need *to listen* to patients explain their perceptions about their sickness or EM and in turn explain their provider.

b. Kleinman (1980, p. 106) suggests asking the following questions to elicit patients' EMs (see Table 5.4 for Kleinman's Explanatory Model Questions):

(1) What do you call your problem? What name does it have?

(2) What do you think has caused your problem?

(3) Why do you think it started when it did?

(4) What does your sickness do to you? How does it work?

(5) How severe is it? Will it have a short or a long course?

(6) What do you fear most about your sickness?

(7) What are the chief problems your sickness has caused for you?

(8) What kind of treatment do you think you should receive?

(9) What are the most important results you hope to receive from the treatment?

c. Helman (2000, p. 85) lists five aspects of EMs for *both clinicians and patients*, aspects that coincide with Kleinman's questions (1980):

(1) Etiology or cause of the condition

(2) Timing and mode of onset of symptoms

(3) Pathophysiological processes involved

(4) Natural history and severity of the illness

(5) Appropriate treatments for the condition

d. Kleinman (1980) developed a mini-ethnographic approach to further explore patients' explanatory models with an altered set of questions (see Table 5.4 for Kleinman's Explanatory Model Questions):

(1) Why me?

(2) Why now?

(3) What is wrong?

(4) How long will it last?

(5) How serious is it?

(6) Who can intervene or treat the condition?

e. Lloyd et al. (1998) used these questions as the basis for developing the Short Explanatory Model Interview (SEMI) with a blend of Kleinman's original (1978, 1980) and 1988 versions and added some additional questions and guidance:

(1) Naming the condition

(2) What causes it?

(3) Is it an illness?

(4) Who do you see about it?

(5) What can you do about it?

(6) What can your doctor do about it?

f. M. G. Weiss et al. (1992) developed the Explanatory Model Interview Catalogue (EMIC):

(1) Patterns of distress

(2) Perceived causes

(3) Disease-specific queries

Table 5.3. Examples of Studies in Which Explanatory Models (EMs) Were Evaluated

Authors (Year)	Purpose	Population	Methods	Conclusions
Aidoo and Harpham (2001)	Comparison of EMs of mental ill health among urban women and local health professionals	Low-income urban women and local providers in Zambia	Qualitative interviews using Kleinman's EM questions as a model for their questions	Women talked about "problems of the mind"; Professionals called this "stress and depression"
McSweeny, Allan, and Mayo (1997)	Address gap in nursing literature that lacks information on how to elicit cultural beliefs	Healthy people after illness and people with a potential health risk condition	In-depth interviews and content analysis using Kleinman's EM framework	Assessing EMs offers ways to explore linkages between beliefs and behaviors
Sumathipala et al. (2008)	Elicit illness perceptions of patients with medically unexplained symptoms (MUS)	68 patients (16-65 years old) with MUS in Sri Lanka	Short Explanatory Model Interviews (SEMI)	The illness perception model uncovered continued distress about persistent symptoms; but most participants did not identify a cause (Western medicine or cultural terminology). The results contributed to development of culturally sensitive interventions
Lynch and Medin (2006)	Explore causal models of heart attack and depression for domain-specific vs. cross-domain beliefs	RNs, RN energy healers, energy healers, undergraduates	Laddering methods based on means–end chain theory (as in market research) to elicit causal models	Energy healers crossed domains between physical and mental beliefs; undergraduates and RNs remained mostly domain specific
Garro (1995)	Explore the EMs about diabetes mellitus (DM) in an Anishinaabe community in Manitoba, Canada	Ojibway adults with DM (females > males) with a mean age of 49 years	Interviews using an open-ended EM framework followed by statements (true/false) about diabetes	Most of the explanations beyond individual dietary choices linked DM to environmental and social change—seen as a disruption in the Anishinaabe way of life
J. M. Anderson (1986)	Analyze families experience with chronically ill child	Anglo-Canadian and immigrant Chinese families	In-depth interviews with parents and observations (parent–child interaction	Immigrant parents saw caretaker role as "looking after" and fostering "contentment"; Anglo-Canadian parents saw caretaker role as "normalization" similar to professionals
Payne-Jackson (1999)	Study patient reports of information regarding management of diabetes	Patients with adult-onset diabetes in Jamaica	In-depth interviews, free listing, tape recordings of doctor–patient appointments	Differences in doctor and patient explanatory models resulted in miscommunication

    (4) Seeking help and treatment

    (5) General illness beliefs

  g. In addition to the term *explanatory models*, a few alternate descriptions of how people describe their illnesses include the following:

    (1) Illness narratives—as in qualitative research

    (2) Illness representations—based on critical theory (Farmer & Good, 1991)

    (3) Illness cognition (Leventhal, Diefenbach, & Leventhal, 1992)

    (4) Cultural formulations (Bucardo, Patterson, & Jeste, 2008)

Table 5.4. Kleinman's Explanatory Model Interview Questions

Interview questions to elicit explanatory models (Kleinman (1980, p. 106)

  1. What do you call your problem? What name does it have?
  2. What do you think has caused your problem?
  3. Why do you think it started when it did?
  4. What does your sickness do to you? How does it work?
  5. How severe is it? Will it have a short or a long course?
  6. What do you fear most about your sickness?
  7. What are the chief problems your sickness has caused for you?
  8. What kind of treatment do you think you should receive? What are the most important results you hope to receive from the treatment?

Mini-ethnographic approach to further explore patients' explanatory models (Kleinman, 1988)

  1. Why me?
  2. Why now?
  3. What is wrong?
  4. How long will it last?
  5. How serious is it?
  6. Who can intervene or treat the condition?

---

5. ***Culture-bound syndromes*** (CBS); also called
    a. Culture-specific disorders (Foster & Anderson 1978),
    b. Culture-bound reactive syndromes (McElroy & Townsend, 1989)
    c. Folk illnesses (Helman, 2000; Rubel, O'Nell, & Collado-Ardon, 1985)
    d. These illnesses usually present as
        (1) "Culturally unique patterns" of behaviors, as in temporary psychosis or phobic states (Kleinman 1980, p. 77)
        (2) Without a "discernible biochemical basis" (McElroy & Townsend, 1989, p. 278)
        (3) Disorders that occur in the context of symbolic meaning, social interaction, and group norms (Kleinman, 1980)
        (4) Created by personal, social, and cultural reactions to adverse situations (Andrews & Boyle, 1999, 2008)
        (5) Some anthropologists argue that some CBS are not as culture bound as previously considered (Ruble et al., 1985; Sumathipala, Siribaddana, & Bhugra, 2004) or incidence will decrease with modernization (McElroy & Townsend, 1989)
        (6) Although CBS and folk illness terminology are often used interchangeably:
            (a) CBS are seen primarily in only one or a few cultures
            (b) Folk illnesses are found in many cultural groups
            (c) Folk illness terminology is seen as a more inclusive term (Weller, Pachter, Trotter, & Baer, 1993)
            (d) Table 5.1 presents a combination of CBS and folk illnesses classified as *Folk Illnesses*
    e. Many CBS and folk illnesses present with somatic symptoms of psychological origin (see Mental Health Beliefs in chapter 6 for further descriptions)
  C. **Meanings of Symptoms and Symptom Management**
    1. The search for the meaning of symptoms and symptom management approaches represent a universal endeavor regardless of cultural and ethnic group. This search for meaning extends beyond CBS and folk illnesses.
        a. ". . . symptoms are grounded in the social and cultural realities of individual patients" (Good & Delvecchio Good, 1981, p. 166).
        b. Patients communicate their symptoms in a variety of ways (Good & Delvecchio Good, 1981; Kisely & Simon, 2006) through
            (1) somatic,
            (2) psychological, or
            (3) interpersonal idioms
        c. When symptoms do not respond to Western medical treatment, providers may characterize patients' symptoms as
            (1) Medically unexplained symptoms (Escobar et al., 2007; Olde Hartman et al., 2008)
            (2) Medically ambiguous symptoms (Karasz, Dempsey, & Fallek, 2007)

        (3) Idiopathic physical symptoms (Escobar, Interian, Diaz-Martinez, & Gara, 2006)

        (4) Somatoform disorders (Kirmayer & Sartorius, 2007)

        (5) Somatic syndromes (Ranjith & Mohan, 2006)

        (6) The World Health Organization (WHO) suggests somatoform disorders may represent a way for specific cultural groups to express psychosocial distress (Isaac et al., 1995)

  2. Individual, family, and cultural approaches to symptom management

     a. Illness is usually first recognized, named, and treated within the family, most often by mothers or grandmothers (Chrisman, 1977; Helman, 1991)

     b. Majority of symptoms dealt with in sequence by

        (1) The sick person

           (a) Notices symptoms, changes in behavior, body appearance or function (Helman, 2000)

           (b) Self-diagnosis (based on their explanatory model)

           (c) Self-treatment with over-the-counter, traditional, and/or folk remedies (Helman, 1991)

           (d) Self-care (Lipson & Steiger, 1996)

        (2) The family based on

           (a) Family recognized patterns/clusters of symptoms

           (b) Underlying family culture (Helman, 1991)

           (c) Most families take responsibility for assuring care for family members across the life span (see this topic below under Sick Role and Role of the Family)

        (3) Health care systems (Kleinman, 1978, 1980; Kleinman et al., 1978, 2006)

           (a) Popular sector: nonprofessional, based on popular culture, family, and social networks

           (b) Professional sector: organized, professional healing and prevention practices (Western, modern scientific medicine, professional indigenous systems, and Ayurvedic medicine)

           (c) Folk sector: nonprofessional sacred, secular, and traditional beliefs

        (4) Simultaneous combinations of all three, the sick person, the family, and the health care system

  3. Managing the symptoms (examples)

     a. Common symptoms, for example, the common cold

        (1) Among five Latin American populations, considerable inter- and intra-agreement occurred regarding causes, symptoms, and treatments of the common cold with views similar to the biomedical perspective, except in the use of the hot/cold system of causality (Baer, Weller, Patcher, et al., 1999)

        (2) In another study comparing physicians and layperson views in south Texas and Guadalajara, Mexico, professional and lay perspectives followed similar explanatory models (Baer, Weller, de Alba, et al., 2008)

     b. Pain (see this topic in chapter 6)

     c. End of life (topic below)

D. Sick Role/Role of the Family

  1. Definitions of sick role

     a. Becoming ill is a process (Helman, 2000):

        (1) Starts with the person recognizing symptoms

        (2) Legitimized by family and/or healer/provider

     b. A socially derived and patterned role with rights and obligations (Parsons, 1951, R. Spector, 2000, 2008)

        (1) Rights: Exemption from

           (a) Normal social roles

           (b) Responsibilities

        (2) Obligations:

           (a) Try to get well

           (b) Seek competent help and treatment

           (c) Acceptable sick role behavior varies among cultural groups, for example, from aggressive to passive (Andrews & Boyle, 1999, 2008)

           (d) Behaviors and perspectives of the sick role are often shaped by what are considered culturally acceptable versus what are thought to be stigmatized (Kleinman, 1980).

  2. Family roles

     a. Over the generations, families develop patterns of behavior to deal with members' illnesses (Helman, 1991)

        (1) Patterns based on

           (a) Underlying culture of origin

        (b) Beliefs about how the body functions
        (c) Explanatory models used within the family
        (d) Power structure within the family
        (e) Family member is responsible for decisions regarding
            i.   When to ignore or treat at home versus seeking professional or folk healer
            ii.   Type of provider
            iii. When to accept or reject treatment
    (2) Family responsibilities toward members are based on beliefs (Helman, 1991) about
        (a) Health and body image
        (b) Gender and generational roles
        (c) Parenting and child-rearing practices
        (d) Lifestyle
        (e) Religious beliefs and practices
        (f) Myths and taboos
        (g) Rituals and family/folk remedies
        (h) Economic and social support structures available

  b. The person who is ill and their family create a dynamic interactive unit that bases decisions on established behavior patterns that reflect their culture of origin and socioeconomic environment.

  c. For example, family life course perceptions can assist families in caregiving and care-receiving roles that enhance the care of older adults in the family as has been shown in Mexican American families (Evans, Crogan, N., Belyea, M., & Coon, 2009).

E. Stigmas and Taboos

1. *Stigma* is a universal cross-cultural phenomenon that involves the stigmatized person and the person(s) applying the stigma label in a dynamic process that results in negative outcomes for both. The recipient of the stigma label suffers the most. Ethnic minority status and racism further complicate the effects of stigma and increase its complexity.

2. Culture-based taboos cover a range of situations and issues, and often serve as interdependent generators or recipients of stigma.

3. Stigmas and taboos occur across the life span and are influenced by gender, age, ethnic identity, religion, culture, and social group membership.

4. Stigma and taboos often complicate health beliefs and practices and the lives of those who suffer illness, leading to reluctance to seek treatment, or avoiding health promoting opportunities.

5. Some illnesses and disabilities serve as the object of stigmatization; HIV/AIDS, visual or hearing impairments, Tourette syndrome are a few examples.

6. Definitions of and commentaries on the stigma concept:

  a. Originating from the Greek word *stigma*, the term refers to an attribute that
    (1) has a discrediting effect on persons with deviant conditions
    (2) is defined by social groups or society in general
    (3) leads to a "moral career"
    (4) requires personal adjustments (Goffman, 1963, pp. 1-5, 32).

  b. E. E. Jones et al. (1984) describe stigma as a relational process that involves
    (1) the social act of stigmatizing, and
    (2) the psychological process by which the individual integrates this social identity.

  c. Stigmatization creates situational social prescriptions and proscriptions for how the stigmatized individual is treated and receives a devalued social identity.

  d. Stigma possesses structural determinants in the form of both intentional and unintentional discrimination, with policy implementations that reduce opportunities for particular groups (L. H. Yang et al., 2007).

  e. Stigma is also viewed as a "moral experience" that requires measurement based on the following factors/processes (L. H. Yang et al., 2007, pp. 1531-1533):
    (1) Spans physical, sociocultural, and emotional domains,
    (2) Is "sociosomatic" with moral–somatic and moral–emotional forms,
    (3) Is intersubjective, and
    (4) Threatens what matters most.

    f. "The burden of stigma follows power differentials, with socially and economically disenfranchised groups being particularly susceptible" (Birbeck, Chomba, Atadzhanov, Mbewe, & Haworth, 2008, p. 168).

    g. Related to stigma concepts and definitions is the concept of self-protection against stigma through, for example avoidance of loss of face:

      (1) among people in China (L. H. Yang & Kleinman, 2008) and

      (2) among people in Japan (Doi, 1986, p. 23)

        (a) *Omote o tateru* "to put up a front" and

        (b) *Omote o tsukurou*" to keep up appearances" or

        (c) *Omote o haru* "to keep up a façade" .

  7. *Taboo definitions*:

    a. A ban or prohibition for the use of words or actions considered socially or culturally objectionable or offensive.

    b. Taboos prescribe and proscribe behaviors for eating, sexual activity, associations with others, birth, end of life, death, and assorted illnesses with perceived stigma (Csikos, Albanese, Busa, Nagy, & Radwany, 2008; Janschewitz, 2008; Kaduszkiewicz, Rontgen, Mossakowski, & van den Bussche, 2008; Kummer, Doren, & Kuhlmev, 2008; Piperata, 2008)

    c. The word *taboo* derives from the Tongan word *tapu* originally meaning "not allowed" or "forbidden" and in modern usage also "sacred" and "holy" (Wikipedia, n.d.)

    d. The religious/spiritual focus combined with the prohibition concept over time may bring social, religious, or legal sanctions for the use of taboo words or behaviors

    e. Taboo topics such as death and dying can have negative health effects. For example, in Hungary, Csikos et al. (2008) found their research participants feared losing autonomy in addition to fear of pain and suffering as reasons for the death and dying taboo. These behaviors can and often do lead to avoidance of seeking care.

  8. *Cultural examples of the impact of stigma/taboos* on the health of individuals and groups:

    a. Loss of face and fears of "moral contamination" can be considered to be a "social death" among people in China with a diagnosis of AIDS or schizophrenia (L. H. Yang & Kleinman, 2008, p. 398).

    b. Dietary taboos and food restrictions in rural Bangladesh can result in malnutrition among pregnant mothers (Shannon, Mahmud, Asfia, & Ali, 2008).

    c. Newman, Williams, Massaquoi, Brown, and Logie (2008) report barriers to HIV prevention among Black women of African and Caribbean descent living in Canada include stigma and cultural disconnections.

    d. A total of 90% of the comments during a focus group with Mexican immigrant women pointed to perceived barriers to care access for illnesses they considered would stigmatize them (Horwitz, Roberts, & Warner, 2008).

    e. African American mental health consumers indicated they initially delayed treatment because of concerns about stigma, and they experienced stigmatizing reactions from others when in treatment (Alvidrez, Snowden, & Kaiser, 2008).

    f. Among aspects of Filipino American culture identified as important for understanding diabetic self-management was participation in storytelling about the stigma associated with diabetes (Finucane & McMullen, 2008).

    g. According to Kalkhoran and Hale (2008), topics such as homosexuality, sex, drug use, and HIV/AIDS are taboo in the Islamic world, thus complicating AIDS education.

F. Gender Identity Related to Health and Illness Beliefs and Practices (see also Adolescence—Rites of Passage and Gender Identity under III. D. below)

  1. *Overview of concepts relevant to the life span*

    a. Components of gender (Helman, 2000, p. 109)

      (1) Genetic gender: based on genotype with male XY and female XX chromosomes

      (2) Somatic gender: based on phenotype (as in physical appearance)

      (3) Psychological gender: based on self-perceptions and behaviors

      (4) Social gender: based on cultural categories and sociocultural prescriptions for behavior and perceptions of "male" and "female" identities

    b. Each cultural and ethnic group assigns gender roles and responsibilities within the family unit and social community

      (1) Parenting roles (Helman, 2000)

(2) Sexual behavior (Andrews & Boyle, 1999, 2008)

(3) Household tasks

(4) Caregiving roles during illness (Tarimo et al., 2008)

(5) Work roles

   c. Gender roles and responsibilities shift and evolve over time depending on sociopolitical and environmental contexts (Bronfenbrenner & Ceci, 1994)

   d. Gender responsibilities often depend on birth order in the family

   e. Personal sexual orientations may alter individual perceptions regarding gender roles that are usually addressed beginning during adolescence (see Adolescence—Rites of Passage below)

   f. Gender roles, issues of equality, and power distribution between the genders receive considerable political and health policy attention in the global arena (Connell, 2005; United Nations, 2000).

   g. Lifelong gender relevant development, experiences, health, and illness interact and are interdependent with culture and society.

(1) Developing racial and gender identity is influenced by local customs, popular culture, and politics (Ibrahim, 1999).

(2) Gender as well as culture and economics influence behavior such as smoking (Stevens & Caan, 2008).

   h. Feminine and masculine perspectives struggle for equality, peace, and safety within households, communities, and nations around the globe (see also the segments on Intimate Partner Violence and Genocide/War in Chapter 6):

(1) The United Nations Security Council unanimously adopted Resolution 1325 to address the disproportionate impact of armed conflict on women and stressed the importance of equal and full participation of women as active agents in peace and security (United Nations, 2000).

(2) Recognition of world-scale contemporary masculine politics (Connell, 2005)

(3) Women with HIV/AIDS in China receive inadequate attention within the Chinese gender role context (Zhou, 2008)

(4) Individuals living with HIV/AIDS in the United States and around the world experience traumatic events and lack of trust in health care systems and governments (Whetten, Reif, Whetten, & Murphy-McMillan, 2008)

(5) Violence against women may be normalized and tolerated in some cultural groups, for example, Jordanian women (Oweis et, al., 2009)

(6) Global, racial, and gender-related issues generate stress around the world and are experienced disproportionately by African American women who have high rates of stress-related illnesses (Woods-Giscombe & Lobel, 2008)

G. Influence of Religious and Spiritual Beliefs and Practices on Health

   1. Overview of concepts and definitions

     a. Spiritual and religious beliefs and practices:

(1) influenced by and intertwined with culture

(2) together they influence health and illness experiences and outcomes

     b. Religion and spirituality terms often used interchangeably but have different meanings (Andrews & Boyle, 1999, p. 381):

(1) "*Religion* refers to an organized system of beliefs concerning the cause, nature, and purpose of the universe . . ." as in the worship of God

(2) "*Spirituality* is born out of each person's unique life experience and his or her personal effort to find purpose and meaning in life."

     c. Religious dimensions that influence beliefs and behaviors vary across formal religious groups (Andrews & Boyle, 1999, p. 397)

(1) Experiential (subjective religious experience)

(2) Ritualistic (religious practices within the specific religion)

(3) Ideological (set of beliefs that require adherence for membership)

(4) Intellectual (sets of beliefs for the cognitive structure of meaning)

(5) Consequential (religiously defined standards of conduct)

     d. Multiple religious groups and organized religions include but are not limited to

(1) Buddhism

(2) Christianity (e.g., Catholic, Protestant, Episcopal, Evangelical)

(3) Hinduism

(4) Islam

(5) Judaism

(6) Mormonism

2. *Spiritual and religious practices* for many believers serve as motivating and organizing factors that govern their lives through individual, family, and organized religious, cultural, and/or social group practices.

   a. Life cycle event observances, celebrations, and rituals (often take place in the home within the family as well as in organized religious settings).

     (1) Birth (e.g., with baptism, circumcision, naming ceremonies)

     (2) Rites of passage (see Adolescence—Rites of Passage below)

     (3) Marriage (formal ceremonies and religious counseling)

     (4) End of life (care of the dying, bereavement, grief and mourning customs, and burial practices—see also End of Life segment below)

   b. Holy day celebrations and festivals

   c. Prayer (individual and group)

     (1) Prayer has been associated with the power to heal, to alleviate illness, and promote good health since ancient times (Narayanasamy & Narayanasamy, 2008)

     (2) Narayanasamy and Narayanasamy (2008) suggest that while empirical studies fail to show conclusive evidence (because of measurement problems) that connects prayer to resolution of illness, prayer is a spiritual activity that compliments health care treatments.

     (3) 1998 National U.S. survey regarding prayer found that 75% of the sample of 2,055 prayed for wellness (McCaffrey, Eisenberg, Legedza, Davis, & Phillips, 2004).

     (4) The 2002 National Health Interview Survey and Alternative Health Supplement data (United States) found 45% of adults prayed for health (Bell et al., 2005).

     (5) The 2004 Survey of Health, Aging, and Retirement in Europe showed a positive relationship between prayer and health outcomes (Hank & Schaan, 2008).

     (6) A 2005 study conducted in Taiwanese hospital units found 75% of patients and family members offered prayers for help (Tzeng & Yin, 2008).

   d. Religious instruction from childhood throughout life

   e. Fasting and food prescriptions and proscriptions

3. *Strong religious and spiritual beliefs influence health and illness behaviors*

   a. Consistent indicators in numerous studies show a strong association between health/healing and spiritual/religious beliefs/behaviors (Koenig, McCullough, & Larson, 2001; Levine, Yoo, Aviv, Ewing, & Au, 2007; Smith, McCullough, & Poll, 2003)

   b. Potentially positive influence examples:

     (1) Spirituality, family communication, shared routines, and rituals seen to enhance family resilience that serve as protective and recovery factors (Black & Lobo, 2008) and contribute to successful aging (Stark-Wroblewski, Edelbaum, & Bello, 2008).

     (2) Health, spirituality, and intergenerational learning and doing among other variables seen to be a supportive worldview ("circle of caring") among First Nations people (Gerlach, 2008).

     (3) Croatian war veterans with posttraumatic stress disorders had significantly lower spiritual well-being and religious well-being scores when compared to a sample of healthy volunteers (Nad, Marcinko, Vuksan-Aeusa, Jakovljevic, & Jakovljevic, 2008).

     (4) In many Asian countries, spiritualism and religion seem to help in the healing process (Chaudhry, 2008)

     (5) Spirituality among Latina and African American breast cancer survivors served as a strong source of comfort and deepening faith, as well as anger at God (Levine et al., 2007).

   c. Potentially negative influence examples:

     (1) Spiritual and religious beliefs, fear and fatalism contribute to dangerous delays in seeking breast cancer screening among African American women (Gullate, 2006)

     (2) Among persons in rural North Carolina living with HIV/AIDS, beliefs that the disease is caused by chance, fate, or God's will may affect adherence to medication (Kemppainen, Kim-Godwin, Reynolds, & Spencer, 2008)

4. *Spiritual care*

   a. Spiritual care is an essential component of holistic care (Andrews & Boyle, 1999, 2008)

   b. Spiritual care can be linked with cultural foci; both require appropriate and respectful assessment, for example, the need to include prayer in the assessment

   c. Consider patients' spirituality as a coping method in the management of chronic illness, pain, and fatigue (Baetz & Bowen, 2008)

   d. Need to create relationships with Lakota Indian patients built on reciprocity and respect for their beliefs about the interrelationship between spirituality and healing (Iron Cloud & Bucko, 2008)

   e. Holistic care for African Americans should include spirituality (Figueroa, Davis, Baker, & Bunch, 2006)

   f. Spirituality and religion are often linked with complementary and alternative medicine by cancer survivors (Hsiao et al., 2008)

5. *Research directions in the spiritual and religion realms* (Williams & Sternthal, 2007)

   a. Careful conceptualization and measurement of these realms

   b. Dimensions of religious participation and psychosocial environment

   c. Define and measure spirituality and religiosity as distinct entities

   d. Design studies to examine cross-cultural comparisons

H. **Summary:** Each of the foregoing topics is intertwined with the others; all interact and are interdependent with cultural issues that face individuals and their families across the life span.

III. BELIEFS AND CARE PRACTICES ACROSS THE LIFE SPAN

A. Birth and Neonatal Care Practices

1. *Population diversity*. The population of the United States is becoming increasingly diverse. Approximately 12% of the U.S. population is foreign born (53% from Latin America, 25% from Asia, 8% from Europe, and the remainder from areas throughout the world (U.S. Department of State, 2004).

   a. This foreign-born population is younger (45% between the ages of 25 and 44 years) compared with 27% of the native born population in that age group. Thus the percentage of foreign-born persons of childbearing age is higher than among native born (U.S. Department of State, 2004). Each year women of childbearing age comprise more than one third of all documented immigrants entering the United States (U.S. Department of Homeland Security, 2007).

   b. Poverty rates are also higher in the foreign-born population, particularly in those from Central America (U.S. Department of State, 2004).

2. *Health care disparities* exist within this diverse population.

   a. Health disparities have been defined in various but similar words: health disparities are differences that may occur in the incidence or prevalence of disease, or in morbidity or mortality.

   b. Health disparities are also differences in the way patients are treated. The Institute of Medicine (2003b) describes health care disparities as "racial or ethnic differences in the quality of healthcare that are not due to access-related factors or clinical needs, preferences and appropriateness of intervention" (p. 32).

   c. Although disparities are often thought of in terms of race and/or ethnicity, disparities may occur between or among any population group, including those that differ in gender, age, economic status, religion and/or sexual preference (Moore, Moos, & Callister, 2010).

   d. Du, Nass, Bergsjo, and Kumar (2009) showed that the resources used to assure healthy babies and maternal health are unequally distributed, particularly in multiethnic countries. Although they studied women in western China, similar findings would exist had the research been done in the United States (Covan, 2009).

3. *Health information*. Shieh, Mays, McDaniel, and Yu (2009) noted that access to information, especially that found on the Internet, is unequally distributed to older mothers and those of minority status having the least access.

   a. Health literacy, that is, the degree to which individuals have the capacity to obtain and use health information, is one variable that impacts the health of all races and ethnicities. Health literacy is more than the ability to read; it is also the ability to gather and process appropriate, relevant information (Moore et al., 2010).

   b. Beyond reading skills, health literacy requires the ability to communicate needs and concerns to health care providers, understand oral instructions, use numbers and basic math skills in order to take medications as prescribed or compute deductibles and co-pays, and the capacity to use the health care system appropriately (North Carolina Institute of Medicine, 2007; U.S. Department of Health and Human Services, 2008).

   c. Some experts have proposed that maternal health literacy is of particular significance because pregnancy may be the initial encounter into the health care system for women with low or marginal health literacy skills. Additionally, a woman's health understanding will impact not only her own health but also that of her fetus and children (Ferguson, 2008; Puchner, 1995; Zarcadoolas, Pleasant, & Greer, 2006).

    d. In addition to language barriers or literacy levels, cultural traditions and beliefs may interfere with the ability to gather and process health information.

      (1) A woman from a patriarchal culture may be unable or unwilling to provide important health information or make treatment decisions without engaging her husband or father.

      (2) A woman from a culture that places high value on respect may indicate that she understands the instructions she has been given when, in fact, she has little understanding. By implying that she understands, she has respected the health care providers' skills and status (Moore et al., 2010).

4. *Cultural causes of disparities* in health care delivery include, but are not limited to

    a. Failure of nurses and other providers to understand the importance of beliefs about health and illness

    b. Unwillingness to coordinate care with traditional healers when appropriate

    c. Lack of minority staff members

    d. Inadequate interpreter services (Moore et al., 2010)

    e. Providers contribute to disparities through bias against minorities, often unconsciously, increased clinical uncertainly when caring for minority patients, and beliefs the provider may have (Institute of Medicine, 2003b)

5. *Disparities among childbearing families*

    a. Latinas who were born in Mexico have lower rates of preterm and low birth weight (LBW) infants than Latinas born in the United States (Page, 2004).

    b. In a study of the effects of acculturation on preterm birth, using English proficiency as a measure of acculturation, Ruiz et al. (2008) found that Hispanic women who were proficient in English (i.e., more acculturated) had a preterm birth rate of 13.95% compared with a rate of 5.8% for women proficient in Spanish (less acculturated).

    c. Mexican-born women are also the least likely of all Hispanic women to receive adequate prenatal care services (National Center for Health Statistics [NCHS], 2007).

    d. Yet the infant mortality and LBW rates for babies born to Mexican-born mothers compared favorably with those of other women with a higher utilization of prenatal care services, lower rates of poverty, and a higher attainment of formal education (Camarota, 2001; NCHS, 2007).

    e. This paradox warrants further examination of the strengths that give this resource-limited immigrant population an advantage during their early years of settlement.

    f. In a study of 49,904 births in Atlanta, Georgia, foreign-born women gave birth to infants with higher mean birth weights and lower rates of preterm birth (Forma, Jamieson, Sanders, & Lindsay, 2003).

    g. Among the greatest reproductive disparities in the United States are preterm birth, infant mortality, and maternal mortality. Preterm birth is lowest among Asian women and highest among African American women. The rate for Hispanic women is only slightly higher than the rate for non-Hispanic White women (Centers for Disease Control and Prevention [CDC], 2007).

    h. The United Staets has an overall maternal mortality rate of 13.1 per 100,000 births, ranking 41st in the world. The U.S. rate for non-Hispanic Whites is 9.3 and for African Americans is 34.5 (CDC, 2007).

    i. Decreasing disparities involves equality in access to care, successful strategies to educate women and their families, diversity and cultural competency of the health care team, and research to better understand the needs of patients from different cultural groups.

6. *Cultural differences in beliefs about health, reproduction, and the status of women.* The ways in which a particular society views this transitional period and manages childbirth depend on the culture's beliefs about health, medical care, reproduction, and the status of women

    a. Within a sociocultural system lies the health and healing belief system, which then defines birth in that culture.

    b. The birth process can then be viewed and assessed from the different components of the childbearing cycle, that is, antepartum (before birth), intrapartum (birth and delivery), postpartum (after birth), and also the newborn period.

    c. Childbearing is a time of transition in any society, and many cultures have particular customs and beliefs that govern and dictate activities during this period (Mattson, Galanti, Lettieri, & Kellogg, 1986).

      (1) Some may be *prescriptive* in nature, where the "rules" are phrased positively and/or describing expectations of accepted behavior, such as wearing special articles of clothing, ceremonies, or recommendations for diet and activity.

(2) Others are *restrictive*, or phrased negatively and limiting choices; these "rules" are usually directed to physical and sexual activity, work and environment, and emotions.

(3) A third area of beliefs is referred to as taboos, which are restrictions that may have serious supernatural consequences.

    (a) Often involve exposure to the moon and sun

    (b) Might refer to witchcraft or avoidance of some types of people (widows, people in mourning)

    (c) Often refer to food choices, activities, and fetal development (Lauderdale, 2008)

d. Pregnancy and childbirth practices in Western society have changed dramatically over the past several decades.

(1) In the United States there has been a trend toward delayed childbearing. Since women in their late 30s and 40s do not become pregnant as easily as when they were younger, there has thus been a growth in the use of reproductive assistance.

(2) In addition, other health issues, such as hypertension and diabetes may have an impact on the pregnancies of older women (Moore et al., 2010).

e. Subcultures within the main society may differ from the predominat culture in prenatal practices, values, and beliefs about childbirth, the roles of women, men, and support networks, and the use of practitioners.

f. A client's religion, age, urban, rural, or regional origin all contribute to cultural differences surrounding the childbearing period.

(1) Large variations exist in the social class, ethnic origin, family network and social support systems of women and their families (Lauderdale, 2008). Women who immigrated from a similar region do not necessarily share similar values and beliefs that influence how they will respond to the childbirth experience (Meleis, 2003).

(2) It is important to always be aware that *within* every group of people, cultural practices will vary.

(3) Examples given should be understand as be generalizations and not stereotypical assumptions about every individual or family of that cultural designation.

7. ***Cultural variations in the intrapartum period.*** Assessment and care needs during the birth and newborn periods

a. Cultural differences may exist in the designated setting for labor and delivery, as well as the appropriate practitioner and support attendants.

b. Most non-Western societies see childbearing as being within the woman's domain.

(1) Support during labor and assistance after delivery and with the neonate are usually provided by the woman's relatives and friends.

(2) It may be unusual for a father from a more traditional society to provide this support and caretaking.

c. Modesty issues can present a challenge to the labor and delivery nurse. Vaginal examinations and a scanty hospital gown may be deeply humiliating and unnerving to Southeast Asian, Orthodox Jewish, Islamic women, and others who value modesty (Moore et al., 2010).

d. Male caregivers may be refused, or may cause distress in Asian, Arab, and many Hispanic groups (Mattson, 2010).

(1) Practices followed by women of Islamic, Chinese, and Asian Indian backgrounds might include strict religious and cultural prohibitions against viewing the woman's body by *either* the husband or any other man (Lauderdale, 2008).

(2) The Muslim woman may request that she wear her head covering during labor and birth, particularly if a male is present (Yosef, 2008).

e. For an Orthodox Jewish woman in labor, the support person of choice may be a woman of her community for reasons of modesty (Lewis, 2003); she may also prefer to have her head covered (Moore et al., 2010).

f. Perceptions of childbirth pain, pain behaviors, and preferences for pain management are culturally bound (Callister, 2006a)

(1) For example, many Asian women are more likely to labor more quietly than women of Arab or Hispanic heritage, who feel "Allah/God needs to know she is suffering" (Kridli, 2002; Mattson, 1992, 2003; Mattson, personal communication/observation, 2008).

(2) Despite these differences, women of *all* cultures should be assessed for and queried about the need for pain medication.

(3) Pain may be perceived as a normal part of giving birth and coping with pain may be viewed as an important maternal achievement.

    (4) Pain may also be viewed as suffering requiring aggressive pharmacological pain management. Mexican women may prefer to avoid epidural analgesia/anesthesia because of concern about slowing labor as well as potential effects on their unborn child.

    (5) Immigrants from developing countries may have lacked the option of pharmacological interventions for previous births and could be resistive to these medications when offered in a highly technological birthing environment in their new country (Moore et al., 2010).

    (6) There are often cultural differences between laboring women and their nurse caregivers related to the application of technology and pain management, creating challenges for both (Carlton, Callister, & Stoneman, 2005).

g. Culturally imposed restrictions and prescriptions for activity during labor, including ambulation and massage.

    (1) Some Hispanic women like to move around and walk, believing that inactivity decreases the amount of amniotic fluid and may cause the fetus to "stick" to the uterus, which may delay giving birth (Moore et al., 2010). They will often come to a hospital for birth in advanced labor, as they have learned, that they will most likely have to remain in bed once there (Mattson, 2010).

    (2) Complementary therapies may include use of herbs, acupressure, massage, meditation, movement, hyrdrotherapy, birthing balls, and position changes to increase comfort and reduce pain.

    (3) Dietary recommendations, including types of teas during labor

       (a) Many Hispanic women prefer to drink *manzanilla* tea, which they believe makes the contractions stronger.

       (b) Asian women would like to drink herbal teas during labor as well (Mattson, 2010).

h. Expected length of labor: Expected interventions if the time is prolonged:

    (1) Despite the growing number of Cesarean births occurring across the world, there are many cultures that are reluctant or genuinely fearful of having a cesarean birth (Callister, 2008; Zlot, Jackson, & Korenbrot, 2005).

    (2) The Hmong view surgery as a violation that releases the soul from the body, thereby weakening it and even causing deformation in the next life (Cheon-Klessig, Camilleri, McElmurry, & Ohlson, 1988)

    (3) In many cultures, the husband, a religious leader, or community/family elders may be called upon to decide the best course of action (Moore et al., 2010).

i. Expected and ideal positions for facilitating pushing and delivery:

    (1) squatting, sitting, side-lying, as opposed to the more usual lithotomy position even with raised head as used in Western institutions

    (2) some women prefer to squat, which opens up the pelvic floor (Moore et al., 2010)

j. Appropriate disposition of placenta and umbilical cord after delivery

    (1) Some cultural groups, particularly the Hmong and Balinese, believe that burying the placenta and umbilical cord in a particular place will bring good fortune to the child and family (Lauderdale, 2008; Mattson, personal communication, 1989).

    (2) Others wish to preserve the cord by drying it, so as to use it medicinally later.

    (3) Parents may want to take the placenta with them to carry out the above activities.

    (4) The preferences of the childbearing family should be honored, if possible, while meeting institutional policies particularly regarding infection control.

k. A transcultural nursing challenge may be the creation of the birthing environment expected by the woman.

    (1) Women entering the foreign "culture" of health care of a highly biotechnological birthing unit may be very anxious and fearful

       (a) they are required to conform to institutional policies and procedures that may be unexpected

       (b) they may experience an invasion of privacy

       (c) they must become the "patient", away from the support of extended female family members

       (d) there may be language barriers

       (e) they will likely experience care from health care providers who are unfamiliar with valued cultural birthing traditions, such as doulas, and *parteras,* and unaccompanied by *promotoras* (Lauderdale, 2008)

    (2) A challenge for the labor and delivery nurse is to look beyond the routine to appreciate the needs and meet the expectations of the women with culturally defined practices. For example, Filippino women value the creation of a peaceful environment to decrease labor pain and facilitate the passage of the child into the outside world (Moore et al., 2010).

8. **Cultural variations in the care of the newborn**
   a. Traditionally, cultures have viewed the birth of a child in two very different ways: an event of great achievement worthy of celebration (i.e., birth of a son), or the birth may be viewed as putting the mother in a state of pollution requiring ritual purification ceremonies for her afterward.
   b. In general, in North American culture, the birth is viewed as an achievement, but not necessarily by the mother, but rather the practitioner who "manages the birth" (Lauderdale, 2008).
   c. Gifts and celebrations that focus on the newborn, rather than the mother, is a departure from the Arab tradition, in which the mother is seen as the "achiever" who has produced this beautiful new baby (Mattson, 2010).
   d. The meaning that parents attach to having a son, daughter, or multiple births varies from culture to culture.
   e. After the baby is born, cultures vary in how they address feeding of the infant, including method and timing of first feeding
      (1) A society's advocacy of breastfeeding varies and many influences must be considered.
      (2) Although American mothers are choosing to breastfeed more often than in the past, immigrants from developing and poorer countries still see bottle-feeding as the modern way to provide nourishment to their infants.
      (3) If the mother has HIV/AIDS, current recommendations in developed countries are to *not* breastfeed (Moran, 2010). However, because of the problem with safe water in developing countries, those mothers *are* told to breastfeed, despite the small chance of HIV transmission through breast milk.
      (4) Several cultural groups, including Hispanic and Arab women, in particular, believe that colostrums is bad for the infant and prefer to bottle-feed until their milk comes in (Mattson, 2010); women born in Mexico believe this but go on to successfully breastfeed once their milk has come in (Moore et al., 2010).
      (5) African American and Latina adolescents identified fear of pain, embarrassment with public exposure, and unease with the act of breastfeeding as significant barriers (Hannon, Willis, Bishop-Townsend, Martinez, & Scrimshaw, 2002).
      (6) An appreciation for the woman's values around modesty first must explore with each woman the is essential for the nurse who is aiming to encourage breastfeeding and facilitate successful latch-on; appropriateness of discussing the breast or exposing it in any way in front of any persons, including female and male relatives (Moore et al., 2010).
   f. Cultural variations in the bathing of the infant, include
      (1) Time of the first bath and appropriate person to do it
      (2) Measures used to protect the infant during the procedure
      (3) Traditional Hispanics believe that both the head and feet should be wet. Water will be placed on the head at the same time that the body is immersed in the bath (Clark, 1978).
   g. Sleeping arrangements and promotion of sleep
      (1) Women often keep the infant physically as close as possible, often sharing the same bed. For example, in Vietnam mothers share the same bed even in the immediate post birth time in the hospital (Mattson, personal communication/observations, 2008).
      (2) This is particularly true if ritual seclusion and limited activity are enforced (Mattson, 2010)
   h. Swaddling practices
      (1) Native Americans may still use cradle boards
      (2) African American, Filipino, and Hispanic women use abdominal binders or "belly bands" over the baby's umbilicus to protect against hernias and injury
      (3) Swaddling the infant is good protection against "bad air" and wind for Hispanics and Southeast Asians in particular (Mattson, 1992, Mattson, 2003)
   i. Circumcision
      (1) Cultures vary greatly in their beliefs about this practice; many Hispanics and Asians do not practice circumcision.
      (2) Ritual circumcision is frequently practiced in traditional Judaism and among followers of Islam
      (3) Jewish traditional circumcision, a *bris*, may be performed by a specially trained Rabbi or a physician while the Rabbi says prayers and is usually performed on the eighth day of life, after the mother and infant go home (DeSevo, 1997; Moore et al., 2010).
      (4) Muslims perform circumcisions anywhere from the 10th to the 70th day of life, while Palestinians circumcise their sons on the 7th day (Moore et al., 2010).

j. Caretaking of the infant at home
  (1) Appropriate caretaker: In some Asian and Asian Indian cultures, it is still considered inappropriate for the mother to care for the child immediately and/or show attention to the child; the grandmother or other female relative perform this task (Choudhry, 1997; Mattson, personal communication/observation, 2008)
  (2) Length of time the infant is allowed to cry before being attended to
    (a) Some cultures expect that the infant will be picked up and attended to (usually breastfed) immediately.
    (b) Others believe that the baby should be allowed to cry for a certain period of time
k. Ritual beautification varies according to cultural tradition and may be done to avoid the "evil eye", often a concern of many families
  (1) Navajo infant girls undergo piercing of their ears and insertion of turquoise earrings to provide protection from evil forces (Kay, 1982).
  (2) Eastern European women may seek to avoid the influence of the evil eye by putting a pin in the baby's bed or stroller.
  (3) Hispanic women may place a black onyx hand in the infant's crib.
  (4) In several cultures, including the Punjabi, a black thread may be tied around the baby's wrist, ankle, or waist to protect the newborn (Moore et al., 2010).
l. Attachment behaviors toward the infant
  (1) Many Asian and Middle Eastern women, in particular, might be seen as exhibiting behavior judged by westerners as maladaptive.
  (2) Asian women may maintain a distance and do not praise their infants because of a fear of evil influences (Mattson, 1992).
  (3) Middle Eastern women may believe the mother is the one deserving of praise for her work in producing the baby (Meleis & Sorrell, 1981).
m. Respecting cultural traditions following the birth of a child is important
  (1) The Muslim father may request to hold his newborn child to chant the Muslim call to prayer in infant's ear (Roberts, 2002).
  (2) Jewish and Muslim mothers in particular should be asked if they want a ritual circumcision rather than having the procedure performed routinely in the hospital; indeed,
  (3) All families should be offered the circumcision procedure, using a trained interpreter if needed to explain and obtain signed consent.
  (4) A transcultural nursing challenge may be a delay in naming of the infant, which is common in many cultures and may present difficulties in the completion of the birth certificate prior to hospital discharge.
n. Care of the preterm and high-risk newborn: Because of disparities in the rate of both prematurity and in certain anomalies, infants from minority populations are at increased risk of needing high risk care.
  (1) For any parent, having their newborn infant in a neonatal intensive care unit (NICU) is an unexpected and frightful experience.
  (2) For parents unfamiliar with Western, high-tech NICUs, the experience is especially shocking.
    (a) This is especially true if the infant is in an NICU where parents are expected to visit frequently to participate in their infants' care.
    (b) If the parents do not speak the language of the health care providers, communication with care providers is severely impaired.
  (3) NICUs usually have liberal visiting hours for the mother and father of the baby only. In cultures where the nuclear family is embedded in an extended family, other members may expect and want to be included.
o. Decision making
  (1) In many cultures, young parents are frequently not the decision makers; thus it is important to understand each family's dynamics.
  (2) In matriarchal American Indian families, the oldest woman in the family may be the ultimate decision maker.
  (3) In Chinese and many other Asian and Arab families, issues must be discussed with the male head of the household (Moore et al, 2010).

p. Parents also bring their own beliefs about infants who need specialized care, whether due to prematurity or a genetic disability.
   (1) The birth of a baby different from the one expected always brings grief, and in every culture there is a search for answers.
   (2) In addition to the scientific reasons for the occurrences, many people have cultural explanations, which include
       (a) God's will or punishment
       (b) Events that shocked the mother during pregnancy, or her behavior during that time
       (c) An angry spirit (Moore et al., 2010)
   (3) The acceptance of a child with a genetic defect in particular varies among cultural groups; physical disease is often viewed as more acceptable than mental disease.
       (a) Among the Hmong, a child is accepted completely without reservations
       (b) In some Mexican families, although a disability may be seen as God's will, it may still be associated with shame
       (c) Parents from groups as diverse as from the Philippines, Ethiopia, and Brazil, as well as those in the United States, talk of God's will as a cause of genetic defects (Moore et al., 2010).
q. A cultural challenge for NICU nurses is explaining and obtaining consent for taking of frequent blood samples. This may be of great concern to some parents, who believe it may weaken their infant and/or lead to hot/cold imbalance (Moore et al., 2010).
r. Another cultural challenge is incorporating specific religious beliefs into the infant's care
   (1) For those of the Jehovah's Witness faith, the practice of receiving blood is not acceptable.
   (2) When infants are critically ill, parents who are Roman Catholic and Episcopalian, among others, may wish their baby to be baptized.
       (a) In the absence of clergy, baptism may be performed by a health care provider or some other person as long as they have the required sacraments (U.S. Catholic Conference, 1994).
       (b) Anointing the baby with holy oil and praying for the baby is also desired by some. In the Roman Catholic faith this is done only by a priest, but in a number of Protestant denominations specially designated lay persons may do so (Moore et al., 2010).
s. Poverty and neonatal outcomes
   (1) The WHO (2004, 2007) estimated that approximately 2 million babies die each year within the first 24 hours of life and that 4 million die within the first month; 26% of newborn deaths are the a result of infections occurring due to the birth.
   (2) Most of the 4 million annual neonatal deaths are preventable
       (a) They occur because of poverty and the lack of resources
       (b) Interventions to save the lives of these babies are possible, but they cannot be implemented owing to lack of infrastructure to provide clean water, sanitation, medical supplies, and well-educated health care professionals (Kenner, Sugrue, & Finkelman, 2007).
   (3) The neonatal death rate is generally a reflection of poverty:
       (a) The microlevel poverty that women and children especially live in around the world.
       (b) The macrolevel or national level of poverty that is prevalent in many parts of the world (Kenner et al., 2007).
   (4) Several organizations are working to improve care for mothers and infants (Kenner et al., 2007; U.N. Population Fund, 2007).
       (a) The United Nations adopted Millennium Development Goals that include reducing maternal and child mortality (WHO, 2004).
       (b) The Council of International Neonatal Nurses (COINN) links researchers to neonatal nurses and provides resources to nurses via international conferences, networking, and supplying materials for nurses to use in their home countries (Kenner et al., 2007).
t. Summary
   (1) Nurses in all settings often serve as "culture brokers." They use "cultural bridging" to work with persons of different cultural groups to help them come to a resolution of differences.
   (2) Both the "emic" (insider's perspective) and the "etic" (outsider's view) are useful in understanding a culture. While it is important to understand how people view their own cultures, an outsider's view can also provide an important platform for understanding (Moore et al., 2010).

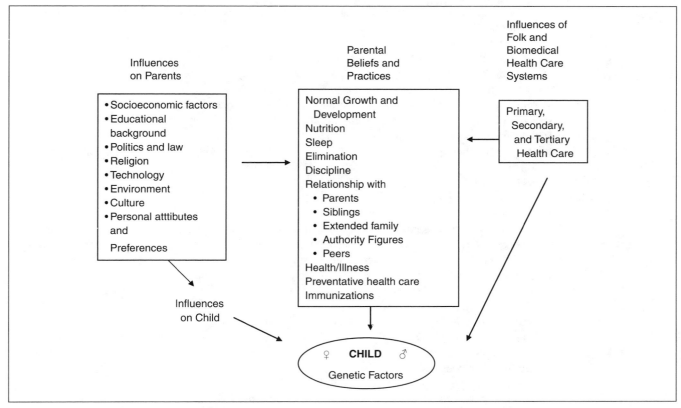

Figure 5.1. Cultural perspectives on child rearing
Source: Andrews and Boyle (2008, p. 117). Reprinted with permission.

     (3) Whether in a maternity or neonatal setting, nurses have an obligation to meet their clients' needs, including assisting them to preserve their cultural pratices as much as possible.

B. Cultural Influencers on Child Care and Parenting Care Health Beliefs and Practices

    1. *Cultures rely on children for their future*, and cultural survival depends on the transmission of values, beliefs, and practices from one generation to the next. All cultural groups provide their offspring with care, nurturance, and socialization.

    2. *Cultural influences on child care and parenting care patterns* (Figure 5.1), includes culture's influences on primary providers of care, health-related cultural beliefs and practices, such as the influence of indigenous/ folk healers and healing systems, and biocultural/ genetic traits of the child (Andrews & Boyle, 2008, figure 6.1, p. 117).

      a. Factors influencing parents' child-rearing beliefs and practices include the following (cf. Leininger, 1991, 1995; Leininger & McFarland, 2002, 2006):

        (1) Socioeconomic factors (e.g., household income, neighborhood, own/rent primary residence)
          (a) culture of poverty
          (b) middle-class culture
          (c) culture of affluence
        (2) Educational background of primary provider(s) of care
        (3) Political and legal factors
        (4) Religious beliefs and practices related to parenting and child rearing held by primary provider(s) of care
        (5) Technological factors
        (6) Environmental factors
      b. Kinship and social factors
        (1) Family constellation
        (2) Assistance with child rearing from siblings and extended family members

(3) Roles/responsibilities of grandparents, aunts, uncles, cousins, and other blood relatives in child care and child rearing

(4) Role of the community in child care and child rearing (e.g., ethnoreligious communities such as Amish)

c. Ethnohistory of child and child's primary provider(s) of care

(1) racial, ethnic, and cultural background(s), including multiple and mixed heritage

(2) Citizenship of primary provider(s) of care

(3) immigration status and level of acculturation of child and primary provider(s) of care

(4) issues of children in bi- and multicultural families, schools, and other settings

d. Individual preferences and personal characteristics of the child's primary provider(s) of care

(1) Parents' socialization, values, beliefs, goals, and behaviors are determined by what their culture defines as good parenting and preferred child behaviors for each gender.

(2) Access to affordable health care

3. *Transcultural perspectives on family*

a. Influences on family structure and function

(1) Types of family structures include nuclear, single-parent, blended, gay/lesbian, transracial or transcultural, and extended, which includes those characterized by kin residence sharing and nonblood members, communal lifestyles arrangements, and related constellations

(2) Family functions include the provision of shelter, comfort, physical, psychological, and emotional security, sense of stability and support, transmission of language, values, beliefs, and customs, and role and gender expectations

b. Transcultural perspectives on normal growth and development

(1) Measurements such as height, weight, head circumference, and chest circumference

(2) Variations in child development

(3) Transcultural perspectives on nutrition and diet

(4) Transcultural perspectives on sleep, including co-sleeping

(5) Transcultural perspectives on elimination and toilet training

c. Transcultural perspectives on parent–child relationships and discipline

d. Transcultural beliefs and practices related to gender

(1) From the moment of birth, all cultures recognize gender differences and begin a differentiated process of socialization to acceptable gender-related behaviors and roles.

(2) For children, gender differences can be identified cross-culturally in six categories of behavior: nurturance, responsibility, obedience, self-reliance, achievement, and independence.

(3) Transcultural differences in gender roles are interconnected with the child's age, ethnicity, religion, education, and socioeconomic background as well as environmental context.

4. *Normal growth and development*

a. Although the growth and development of infants and children is similar in all cultures, important racial, ethnic, and cultural differences exist.

b. From the moment of conception the developmental processes of the human life cycle take place in a cultural context.

c. Throughout life culture exerts an all-pervasive influence on the developing infant, child, and adolescent.

d. Culture universals (Garcia Coll, 2004; Harkness, 2008; Pan, 2008; Quintana et al., 2006).

(1) There is transcultural similarity in the sequence and timing of *developmental milestones.*

(2) Smiling, separation anxiety, and language acquisition occur in a similar time frame and follow a common sequence or order regardless of the child's racial, ethnic, or cultural background.

(3) Human functioning cannot be separated from the cultural context and environment in which children develop.

(4) Certain *growth patterns* can be recognized across cultural boundaries.

(5) Regardless of culture there is a pattern of general-to-specific abilities, from the center of the body to the extremities (proximal-to-distal development), and from the head to the toes (cephalocaudal development).

(6) In all cultures, adult head size is reached by the age of 5 years, whereas the remainder of the body continues to grow through adolescence.

(7) In all cultures, physiologic maturation of organs such as those in the renal, respiratory, and circulatory systems occurs early in infancy and childhood whereas maturation of the central nervous system continues beyond childhood.

e. Culture specifics (LeVine et al., 1996; Overfield, 1995; Pan, 2008; Quintana et al., 2006)

(1) Not all developmental theories formulated on the basis of observations with Western children have transcultural generalizability (Garcia Coll, 2004; LeVine et al., 1996; Overfield, 1995).

(2) Transcultural and transnational investigations that have tested several classic Western theories such as the stages of child development, family role relations, family systems, and patterns of mother–infant attachment have raised questions about their validity across cultures.

(3) Transcultural comparative investigations of growth patterns reveal that, in some cultures, the Western developmental pattern of sitting–creeping–crawling–standing–walking is not followed.

(4) In Bali, infants go from sitting to squatting to standing to walking.

(5) Hopi Indian children begin walking, on average, about 1½ months later than Western Anglo children.

(6) Other culture specifics in child growth patterns

(a) Overall, Native American and First Nation Peoples of Canada have a larger number of infants weighing 4,000 grams or more at birth—believed to be associated with higher incidence of diabetes mellitus in Native populations.

(b) Tooth eruption occurs earlier in Asian and African American children than in their White counterparts.

(c) Some populations are shorter or taller than others during various periods of growth and development, for example, African American infants are 0.75 inches shorter than White infants.

(d) At 6 years of age, African American children are taller than Whites, but White boys catch up by age 9 or 10; White girls catch up with their African American counterparts by age 14 or 15.

(e) By adulthood, Whites and African Americans achieve approximately the same average height.

(f) Sitting/standing height ratios vary, for example, African and African American children have longer legs in proportion to height than Whites, Asians, American Indians, and Mexicans.

(7) Infant attachment: Cross-national research reveals significant variation in infant attachment

(a) German mothers expect very early autonomy in the child and have few physical interventions while the child is playing alone.

(b) Japanese mothers allow very few mother–child separations.

(c) Mothers of Puerto Rican and Dominican Republic cultures emphasize close mother-child relationships and demonstrate more verbal and physical expressions of affection.

5. ***Transcultural perspectives on parent–child relationships*** (Kazura, 2000; Lamb & Lewis, 2004)

a. In some cultures, both parents assume responsibility for the care of children.

b. In other cultures, the relationship with the mother is primary and the father remains somewhat distant.

c. When members of the extended family raise children, the role of the biological parents tend to be different from families with other types of consellations (e.g., nuclear or single-parent structures).

d. Some cultures encourage children to participate in family decision making and to discuss significant family matters with their care providers, for example, some African American families encourage children to express opinions verbally and to take an active role in all family activities, whereas Japanese, Chinese, and many other Asian cultures and subcultures encourage children to be less vocal (Sperry & Sperry, 2000).

e. Some cultures value respectful, deferential behavior toward adults, who are respected for their experience, age, and wisdom.

6. ***Transcultural perspectives on play*** (Edwards, 2000; Goencue, Mistry, Artin Göncü, Mistry, & Mosier, 2000; Taylor & Carlson, 2000; Thyssen, 2003; Von Klitzing, Kelsay, Emde, Robinson, & Schmitz, 2000)

a. In all cultures, play is an integral component of normal growth and development

b. Play prepares children for their future adolescent and adult development, including culturally acceptable behaviors and social roles

c. Toys and encouragement from parents and other care providers foster children's engagement in play

d. Some developmental experts (Piaget, 1962) have delineated play into three major periods, but generalizability to all cultures had not yet been verified

(1) *Imitation and practice* are the earliest form of play, usually occurring during the sensory-motor period from birth to approximately 24 months.

(2) *Symbolic play* occurs around 3 to 5 years of age when there is assimilation or distortion of reality and the child attributes an identity to an absent object or person, for example, imaginary playmate (Piaget, 1962; Taylor & Carlson, 2000).

(3) *Games with rules* is the last stage in play and usually occurs around 7 years of age when children begin to think logically and concretely and understand that rules are supposed to be adhered to; it usually takes several more years before children truly abide by the rules without modifying them or "cheating."

  e. Significant gender differences in play exist for boys and girls in all cultures around the world

7. Discipline

  a. Discipline varies widely among cultures and may involve the use of mild, moderate, or severe physical or corporal punishment; verbal guidance, advice, and admonitions; temporary removal of privileges; providing rewards for desired behaviors; social separation or isolation from others or removal of the child from a social setting (e.g., "time out"); and related strategies employed by the child's primary provider(s) of care.

  b. Parents may share responsibility for disciplining children, for example, in most Western cultures. The mother or other female might be expected to provide discipline, for instance, in many African, Middle Eastern, and Asian cultures, whereas the father and other male relatives remain distant.

  c. In many cultures, boys are permitted more freedom than girls of the same age and are permitted to be farther distances away from care providers during play

8. Child abuse versus cultural child-rearing practices

  a. Child abuse and neglect have been documented throughout human history and are known across cultures.

  b. *International attention to child maltreatment* emerged in the late 1970s. The International Society for the Prevention of Child Abuse and Neglect (ISPCAN) has held international congresses and regional meetings to explore physical abuse and neglect, sexual molestation, child prostitution, nutritional deprivation, emotional maltreatment, and institutional abuse from a cross-national perspective.

  c. Cross-cultural and transnational variability in child-rearing beliefs and practices has created a dilemma that makes the establishment of a universal standard for optimal child care, as well as definitions of child abuse and neglect, extremely difficult.

  d. Korbin (1991) has identified three levels in formulating culturally appropriate definitions of child maltreatment:

    (1) *Cultural differences in child-rearing practices and beliefs*

      (a) In Turkey and many Middle Eastern cultures, despite warm temperatures, infants are covered with multiple layers of clothing and might be observed to sweat profusely because parents believe that young children become chilled easily and die of exposure to the cold.

      (b) Many African nations continue to practice rites of initiation for boys and girls, usually at the time of puberty. In some cases, ritual circumcision—of both boys and girls—is performed without anesthesia, and the ability to endure the associated pain is considered to be a manifestation of the maturity expected of an adult.

    (2) *Idiosyncratic abuse or neglect* signals a departure from one's cultural continuum of culturally acceptable behavior.

      (a) Some societies (Turkish, Mexican, and others) permit fondling of the genitals of infants and young children to soothe them or encourage sleep.

      (b) However, such fondling of older children or for the sexual gratification of adults would fall outside of the acceptable cultural continuum.

    (3) *Societal harm to children* is often interconnected with societal conditions.

      (a) Examples of social harm include poverty, inadequate housing, poor maternal and child health care, and lack of nutritional resources, which either contribute powerfully to child maltreatment or are considered maltreatment in and of themselves.

      (b) African American children are three times as likely as White children to die of child abuse, but considerable disagreement exists about whether these racial differences exist independently of socioeconomic factors such as income and employment status.

9. Language and communication (Grant, Luxford, & Darbyshire, 2005)

  a. Developmental considerations and language acquisition

  b. Literacy levels of primary providers of care and their children

10. Transcultural perspectives on well-child care (Schor, 2004)

  a. An ideal well-child care system should accommodate the parents' communication needs, values, preferences, expectations, and cultural health-related beliefs and practices.

b. Children and families should have access to language and other cultural interpretation services in cases where a different language is spoken at home.

c. Some well-child care experts have recommended offering some components of well-child care in sites such as daycare centers, churches, or homes.

d. Some families might find community settings more familiar or comfortable than health clinics or offices of professional health care providers.

e. Health care teams should include family members and indigenous, folk, or cultural healers who are familiar with the beliefs and practices of the child's parents.

f. Components

   (1) *Immunizations:* The decision to immunize infants and children is complex, multifaceted, and interwoven with cultural beliefs and practices, accessibility, and affordability of vaccines

   (2) *Diet and nutrition in infancy and childhood*

      (a) Cultural definitions of food

      (b) Food and meal preparation

      (c) Age-appropriate diets for infants and children from different cultures

g. Transcultural gender and cultural identity considerations

11. ***Transcultural perspectives on disease and illness in infancy and childhood***

a. *Transcultural perspectives on the health assessment* of infants and children

   (1) A comprehensive cultural assessment provides the foundation for culturally competent and culturally congruent nursing and health care for infants and children (Andrews & Boyle, 2008; Giger & Davidhizar, 2008; Leininger, 1991, 1995; Leininger & McFarland, 2002, 2006; Purnell & Paulanka, 2008; R. Spector, 2008).

b. *Transcultural perspectives on the physical examination of infants and children* (Andrews & Boyle, 2008)

   (1) Nurses frequently encounter normal biocultural variations when examining infants and children from different racial and ethnic backgrounds.

   (2) These variations include differences in height/length, weight, vital signs, body proportions, general appearance, skin, eyes, ears, mouth, and musculoskeletal system.

   (3) There is also evidence that biocultural variations occur in some laboratory test results such as measurement of hemoglobin, hematocrit, serum transferrin, lecithin/sphyngomyelin ratio, and blood glucose.

   (4) Similarly, the multiple-marker screening test and two tests of amniotic fluid constituents (used to screen for potential fetal abnormalities) reveal differences between African, Asian, and Caucasian women.

c. *Biocultural variations in assessing disease/illness in infants and children* (Andrews & Boyle, 2008)

   (1) When assessing clinical manifestations of disease, nurses often encounter differences related to the skin pigmentation of infants and children.

   (2) Special skill is needed to distinguish evidence of cyanosis, jaundice, pallor, erythema, petecchiae, and ecchymoses in lightly versus darkly pigmented infants and children.

   (3) Care needs to be taken to differentiate normal biocultural variations, such as, Mongolian spots from bruises or scratches or confusing manifestations of certain indigenous or folk healing practices, such as is, coining or cupping practiced by many Asian cultures, with child abuse

d. *Genetic traits or disorders affecting infants and children from diverse ethnic and population groups*

   (1) There is extensive evidence that certain genetic traits and disorders tend to have a higher prevalence in some population groups, which provides nurses and other health care professionals with useful information when assessing infants and children from diverse backgrounds.

   (2) Table 5.5 summarizes the distribution of selected genetic traits and disorders by population or ethnic group.

e. *Cultural beliefs about the causes of disease and illness in children:* Classic paradigms include biomedical/scientific, holistic/naturalistic, and magicoreligious causes

f. *Transcultural perspectives on children's mental health*

   (1) Major mental disorders such as schizophrenia, bipolar disorder, depression, and panic disorder are found world-wide, across all racial and ethnic groups.

   (2) According to the U.S. Surgeon General, in the United States, the overall annual prevalence of mental disorders in children is about 21% regardless of race or ethnicity (http://mentalhealthsamhsa.gov/cre).

Table 5.5. Distribution of Selected Genetic Traits and Disorders by Population or Ethnic Group

Ethnic Group or Population	Genetic or Multifactorial Disorder Present in Relatively High Frequency
Africans/ African Americans	Sickle cell anemia
	Hemoglobin C disease
	Hereditarypersistence of hemoglobin F
	G6PD deficiency, African type
	Lactase deficiency
	Beta-thalassemia
Aland Islanders	Ocular albinism (Forsius-Eriksson type)
Amish	Limb girdle muscular dystrophy (Indiana--Adams & Allen Counties)
	Pyruvate kinase deficiency (Ohio—Mifflin county)
	Hemophilia B (PA—Holmes county)
Armenians	Familial Mediterranean fever
	Familial paroxysmal polyserositis
Burmese	Hemoglobin E disease
Chinese	Alpha-thalassemia
	G6PD deficiency, Chinese type
	Lactase deficiency
Costa Ricans	Malignant osteopetrosis or Albers-Schonberg disease
Danes	Krabbe disease
Druze	Alkaptonuria
English	Cystic fibrosis
	Hereditary amyloidosis, type III
Eskimos	Congenital adrenal hyperplasia
	Pseudocholinesterase deficiency
	Methemoglobinemia
French Canadians (Quebec)	Tyrosinemia
	Morqulo syndrome
Finns	Congenital nephrosis
	Generalized amyloidosis syndrome, V
	Polycystic liver disease
	Retinoschisis
	Aspartylglycoasaminuria
	Diastrophic dwarfism
Greeks	Beta-thalassemia
	Sickle cell anemia
	G6PD deficiency
	Familial Mediterranean fever
Gypsies (Czech)	Congenital glaucoma
Hopi Indians	Tyrosinase-positive albinism
Icelanders	Phenylketonuria
Indians/Pakistanis	Ichthyosis vulgaris
	G6PD deficiency, Mediterranean type
Irish	Phenylketonuria
	Neural tube defects such as spina bifida
Iranians	Dubin-Johnson syndrome
Iraqis	Ichthyosis vulgaris
Italians	Beta-thalassemia
	Sickle cell anemia
	G6PD deficiency
	Familial Mediterranean fever
Japanese	Acatalasemia
	Cleft lip/palate
	Oguchi disease

(continued)

Table 5.5. (Continued)

Ethnic Group or Population	Genetic or Multifactorial Disorder Present in Relatively High Frequency
Jews	
Ashkenazi Jews	Tay-Sachs disease (infantile)
	Niemann-Pick disease (infantile)
	Gaucher disease (adult type)
	Canavan disease
	Familial dysautonomia (Riley-Day syndrome)
	Bloom syndrome
	Torsion dystonia
	Factor XI (PTA) deficiency
Habbanite Jews	Metachromatic leukodystrophy
Karaite Jews	Werdnig-Hoffman disease
Sephardi Jews	Familial Mediterranean fever
	Ataxia-telangiectasia (Morocco)
	Cystinuria (Libya)
	Glycogen storage disease III (Morocco)
Lapps	Congenital dislocation of hip
Lebanese	Dyggve-Melchoir-Clausen syndrome
Mennonites, Old Order	Maple syrup urine disease
Mexicans	Cystic fibrosis
	Familial combined hyperlipidemia
	Hereditary peripheral neuropathies
	Muscular dystrophies
	Limb malformations
Navaho Indians	Ear anomalies
Polynesians	Clubfoot
Poles	Phenylketonuria
Portuguese	Joseph disease
Nova Scotia Acadians	Niemann-Pick disease, type D
Saudi Arabians	Metachromatic leukodystrophy
Scandinavians	Cholestasis-lymphedema (Norwegians)
	Krabbe disease (Danes, Norwegians, Swedes)
	Sjögren-Larsson syndrome (Swedes)
	Phenylketonuria (Danes, Norwegians, Swedes)
Scots	Phenylketonuria
	Cystic fibrosis
	Hereditary amyloidosis, type III
Thais	Lactase deficiency, adult
	Hemoglobin E disease
	Alpha-thalassemia
Yemenis	Phenylketonuria
Zuni Indians	Tyrosinase-positive albinism

Sources: Jewish Genetic Disorders. African Ancestry (2003); American Anthropological Association (2004); Bamshad, et al.(2004); Burchard et al. (2003), Cohen (1984), Phimister (2003), Plapp, Hamilton, and Garg (2003), Prevalence and incidence of maple syrup urine disease. Risch et al. (2002), Shriver et al. (2003), Tishkoff and Verrelli (2003), Sickle Cell Disease (2007).

    (3) Mental health and mental illness are culturally defined.

    (4) Members of a society collectively interpret children's behaviors as abnormal or aberrant at various chronological ages and stages of the child's development.

  12. *Global perspectives on children's health*

    a. *UNICEF's Rights of Children*: Marked the first time, during an international convention, children were identified as citizens with definable rights (UNICEF, 2002).

      (1) The inherent right to life

(2) The right to a name at birth

(3) The right to enter or leave any country for purposes of maintaining the parent-child relationship

(4) The right to express his or her opinion freely, and have that opinion taken into account in any matter affecting the child

(5) The right to meet with others and join or form associations

(6) The right to the highest standard of health and medical care attainable

(7) The right to primary and secondary education

(8) The right to be protected from work that threatens his or her health, education, or development

(9) The right to be protected from sexual exploitation and abuse, including prostitution and involvement in pornography

(10) The right to be protected from torture, cruel treatment, unlawful arrest, or deprivation of liberty

(11) The right to be protected from recruitment into the armed forces below the age of 15.

b. *Global perspectives on child morbidity and mortality*

(1) UNICEF's recent report titled "State of the World's Children 2008: Child Survival" examines the state of child survival and primary health care for children, with a strong emphasis on trends in child mortality.

(a) It appraises the lessons learned in child survival over the past century.

(b) The centerpiece of the report looks at several of the most promising approaches used in countries and districts that have employed successful strategies for improving child survival (UNICEF, 2008).

(2) Major causes of child mortality worldwide

(a) A total of 73% of the 10.9 million child deaths each year are the result of six causes: pneumonia, diarrhea, malaria, neonatal sepsis, preterm delivery, and asphyxia at birth.

(b) Malnutrition contributes to more than one half of all deaths. A total of 75% of deaths of children younger than 5 years occur in Africa (WHO, 2008).

13. ***Contributions of transcultural nursing to improved health and well-being of infants and children***. The reader is encouraged to conduct a search for electronic and print resources on topics such as the following:

a. Child care and parenting care beliefs and practices

b. Evidence-based and best practices in the care of infants and children from diverse cultures

c. The reader is encouraged to search the *Journal of Transcultural Nursing, Journal of Cultural Diversity*, and related publications for current research, and evidence-based and best practices from a transcultural nursing and health care perspective.

C. **Adolescence:** An intense developmental journey in the life course where rites of passage, developmental tasks, gender and sexual identity, and adaptation to emerging and continuing relationships challenge adolescents, their family, and their sociocultural worlds.

1. *Rites of Passage: Definitions and Agendas*

a. Rites of passage characterize the interval between childhood and adulthood; alternate terms describe this developmental stage (Markstrom & Iborra, 2003):

(1) Liminality (marginal, being on a threshold, a ritual process)

(2) Betwixt and between

b. This time of transition incorporates

(1) Puberty with associated physiological, psychological, social, and cultural components

(2) Physical growth and development

(3) Transition from one set of obligations and roles to another

(4) An interval of psychosocial moratorium for establishing ego identity before taking adult responsibility (Hashimoto, 1992).

c. Adolescent developmental tasks (Masten, 1994)

(1) Learning to adjust and cope with puberty and body image changes

(2) Moving into the peer sphere and away from the intense family involvement of earlier childhood

(3) Developing a coherent identity

(4) Three universal tasks (Greenfield, Keller, Fuligni, & Maynard, 2003):

(a) relationship formation

(b) knowledge acquisition

(c) balance between autonomy and relatedness (cultural pathways of independence and interdependence)

   d. Cultural, social, and religious influence on adolescent rites of passage

     (1) Traditional recognition of passage between childhood and adulthood share some commonalities across cultural groups through

       (a) Initiation rites and rituals

       (b) Ceremonies of celebration

       (c) Enculturation and education for assuming responsible adult roles (provided by families, cultural and religious groups, formal public and private educational institutions)

     (2) Basic cross-cultural rites and ritual elements (Delaney, 1995; Munthali & Zulu, 2007):

       (a) Separation from the group (less common in current practice)

       (b) Instructional preparation by an elder

       (c) Formal and informal adolescent tasks, quests, cleansing, and/or self-reflective leaning and initiation rituals

       (d) Ceremonial welcome back into society as an adult

     (3) Cultural and religious rite and ritual examples

       (a) Confirmation ceremonies specific to religious groups

       (b) Bar and Bat Mitzvah (Blumenkrantz & Gavazzi, 1993; Marcus, 2004)

       (c) Ceremonial male and female circumcision (see this topic below).

       (d) Navajo Kinaalda ceremony for girls (menarche cues the initiation of the ceremony; Markstrom & Iborra, 2003)

       (e) *Iria* (fattening of African Okrika girls 14-16 years of age; Delaney, 1995)

       (f) *The Vision Quest* (seeking personal relationship with a guardian spirit among *Algonkain*-speaking groups such as the *Ojibwa* (Merkur, 2002); also described as a "journey inward" (Martin, 1996)

       (g) *Cemaasiit*—a mythical beast that frightens secluded initiates in passage ceremony for male and female adolescents 14 to 16 years of age among the *Okiek*, a tribe in Kenya (Delaney, 1995)

     (4) Current trends in the practice of some ceremonial rites

       (a) Many traditional ritual rites of passage ". . . have given way to a more vague and meaningless set of adolescent expectations and affirmations" (Quinn, Newfield, & Protinsky, 1985, p. 101)

       (b) Some rituals such as circumcision have been shown to result in lingering complications, even death (Schmid & Dick, 2008; WHO, 2008; see also circumcision topic below)

       (c) Some aspects of cultural rituals employed as motivating components in health education interventions with specific ethnic groups (see Adolescent Risk Behavior segment below)

     (5) Environmental and social issues that may alter the ideal transition

       (a) Health disparities, issues of stigma, discrimination, and racism

       (b) Risk behaviors among adolescents (see risk topic below)

       (c) Altered modern family lifestyle enculturation functions with increased uncertainty among adolescents and parents about their roles (Quinn et al., 1985)

       (d) Accelerated physical maturation (Quinn et al., 1985)

     (6) Approaches to counteract negative influences and promote cultural integrity focused on empowering adolescents and families to achieve healthier lifestyles by promoting culture-relevant rituals as part of the education process:

       (a) Young Empowered Sisters (YES!; Thomas, Davidson, & McAdoo, 2008)

       (b) Africentric Youth and Family Rites of Passage Program (Harvey & Hill, 2004)

       (c) The Navajo Kinaalda ceremony for girls (Markstrom & Iborra, 2003)

       (d) Preparing young people for adolescence and responsible sexual and reproductive behavior in Malawi (Munthali & Zulu, 2007)

  2. *Gender Identity and Sexual Orientation* (see also Young Adult—Gender Identity segment below)

  "I think what is happening to me is so wonderful, and not only what can be seen on my body, but what is taking place inside." (Frank, 1952). Hidden away during World War II, Anne Frank expressed in her diary what she could not talk about with her family: the universal complexity of her feelings as she experienced her passage from childhood to the realization of her gender identity.

   a. Gender identity and sexual orientation are linked in the context of the rites of passage and the developmental phase of identity formation as adolescents ask "who am I?"

     (1) Integration of intellectual, skill, and psychosexual development take place in the form of "ego identity" (Erikson, 1963, p. 261)

(2) Gender identity linked with self-image as adolescents ask themselves, "What am I like . . . what should I become?" (Rosenberg, 1989, p. 3)

(3) ". . . increasing body awareness is linked to the individual's need to develop the series of symbolic skins characteristic of their own culture or social group" (Helman, 2000, p. 16).

b. Adolescent perceptions of their gender and culture identity influence their behaviors in many different arenas, for example,

(1) Intellectual arena

(a) Guiso, Monte, Sapienza, & Zingales (2008) used findings from the 2003 Programme for International Student Assessment (PISA) that includes data from 276,165 students aged 15 years in 40 countries to assess the importance of cultural and biological explanations for the gender gap in math scores (boys scoring higher than girls). They found the gender gap in math scores disappears in those countries with cultures that have more gender equality.

(b) In the same study, girls scored higher than boys in reading (Guiso et al., 2008).

(c) Mello (2008) found both genders (females > males) with high occupational expectations in adolescence had higher occupational attainment in adulthood

(2) Gender role arena

(a) Cultural norms regarding sexual behavior for each gender (Helman, 2000)

    i.   Can be viewed as positive mechanisms for organization of cooperative roles

    ii.   These norms also can often create situations of inequality between the genders with the distribution of power slanted to males (Connell, 2005)

    iii. Culture-generated gender inequality can result in health disparities, for example, the higher rate of HIV/AIDS among 13- to 29-year-old African American females (CDC, 2008; Kerrigan, Andrinopoulos, Chung, Glass, & Ellen, 2008)

(b) Hyperfeminine thinking: definition of self based on relationships with males (Murnen & Byrne, 1991)

    i.   Primary concern for maintaining relationship with male

    ii.   Use physical/sexual attraction

    iii. Prefer traditional male sexual behaviors (see also Adolescent Risk Behavior content below).

(c) Aggressive behaviors

    i.   Based on socialization for masculine gender prowess, some adolescent males living in poverty and dead-end ethnic neighborhoods may turn to gangs (for camaraderie or safety) and/or sexually aggressive behaviors with multiple partners (Kerrigan et al., 2008; see also Adolescent Risk Behavior content below).

    ii.   Traditionally, girls exhibited less aggressive behavior than boys; however, Brown and Tappan (2008) found a trend for fighting among early adolescent girls in several sociocultural groups representing a complex interrelationship between personal and social identity.

    iii. Schoolgirls in another study described their experiences with disrespect, dismissal, and refusal of the right to express their anger (van Daalen-Smith, 2008)

(3) Race and ethnicity arena

(a) "The black teenager is an endangered species and there's a lot of very scary, life-threatening things waiting for my children" (Konner, 1991, p. 353, quoting an African American mother).

(b) Ibrahim (1999, p. 351) suggests that Black English Rap and Hip-Hop serve as rituals to express political perspectives, as moments of identification, or a way of saying, "I too am Black or "I too desire and identify with Blackness"

(c) Issues of health disparities related to gender and ethnicity: For example, the highest incidence of new HIV infections in 2006 occurred among African American females (61%—of those the highest incidence was among the 13-29-years age group at 32%; CDC, 2008).

c. Adolescent sexual identity and orientation

(1) Same-gender attraction awareness:

(a) 13 years of age for gay males

(b) 16 years of age for lesbians

(2) Same-gender self-designation:

(a) 14 years of age for gay males

(b) 21 years of age for lesbians

(3) In the Growing Up Today Study conducted in the United States (Austin, et al., 2004):
    (a) 92% of 10,685 adolescent girls and boys (12-17 years of age) described themselves as heterosexual
    (b) 5% mostly heterosexual
    (c) 1% lesbian/gay/bisexual
    (d) 2% unsure

(4) Same-gender sexual orientation and health:
    (a) Associated with alcohol use at younger ages (Corlis, Rosario, Wypi, Fisher, & Austin, 2008; Rosario, 2008)
    (b) Bisexual adolescents in one study reported less family and school connectedness than heterosexual adolescents (Saewyc et al., 2008)
    (c) Based on a large-scale high school youth survey, Busseri, Willoughby, Chalmers, and Bogaert (2008) found more high-risk involvement among same sex (SSA) and bisexual (BSA) attracted youths but suggest that these disparities may originate from the intra/interpersonal and sociocultural challenges faced by youths classified as BSA/SSA.

(5) Gender identity and mental health
    (a) The *Diagnostic and Statistical Manual of Mental Disorders*, Fourth Edition (*DSM-IV*) includes diagnostic criteria for "... gender identity disorder" (American Psychiatric Association, 1994, p. 532) with two primary categories:
        i. strong, persistent cross-gender identification
        ii. persistent discomfort with his/her sex or a sense of inappropriateness of the gender role of that sex
        iii. Based on an extensive review of the literature, Wilson, Griffin, and Wren (2002, pp. 335, 348) suggest the term *atypical gender identity organization* (Di Ceglie, 1998) rather than labeling as pathological behavior that may be a normal developmental pathway.

d. Adolescent gender, socioeconomic status, and health
  (1) Disabilities, particularly those that alter physical body image may interfere with normal psychosexual development for adolescents of both genders
  (2) Mental health disorders may present with altered symptom patterns; for example, manifestations of depression may include acting out or risky behaviors such as binge drinking or early initiation of cigarette smoking (Hutchinson, Richardson, & Bottorff, 2008)
  (3) Overweight and obesity in adolescence can lead to increased cardiovascular risk (high blood pressure and cholesterol female > male) by early young adulthood (Ford, Nonnemaker, & Wirth, 2008)
  (4) Duration of homelessness lasting more than 1 year resulted in lower levels of perceived health status for females and greater sexual self-care behaviors (Rew, Grady, Whittaker, & Bowman, 2008).
  (5) Genetic disorders may create added stress during adolescent gender identify formation (see, for example, Sickle Cell Anemia content below).

e. Gender-relevant interventions and adolescent education interventions (see Adolescent Risk and Cross-Generational Communication content below)

3. *Circumcision During Adolescence*

a. Primarily serves as a rite of male and female passage that is rooted in both cultural and religious traditions among some groups and varies in participation/nonparticipation, particular procedures, and ascribed meanings across cultures and religions.

b. Male circumcision
  (1) One of the oldest surgical procedures traced back to around 2300 BC through Egyptian tomb wall paintings (WHO & UNAIDS, 2007)
  (2) A total of 30% to 34% of men worldwide circumcised (H. A. Weiss et al., 2008)
  (3) Most often performed in conjunction with ritual rites of passage during adolescence for cultural or religious reasons (Schmid & Dick, 2008; WHO, 2007b)
    (a) Circumcision grounded in religion:
        i. Judaism: Jewish male infants on eighth day of life
        ii. Islam: Muslim practice confirms relationship with God: *tahera* (purification)
        iii. "Coptic Christians in Egypt and Ethiopian Orthodox Christians ... retain some features of early Christianity including male circumcision" (WHO, 2007b, p. 9)
        iv. Most other Christian groups do not prescribe or proscribe circumcision

      (b) Circumcision grounded in ethnicity: A major global determinant (WHO, 2007a) with varied percentages practicing circumcision, for example
         i.   Sub-Saharan Africa
         ii. Aboriginal Australasians
         iii. Aztecs and Mayans in the Americas
         iv Some Pacific Islands

(4) Male circumcision for HIV prevention (Bailey, Egesah, & Rosenberg, 2008; H. A. Weiss et al., 2008)
      (a) Male circumcision found to reduce the risk of HIV by about 60% (based on observational projects and randomized controlled clinical trials in sub-Saharan Africa)
      (b) Thus, male circumcision as an intervention in high HIV prevalence regions could reduce risk for infection.

(5) Access to safe male circumcision services
      (a) Many circumcisions performed as part of traditional rituals by poorly trained practitioners using unsterile knives (Ndiwane, 2008) that result in high rates of complications (35.2% contrasted with 17.7% in medical settings; Bailey et al., 2008)
      (b) Preference in sub-Saharan Africa for circumcision of sons in formal health care settings (Westercamp & Bailey, 2007)
      (c) Needed are (Bailey et al., 2008; Schmid & Dick, 2008):
         i.   Training/supervision of traditional practitioners
         ii. Hygienic settings
         iii. Up-to-date instruments
         iv. Adequate expendable supplies

c. Female circumcision: A traditional cultural and religious surgical procedure, with complex terminology, controversial perspectives, and international debate, that dates back to the second century BC (Andrews and Boyle, 1999, 2008)

(1) Alternative terms:
      (a) *Female genital mutilation* (FGM; WHO, 2008) classification:
         i.   Type I: partial/total excision of prepuce with/without clitoris (*sunna*)
         ii. Type II: partial/total excision of clitoris and labia minora with/without labia majora
         iii. Type III: Excision of part/all of external genitalia with narrowing of vaginal orifice, with/without clitoridectomy (infibulation)
         iv. Type IV: Unclassified other procedures for nonmedical purposes
      (b) *Female genital cutting* (FGC): a collective term given to traditional practices in removal of part or all of external genitalia (Tag-Eldin et al., 2008)
      (c) *Female genital modification*: elongation of labia minora and use of local botanicals (Rwandan example; Koster & Price, 2008)
         i.   Suggested alternative term from WHO–Type IV
         ii. Considered to have less powerful negative connotations than FGM
         iii. Rwandan women consider this modification a positive in their lives
      (d) *Restoration*: restoring the integrity of the hymen (hymenoplasty) in consenting adult women in cultures valuing virginity (O'Connor, 2008)

(2) Incidence and prevalence:
      (a) Global estimates: 100 to 140 million girls and women circumcised (WHO, 2008) with more than 74 million in Africa; and 12 million African girls 10 to 14 years of age (Yoder & Khan, 2008)
      (b) Africa, some countries in Asia, the Middle East and in immigrant communities in North America and Europe
      (c) Conducted at infancy or during adolescence as a rite of passage as well as during adulthood
      (d) Incidence of FMG decreasing in some countries (e.g., Kenya; Livermore, Monteiro, & Rymer, 2007)

(3) Cultural/religious perspectives:
      (a) Deeply rooted tradition (Andrews & Boyle, 1999, 2008):
         i.   generally viewed as an important preparation of young girls for womanhood
         ii. women not circumcised seen as unclean, not marriageable

(b) In Nigeria (WHO, 2007a) based on
    i.   Custom and tradition
    ii.   Family honor
    iii. Hygiene
    iv   Protection of virginity
    v.   Increases matrimonial opportunities
(c) Rwanda (Koster & Price, 2008)
    i.   Elongation of labia minora seen to increase male and female pleasure
    ii.   "modification" the preferred term instead of "mutilation"
(d) Many cultural groups oppose formalizing female circumcision in medical systems.

(4) World Health Organization and related agencies' perspectives:
(a) Human rights perspective: FGM/FGC seen as discrimination against women that promotes inequality between women and men (WHO, 1997)
(b) Concerns:
    i.   often performed with unsterilized instruments
    ii.   by designated village woman
    iii. assistants and/or family hold the girl to prevent struggling
    iv. local herbs, hot ashes, cow dung mixtures used to stop bleeding
(c) Complications
    i.   Severe pain
    ii.   Heavy bleeding
    iii   Shock
    iv   Injury to urethra, vagina, perineum, or rectum
    v.   Infections
    vi. Possible difficult menstruation and/or childbirth
    vii. Genitourinary problems
    viii. Occasionally death

(5) Ethical and human rights recommendations and actions:
(a) Islamic ruling: female circumcision not legitimate under Islamic law (Lutfi & Al-Sabbagh, 1996).
(b) Kenyan government outlawed FGM in 2001 (Livermore et al., 2007)
(c) Elimination of FGM recommended by multiple agencies (WHO, 2008).

4. *Child Abuse During Adolescence* (see also the Child Care/Parenting segment above and the Intimate Partner Violence segment in Chapter 6)
a. Definition for child maltreatment: Child Abuse Prevention and Treatment Act identifies four types (CDC, n.d.)
  (1) Physical abuse
  (2) Neglect
  (3) Sexual abuse
  (4) Emotional abuse
b. Statistics:
  (1) In 2000, ~57,000 children younger than 15 years of age suffered fatal abuse (WHO, 2002a).
  (2) In 2000, ~199,000 global youth homicides; ". . . an average of 565 children, adolescents, and young adults aged 10 to 29 years die each day as a result of interpersonal violence." (WHO, 2002b, p. 25)
  (3) In 2002, ~1,400 children younger than 18 years in the United States died from maltreatment (CDC, n.d.)
  (4) In the same year, ~896,000 children identified as abused by U.S. state and local child protective services (CDC, n.d.)
  (5) In 2002, 93% men and 79% women (aged 15-45 years) in Guatemala reported that they received some kind of parental punishment when children (verbal most common then beatings; CDC, 2001)
  (6) Among 6,592 high school students in southern China, 78.3% reported parental psychological aggression, 23.2% corporal punishment, and 15.1% severe maltreatment within the past 6 months (Leung, Wong, Chen, & Tang, 2008)
  (7) A total of 30% of female adolescents and young adult women aged 14 to 23 years reported an unwanted sexual experience in the past year (Rickert, Wiemann, Vaughan, & White, 2004)
  (8) "1 in 11 adolescents reports being a victim of physical dating violence" (CDC, 2006)

c. The trauma of abuse occurring earlier in childhood as well as during the adolescent years has lasting effects that continue in many forms through the teen years and beyond
  (1) Health consequences of abuse (WHO, 2002a)
    (a) Physical
        i.   injuries (brain, abdominal, central nervous system)
        ii. lacerations, bruises
        iii. fractures
        iv. disabilities
    (b) Psychological and behavioral
        i.   substance abuse
        ii. cognitive impairment
        iii. depression
        iv. developmental delays
        v.   suicidal behaviors
    (c) Sexual
        i.   sexually transmitted infections, HIV/AIDS
        ii. unwanted pregnancy
        iii. sexual dysfunction
  (2) Child and adolescent abuse seen as a pathway to future victimization (child to adolescent to adult; Fargo, 2008).
  (3) Lesser, Koniak-Griffin, Gonzalez-Figueroa, Huang, and Cumberland (2007) found a relationship between child abuse history and adolescent high risk behaviors in Latino adolescent parents (see Adolescent Risk content below for an intervention project that uses these parents' desire to protect their children from experiences they suffered).
  (4) Behavioral and emotional consequences of child abuse can be found in the extended incidents of emotional instability, depression, and aggressive behaviors long after abusive events occur (Stirling & Amaya-Jackson, 2008).
  (5) Posttraumatic stress disorder (PTSD) is an underdiagnosed disorder among adolescents with severe behavioral and emotional disorders (Mueser & Taub, 2008).
  (6) PTSD implicated in adolescent suicidal behavior (Sher, 2008).
  (7) Binge drinking (Shin, Edwards, & Heeren, 2008) and self-injurious behaviors (Yates, Carlson, & Egeland, 2008) seen to be linked to child abuse and neglect.
d. Adolescents who have experienced abuse, lived in violent environments, or endured "wounded relationships" often experience subsequent violence as perpetrators and/or victims (Biering, 2007; Oscós-Sánchez & Lesser, 2007).
  (1) Biering (2007) elicited explanatory models from male and female adolescents in an Iceland treatment home, from parents and from caregivers providing treatment. Painful life experiences seen as causation by all four groups.
  (2) Latino youths in a south Texas long-term juvenile correctional treatment center described wounded relationships as a major factor precipitating the "low point" preceding subsequent violent behavior (Oscós-Sánchez & Lesser, 2007).
  (3) Each of these studies with youths in different parts of the world suggests foci for intervention strategies.
e. Assessment and treatment of abused adolescents require
  (1) Careful examinations to assess trauma and ongoing vigilance (Adams, 2001, 2008)
  (2) Standardization of training for health care professionals (Adams, 2008)
  (3) Attentiveness to parent–child interactions
  (4) Evaluation of emotional and behavioral disorders to assess for potential abuse (Stirling & Amaya-Jackson, 2008)
  (5) Interventions that begin with discovery and discussion of explanatory models and incorporate cultural beliefs and practices in the intervention design (Biering, 2007; Lesser et al., 2007; Oscós-Sánchez & Lesser, 2007)

5. ***Sickle Cell Anemia:*** An example of one of many genetic disorders affecting adolescents among particular ethnic groups

a. Definitions:
   (1) A blood-related disorder affecting the hemoglobin molecule in the red blood cells that delivers oxygen to cells throughout the body (WHO, n.d.)
   (2) A hemoglobinopathy that produces the hemoglobin S by substituting amino acid valine in the y-globin chain (Ferri, 2008).
   (3) Red blood cells assume a sickle shape with exposure to lower oxygen tension (Ferri, 2008)
   (4) Sickle cell disease (SCD) hemoglobin S inherited from both parents
   (5) Sickle cell trait (SCT) the defective S gene inherited from only one parent
b. Epidemiology (Ferri, 2008):
   (1) Sickle cell hemoglobin S genetically transmitted by an autosomal recessive gene.
   (2) Found mostly in Blacks
   (3) Affects all age groups from birth through adulthood
   (4) Both genders affected
c. Prevalence and global distribution
   (1) SCD—globally the most common single gene disorder (Inati et al., 2007)
   (2) One in 500 African American and 1 in 1,000 to 1,400 Hispanic American births (WHO, n.d.)
   (3) Affects millions globally—especially common among people with ancestors from (WHO, n.d.)
       (a) Sub-Saharan Africa
       (b) South America
       (c) Cuba
       (d) Central America
       (e) Saudi Arabia
       (f) India
       (g) Mediterranean countries (e.g., Turkey, Greece, Italy)
   (4) SCD—Italy's most frequent hemoglobinopahty (Colombatti et al., 2008)
d. Presentation (Ferri, 2008):
   (1) Painful crises caused by ischemic tissue injury
   (2) Due to obstruction of blood flow by sickled red blood cells
   (3) Diagnosed with blood test—hemoglobin electrophoresis
   (4) Bones most common pain site
   (5) Abdominal pain
e. Complications (Ferri, 2008)
   (1) Pneumonia
   (2) Acute chest pain
   (3) Musculoskeletal and skin abnormalities
   (4) Neurologic abnormalities
   (5) Infections
   (6) Severe splenomegaly—resulting from sequestration of sickled cells
f. Issues and challenges for adolescents
   (1) Adjustment during transition from pediatric to adult health care (Anie & Telfair, 2005)
   (2) Depression (Jenerette, Funk, & Murdaugh, 2005; Laurence, George, & Woods, 2006)
   (3) Health-related quality of life (HRQL)
       (a) Palermo, Riley, and Mitchell (2008) found neighborhood socioeconomic distress diminished physical HRQL
       (b) Barakat, Patterson, Daniel, and Dampier (2008) had similar findings and in addition discovered concomitant with pain, the internalizing of symptoms and family variables affected HRQL.
g. Culturally focused family centered interventions
   (1) Family-focused culturally relevant disease management interventions for adolescents recommended to address issues associated with SCD (Barakat et al., 2008; Schwartz, Radcliffe, & Barakat, 2007)
   (2) Religion and spirituality based beliefs to modulate the pain experience among African Americans (Harrison et al., 2005).
   (3) Parent support groups (see WHO Genomic Resource Center)

(4) SCD detection and management foci in a community setting could serve to empower communities as well as help patients and families to make informed decisions and serve to stimulate desire for genetic counseling (Treadwell, McClough, &Vichinsky, 2006).

6. *Adolescent Risk Behaviors*

   a. Adolescent perceptions of risk

   (1) For teens in one detention setting, the term *risk* was not common, instead they talked about what they considered dangerous in their neighborhoods—gangs, drugs, and violence (N. L. R. Anderson, Nyamathi, McAvoy, Conde, & Casey, 2001)

   (2) These teens ". . . considered that problems arose in their lives (leading to gangs, drugs, violence) when they discovered they could not trust someone or felt they were being disrespected" (N. L. R. Anderson et al., 2001, p. 349).

   (3) Among a group of Vietnamese injection drug users 16 years of age and older, cultural characteristics influenced their vulnerability: trust/obligation, stoicism, importance of "face," and beliefs in fate (Ho & Maher, 2008)

   (4) Perceived barriers to accessing services in this group: stigma, discrimination, worry about confidentiality, long waits, language and financial issues (Ho & Maher, 2008)

   (5) Gender norms for rural Nigerian male youths characterize male sexuality as naturally dominant and aggressive; associate maleness with power and leadership, emphasize sexual potency (Izugbara, 2008).

   (6) Youths in Nicaragua aged 15 to 24 years described perceptions that differed between males and females: 83% of males stated they were encouraged to engage in premarital sex; females described more negative attitudes and were more frequently discouraged by parents from engaging in sex (Rani, Figueroa, & Ainsle, 2003)

   (7) African American adolescents perceived their vulnerability to HIV/AIDS as: image, the music/drug culture, and peer pressure (Glen & Wilson, 2008).

   (8) Urban adolescent school girls in South Delhi, India (McManus & Dhar, 2008):

   (a) >1/3 did not understand signs/symptoms of sexually transmitted infections

   (b) 30% thought HIV/AIDS can be cured

   (c) 49% said condoms should not be available to youths

   (d) 41% were confused whether the contraceptive pill did or did not protect against HIV

   (9) Male adolescents in juvenile detention considered that substance use is like a "natural life" only requiring a decision to use (N. L. R. Anderson, 1999, p. 659):

   (a) the first time

   (b) if an addictive substance

   (c) after the age of 21 years

   b. Societal perceptions of risk antecedents (Panel on High Risk Youth, 1993).

   (1) Societal concerns regarding adolescents usually focus on the behavior of the adolescent

   (2) The Panel of High Risk Youth (1993) determined to focus on the ". . . profound influence that settings have on the behavior and development of adolescents" (p. 1) rather than the traditional focus on characteristics of adolescents and their families.

   (3) Thus, more attention should be addressed to environmental contexts of the school milieu, the neighborhoods where teens live, their socioeconomic status, and expectations for future employment

   c. Types of risk

   (1) STIs and HIV

   (2) Adolescent pregnancy

   (3) Substance use/abuse

   (4) Violence (perpetrators and victims)

   (5) Gang membership/activities

   (6) School drop out

   (7) Suicidal and self-mutilation behaviors

   d. Risk factors—antecedent to risk behavior

   (1) Future uncertainty

   (2) Depression

   (3) Stress (Vazsony et al., 2008)

   (4) Neighborhood problems (N. L. R. Anderson et al., 2001)

(5) Deviant friends and peer pressure (Duncan, Duncan, & Strycker, 2000)

(6) Socio-economic pressures (Panel on High Risk Youth, 1993).

(7) Gender bias (Magado & Agwamda, 2008)

(8) History of preadolescent abuse (Salzinger, Rosario, Feldman, & Ng-Mak, 2007)

(9) Chronic illness (Suris, Michaud, Akre, & Sawyer, 2008).

e. Protective factors

(1) Peer attachment

(2) Family attachment

(3) School attachment (Jessor & Jessor, 1977)

(4) Family time

(5) Family support (Duncan, Duncan, & Strycker, 2000)

(6) Higher socioeconomic status

(7) Educational attainment

(8) Communication with parents

(9) Mother's higher educational attainment (Magadi & Agwanda, 2008).

f. Intervention examples and strategy recommendations

(1) Adolescents in juvenile detention asked for programs led by an adult they could trust, someone who "really understands and listens . . . someone that would really care about you . . ." who would put aside their own problems and give their time" (N. L. R. Anderson, 1994, p. 312).

(2) *Respecting and Protecting Our Relationships: A Community Research HIV Prevention Program for Teen Fathers and Mothers* based on "Healing the Wounded Spirit" framework focuses on healing and strengthening relationships (Lesser et al., 2005)

(3) Based on a pilot intervention *My Sister, Myself,* Shambley-Ebron (2008) recommends culture and gender-based foci for HIV/AIDS prevention programs

(4) *Stepping Stones,* a 50-hour intervention using participatory learning approaches with a large sample of men and women aged 15 to 26 yeras in the Eastern Cape province of South Africa improved risk behaviors among men, and lowered their reports of IPV perpetrations, and reported fewer transactional sex and drinking problems (Jewkes et al., 2008).

(5) *Exploring the World of Adolescents,* a gender-specific program developed for adolescents in Vietnam used capacity building and participatory strategies for program development (Lerdboon et al., 2008).

(6) Koniak-Griffin et al. (2008) conducted a couple-focused theory–based HIV prevention program for adolescent mothers and their partners that resulted at 6 month evaluation in signs of significant reduction in unprotected sex and increased intention to use condoms.

(7) *Familias en Acción* a community-based participatory action research project is based on an environment of trust and active community participation in the conduct and evaluation of a successful violence prevention program (Oscós-Sánchez, Lesser, & Kelly, 2008).

g. Policy recommendations

(1) Empowerment for teenagers and families (N. L. R. Anderson & Kagawa-Singer, 1996)

(a) Identify strengths such as within-group solidarity that can be harnessed for risk protection

(b) Involve adolescents in the design of interventions using participatory research and community partnership strategies.

(c) Assist parents and teens to learn how to listen to each other

(2) An agenda and framework for research (Panel on High Risk Youth, 1993)

(a) Achieve greater understanding by studying adolescent and community everyday life

(b) Study the interactions in multiple settings

(c) Support long-term, longitudinal studies and interventions that follow individual development over time

(d) Assess adolescent and community attributes

7. *Cross-Generational Enculturation/Acculturation*

a. Dimensions of parent/adolescent communication

(1) Parents and adolescents interact with each other each from their own perspective, developmental stage, and experience base

(2) Adolescent developmental tasks of separating from parents mean they push the limits and rebel against parents' rules

(3) Age, ethnicity, gender, socioeconomic factors, and religious beliefs all influence the dynamic interactions between parents and children

b. Parent/adolescent communication effectiveness can be positively influenced by willingness of both to:
(1) Listen
(2) State biases
(3) Discuss beliefs and explanatory models
(4) Work out differences
(5) Find common ground
(6) Try alternative solutions to conflict
(7) Establish appropriate power differential with the parent retaining authority
(8) Establish boundaries that stretch as the adolescent matures
(9) Recognize that conflict is a normal part of this developmental phase for both adolescent and parent.

c. Risk prevention assessment, programs and interventions that focus on or employ parent-teen communication and cooperative efforts
(1) *Parent–Adolescent Relationship Education (PARE)* increased parental rules about having sex and other risky behaviors and enhanced adolescent self-control with increased prevention knowledge (Lederman, Chan, & Roberts-Gray, 2008).
(2) Schouten, van den Putte, Pasmans, and Meeuwesen (2006) explored adolescent beliefs and perceived behavioral control to assess the amount of parent–adolescent communication about sexuality.
(3) Parent effectiveness beliefs related directly to their communication with their teens with minority, politically conservative and low-income parents reporting lower effectiveness beliefs than other parent groups (Swain, Ackerman, & Ackerman, 2006).
(4) Parents and adolescents who participated in the *Check Point Program* to promote parental management of teen driving, reported significantly greater limits on teen driving (Simons-Morton, Hartos, & Leaf, 2002).
(5) Adu-Mireku (2003) evaluated the relationship between family communications and HIV/AIDS and sexual activity and condom use with a group of secondary school students in Accra, Ghana and found that communication about HIV/AIDS increased the odds of using a condom.

8. *Summary:* Adolescence, a time of transition and change, provides opportunities for adolescents, their families and the community to assure the best outcomes. Culture, ethnicity, socioeconomic factors, and the neighborhood environmental context influence the outcomes of this important developmental journey.

D. **Young Adult through Middle-Aged Health Care Practices**
1. *Gender/Sexual Identity and Sexual Orientation*: These biopsychosocial constructs are strongly influenced by cultural norms and identity. Racial, ethnic, and socioeconomic differences provide added sources of diversity and in some cases, susceptibility to risk.
a. *Gender role expectations or stereotyping*–cultural and ethnic definitions of male and female sex roles may constrict individual self-expression and limit one's rights in society
b. *Gender/sexual identity terminology*—(see Table 5.6). Lay terminology is variable, linked with particular age, ethnic and sexual minority groups. Terms casually used by persons within the population may be perceived as offensive if used by an "outsider."
c. *Gender-based populations*—Women's and men's health care are relatively recent conceptual and practice frameworks addressing the historically male gender-biased approaches to health promotion and treatment of a wide range of general medical conditions. Also refer to gender-specific conditions. During young adult through menopause, women more regularly seek reproductive health–related services and individual health care services, compared with less frequent utilization by men.
(1) Women's health
(a) conceptual origins based in feminism (1970s-1980s)
(b) reproductive health and empowered decision making—contraception, pregnancy, sexuality, menarche through menopause, sexual health promotion
(c) full spectrum of health and medical conditions identifying and integrating understanding of gender-specific responses to health needs and illness
(d) developmental

Table 5.6. Glossary of Terms Related to Gender, Sexuality, and Sexual Orientation

Term	Definition
Gender	The collection of characteristics culturally associated with being "male," and "female," often seen as categorical, rather than a continuum. Gender identity refers to one's sense of oneself as male, female, or transgender
Sexual orientation	Sexual orientation refers to an enduring pattern of emotional, romantic, and/or sexual attractions to men, women, or both sexes. Sexual orientation also refers to a person's sense of identity based on those attractions, related behaviors, and membership in a community of others who share those attractions. Three sexual orientations are commonly recognized: homosexual, attraction to individuals of one's own gender; heterosexual, attraction to individuals of the other gender; bisexual, attractions to members of either gender. Persons with a homosexual orientation are sometimes referred to as gay (both men and women) or lesbian (women only). Sexual orientation differs from sexual behavior because it refers to feelings and self-concept. Persons may or may not express their sexual orientation in their behaviors. (American Psychological Association, 2008) Copyright 2008 American Psychological Association
Sexual minority	Population of gay, lesbian, bisexual, and transgender people whose sexual orientation, behaviors, and/or attraction are perceived to be in contrast to the majority population of heterosexuals
Sexual health	"A state of physical, emotional, mental and social well being related to sexuality, not merely the absence of disease, dysfunction or infirmity. Sexual health requires a positive and respectful approach to sexuality and sexual relationships, as well as the possibility of having pleasurable and safe sexual experiences, free of coercion, discrimination and violence" (WHO, 2006)
Sex	A person's sexual characteristics (including anatomical, chromosomal, hormonal, and/or physiological) as male, female, both, or neither. Transgender people and people with intersex conditions may have sexual characteristics that do not entirely align with the typical definition of "male" or "female"
Transgender	An umbrella term used to describe people whose gender identity (sense of themselves as male or female) or gender expression differs from that usually associated with their birth sex. Many transgender people live part-time or full-time as members of the other gender. Broadly speaking, anyone whose identity, appearance, or behavior falls outside of conventional gender norms can be described as transgender. However, not everyone whose appearance or behavior is gender-atypical will identify as a transgender person. (American Psychological Association, 2006) Copyright 2006 American Psychological Association
Intersex	Refers to a variety of conditions in which a person has reproductive or sexual characteristics that do not fit the typical definition of "male" or "female"
Heterosexism	The assumption that heterosexuality is the "norm" and other sexual orientations are deviant. Often, homosexuality is viewed as being in opposition to heterosexuality, rendering bisexuality invisible and irrelevant
Academic/professional terms with a behavioral health risk focus	MSM: men who have sex with men MSMW: men who have sex with men and women (including transgender people) WSW: women who have sex with women WSMW: women who have sex with men and women (including transgender people)

(2) Men's health—more recent framework, a corollary response to address men's similar need for gender specific care in areas of reproductive (genitourinary) function, as well as specific behavioral and high-risk areas

(3) Lesbian, gay, bisexual, and transgender (LGBT)—refers to affective, sexual, and behavioral aspects of sexual orientation (lesbian, gay, bisexual) and gender identity (transgender). Sexual minority status is associated with its own unique set of stressors (Meyer, 2003), challenges and strengths

    (a) Sexual minorities (men who have sex with men [MSM], women who have sex with women [WSW], LGBT people) are at greater risk of experiencing mental and physical health problems.

    (b) Societal homophobia, marginalization, and discrimination present threats to health through

        i. Covering, passing, and other behaviors that deny one's authentic self can result in social restrictions of civil rights (Yoshino, 2007).

        ii. Cultural, social, and legal restrictions interfere with family function and obtaining other sources of social support:

            (aa) disruption of ties with family of origin

            (ab) barriers to family formation (adoption, foster care, civil marriage, domestic partnerships) (ac) lack of access to federal and most state-level benefits (such as Social Security, inheritance, health insurance) available to heterosexual couples and families

   iii. Delays in seeking health care due to
- (aa) inaccurate perceptions of risk, for example, lesbians at risk for cervical cancer
- (ab) lack of insurance, regular trusted health care provider
- (ac) perceived risk of discrimination by health care provider

   iv. Concealment of sexual orientation. Readily available social support may be better utilized by those open about their sexual orientation (Ullrich, Lutgendorf, & Stapleton, 2003).

   v. Stress
- (aa) Coming out
- (ab) Chronic stress related to discrimination
- (ac) Racial or ethnic minority status

   vi. LGBT cultural strengths
- (aa) Shared meanings
- (ab) Recognizable artistic expressions
- (ac) Sense of community
- (ad) Social roles and expectations
- (ae) Group identity and visibility

   vii. LGBT culture from a sociopolitical perspective
- (aa) Stigma and alienation
- (ab) Disenfranchisement and heterosexism
- (ac) Civil rights and discrimination
- (ad) Discrimination related to gender, gender identity, and sexual orientation is illegal in some states
- (ae) Areas of evolving law include family (domestic partnership and marriage, foster parenting and adoption, custody, and visitation), hate crimes

d. Sexual and reproductive health (SRH)—population oriented, inclusive coverage of sexuality and reproductive health topics affecting men and women, considering developmental, social, behavioral, and biologic factors.
- (1) Pregnancy, contraception, abortion, preconception
- (2) Sexual health promotion, treatment of sexual dysfunction
- (3) Prevention and treatment of sexually transmitted infections (STIs), reproductive tract cancers (WHO, 2009)
- (4) Urologic and gynecologic conditions
- (5) Reproductive health and environment, fertility

e. Global perspective and social determinants of SRH. The World Health Organization is a leading resource for information and policy development (http://www.who.int/reproductivehealth/en/).
- (1) Low socioeconomic status and limited resources
- (2) Social justice, gender equity, and human rights
- (3) Violence, abuse, and sexual violence
- (4) Involvement of males to partner in improved sexual health

f. Health disparity—defined as avoidable and unjust health status differences (Adler & Rehkopf, 2008) due to systematic sources of discrimination within society and the health care system, including health care providers. Gender bias (against women), sexual and racial minority status, and discrimination all contribute to significant health disparities. Males suffer effects of differential health risks related to gender role and social expectations of masculinity (Courtenay, 2000). Disparities related to
- (1) gender differentiated behaviors (smoking, alcohol, and illicit drug use)
- (2) unprotected sex
- (3) unhealthy nutrition and exercise
- (4) violence
- (5) response to common health problems (cardiovascular, cancers, STIs, depression)

g. Male health disparities and indicators
- (1) Increased adult mortality from violence and automobile accidents, and remains more common among African Americans.

(2) Higher rate of tobacco use among men, even more common among men with lower education levels, (Mensah, Mokdad, Ford, Greenlund, & Croft, 2005).

(3) Less likely to have a usual source of health care compared to women (74% vs. 82%), despite similar levels of health insurance (83% male vs. 85% female lack coverage; National Health Interview Survey, 2002).

(4) Syphilis rate higher in males

(5) African American males experience increased morbidity and mortality from prostate cancer

h. Female health disparities:

(1) Undetected cardiac disease, thyroid dysfunction and depression

(2) Providers fail to understand "a typical" presentation of cardiovascular, endocrine problems

(3) Women 25 years and younger have three times the Chlamydia rate, of older women and is more common among African Americans.

(4) Increased HIV infection among racial minority women

(5) Although White women are 70% more likely to develop endometrial cancer, African Americans are more likely to die from it.

i. Sexual orientation, MSM and WSW health disparities (Mays, Yancey, Cochran, Weber, & Fielding, 2002; Meyer, 2003).

(1) Women—lesbian, WSW (Diamant, Wold, Spritzer, & Gelberg, 2000; Mravcak, 2006)

(a) Obesity, possible higher incidence of breast and endometrial cancer

(b) Tobacco addiction

(c) Alcohol abuse (Cochran, Keenan, Schober, & Mays, 2000)

(d) Depression, anxiety, and stress

(2) Men—gay, MSM

(a) 20% of MSMs are HIV positive (CDC, 2009).

(b) 72% of new HIV infections in males are MSM transmitted (Prejean, Song, An, & Hall, 2008)

j. Transgender health disparities

(1) Sexual and physical victimization, including hate crimes. More prevalent in minority transgender, especially male-to-female transgenders

(2) HIV/AIDS

(3) Depression and suicide

(4) Poor access and limited insurance coverage for trans health care

k. Sexual minority families

(1) Family of origin

(2) Coming out–families beneficial source of support

(3) Adult relationships

(a) Civil unions and marriage

(b) Domestic partnerships

(4) Pathways to parenthood

(a) Surrogacy

(b) Donor insemination

(c) Adoption

(d) Foster parenting

(5) Gay and lesbian parenting (Golombok et al., 2003; Weber, 2008)—No differences among children in

(a) Sexual or gender identity

(b) Personality traits

(c) Intelligence

l. LGBT culturally competent health providers/setting characterized by

(1) Sexual history—ask clearly and inclusively

(2) Avoid forced gender terms, avoid heterosexist assumptions

(3) Ask questions for clarity

(4) Have information resources available for families

(5) Institutional policies and procedures to promote equality and avoid discrimination

m. Nursing interventions based on culturally competent assessment of unique and population specific factors related to behaviors, health, and illness management.

(1) Health promotion—strengthening individuals and families

(a) addressing gender differences (biobehavioral and social)

(b) based within sexual minority communities

(c) increasing access to LGBT-friendly health care services in non-metropolitan areas.

(2) Population based interventions

(3) Education of health professionals to increase cultural competence in communication, build trust and gain increased knowledge of specific health care needs, eliminate health care

(4) Advocacy to insure LGBT welcomed and overtly included in health care environment

2. ***Reproduction, Pregnancy, and Postpartum:*** Childbearing is a time of transition and social celebration in any society, reflecting a realignment of existing cultural roles and responsibilities and states. The different ways in which a particular society views this period are dependent on the culture's beliefs about health, medical care, reproduction, and the status of women (Dickason, Silverman, & Schult, 1994).

a. A number of factors have contributed to the changes in childbirth in Western society:

(1) Increase in number of women in the work force

(2) Advances in reproductive technology

(3) Alternative therapies

(4) Increased health information available to consumers

(5) Influx of immigrants and refugees (Tiedje, 2000)

b. Dominant medical practices in the United States and Canada include the use of various state of the art technologies, and include formal prenatal care and delivery in a hospital (or sometimes a free-standing birthing center)

c. Subcultures within the United States and Canada have very different practices, values, and beliefs about pregnancy and childbirth; great variations exist in the social class, ethnic origin, family structure and social support networks of women, men, and families (see previous discussion of social determinants of health and health care during this period).

d. Reproduction and pregnancy

(1) A woman's fertility varies on several physical factors as well as cultural and social variables, including

(a) marriage and residence patterns

(b) diet

(c) religion

(d) the availability of abortion

(e) incidence of sexually transmitted infections

(f) regulation of birth intervals by cultural or artificial means (Lauderdale, 2008).

(2) Cultural and religious beliefs can impact desired family size, interpregnancy intervals, and contraceptive choices (Purnell & Paulanka, 2008).

(3) While little research exists on the fertility control practices of diverse ethnic, cultural, and racial groups (Purnell & Paulanka, 2008), more is known about the positions of various religions. The religious beliefs of some cultural groups might affect their use of fertility controls such as abortion or artificial regulation of conception

(a) Roman Catholics might follow church advice against artificial control of conception; natural family planning (the "rhythm method"), abstinence, and coitus interruptus are the only church-approved choices (Schenker & Rabenou, 1993; Srikanthan & Reid, 2008).

(b) Orthodox Judaism, however, prohibits these same choices because they conflict with basic religious tenets (Srikanthan & Reid, 2008).

(c) In general, Islamic and Protestant teachings do not prohibit hormonal contraceptives, but fundamentalist interpretations result in some believing that the use of any contraception violates God's intentions (Srikanthan & Reid, 2008).

(d) The religious teachings of Hinduism and Buddhism lack any prohibitions against contraception (Schenker & Rabenou, 1993; Srikanthan & Reid, 2008).

(e) Mormon families might follow their church's teaching about a spiritual responsibility to have large families (Andrews & Hanson, 2003).

(f) Religion is a powerful influence on sexual attitudes and behaviors and often establishes a society's orientation to sexuality (Moore et al., 2010). When a particular religion is practiced by a majority of people in a society, or by a powerful minority, it helps to create culture, even for those who do not adhere to the specific religion (Family Planning Association of United Kingdom, 2004).

(g) However, attempts to predict attitudes and behaviors based on a specific religious affiliation may result in false assumptions.

    i.   It is common to differentiate adherents to Islam, Christianity, and Judaism by whether they practice more conservative or liberal interpretations of their holy books and teachers.

    ii.   Within faiths there are likely differences in how teachings about procreation and contraception are viewed.

    iii.   It is imperative to realize that all people from one country, one neighborhood, or one faith do not share one culture or a single set of religious beliefs (Moore et al., 2010).

(h) In the United States, recent studies have found that religious affiliation plays little or no role in determining individual contracepting behaviors (R. Jones, Darroch, & Singh, 2005; Kramer, Hogue, & Gaydos, 2007).

    i.   Contraceptive use and method of choice is more reflective of gender roles, access to contraception and personal values regarding ideal family size than religion or cultural influences (Schenker, 2000; Srikanthan & Reid, 2008)

    ii.   This may or may not also reflect immigrants' acculturation, as no longitudinal studies were found that examined family planning desires and practices over time It has been postulated that when faced with the challenges of acculturation, women may "anchor more strongly to traditional religious and cultural expectations with respect to family, sexuality and fertility" (Srikanthan & Reid, 2008, p. 136; see work cited later by Van Rooij, Van Balen, & Hermanns, 2004, about Turkish migrants in The Netherlands and infertility).

(4) Studies regarding the parenthood motives of people (the desire to have a child) show a wide variety in motives, and the importance people attach to these motives (Van Balen & Inhorn, 2002). These authors divide the many reasons into two types, social and individual:

(a) social parenthood motives—motives include

    i.   social power reasons—having children gives status or adult identity

    ii.   continuation motives—desire for immortality through children, continuation of family name

    iii.   social pressure motives—implicit and explicit expectations of the cultural and/or religious group to have children

    iv.   economical reasons—children contribute to family survival through labor or care of parents

(b) individual motives are related to:

    i.   the child—joy that children bring and the unique relationship with the child as parent

    ii.   feelings for and about the partner

    iii.   biological urge and having children as family fulfillment

(c) Individual motives appear to be present in most cultures, but differences exist across cultures in regard to social motives (Van Balen & Inhorn, 2002).

    i.   As shown in several studies, these differences can be related to variation in

        (aa)   cultural variables such as degree of pronatalist norms (importance of children), position of men and women, family structure

        (ab)   religion

        (ac)   economic welfare

        (ad)   demographic variables (Colpin, DeMunter, & Vandemeulebroecke, 1998; Kagitcibasi & Ataca, 2005; Schenker, 2000; Trommsdorff, Kim, & Nauck, 2005; Van Balen & Inhorn, 2002).

    ii.   Studies about the desire for a child and the desire for children in Turkey demonstrate both high individual motives as well as high social importance (Ataca & Sunar, 1999; Kagitcibasi & Ataca, 2005).

        (aa)   Having children is the social norm, functions for men as a proof of manhood and provides status for both men and women (Guz, Ozkan, Sarisoy, Yank, & Yanik, 2003; Hortacsu, 1999)

        (ab)   Turkish men and women also marry relatively early and have children early in the marriage (Ataca, Kagitcibasi, & Diri, 2005).

> (ac) This strong pronatalist norm might be related to the strong influence of Islam on procreation and to traditional patriarchal cultural beliefs in this area (Schenker, 2000; Van Rooij, Van Balen, & Hermanns, 2004).
>
> (ad) Additionally, this norm might be related to the relatively moderate economical welfare (WHO, 2005); in rural areas, especially, having children can provide income.
>
> iii. Van Rooij, Van Balen, and Hermanns (2006) compared parenthood motives of Turkish migrants in the Netherlands and Dutch men and women, particularly in relation to adaptation of the migrants to the Dutch culture.
>
> (aa) Social motives were more important to Turkish migrants than to indigenous Dutch.
>
> (ab) These differences are less if people are more culturally adapted to life in the Netherlands.

(d) An essential component of transcultural nursing care during the reproductive stage of a woman's life would be an assessment of these features and the role they play in the parents' desire for and acceptance of treatment and/or interventions for infertility. Each of the major religions has specific doctrine about the use of infertility treatments.

  i. Judaism allows the practice of all techniques of assisted reproduction as long as the oocyte and spermatozoon are from the husband and wife

  ii. In vitro fertilization and embryo transfer are acceptable in Islam although they can be performed only for a husband and wife

  iii. Whereas assisted reproduction is not accepted by the Roman Catholic church, it may be consistent with the doctrine of various Protestant denominations (Schenker, 2005).

(5) The ability to control fertility successfully also requires an understanding of the menstrual cycle and the times and conditions under which pregnancy might or might not occur.

(6) Competent preconception care also includes assessment of genetic risks so that parents have the opportunity to make informed decisions about various reproductive options.

(a) Couples found to be at risk prior to conception for having a child with a genetic disorder have several reproductive options:

  i. choosing to not become pregnant

  ii. accepting the risk

  iii. choosing to have prenatal diagnosis after conception to determine if the child is affected

  iv. using artificial insemination or oocyte donation to avoid passing on the mutant gene

  v. undergoing preimplantation diagnosis (Moore et al., 2010)

(b) Each couple should be assessed appropriately and in a culturally sensitive manner; clinical care should not result in some segments of the population receiving a different level of attention to genetic risks because of preconceived notions about the patient's values, low health literacy or language barriers (Moore et al., 2010)

(c) Common genetic diseases for various population groups:

  i. Arabs/Middle Easterners: thalassemias, sickle cell disease, and glucose-6 phosphate dehydrogenase deficiency (G6PD)

  ii. Asian/Pacific Islanders: thalassemias, cleft lip/palate, and G6PD

  iii. African Americans are at increased risk for sickle cell disease, G6PD, hemoglobin C disease, and beta-thalassemia

  iv. Depending on which specific ethnicity to which those of the White race or American/European ethnicities belong, there are various disorders to which they are susceptible: cystic fibrosis, dwarfism, phenylkenonuria (PKU), Tay-Sachs disease, hemophilia, and neural tube defects

  v. Hispanic groups often demonstrate a higher incidence of cleft lip/palate

  vi. Native Americans/Alaskan natives are at higher risk for ear anomalies, albinism, and adrenal hyperplasia (specific to various nations; see tables in Purnell & Paulanka, 2008; Moore et al., 2010; various maternity textbooks have more complete lists and discussion)

(7) Kay's (1982) areas of assessment during antepartum (pregnancy) and postpartum. The following are areas to address:

(a) Determinants of the society's acceptance of the pregnancy
   i.   acceptable age
   ii. marriage requirements
   iii. acceptable father
   iv. pregnancy frequency
(b) Consideration of pregnancy as a state of illness or health
   i.   Western providers tend to view pregnancy as a physiologic state that at any moment will become pathologic;
   ii. Many cultural groups perceive pregnancy as a normal physiologic process or state, and don't believe that pregnant women are ill or in need of "curative services". These women often delay or do not receive any prenatal care from a health care provider (Lauderdale, 2008).
      (aa) Latinos in particular consider pregnancy a natural condition that usually doesn't require medical care, unless there is a problem, until late in the pregnancy. However, the mother and fetus are vulnerable to outside influences and will take protective measures if necessary (Mattson, 2003).
      (ab) In one study, Amish women used perinatal care based on their beliefs about pregnancy and childbirth, and in relation to cost, transportation, and child care. The women initiated prenatal care earlier for first pregnancies, and later with subsequent ones, knowing that pregnancy was a "nonproblematic" condition. They did seek immediate attention if a serious problem arose, e.g. bleeding (Campanella, Korbin, & Acheson, 1993).
(c) Prenatal testing for a variety of disorders is common in the United States. Cultures vary in how the occurrence of genetic or other conditions is explained.
   i.   Many Eastern Indians, and those who believe in karma, think that hereditary and congenital problems are caused by the actions of that person in a prior life (Lipson & Dibble, 2005). People with this belief see no value in prenatal testing.
   ii. In other cultures, hearing about the possibility of genetic diseases or the likelihood of complications from procedures such as amniocentesis is considered prophetic; Mexican immigrants may believe that if they discuss the possibility of a genetic condition, they will "get it" from the health care provider.
   iii. In some cultures, positive findings from prenatal diagnostic testing or giving birth to an abnormal infant can result in negative consequences for the woman (Moore et al., 2010).
   iv. The nurse's role around prenatal testing is to facilitate informed choices by the woman and her family if appropriate (Moore et al., 2010)
   v.   Complicating informed decision making around prenatal testing is that it requires a level of health literacy that is not always found among women who may not be fluent in the language of the nurse or health care provider. The conversation must include time to appreciate what the woman understands, what she wants to do (including postponing the decision), and what the results would mean to her (Moore et al., 2010).
(d) Behavioral expectations during pregnancy:
   i.   Dietary prescriptions or restrictions
      aa. Food has symbolic as well as health connotations, which are generally culturally determined. An important example is the tradition in many cultures, including Latino, Asian, and Arabic, of adherence to the hot or cold theory of health and diet.
         (i)   This theory describes the intrinsic properties of foods, beverages, medicines and their effects on the body
         (ii) Health is maintained through a balance of these forces
         (iii) If an imbalance occurs, illness results (Andrews, 1989).
         (iv) To produce balance (and restore or maintain health), illness and conditions such as pregnancy are treated with substances having the opposite property of the illness (i.e., pregnancy is considered to be a "hot" state; thus, any treatments must be of a "cold" nature. The woman loses this heat at delivery, so in the postpartum period, she is considered "cold" and must be protected with "hot" or "warm" treatments and substances.

      (aa) Temperature and spiciness do not determine classification

      (ab) Generally, warm or hot foods are believed to be easier to digest than cold or cool foods

          (v) In the Mexican culture, women are encouraged to ingest "hot" foods throughout the pregnancy, whereas in the Vietnamese culture, women are encouraged to move from "hot" foods in the first two trimesters to "cold" foods in the final weeks of pregnancy (Moore et al., 2010).

         (vi) It is important to know that a 'cold" condition in one culture may be a "hot" condition in another and that the foods needed to balance the condition are based on the foods available within the specific country of origin. (Moore et al., 2010)

        (vii) These properties of hot and cold are also part of the *yin–yang* belief system prevalent among Asian approaches to health and diet (Andrews, 1989).

ab. Another somewhat unfamiliar practice is that of pica, or the ingestion of nonfood substances, especially clay or starch.

          (i) Some Hispanic women prefer the solid milk of magnesia, whereas others eat the ice or frost that forms inside refrigerator/freezer units (Boyle & Mackey, 1999).

         (ii) Pica may be practiced by African American women, often in the rural southern United States and by women of lower socioeconomic levels

        (iii) There are many explanations for why this occurs, some with cultural implications

    (aa) A result of an iron deficiency, which leads to the craving

    (ab) A carryover from behaviors practiced in Africa

    (ac) Geissler et al. (1999) found a high prevalence of geophagy among pregnant women in Kenya, and a strong association of geophagy, anemia, and iron depletion. They found that of the 52 women observed, 73% ate soil regularly; they mainly ate the soil from walls of houses. They made associations between soil-eating, the condition of the blood and certain bodily states, including pregnancy.

ac. Fasting is an important religious observance for followers of Islam. Fasting during the month of Ramadan is one of the five pillars of faith for Muslims.

          (i) The fast requires abstaining from food, drink, sexual activity, and smoking from sunrise to sunset for 29 or 30 days.

         (ii) It is compulsory for every Muslim who has reached puberty, with certain exceptions for those who are sick, menstruating, traveling, elderly, or unable to understand the purposes of the fast (Cross-Sudworth, 2007).

        (iii) The *Qu'ran* does not specifically exempt pregnant or breastfeeding women, although most Muslims believe that a pregnant woman can be exempted if she is ill, or the fetus is compromised (Cross-Sudworth, 2007).

        (iv) It has been reported that 60% to 90% of pregnant Muslims living in the United States fast and that immigrant populations are more likely to participate in the fast than American-born Muslims (Robinson & Raisler, 2005).

         (v) Little research exists that fully explores the impact of fasting every day for a month on pregnancy outcomes, but one analyst suggested that Ramadan fasting in healthy women has no effect on the weight of the offspring (Cross-Sudworth, 2007).

ii. Activity restrictions or prescriptions, including the use of massage as a treatment for the various symptoms experienced during pregnancy; many people believe that the activities of the mother influence the outcome of pregnancy and their well-being of the newborn.

    aa. Positive or prescriptive beliefs might include wearing special articles of clothing, performing certain ceremonies that act as blessings, continuing sexual activity, continuing daily shampoos and baths (Lauderdale, 2008)

    ab. Negative or restrictive beliefs include activity and work (don't reach over your head, don't sew, avoid heavy work, and get frequent rest), sexual activity (avoid especially in third trimester) and environmental effects (avoid weddings or funerals, or people in mourning, especially those who have lost children; avoid cold air/drafts)

    ac. Taboos, or restrictions that may have supernatural consequences or connections, include avoidance of baby showers and avoiding persons who could cast a spell. Avoiding moonlight and eclipses, saying the baby's name before a naming ceremony and not having your picture taken are also taboos (Lauderdale, 2008; Mattson, 2000; Waxler-Morrison, Andrews, & Richardson, 1990).

iii. Expression of emotions, including anger, fear, and anxiety

    aa. Many Pueblo and Navajo Indians, Mexicans and Japanese believe the mother should remain happy to bring the baby joy and good fortune (Waxler-Morrison et al., 1990).

    ab. Some Hispanics believe experiencing *susto* in pregnancy is bad for the mother and baby (Mattson, 2003).

    ac. One major consideration at this time is intimate partner violence (IPV) that may escalate or begin during pregnancy

        (i) IPV of pregnant women has been associated with adverse pregnancy outcomes for both mother and infant (Taggart & Mattson, 1996).

        (ii) In addition to direct injury, many women delay seeking prenatal care due to overt signs of abuse or prevention by the partner (Taggart & Mattson, 1996).

        (iii) An abused pregnant woman has a greater risk of delivering a low birth weight (LBW) infant; studies suggest that physical and sexual abuse predict poor health during pregnancy and the postpartum period (Lauderdale, 2008).

        (iv) For women who self-identify as ethnic minorities the degree of acculturation or assimilation into the dominant culture must be taken into consideration when assessing or determining a woman's risk for abuse, since it indicates to what degree the woman has taken on those values and customs (Mattson & Rodriguez, 1999).

        (v) Conflicting data exist about IPV in different groups, with some studies indicating higher levels and/or severity of abuse in some cultures versus others (see additional bibliography for citations).

    ad. Depression has also been identified in pregnant immigrant women. According to Diaz, Le, Cooper, and Munoz (2007), interpersonal factors (marital quality and social support) are among the risk factors that predisposed 69 low-income, mostly immigrant Latina mothers to mood disturbances. The authors suggest targeting social support and marital quality in preventive interventions for perinatal depression in Latinas.

    ae. Likewise, Zelkowitz et al. (2004), examined psychosocial risk factors for depressive symptomatology in 119 pregnant immigrant women in Montreal, Canada. In this sample, depressive symptoms were associated with poorer functional status and more somatic symptoms. Depressed women reported a lack of social support, more stressful life events and poorer marital adjustment. They concluded that transitions associated with migration may place pregnant immigrant women at high risk for depression.

iv. Biological variations appear in certain ethnic groups that can have an effect on the pregnancy, the mother, or the newborn

    aa. African Americans and others of Mediterranean descent may have sickle cell disease

    ab. Native Americans and Hispanics are susceptible to diabetes mellitus

    ac. Jewish populations from Europe (Ashkenazi) carry the traits for Tay-Sachs and Gaucher's diseases

    ad. Greek and Southeast Asian women can present with thalassemias, along with women of Arab/Eastern Mediterranean descent.

    ae. Amish women may have PKU, and infant boys may have hemophilia B (Moore & Moos, 2003).

(e) Many cultures consider the postpartum period to be one of increased vulnerability for both mother and infant; dietary and activity prescriptions are common at this time and might be in conflict with the usual Western methods of obstetric care (Mattson, 2004). Postpartum practices exist to provide social support, adaptation to the maternal role, care of the newborn and physical recovery (Moore et al., 2010).

i. Activity restrictions and prescriptions

    aa. One way to protect against danger is for the mother to remain quietly in bed, without activity to disturb her

        (i) Hispanic women may observe *cuarenta*, or a 40-day rest period.

        (ii) Laotian postpartum women stay home near heat for 30 days to "dry up the womb" (Moore et al., 2010).

ab. This includes restrictions on
(i) Ambulating
(ii) Bathing (especially showering)
(iii) Infant caretaking
(iv) Other activities seen as normal from a Western medical perspective

ac. In some cultures, women are considered to be in a state of impurity during the puerperium, which often coincides with the period of lochial flow. Common behaviors include
(i) Seclusion and avoidance of contact with others
(ii) Avoidance of sexual relations (Lauderdale, 2008).
(iii) Restitution of physical balance and purification might occur through many mechanisms, including
(aa) Dietary restrictions
(ab) Ritual baths
(ac) Seclusion for specified period of time
(ad) Restriction of certain activities
(ae) Other ceremonial events (in medieval times a woman could not attend church until the lochial flow had stopped and she was officially "churched or cleansed" by being blessed by the priest (Horn, 1981; Lauderdale, 2008; Mattson, personal communication).

ad. Culturally bound practices are many
(i) On Eastern European and Scandinavian mother/baby hospital units postpartum women come together in a common dining room for their meals, which may foster communication provide social support for first time mothers especially, and overcome feelings of isolation.
(ii) Korean postpartum women may traditionally be cared for by their mother-in-law (Moore, et al, 2010).
(iii) Chinese women practice *zuoyuezi*, or "doing the month" to promote maternal/newborn health. Women believe that not following this practice could have long-term adverse effects on their health (Callister, 2006b; N. Cheung et al., 2006).
(iv) Punjabi women may practice *jholabharai*, returning to their mother's home in preparation for the upcoming birth and rest for 40 days afterward, viewed as necessary for maternal recovery (Grewal, Bhagat, & Balneaves, 2008), which is similar to the Japanese practice of *satorgarir bunben* (Yoshida, Yamashita, Ueda, & Tashiro, 2001).

ii. Dietary restrictions and prescriptions
aa. Many of the same requirements based on a theory of hot and cold apply to the postpartum period as well.
ab. The puerperium is a cold time (as heat was lost at delivery), so foods should be hot in nature; women will avoid fruits and vegetables that are considered cold.
ac. Women often prefer a hot drink after delivery rather than a cold one which is usually offered in western hospitals.

iii. Appropriateness of therapeutic heat and cold
aa. Western practitioners usually use cold packs or sitz baths for perineal comfort and healing.
ab. These practices are not acceptable to women from many cultures.
(i) Cold air and water are often believed to be harmful.
(ii) These entities are believed to cause uterine problems and even infertility when they enter the uterus through the vagina (Greener, 1989).

iv. Expression of emotions
aa. Postpartum depression (PPD) seems to occur in most cultures throughout the world.
ab. Risk factors are similar, but some specific to particular cultures may include
(i) Higher value placed on birth of a male child
(ii) The family's immigrant or refugee status
(iii) Distress from not being able to practice expected postpartum rituals
(iv) Lack of an effective social support system (Chaudron et al., 2005).

(v) Zelkowitz et al. (2008) explored changes in mental health and functional status beginning in pregnancy to two months postpartum in 106 childbearing immigrant women in Montreal, Quebec, Canada. In looking at three sets of variables in relation to postpartum depression (1) prenatal depression, worries, and somatic symptoms; (2) social relationships; and (3) factors related to migration, they found that almost 38% of the women scored above the cutoff point of 12 on the Edinburgh Postnatal Depression Scale (EDPS). Prenatal depressive and somatic symptoms as well as marital quality (social relationships) were the best predictors of postpartum depression (PPD). Women who were not depressed prenatally, but reported postpartum depressive symptoms showed several predisposing risk factors during pregnancy: many somatic complaints, high perinatal anxiety, and premigraton stress.

ac. Reporting of the phenomenon in non-Western culture may be hindered by culturally unacceptable labeling of the disorder, variance of symptoms from group to group, or differences in diagnostic standards (Lauderdale, 2008).

ad. Women may report somatic symptoms rather than psychological ones, especially in cultures that have no name or definition for PPD, such as the Korean and other Asian cultures (Posmontier & Horowitz, 2004).

ae. A challenge for transcultural nurses is to have an understanding of the many ways that mothers perceive, explain and report symptoms of PPD. If the mother does not return for a 6-week check up, brief maternal screening for PPD can be conducted during well-child visits in pediatric settings (Feinberg et al., 2006; Olson, Dietrich, Prazar, & Hurley, 2006).

af. Women need supportive postpartum care that recognizes the importance of the sociocultural context of women's lives, attends to maternal health and postpartum recovery, and generates strategies to enhance social support and reduce isolation.

    (i) The Hispanic Labor Friends Initiative is an innovative program that can make a difference for Hispanic immigrant childbearing women.

    (ii) This organization assigns a "friend" to assist the pregnant woman during the third trimester of pregnancy, during labor and birth and in the early postpartum period (Hazard, Callister, Birkhead, & Nichols, 2009).

e. Summary:

  (1) Cultural competency is a journey for both individuals and organizations.

    (a) The journey involves introspection to identify current attitudes toward persons that are different from oneself; the discovery and acquisition of knowledge; and the development of specific skills.

    (b) Foronda (2008) described cultural sensitivity as "employing one's knowledge, consideration, understanding, and respect, and requires each nurse to have a plan for how to grow as a culturally competent provider" (p. 208).

    (c) The plan must extend beyond the search and use of a specific book on culture because no one reference can possibly address the needs of every woman (Moore et al., 2010).

  (2) Cultural relevance is an essential component of providing meaningful and acceptable perinatal care.

    (a) Some individuals do not recognize differences in their clients; this devalues the client's beliefs, because it fails to recognize that these differences are valid and important.

    (b) Other nurses may exhibit ethnocentrism; they recognize differences are present, but believe their ways are superior (Moore et al., 2010).

  (3) A culturally competent nurse acknowledges differences between people as valuable and both seeks to understand the perspectives of those who are different and modifies her own practice to accommodate those differences.

  (4) Nurses in the United States care for an increasingly diverse population of childbearing women and families. Concepts related to culture, health care disparities, and cultural competence provide a framework for understanding the role of culture and cultural competence throughout the childbearing cycle.

3. Acute Illness and Trauma in Adulthood

a. Suffering, the beginning point of caring, is linked with all of human existence. Caring expressed in compassion, can alleviate suffering (Lindholm & Eriksson, 1993).

b. Acute illness and trauma inflict culturally defined suffering for patients, families, and caregivers.

   c. Three questions, according to Lindholm and Eriksson (1993), provide a starting point for the alleviation of suffering:
      (1) How does the patient describe his or her suffering?
      (2) How does the nurse describe the patient's suffering?
      (3) What is the opinion of both patient and nurse on how to alleviate the suffering?
   d. R. Spector (2008) suggests assessing the cultural phenomena affecting health by using Giger and Davidhizar's Transcultural Assessment model (Giger & Davidhizar, 2004, pp. 10-12) in order to discover culturally appropriate ways of caring for the patient.
      (1) The model is adaptable to many health care disciplines and educational levels (Davidhizar, Bechtel, & Giger, 1998).
      (2) It is particularly appropriate in the acute care setting where the patient may be too ill to participate in a lengthy interview, but caregivers can collect much data through observation.
   e. General guidelines for both nurses and acute care facilities in working with culturally diverse patients.
      (1) Culturally diverse families and their hospitalized relatives
         (a) Many cultures require families to remain with ill/hospitalized family member.
         (b) Illness is family affair
         (c) Share care giver role with nurses
         (d) Need comfort with level of access to family member
         (e) Lack of/need for qualified interpreters
         (f) Suggestions for nurses
            i. Consider racial and ethnic differences is physical assessment
            ii. Assess social, psychological, world view, and cultural needs with a cultural assessment tool
            iii. Avoid stereotyping
            iv. Include family and all stakeholders in plan of care
            v. Consider exceptions to hospital visiting policy
            vi. Negotiate family helping role
            vii. Schedule professional interpreters (Cioffi, 2006; Meddings & Haith-Cooper, 2008)
            viii. Adjust staffing levels to avoid haste (Cioffi, 2006)
            ix. Employ cultural sensitivity to all aspects of care (Cioffi, 2006; Meddings & Haith-Cooper, 2008)
            x. Nondisclosure or obtaining informed consent may require extra time. Family physician can be of great assistance
         (g) Suggestions for acute care facilities (Whitman & Davis, 2008)
            i. Health care personnel understanding of different cultures served
            ii. Awareness of similarities and differences among cultures in values, beliefs, and practices
            iii. Respect diversity
            iv. Consider modifying practices to improve care
            v. Work to remove communication barriers
            vi. Adopt the *National Standards for Culturally and Linguistically Appropriate Services in Health Care*, March 2001 (U.S. Department of Health and Human Service. 2001)
            vii. Use a variety of language access services: telephone, professional interpreters, printed material
            viii. Support from all levels of management
            ix. Specific person or department responsible for promoting and supporting cultural competence
            x. Multidisciplinary committee or task force (Whitman & Davis, 2008)
      (2) Ethical considerations (Meddings & Haith-Cooper, 2008)
         (a) Autonomy—a Western value
            i. Challenge when autonomy/individualism clashes with paternalism/group
            ii. Communication barriers when patient does not speak same language as health care provider
            iii. Informed consent presents cultural and legal challenges
         (b) Beneficence and non-maleficence
            i. Communication difficulties affect care
            ii. Anger/frustration may develop because of inability to communicate
            iii. Patient may feel vulnerable and inadequate
            iv. Cultural context and nonverbal cues missed may lead to diminished quality of care

(c) Justice
    i.   Equal treatment is not necessarily just treatment
    ii.   Right to access culturally sensitive forms of screening and treatment
    iii. Fair distribution of services (Meddings & Haith-Cooper, 2008)

(3) Application of general guidelines to one example: Hospitalized patient of the Islamic faith. Islam is a religion and has cultural variations and differences just as other religions. Therefore, it is essential to consider the patient's cultural origins as well as the degree of adherence to religious practice. Similarities are found within the unity of Islam that may assist nurses in providing care.

  (a) Prayer five times a day (Leininger & McFarland, 2002; McKennis, 1999)
    i.   Assist patient to face toward Mecca
    ii.   Provide water for ritual cleansing
    iii. Provide privacy for prayer time
    iv. Adjust care schedules when possible to accommodate patient's desire to pray

  (b) Ramadan, the month of fasting during daylight hours (Leininger & McFarland, 2002; McKennis, 1999)
    i.   Hospitalized adult may attempt fasting even though excused from the practice because of ill health
    ii.   May need to adjust medication schedules to avoid missed doses and serious consequences (Leininger & McFarland, 2002; McKennis, 1999)
    iii. Careful observance for signs and symptoms of dehydration

  (c) Dietary requirements
    i.   Consult with patient for preferences
    ii.   No alcohol, pork or pork products, e.g. in heparin or porcine heart valves
    iii. Prefer food that is halal; Kosher is acceptable (Leininger & McFarland, 2002; McKennis, 1999)
    iv. Based on patient's condition, consider asking family to bring some favorite foods from home

  (d) Modesty
    i.   Expected of both male and female patients
    ii.   Female modesty linked to chastity and family honor; do not expose body unnecessarily
    iii. May wish to maintain head covering (hijab)
    iv. Prefer same-sex caregivers
    v.   Husband may want to remain with wife during an examination, especially if provider is male
    vi. May avoid eye contact (Leininger & McFarland, 2002; McKennis, 1999)

  (e) Illness and dying
    i.   May understand scientific basis for illness, but believe it is fate or will of Allah if afflicted
    ii.   Repression of emotions is common
    iii. Family may choose not to tell patient of terminal diagnosis
    iv. Dying person may wish to face Mecca; family member may whisper call to prayer in ear
    v.   Death is generally not spoken of or planned for; to do so brings it about
    vi. Islamic law does not forbid organ transplantation, but it remains controversial among followers due to belief that body belongs to Allah
    vii. Body of deceased prepared for burial by a Muslim according to ritual (Leininger & McFarland, 2002; McKennis, 1999)
    viii. Embalming is not done unless demanded by law (Leininger & McFarland, 2002; McKennis, 1999)

  (f) Ethical Issues
    i.   Paternalistic social structure that may make obtaining informed consent a challenge for female older than 18 years of age
    ii.   Discussion of advanced directives is problematic; Muslims usually do not plan for death
    iii. Individualized approach: consider ethnic identity, adherence to religion, age, illness, and prognosis
    iv. Consider involving ethics committee
    v.   Professional interpreter may be needed
    vi. Charms or amulets may be present; do not remove

      vii. Do not shave a man's beard unless absolutely necessary and the need has been thoroughly explained by the physician. For a traditional man, beard is linked to honor; shaving is a shame and dishonor (Leininger & McFarland, 2002; McKennis, 1999)

   (g) Family and visiting

      i. Usually families are large with many extended members

      ii. Visiting the sick is a mandatory religious and social obligation for family and friends. Not visiting may result in severance of relationships

      iii. Nurses should try to accommodate and facilitate this important cultural need (Leininger & McFarland, 2002)

f. Specific examples of acute illnesses with high mortality and morbidity among minority populations (Davidson, 2007)

   (1) Coronary heart disease (CHD) Example: Asian Indians

     (a) Asian Indians are the fastest growing group of immigrants in the United States and are identified with cultures from Bangladesh, Sri Lanka, Nepal, and Pakistan.

     (b) Asian Indians have a higher mortality rate due to CHD than any other population in the United States, England, South Africa, Trinidad, West Indies, Malaysia, and Uganda.

     (c) Death from CHD occurs at a younger age for South Asians (Mathews & Zachariah, 2008).

     (d) Risk factors for Asian Indians and CHD

       i. Compared with majority populations, south Asians present with increased incidence of diabetes, obesity, insulin resistance, and elevated lipoprotein (a) levels.

       ii. Intake history may reveal dietary changes since immigration to a new country as well as decreased physical activity, and a higher caloric intake.

       iii. Fried foods are preferred by people from southern India, whereas those from the north tend to consume more butter or margarine and sweets. Diets with an excess consumption of dairy and butter with low fiber intake are common among Asian Indian vegetarians.

       iv. Muslims may have symbolic jewelry of an eye or a blue hand with an eye. This is protection to ward-off the bad eye or evil eye. It is important that this item not be removed unless absolutely necessary. If it must be taken off, return it to the patient as soon as possible (R. Spector, 2008).

   (2) Breast cancer: Lessons from some patients—Nordic (Sweden and Finland), Punjabi immigrants to Canada

     (a) Nordic experience of breast cancer viewed as causing suffering in women across all dimensions of life (Arman, Rehnsfeldt, Lindholm, Hamrin, & Eriksson, 2004)

     (b) Eriksson says suffering can change focus from the diagnosis and symptoms to suffering within an ontological dimension. Human dignity is violated by suffering implying loss and dying, but also new life and reconciliation are possible.

     (c) Nordic culture sees cancer as a phenomenon with overtones of death that causes the patient to consider existential questions (Arman et al., 2004)

     (d) "Suffering related to care" is part of Eriksson's theory on caring

       i. Dignity of patients can be violated by not believing them or taking them seriously

       ii. Caregivers use their authority to make decisions for the patient on what they think is best

       iii. Neglect of care occurs when caring dimension is missing; lack of caring results in undesirable care (Arman, et al., 2004)

     (e) Suffering related to health care often results when health care professional and patient are in close contact in an ethical relationship. Suffering increases when

       i. A caring relationship does not develop

       ii. Patient not treated as a unique human being

       iii. Patient not given enough time or information

       iv. Care giver hides behind culture and routine of health care

       v. Care giver does not risk being open to patient

       vi. Biomedical values upheld in disregard for caring values

       vii. Breast cancer patient does not feel like she is being treated as a whole person

         aa. Mental and spiritual experiences are ignored

         ab. Patient is treated as though she is emotionally unstable

         ac. Patient is made to feel ashamed of her emotional and spiritual suffering

        viii. Cry for help to understand life and death not heard (Arman et al., 2004)

    (f) Care givers must demonstrate charity and compassion in their basic attitude toward life or risk being a barrier to alleviating patient suffering (Arman et al., 2004)

    (g) Punjabi immigrants in Canada: Listening to stories of patients' experiences with breast cancer may aid understanding for health care providers. Telling stories may help patients make sense of their lives. Cultural norms, values, and beliefs influence patients' stories. Treatment decisions should be examined within cultural contexts (Howard, Bottorff, Balneaves, & Grewal, 2007).

        i. Focus on collective rather than individual

        ii. Focus on experiences associated with breast cancer rather than identifying self as a breast cancer survivor

        iii. Avoided attaching significance to the breast, concerned with cancer as life-threatening disease

        iv. Expectation of strong family support during diagnosis and treatment

        v. May combine traditional treatments with western medical care

        vi. Various descriptions of breast cancer and treatment

            aa. Getting through a family crisis; survival was a family accomplishment; described treatment as a collective family experience

            ab. Just another health problem

            ac. Never ending pain and suffering emotionally and physically for entire family

            ad. Detailed descriptions of difficulties of treatment

            ae. Some very stoic

            af. Part of their karma (reflection on present or past lives) and kismet (fate); took comfort in religion; spiritual journey for personal change

            ag. Intensely emotional, including shock and disbelief

            ah. Cancer diagnosis seen as social stigma (Howard et al., 2007)

        vii. Deferring to family for decisions about treatment choices consistent with Punjabi gender role for women

        viii. Family presence essential throughout

        ix. Punjabi women usually reluctant to discuss health issues outside family (Howard et al., 2007)

g. Trauma

    (1) All trauma is essentially historical whether it is injury from an accident as in a motor vehicle crash, long-term mass trauma such as colonialism, slavery, war, genocide, or forced suppression of cultural expression (Sotero, 2006), terrorism trauma like the attack of 9/11 (Marshall & Suh, 2003), or trauma caused by natural disaster like a tsunami or earthquake (Thirumurthy, Uma, and Muthuram, 2008).

    (2) Historical trauma may affect health disparities and disease prevalence several generations after the original occurrence (Sotero, 2006).

    (3) When a patient is admitted with traumatic injury, general appropriate culture care needs to be accomplished. The care giver must recognize that any patient with illness or traumatic injury could also be suffering from historical trauma that could be a root cause of the acute problem or affect the plan of care.

    (a) The trauma is felt by the entire population that is targeted resulting in physical, psychological, social, and economic disparities that last for generations.

    (b) The stresses created have been associated with impairment of the nervous system, the hypothalamic–pituitary–adrenal axis. Cardiovascular, metabolic, and immune systems are also affected. Diabetes, hypertension, and cardiovascular disease may result.

    (c) Holocaust survivors, Palestinian, Russian, African American, Native American, Cambodian populations have children with documented posttraumatic stress disorder (PTSD) responses. There are psychological, social, and physical responses.

    (d) The subordination of indigenous populations by a dominant group has been described as producing a "soul wound" (Sotero, 2006; Struthers & Lowe, 2003).

    (e) The clinician caring for the patient with an acute illness or trauma may need the assistance of social and psychological caregivers to meet the needs of the patient also suffering with historical trauma (Marshall & Suh, 2003).

h. Summary: There are many general recommendations for culture care that the acute care provider needs to consider. No one can be an expert on all cultures. Developing personal and unit resources can be of great assistance in delivering meaningful care to diverse populations. The following are some websites that offer additional excellent information related to culture care.

(1) http://www.stanford.edu/group/ethnoger/module_three.html

(2) http://www.snrs.org/publications/SOJNR_articles/iss07vol02.htm

(3) http://www.kaisernetwork.org/daily_reports/rep_index.cfm?DR_ID=50676

(4) http://www.biomedcentral.com/1472-6831/8/26

4. ***Sexually Transmitted Illness***

   a. Sexually transmitted illness has a major global impact.

     (1) According to the Centers for Disease Control and Prevention (CDC), sexually transmitted infections (STIs) are a group of contagious diseases most commonly transmitted through close intimate contact, including vaginal, anal, and oral sex. Although most of the transmission has been through sexual contact, vertical transmission from mother to baby is also possible. (CDC, 2007).

     (2) Pathogens causing STIs include a wide spectrum of organisms, including bacteria and viruses. Syphilis, gonorrhea, and chancroid are the most common sexually transmitted diseases; however, a wide variety of other diseases are also sexually transmissible, including chlamydial infection, trichomoniasis, genital warts, HIV infection, and hepatitis B infection (CDC, 2007).

     (3) Despite recent advances in treatment and prevention efforts, STIs, including HIV/AIDS, continue to pose a serious international threat to public health (Tillerson, 2008). Extensive research has been directed toward this important issue both nationally and internationally.

     (4) STIs are a major cause of acute illness, infection, long-term disability and death with severe medical and psychological consequences for millions of men, women, and infants worldwide (Nelson & Woodward, 2006).

     (5) The WHO estimates that 340 million new cases of curable STIs due to gonorrhea and trichomoniasis occur throughout the world every year. The largest number of new infections occurs annually in Southeast Asia, followed by sub-Saharan Africa, Latin American, and the Caribbean (WHO, 2007c).

     (6) Millions of viral STIs, including HIV, human herpes virus, human papilloma virus, and hepatitis B occur annually (WHO, 2007b).

     (7) The global epidemic of HIV/AIDS is stabilizing but remains at an unacceptable high rate. The Joint United Nations Programme on HIV/AIDS reports that 33 million persons were living with HIV disease in 2007, with the highest country prevalence rates in sub-Saharan Africa. A total of 22 million adults and children are currently living with HIV/AIDS in sub-Saharan Africa. Women account for 50% of all persons living with HIV/AIDS worldwide, with 59% in sub-Saran Africa (UNAIDS, 2008).

     (8) The greatest burden for STIs is in the developing world; however, industrialized nations can be expected to experience an increased burden of the disease because of the prevalence of non-curable viral infections, increased travel, and trends in sexual behavior (WHO, 2007b).

   b. Complex arrays of factors affect engagement in care and treatment for sexually transmitted illness.

     (1) Although newer treatments have helped to reduce the consequences of infection, persons who need care and treatment, as well as those at high risk for STI/HIV, do not always seek or accept medical care. Many are sporadic users of care, often missing appointments or dropping out of care for periods of time.

       (a) In the United States, where efforts to expand access to care and treatment are underway, one third of persons who know their HIV status are not receiving or actively participating in medical care to treat their HIV infection (Tobias et al., 2007).

       (b) A substantial number of females with symptoms of gonococcal and chlamydial infections delay STI-related care seeking (Cunningham, Kerrigan, Pillay, & Ellen, 2005; Turner et al., 2002).

     (2) Critical factors that influence health-seeking behaviors in STI/HIV include individual characteristics, behaviors and attitudes of health care providers, sociodemographic factors, and health care system factors (Whetten et al., 2008).

       (a) *Individual characteristics* can become barriers to STI/HIV prevention and use of health care services.

         i. Stigma and shame associated with STI/HIV are important barriers to diagnosis and treatment services (Arkell, Osborn, Ivens, & King, 2006; Fortenberry et al., 2001; Fortenberry et al., 2002; Rusch et al., 2008).

         ii. Health-related beliefs and knowledge about STI/HIV affect health-seeking behaviors in patients with STI/HIV (Crepaz, Hart, & Marks, 2004; Meyer-Weitz, Redduy, Van den Borne, Kok, & Pietersen, 2000; Reynolds et al., 2004).

    aa.   Persons may have misperceptions about being able to control circumstances over acquiring STI/HIV. Examples include the following:

(i)   HIV may be viewed as "God's punishment" (Kemppainen et al., 2008).

(ii)   HIV may be attributed to chance or "bad luck" (Kemppainen et al., 2008)

(iii)   Feelings of fatalism are prevalent, especially in Hispanic/Latino populations (Tobias et al., 2007).

(iv)   Only women who engage in sexual risk-taking behaviors need to obtain Papaniculou (PAP) smears (Ackerson & Greterback, 2007)

(v)   Not knowing a diagnosis is "better" than knowing (Ackerson & Greterbeck, 2007).

(vi)   Treatment is not needed unless symptoms are present.

(vii)   Treatment is worse than the disease (Ackerson & Greterbeck, 2007).

(viii)   Little can be done to reduce risk for STD/HIV.

    ab.   Despite the high prevalence rates, many young adult men and women know very little about STI (Baer, Allen, & Braun, 2004; Lambert, 2001).

    iii.   Cultural values, gender roles, and norms influence differences in sexual behaviors (Schwartz & Rubel, 2005).

    iv.   Concerns about confidentiality and privacy serve as barriers to care and treatment (Tobias et al., 2007).

    v.   Low literacy appears to pose a barrier to care and treatment for STI (Fortenbery et al., 2001).

    vi.   Since STI/HIV disorders are frequently asymptomatic, individuals may not be aware of their disease (Tobias et al., 2007).

    vii.   Recent research generated by the HIV epidemic revealed the linkage between mental health disorders, partner violence, depression, childhood sexual abuse, and STI/HIV prevalence (Erbelding, Hutton, Zenilman, Hunt, & Lyketsos, 2004).

    viii.   Addictions to alcohol, cocaine or injection drugs, sex, gambling may create barriers to STI/HIV treatment.

(b)   *Behaviors and attitudes of health care providers* play a key role in STI/HIV health care utilization.

    i.   Many persons with STI/HIV have experienced actual or perceived discrimination in health care settings (Sohler, Li, & Cunningham, 2007).

    ii.   Personal attitudes, beliefs, biases, and behaviors of health care providers may consciously or unconsciously influence communication and patient–provider relationships (Dominquez, 2006).

    iii.   Cross-cultural miscommunication may hinder access to care.

    iv.   Lack of trust in a health care provider can become a barrier to appropriate use of medical services.

    aa.   Persons report a lower mistrust with providers of their own race/ethnicity (Sohler et al., 2007).

    ab.   Increased trust in a health care provider is associated with improved adherence to treatment, increased outpatient clinic visits, fewer emergency room visits, and improved physical and mental health (Whetten et al., 2008)

(c)   Health disparities in STI/HIV are linked to a complex blend of *social and economic factors* (CDC, 2008a).

    i.   Social determinants include poverty, unequal access to health care, lack of education, stigma, and racism (CDC, 2008a).

    ii.   Persons with STI/HIV may postpone or go without care because of basic survival needs (Tobias et al., 2007).

    iii.   Physical locations such as prisons, and social networks, especially sexual networks, within which people interact may also promote health risk behaviors and account for some health disparities.

    iv.   Financial barriers to care include lack of insurance, underinsurance, or the cost of obtaining services (Tobias et al., 2007).

(d)   *Health care system factors* may serve as barriers to SDI/HIV treatment.

    i.   Many persons with STI/HIV have insufficient access to medications for treatment of STD/HIV (Gebo et al., 2005).

      ii. A vast body of evidence shows that minorities, regardless of income or insurance, do not received the same quality of care as Caucasian counterparts (Aliance for Health Reform, 2006; Institute of Medicine, 2003b; Sohler et al., 2007).

      iii. Unavailable or inconveniently located services serve as a barrier to STI/HIV care (Tobias et al., 2007).

      iv. Health care access and quality varies widely among populations and is less available in higher STI-risk areas.

  c. Although STIs affect persons in all groups, racial and ethnic minority groups continue to account for a disproportionate percentage of new STD/HIV cases.

    (1) Racial and ethnic minority groups are more likely than Caucasian counterparts to face multiple challenges associated with risk for contracting STDs (CDC, 2008a).

    (2) Health disparities in STI/HIV are linked to a complex blend of social and economic determinants, including poverty, unequal access to health care, lower levels of education, stigma and racism (Division of STD Prevention [DSTDP], 2007; Steele, Melendez-Morales, Campoluci, DeLuca, & Dean, 2007).

    (3) Physical locations such as prisons, and social networks, especially sexual networks, within which people interact may also promote health risk behaviors and account for some health disparities.

      (a) Blacks/African Americans are the most severely affected racial/ethnic group in the United States (CDC, 2008c; DSTDP, 2007).

        i. STI disparities are greatest for gonorrhea and congenital syphilis but also high for Chlamydia and adult syphilis (DSTDP, 2007).

        ii. African American women have higher prevalence rates of human papilloma virus (HPV) and are 50% more likely to die from HPV-related cervical cancer than Caucasian counterparts (DSTDP, 2007).

        iii. A total of 46% of the persons living with HIV are Black (CDC, 2008c).

        iv. The HIV diagnosis rate for Black females is19 times higher than the rate for Caucasian females (CDC, 2008b).

        v. Research findings reflect a shortened survival time in African Americans after an AIDS diagnosis (Hall, Byers, Ling, & Espinoza, 2007).

        vi. Disparities in STI/HIV prevalence for African Americans have multiple interrelated causes (CDC, 2008b).

          aa. Contextual factors such as racial and economic oppression, high rates of incarceration, and drug abuse play an important role in sexual partnering decisions (DSTDP, 2007).

          ab. Sexual partners frequently conceal injection drug use and crack/cocaine use (Gilbert, 2003).

          ac. High risk sexual acts frequently occur while using drugs (Gilbert, 2003)

          ad. Women may engage in high risk sexual activities to meet survival requirements (Mallory & Stern, 2000).

          ae. Increased rates of incarceration among Black males affect sexual partnering decisions. In-prison sex partners from high-HIV prevalence pools are common and, once released, high-risk males return to low-risk partners (DSTDP, 2007).

          af. Black men who hide their bisexuality (living on "The Down Low") may place women at risk for STI/HIV (Ford, Whetten, Hall, Kaufman, & Thrasher, 2007).

          ag. Concurrent sexual partnerships are widespread among unmarried persons (CDC, 2008b).

          ah. High incidence of sexual and physical violence place women at high-risk for STI/HIV (Laughton et al., 2007).

          ai. Unlike other groups, African Americans need not engage in high-risk behaviors to be at risk for contracting STI/HIV due to the greater prevalence of STI/HIV in African American communities (DSTDP, 2007).

          aj. African American women are less likely to use information about HPV to reduce risk and prevent cervical cancer (Scarinci, Garces-Palacio, & Partridge, 2007).

          ak. Poor African Americans tend to mistrust the health care system and are skeptical of receiving adequate treatment because of the legacies of racism and discrimination (DSTDP, 2007).

  (b) STI/HIV remains a serious threat for the Hispanic/Latino population (CDC, 2008b)

     i. Hispanic/Latino women have the highest rates of HPV infection and the highest HPV-related cervical cancer in the United States.

     ii. A total of 18% of new HIV infections occur in Hispanics (CDC, 2008b).

     iii. HIV/AIDS rates for Hispanic women are four times higher than for Caucasian women (CDC, 2008c).

     iv. Heterosexual contact is the principal mode of HIV transmission in Hispanic/Latino women.

     v. Hispanic/Latino women are more likely to acquire HIV because of high rates of STIs.

     vi. Health outcomes in STI/HIV differ by country of birth (Solorio, Currier, & Cunningham, 2004).

       aa. A shorter period of a conversion from HIV to AIDS interval is more common among Mexican-born Hispanics than U.S.-born Hispanics.

       ab. Hispanics born in Puerto Rico are more likely to contract HIV infection by injection drug use.

     vii. Effects of migration and varying levels of acculturation impact STD/HIV transmission.

       aa. Immigrant Latinas are vulnerable to social isolation.

       ab. The incidence of IPV is higher in the United States than in Latin American countries (Weidel, Provencio-Vasquez, Watson, & Gonzalez-Guarda, 2008).

       ac. Strong family support networks are weakened as a result of migration.

       ad. There is a lack of a single Hispanic culture in the United States.

       ae. Mexican migrant men are unlikely to disclose bisexual behavior or HIV status to female partners or family (Solorio et al., 2004).

     viii. Gender inequality in male–female relationships represents a major cultural factor in the transmission of STI/HIV (DeSantis & Patsdaughter, 2008).

     ix. Aspects of the Hispanic culture can make the negotiation of safer sex difficult (Marin, 2003).

       aa. Machismo, masculinity that is influenced by power and dominance, is a traditional male gender role. Sexual coercion is common in Hispanic men who endorse this belief, along with physical and emotional abuse of sexual partners (Caceres, Marin, & Hudes, 2000; Marin, 2003).

       ab. Marianisma is a cultural view of women that includes saintliness, submissiveness to male partners, and self-sacrifice. Hispanic women may feel disempowered in relationships with their partners, and also may have difficulty negotiating skills for sexual safety (Marin, 2003; Peragallo et al., 2005)

       ac. Simpatia is the importance of maintaining nonconfrontational behavior. Women are encouraged to acquiesce, and both genders are uncomfortable in a discussion of sex (Marin, 2003).

     x. In Hispanic communities, homophobia is seriously stigmatized. High levels of experienced homophobia and racism have been associated with increased levels of risky sexual behavior, as well as depression and suicidal thoughts (Diaz, Ayala, Bein, Henne, & Marin, 2001).

     xi. Sexual activity is initiated early and multiple sex partners are frequent.

  (c) In recent years, rates of STI/HIV among Asians and Pacific Islanders have steadily increased (CDC, 2008b).

     i. The number of AIDS diagnoses among Asians and Pacific Islanders increased from 0.6% to 1.1% (CDC, 2008b).

     ii. Unlike other groups, there has been an increase in the number of cases of syphilis (U.S. Department of Health and Human Services, 2009).

     iii High-risk heterosexual contacts are the primary way that Asian and Pacific Islander women become infected with HIV/AIDS (CDC, 2008b).

     iv. Culturally embedded sexual attitudes and behaviors of Asian and Pacific Islanders have significant implications for STI/HIV care (Bhattacharya, 2004).

       aa. Asian/Pacific Islanders delay in engaging in SDI/HIV-related services and are the least likely of all ethnicities to discuss STIs with their health care provider (Chin, Kang, Kim, Martinez, & Eckholdt, 2006; National Asian Women's Health Organization, 2000).

       ab. Expressions of sexuality outside of marriage are considered highly inappropriate, regardless of the Asian culture (Okazaki, 2002).

ac. Many Asian cultural traditions place emphasis on strict moral and social conduct, and modesty and restrained sexuality are valued (Okazaki, 2002).

ad. Rates of Pap tests and clinical breast examination are extremely low, especially among recent immigrants to the United States (Okazaki, 2002; Tu, Taplin, Barlow, & Boyko, 1999; Yu, Kim, Chen, & Brintnall, 2001).

ae. Asian American victims of sexual abuse or assault are extremely reluctant to disclose the violence to providers.

af. One quarter of Asian Americans and Pacific Islanders have never visited a health care provider for STI education or a gynecological exam.

v. Divergent cultural values and languages present barriers for Asian/Pacific Islanders seeking health care for SDI/HIV (Chin et al., 2006).

vi. Many Asian Americans and Pacific Islanders maintain beliefs that they are unaffected by STI/HIV and that preventive care is unnecessary (National Asian Women's Organization, 2000).

vii. Health care decision making in HIV/AIDS for south Asians is more collective with the family than with individuals (Bhattacharya, 2004).

viii. Seeking health care for HIV/AIDS can bring shame on families or a community.

d. STI/HIV prevention and control strategies in racial and ethnic communities face important challenges.

(1) Despite increasing public health efforts aimed at preventing STI/HIV, rates of STI/HIV continue to rise among minority and vulnerable populations (CDC, 2007). The persistence of STI/HIV disparities indicates that many current strategies are not achieving impact in these communities (Barrow et al., 2008).

(2) Members of racial and ethnic population groups frequently do not have comprehensive and correct information about STI/HIV to promote risk reduction behaviors. In addition, cultural and economic based factors continue to impact the effectiveness of many prevention strategies (Barrow et al., 2008).

(3) Despite their potential, behavioral interventions aimed at individuals have had only modest effects for members of minority races and ethnicities (Cohen, Wu, & Farley, 2006).

(4) Culturally tailored education programs that allow community members to define their own needs and identify opportunities for STI/HIV testing and prevention services are key to reducing new infections (CDC, 2008c).

(a) Community-based participatory models engage community members and health care providers and researchers in a collaborative process designed to reach a broader population more effectively. This approach also has a more meaningful and sustainable impact over time (Ammerman & Tajik, 2005).

i. Messages should personalize risk by focusing on accurate risk assessment.

ii. Community spokespersons are used to disseminate prevention messages.

iii. Communication is centered on cultural experiences.

iv. Prevention efforts should be located within the communities being targeted.

v. Proactive and participatory skill building activities provide an outlet for acceptance and peer support.

(b) Prevention initiatives must include both men and women (Russell, Alexander, & Corbo, 2000).

(c) Partner services can be an effective tool for reducing STI rates and preventing adverse outcomes of STI/HIV when offered in a culturally sensitive manner (Barrow et al., 2008; WHO, 2007b).

i. Patient–provider relationships are a key element in providing effective partner services.

aa. Providers need to ensure confidentiality and build rapport with the patient (Barrow et al., 2008).

ab. Be nonjudgmental.

ac. Accept the patient's right of self-determination.

ad. Respect the patient's worth, dignity, and problem-solving ability.

ae. Counsel partners in private settings.

af. Avoid disclosing the patient's name to a sexual partner (Barrow et al., 2008).

ii. Sexual partner notification includes three main approaches.

aa. Health care personnel can notify exposed partners through in-person meetings (WHO, 2007c).

ab. Index patients may notify their sexual partners and can be supplied with medications to deliver to their sexual partners (WHO, 2007c).

ac. Index patients agree to notify partners, with the understanding that health care providers will notify sexual partners who do not present for treatment by a given time.

(d) STI/HIV prevention programs must engage the target audience to achieve a positive result (Barrow et al., 2008).

i. Special efforts should be made to overcome the historical mistrust of health care providers when promoting STD/HIV prevention among African Americans (Scarinci et al., 2007).

ii. Prevention programs should be flexible in design to accommodate competing demands of busy life circumstances or inconsistent weekly personal schedules (multiple jobs or inconsistent work schedules, maintaining households, caring for relatives).

iii. Education programs for Hispanic/Latinos should incorporate traditional roles and cultural concepts that influence health-seeking behaviors.

aa. Emphasize the traditional role of caretaking.

ab. Encourage participants to take an active role in teaching STI/HIV prevention measures to their families (Russell et al., 2000).

ac. Be aware that Hispanic/Latino patients find it difficult to be open and comfortable in talking about body functions (Russell et al., 2000).

ad. Promote positive aspects of culturally ascribed ideas for men (machismo) and women (marianismo; Gonzalez-Guarda, Peragallo, Urrutia, Vasquez, & Mitrani, 2008).

iv. Since the population of Asian Americans and Pacific Islanders is so diverse, culturally and linguistically appropriate health care and services are an essential component of STI/HIV prevention (National Asian Women's Organization, 2000).

v. Understand gender roles and the level of acculturation in planning interventions for many target groups, including refugees, asylees, and immigrants (Weidel et al., 2008).

vi. South Asian immigrants to the United States may delay or not seek health care because of their lack of knowledge about access to health care systems (Bhattacharya, 2004).

e. Clinical practice implications for providers

(1) Provide routine screening services for at-risk individuals since most women and many men with bacterial STIs do not experience symptoms or may not recognize them (Barrow et al., 2008).

(2) Assess knowledge and health beliefs about STI/HIV.

(3) Discuss the association between STI and HIV/AIDS.

(4) Provide counsel about the impact of chronic STIs on fertility.

(5) Recognize the importance of spirituality in self-managing physical and psychological symptoms of STI/HIV in African Americans (Coleman et al., 2006).

(6) Provide education about STIs (including HPV) and the link between HPV infection and cervical cancer.

(7) Assess readiness for behavior change related to risk reduction.

(8) Address interwoven STI/HIV, substance abuse, and IPV simultaneously (Gonzalez-Guarda et al., 2008).

(9) Diminish barriers to receipt of mental health or substance abuse treatment (Tobias et al., 2007).

(10) Examine the supportive role of partners and family. Include partners and family members in counseling, testing, and treatment as indicated (Scarinci et al., 2007).

(11) Since STI and HIV epidemics are interdependent, improved STI treatment may contribute substantially to HIV prevention (Sagani, Rutherford, & Wilkinson, 2004).

5. *Living With Disability**

a. The context of disability includes culture, health disparities and poverty.

(1) There are links between cultural competence and disability disparities (see Table 5.7).

(2) In the United States, 40% of disabled adults* reported being in fair or poor health compared to 10% of those without disabilities.

(3) Fair or poor health is more common among Hispanics (50%) and American Indians/Alaskan Natives (55%) who are disabled (CDC, 2008a).

(4) This segment's emphasis is on disability as a subculture in social, legal, national, and economic contexts rather than on values and practices related to disability in various cultures.

b. Demographics

Table 5.7. Approaches to Disability[a] in 35 Cultural Groups[b]

Afghans: Believed to be will of Allah. Family member not discriminated against; parents or eldest sibling care for him/her

African Americans: Physical and developmental disabilities believed to be God's will, but attitude varies by education. Family members and friends care for disabled member in a nonjudgmental manner, usually at home. Family seeks adult day care and respite care to cope with the disability; institutionalization usually last resort

American Indians/Alaskan Natives: Varies, depends on the context and individual experiences with disabilities. Sometimes believed to have occurred for an unknown reason. Persons with disabilities generally integrated in the community. Health care providers should cautiously discuss disability in terms of meaning and degree of function

Arabs: Disability a stigma, family member shielded from public view. In extended family, treated sympathetically. Overindulgent care may interfere with development and healthy self-care

Brazilians: Family may view disabilities as divine punishment or a "cross to bear." Tend to confine disabled member to home, fearing possible public humiliation. Children usually do not attend regular school classes at school and parents not accustomed to "mainstreaming"

Cambodians: Immediate family accepts and cares for, and the community watches over, persons with disabilities

Caribbeans: Disability often viewed as a "defect," something to be ashamed of. Disabled persons less inclined to engage in social events or outings. Families feel responsible to care for their own; disinclined to institutionalize, unless family employment necessitates

Central Americans: Family fully accepts a member's disability and cares for him/her at home. "Such is life" (*asi es la vida*) is a common response

Chinese: If possible, family member receives care at home. May not be taken out in public because of shame. Willing to undergo rehabilitation or receive other necessary services

Colombians: Less educated may attribute disability to supernatural causes. Family usually cares for disabled member, typically confined to the home. If obvious physical deformity, member faces stigma

Cubans: View persons as unfortunate and perhaps deserving the disability. Often blamed on family or personal misconduct or behavior. Frequently conceal and do not mention family member who usually receives care at home if possible

Dominicans: View some disabilities as punishment for a sin committed against God. Family does not take disabled disability out in public. Some families consider him/her an embarrassment

East Indians: Disability believed to occur with God's knowledge. Person accepts and lives with disability. Parents and/or family members love and care for him/her. In India, traditionally kept at home; sometimes institutionalized (orphanages). Immigrants to other countries effectively seek and use resources to help family member live independently

Ethiopians and Eritreans: Disability highly stigmatized. Family cares for member, but he/she is not visible when strangers visit nor taken out in public

Filipinos: Accepted as God's will and family member treated with kindness and pity, especially elderly. Relatives often help member with chores, considered a worthy sacrifice in the eyes of God; turning one's back considered cruel and can cause misfortune

Germans: Generally accept physically disabled and they participate in public life. Amish and German Baptists in the United States attribute disabilities to "God's will." Amish have special schools for children. Care of disabled persons is community's responsibility

Greeks: Disability a routine part of family life and of family member's role as caretaker. Family member attends church, is part of the community, and family may enroll him/her in life-skills or related programs

Haitians: View having disabled child as punishment or caused by a supernatural force, but disability not viewed as shameful. Mother may feel guilty and wonder why she deserves punishment. Parents try to determine if the disability is due to the influence of a neglected or malicious powerful spirit; placate with prayer services or voodoo ceremony or may seek medical care. Similar for adults who become disabled. Family member is loved, sheltered, and cared for at home

Hawaiians: Traditionally were outcasts. Now families care for relatives with disabilities and accept them as active community members

Hmong: High value on functioning normally and being healthy and whole. Although disabilities are stigmatized, family members are well cared for. Disabled members, including those who need assistive devices, stay home and do not participate in community events. A child may not be marriageable

Iranians: Disability due to God's will and an act of nature. Do not discriminate against disabled persons since war created many physically and psychologically disabled veterans. Family members care for person but may institutionalize someone with severe mental or physical disability

Irish: High value on independence and value those who attempt to overcome adversity. Community is compassionate and does not stigmatize disabled persons. Family willing to care for member at home. Refer him/her to programs that encourage personal development and independence

Italians: Family's duty to care for member at home. Physical disability more accepted than mental illness or HIV/AIDS. Rarely share information about disabled family member outside the family and may conceal him/her from society

Japanese: Older and more traditional Japanese tend to view disabilities as shameful or disgraceful. May believe disability is punishment for something one did in his/her life or something a family member has done. If a disability is not overtly visible, attempt to conceal it from others. Younger generations and immigrants to the United States more accepting and proactive

Koreans: Traditionally may view disability at birth as punishment for ancestors' sins or accident and family's misfortune. In past, disabled people were publicly ridiculed. Although negative attitudes have lessened still consider disability a family stigma

(continued)

Table 5.7. (continued)

Mexicans: More traditional or religious persons view disability as a fate to be accepted. Immigrants acculturated to the United States may view it as a challenge to be overcome. Disabilities remain stigmatized; family may conceal a disabled member

Nigerians: Strong stigma associated with disabilities, attributed to evil spirits or punishment by the gods. Family members care for member, who outsiders rarely see; involvement outside the family is limited

Pakistanis: Limited understanding of disability. Disabled family member often feels undervalued, not respected, and forced into a passive role within family. Parents may regard disability as tragedy, with implications for their future and child's development and family life. Consider disabled persons to be free of sin. Some families believe it a blessing to care for a disabled member

Polish: Accept disabilities as God's will for the person and family. Value family loyalty and family loves/cares for disabled member, takes him/her out with family. Home care as long as possible, accepting institutionalization when no longer possible but family continues providing support

Puerto Ricans: May blame a baby's disabling condition on mother's lack of self-care, working during pregnancy, or personal suffering. People generally caring and helpful. Some families initially hide physically disabled children; less likely to hide adults, especially older family members or parents. Prefer to care for members at home. Children attend school and outdoor programs

Roma: Generally tolerant. Accept disability as bad luck

Russians: Family accepts disability without stigma or shame. Some highly supportive families take family member out in public

Samoans: Accept disabled family member, care for him/her at home unless care becomes unmanageable. Accept disabilities as part of life, no stigma although some may joke about disability. Although family members may help, Samoan culture encourages member to be independent and freely participate in daily activities

Vietnamese: Many physically disabled from war. Families and government treat and care for them well, resources permitting. Society may stigmatize those with mental disabilities because of jeopardy to relatives' ability to find marriage partners

Yugoslavians (former): View disability as God's will; some families feel shame and guilt, isolate themselves. Mostly take good care of disabled member. People generally do not discriminate against disabled people but some pity them

Source: Adapted from Lipson and Dibble (2005). Reprinted with permission.

a. "Disabled person" is used here for brevity.

b. Table is oriented to cultural groups and immigrants in the United States who vary widely, based on education and acculturation. Descriptions may reflect some home country attitudes.

(1) About 10% of the world's population lives with a disability.
   (a) A total of 80% of persons with disabilities live in developing countries, according to the United Nations Development Program (UNDP).
   (b) The World Bank estimates that 20% of the world's poorest people have some kind of disability, and tend to be regarded in their own communities as the most disadvantaged (http://www.disabled-world.com/disability/statistics/). People in this largest minority group have reduced access to education, full employment and other resources.
(2) It is difficult to compare disability percentages between countries because of relatively recent interest in many developing countries.
   (a) Incidence, causes and typology of disability are rarely available.
   (b) South Africa now includes questions on disability in the national census; other country estimates are based on data collected for various purposes.
   (c) There are variations in sampling (total population, adult or working age), the definition of disability, and cultural constraints. For example, a 2.5% incidence in India is considered a major underestimate because of avoidance in declaring a disability due to the stigma. (http://www.globalride-sf.org/images/DFID.pdf)
c. Disability and civil rights legislation
   (1) In December 2006, the United Nations Department of Economic and Social Affairs and Office of the High Commissioner for Human Rights adopted the Convention on the Rights of Persons with Disabilities, a worldwide effort to (i) to support the full and effective participation of persons with disabilities in social life and development; (ii) to advance the rights and protect the dignity of persons with disabilities; and (iii) to promote equal access to employment, education, information, goods, and services.
   (2) National policies are in place in 59 countries according to the Disability Rights Education & Defense Fund Education (see Resources). The policy titles include such words as human rights, discrimination, protection, treatment, support, rehabilitation and special educational needs, and equal status, rights, opportunities, and employment.
   (3) Example: European Union (EU) policy objectives:

    (a) To promote equal rights for people with disabilities; to combat social exclusion

    (b) Article 15 of the European Social Charter notes the "right of persons with disabilities to independence, social integration and participation in the life of the community"

    (c) Pillars of the EU disability strategy: (http://www.eaie.org/DIW)

       i. EU antidiscrimination legislation and measures: Using legislation to protect disabled persons from discrimination

       ii. Mainstreaming of disability issues: To facilitate active inclusion of disabled people

       iii. Accessibility: To facilitate active inclusion of disabled people

       iv. Mobilizing stakeholders through dialogue: Through regular meetings with all parties (stakeholders, disabled persons, civil society representatives)

(4) Example: The U.S. *Americans with Disabilities Act* (ADA). Passed in 1990, the ADA (Job Accommodations Network, 1997) aims to make society more accessible to people with disabilities:

    (a) employers must provide reasonable accommodations;

    (b) public services must ensure accessibility to government instrumentalities and transportation systems;

    (c) new construction of public buildings must be accessible and barriers must be removed in existing facilities;

    (d) telecommunications (TTY or other devices) should be available to deaf or persons with hearing impairment; and

    (e) prohibition of coercion, threat or retaliation against people with disabilities or those attempting to help those who assert their rights under the ADA.

    (f) A recent national civil rights bill expands the definition of disability, making it easier for people to prove discrimination in the workplace if they have hidden disabilities or those that are episodic or in remission (Pear, 2008).

d. Types of disabilities: congenital or acquired by illness or injury after birth.

    (1) Physical: anatomical loss or limitations, musculoskeletal, neurological, respiratory or cardiovascular chronic disease/illness.

    (2) Sensory: hearing loss, deafness, vision loss, blindness, deaf-blindness.

    (3) Cognitive, intellectual, or developmental: arrested or incomplete development of the mind characterized by impairment of skills and overall intelligence in areas such as cognition, language, and motor and social abilities (WHO, 2007d).

    (4) Learning: neurological disorder that affects the brain's ability to receive, process, store and respond to information, causing difficulty acquiring academic skills in a person of at least average intelligence.

    (5) Traumatic brain injury: can affect cognition, language, memory, attention, reasoning, judgment, problem solving, information processing, or motor abilities.

    (6) Emotional, behavioral, or mental: can affect thinking, learning, sleeping, and relationships.

    (7) Speech and language: can impair language, voice or eating, difficulty speaking understandably, for example, cerebral palsy or stuttering, or difficulty understanding language, for example, autism, mental retardation.

e. Definitions and disability models

    (1) According to the Americans with Disabilities Act (ADA), a disability is a physical or mental impairment in an individual that limits one or more major life activities. A handicap is a social or other disadvantage stemming from or related to the disability.

    (2) The *medical model* focuses on biological and functional impairments in *individuals.* The *social model* emphasizes the social–political–economic–environmental *context* in which people with disabilities live, focusing on barriers to full participation rather than individual impairments.

       (a) If the environment were adjusted to the varying capacities of all persons, people with disabilities might not be considered a subculture or minority group.

       (b) Most research on people with disabilities assumes the irrelevance of the social experiences of culture, ethnicity, race, social class, gender, and sexual orientation.

f. Life issues

    (1) Culture and stigma. The concept of disability must be viewed within a cultural context. Some cultures recognize "blind, lame, and slow people" but do not lump them into a single category of disability.

Instead, cultural groups may view personal qualities as disabling or enabling based on valued personal characteristics and ability to carry on normal roles in the group, for example, in Taureg society, illegitimate birth, excessive freckles, absent-mindedness, flabby buttocks, and so on are disabling conditions (Ingstad & Whyte, 1995, p. 6).

(a) Disability and rehabilitation concepts were generated in Northern Europe and North America, which value independence and autonomy. The Independent Living Movement fosters self-determination through Centers for Independent Living (CILs). Whereas the first CIL started in Berkeley, California, in 1973, there was a similar movement in Western Europe in the 1960s and 1970s. In addition to numerous CILs in the United States, there are many in Europe, Canada, Africa, and South America.

(b) People in cultural groups that value interdependence more than they value autonomy may take for granted that family and community will take care of people with disabilities; may not see a need for rehabilitation or community programs. See Table 5.7 for 35 brief cultural group descriptions "causes" of disability and family values regarding care and stigma. Also see Leavitt (2006) on disabilities across cultures.

(c) Stigma and marginalization are rife: "For centuries, people with disabilities have been an oppressed and repressed group . . . isolated, incarcerated, observed, written about, operated on, instructed, implanted, regulated, treated, institutionalized, and controlled to a degree probably unequal to that experienced by any other minority group" (Davis, 1997).

(2) Income, work, and education

(a) People with disabilities generally have lower income and less health insurance coverage, participate less in regular education, have a lower high school completion rate, and are less employed than the U.S. national average.

(b) Other countries have similar disparities. Example: 16% of the overall EU working age population is disabled; only 50% of disabled persons are employed, compared to 68% of non disabled persons. Only 15.9% of these working disabled persons are provided with some assistance at work, though 43.7% of respondents in a survey believe that they could work if the were given adequate assistance (http://www.eaie.org/DIW)

(3) Parenting: Historic public bias against disabled people bearing and raising children; attitudes are changing with activism and public education.

(a) Some people with disabilities have more difficulty with pregnancy, birth, or child rearing associated with lack of accessible clinical services and professional knowledge (Rogers, 2006).

(b) Some social service providers doubt people's "ability" to be good parents (Lipson & Rogers, 2000a). Type and severity of disability influence need for assistance, for example, agencies like Through the Looking Glass (http://lookingglass.org/index.php).

g. Disability subcultures and status

(1) Types of support

(a) *Pan-disability activists*

i. They may not support organizations that focus on particular disabilities or diseases because they are based on the medical model and support condition-centered research.

ii. These activists strongly advocate for equal access to buildings, jobs, and education; resist being pitied, defined, or controlled by medical/rehabilitation professionals and the public; and embrace disability as a normal and acceptable way of being.

(b) *Specific disability organizations* often raise funds and sponsor support groups.

i. They focus on a chronic disease or type of injury, for example, cerebral palsy.

ii. Influenced by language, the "Deaf Culture" is the strongest subculture; people are socialized into Deaf Culture from infancy or early childhood, often through education. They share world view, behaviors, and norms.

(2) Apparent *status hierarchy* of disabilities mirrors that of the broader society. People with higher status disabilities may experience less stigma and marginalization than those with lower status disabilities.

(a) *Higher status:*

i. Disability activist leaders, often wheelchair users with post-polio syndrome or spinal cord injury

ii. Common disabilities, for example, heart disease or vision impairment.

    (b) *Lower status:*
        i. Developmental disabilities, mental illness, severe movement or speech disorders (Lipson & Rogers, 2000b).
        ii. Medically contested conditions, rarely recognized in developing countries, such as multiple chemical sensitivities (MCS), fibromyalgia, chronic fatigue syndrome, and Gulf War syndrome, which may severely impact many areas of life.
        iii. Typically acquired and often overlapping, people with these hidden disabilities face social stigma and disbelief, partly related to ongoing medical debate on physiological versus psychological etiology (Lipson, 2004).

h. Health care and social service providers: Educational and practice issues
  (1) Health professional curricula and continuing education
    (a) Must be broader than the medical model, with a focus on *living with disability*, not just information on disabling conditions.
    (b) Teach that people are disabled within a cultural context that frames the *meaning* of their experiences.
        i. Older Japanese and Korean immigrants in the United States may view disability as shameful, a family stigma, or punishment for what the individual or a family member has done; they may attempt to conceal the disability.
        ii. Samoans accept disability as part of life and care for disabled family member at home; they encourage him or her to be independent and freely participate in daily activities (Lipson & Dibble, 2005).
  (2) Cultural competence
    (a) With the help of disability and cultural community leaders, tailor health and social service programs so that they are based on the needs, communication styles and values of the population to be served.
    (b) Program example: New Zealand Disability Strategy (NZDS) implemented to promote participation of disabled Maori (Wiley, 2009).
        i. This year-long outcome evaluation collected data via 34 semistructured interviews with ministry officials, service provider organizations, Maori consumers with disabilities, and caregivers.
        ii. Themes included conflict between indigenous worldviews framed within a mainstream service paradigm, accountability, perceived levels of cultural competency, and need for collaboration across sectors and information exchange.
        iii. Despite shortcomings, NZDS provides lessons for culturally appropriate, effective disability services; increased coordination and collaboration, staff training, indigenous service provider resources, information distribution and community engagement. These will allow indigenous peoples with disabilities to participate in society while fully acknowledging their heritage.
  (3) Nursing and other clinical considerations
    (a) Accessible clinical settings and materials, for example,
        i. door width to accommodate wheelchairs and walkers
        ii. wheelchair ramps
        iii. height-adjustable examination tables
        iv. fragrance-free personnel and indoor air
        vi. large font for printed instructions and materials
        vii. sign interpreters
        viii. Braille materials and signage
        ix. audio-taped, and onsite computer health education materials, outreach programs
    (b) Terminology: there are national, cultural, and individual preferences.
        i. Ask clients how they refer to themselves and use their language. People with disabilities may view supposedly "politically correct" euphemisms such as "differently abled" or "physically challenged" as trivializing and demeaning.
        ii. "People first" language puts the person before the disability and uses active rather than passive voice. It avoids implying that the disability is the person's whole identity, for example, "he *has* autism" instead of "he *is* autistic," or "I *use* a wheelchair—I am *not* wheelchair *bound.*"
        iii. Popular in North America, "people first" is resisted by British disabled peoples' movement in which "disabled people" is preferred because of emphasis on the structural/cultural location of disability and social oppression, manifested in discriminatory practices (Priestly, 2001).

    (c) Examine own experiences, perceptions, and biases.

        i. Some people with disabilities call themselves "an equal opportunity minority—everyone is a potential member," or designate those without disabilities "temporarily abled." May threaten and reduce identification with disabled people.

        ii. Good care requires self-awareness and knowledge of own cultural baggage (Lipson & Dibble, 2005) because unexamined biases will emerge in remarks or nonverbal communication that disrespect clients and further undermine their trust in the health care system.

    (d) Respect and trust:

        i. Some disability activists are hostile to health care providers who medicalize their situations and do not recognize that many limitations are due to lack of effort to remedy social and physical environments.

        ii. Some providers do not trust people with disabilities to competently carry out ordinary tasks and, in effect, "put them under the microscope."

        iii. Avoid a medicocentric approach

        iv. Encourage clients to take the lead in guiding their care from their own perspective and experience.

    (e) Individuality:

        i. Focus on the individual rather than diagnosis

        ii. Age of disability onset influences identity formation; congenital or early onset may reduce the opportunity to be socialized into mainstream culture

        iii. Wide range of experiences within developmental, psychiatric, and physical disabilities and within each disabling condition

        iv. Severity/ stability/changeability of a disability shapes the person's life and others' responses

        v. Consider: Who is the individual's reference group? Does he or she primarily socialize with people who are disabled, nondisabled, or both?

    (f) Advocacy: in health care/social service agencies, support decreasing physical, social, and attitudinal barriers faced by people with disabilities; institute and educate about universal design.

    (g) Research and community participation.

        i. Follow the lead of the Independent Living Movement by replacing paternalistic research approaches with participatory action research.

        ii. Disabled people should guide relevant research questions and methods that can result in better education of health and social service professionals.

        iii. Visual research methods, in which people with disabilities use cameras to depict problematic images and effective approaches, can be particularly enlightening (Lorenz & Kolb 2009).

        i. Summary

(1) People with disabilities are the world's largest minority population. Rather than relying on the medical model, health and social service providers should view living with disability within its complex context, which for each individual, is a combination of cultural and national background, social and economic status, the built environment, and barriers to full community participation imposed by social marginalization and stigma.

(2) Since the 1970s, international and country-wide organizations have attempted to reduce barriers and promote equal rights and access to work, education, protection, treatment and rehabilitation, and self-determination.

(3) Health and social service providers have a mandate to support international, national, and local efforts to provide accessible, respectful, and individualized care that supports the life goals of individuals with disabilities.

(4) The Hesperian Foundation's statement provides a good summation: "Disability must first be defined as it is experienced by all disabled people, regardless of age and gender, including those with sensory, physical and intellectual impairment and mental health difficulties. Then, with this shared understanding, an assessment can be made of how well disabled people are being supported within mainstream agendas for health and well-being, the fight against global poverty and the human rights agenda." (http://www.hesperian.info/assets/GHW/C2.pdf)

(5) *Both terms, "people with disabilities" and "disabled people," are used in this segment in recognition of individual choice in how people identify themselves. The choice may be influenced by culture,

subculture, and national origin as well as identification with the disability activism and independent living movements.

E. **Older Adults** (Gerontology)

1. ***Cultural Influences on Aging and Older Adults***

   a. Culture influences how we view the aging process, how we deal with crisis and illness, as well as use of traditional and biomedical sources of health care.

   b. Older adults may blend traditional and popular beliefs about the causes of illness (McKenna, 2008).

   c. The degree of acculturation of persons from similar backgrounds varies along a broad spectrum and care should be given to avoid stereotyping (Ethnogeriatrics Committee of the American Geriatrics Society, 2004).

   d. Quality of life is measured by the level of physical functioning, life satisfaction, and happiness (McKenna, 2008).

   e. Lifelong eating habits developed from tradition, ethnicity, and religion influence food intake (Krebs-Smith et al., 1995).

   f. Information regarding religion and spirituality assist with the understanding of an ethnic older adult's health care needs (McBride, 2008).

   g. End-of-life care options need to consider the patient's values and culture; some cultures believe that patients should not be informed of a terminal diagnosis (Ethnogeriatrics Committee of the American Geriatrics Society, 2004).

2. ***Caring Practices***

   a. Definitions:

      (1) Older adult (elder): age 65 years and older

      (2) Oldest old: age 80 years and older

      (3) Definitions of "being old" and stereotypes associated vary for each group and depend on an individual's place of birth, migrant status, and level of acculturation (F. M. Yang & Levkoff, 2005)

      (4) Gerontology (geriatrics): the multidisciplinary study of the physical, psychological, and social change in people as they age

      (5) Ethnogeriatrics: the study of disease, disabilities, and the care of ethnic older adult (Ebersole, Hess, Touhy, & Jett, 2001)

      (6) Cultural competence in gerontology (geriatrics): Ability to deliver health care to older adults with the acknowledgement of the role of culture (McBride, 2008)

      (7) Care practices: family and cultural beliefs related to the care of the older adult

      (8) Provider: those who care for an older adult

      (9) Spirituality: "all behaviors that give meaning to life and provide strength to the individual" (Purnell, 2008, p. 45)

      (10) Older adult (elder) abuse: intentional acts by a caregiver or "trusted" person that lead to harm of an elder (National Center of Elder Abuse, 2005)

   b. Epidemiological factors and aging:

      (1) In the United States, one in five people will be age 65 years and older by 2030 (U.S. Census Bureau, 2005); cultural diversity in this group continues to grow (Ethnogeriatrics Committee of the American Geriatrics Society, 2004); by 2050, the proportion of elderly will increase to 23% Caucasian, 14% African Americans, 13% American Indians, Eskimos, and Aleuts, 15% Asians and Pacific Islanders, 14% Hispanics, and 21% other (U.S. Census Bureau, 2008); one in four people age 65 years and older in the U.S. will be of minority descent (Angel & Hogan, 2004).

      (2) Half of the aging population lives in developed countries, and developing countries are expected to increase their numbers from 59% to 71% (Administration on Aging, 2009; Kinsella & Velkoff, 2001); the world's older population is growing by an unprecedented 800,000 a month; more than one third of the world's oldest people (80 years and older) live in three countries: China (11.5 million), the United States (9.2 million), and India (6.2 million; U.S. Census Bureau, 2009).

      (3) Globally, fertility and mortality is declining resulting in the aging of the population; aging will be universal phenomena in all regions of the world in future decades (Bongaarts & Zimmer, 2002; United Nations, 1998).

(4) Approximately 200 million people live outside of their birth country. There are 19 million refugees globally; major challenges exist for dealing with human displacement (Amnesty International, n.d.; UN Refugee Agency, 2008). There is a need to take into account the different needs of the displaced ethnic elder when formulating policies and social programs. Immigrants and refugees should be fully involved in all stages of problem resolution and prevention. Interagency national and international cooperation is needed (International Federation of Social Workers, 1998).

(5) The growing population of older adults will be felt throughout the global economy and will challenge health care providers, governments, and society (Flesner, 2004).

c. Older adult epidemiological gender factors:

(1) In most parts of the world, women live longer than men; the disparity varies between 9 years or more in countries such as Sweden and the United States to no difference or higher life expectancy for men in countries such as Zimbabwe and Uganda (de Blij, 2009).

(2) Internationally, women dominate the older adult population; globally, in developing counties female life expectancy is 80 years and older while in developing countries the norm is 70 to 79 years (U.S. Census Bureau, 1998, 2000)

(3) Life expectancy at birth is 80.4 years for women and 75.2 years for men in the United States. In developed nations, range of life expectancy at age 65 years is 12% for both men and women (Health U.S., 2008; Kinsella & Tauber, 1993).

(4) Globally, the oldest old are mostly women, are the fastest growing group, and are more likely to have health care issues and need services; the proportion of oldest old women is expected to increase in developing countries; by 2015 the majority of the oldest old will reside in developing countries (Flesner, 2004; Kinsella & Gist, 1995; Velkoff & Lawson, 1998).

d. Older adult epidemiological financial factors:

(1) Cost of health care for the older adult will rise as the population increases; countries that have long-term care included in public health programs have higher per capita expenditures; per capital health expenditures for the elderly ranges from 1.4 (Portugal) to 3.1 (United States) to 6.0 (Australia; Flesner, 2004; OECD, 2001)

(2) Cross-national data comparisons of institutional elders are difficult to calculate because of inconsistent data and differences between countries (Flesner, 2004).

(3) The percentage of older adults' instutionalized internationally range from 0.2% (Turkey) to 5.7% (United States) to 8.8% (Netherlands); while this model is not popular outside of Europe and North America, as the numbers of the aging increase, developing countries may look at long-term care models in the future (Flesner, 2004).

(4) Poverty levels are the highest among adult populations (Andrew & Boyle, 2008); 40% live on incomes only twice the national poverty level (Glasmeier, 2005); poverty rates vary among subgroups of the older population with women being 16% more likely than elderly men to be poor and elderly African American women being 38% more likely than African American men (27%) to be poor (U.S. Census Bureau, 2008).

e. Health seeking

(1) Health care seeking practices are influenced by life experiences, health status, family support, and socioeconomic status (Zunker, Rutt, & Meza, 2005).

(2) A total of 40% of the visits to health care provider involve a companion, most likely an adult daughter (Coupland & Coupland, 2001)

(3) The living situation of the older adult is a determinant of well-being; support of family is an important factor in the developing world (Population Council, 2006).

(4) Mistrust of health care providers may be a result of past trauma (oppression or persecution; McBride, 2008).

3. **Chronic Illnesses**

a. Statistical data

(1) Globally, the leading cause of death is chronic and degenerative illness (U.S. Department of Health and Human Services, 2003); in 2001, the leading cause of death in developed countries was cardiovascular disease, cancer, and respiratory diseases; in 2001, the leading cause of death in undeveloped countries was infectious and parasitic diseases, and respiratory infections (WHO, 2002)

(2) In the United States, 80% of all older adults have at least one chronic illness, and 50% have at least two (U.S. Department of Health and Human Services, 2003); diabetes affects 18.7% with the largest increase expected in those aged 75 years and older; Alzheimer's disease doubles every 5 years after 65 years of age; after 85 years of age 47% have degenerative and debilitating disease (National Center for Chronic Disease, 1999).

(3) A common myth is that the majority of elders suffer from chronic illness, physical disability, and mental loss; although the rates increase with age, they differ across health indicators for minorities and Caucasians (Levy & Langer, 1994; Palmore, 1990; F. M. Yang & Levkoff, 2005).

(4) Vulnerable populations (uninsured, immigrants, refugees, poor) are at the greatest risk for developing health problems (Van Zandt, Sloan, & Wilkins, 2008).

(5) Older ethnic adults face greater disadvantages in health status and life expectancy compared to those who are younger and Caucasian.

(6) A total of 20% of elders have disabling conditions; culture influences how functional disabilities are perceived and when assistance is needed (Freedman, Martin, & Schoeni, 2002; U.S. Department of Health and Human Services, 2003).

(7) In the United States, the leading causes of death in older ethnic persons varies widely by race and ethnicity for example, in 2000-2001, 65% of African Americans had hypertension compared with 49% of Hispanics and 47% of Caucasians, and 22% of Caucasians had some form of cancer compared with 10% of Hispanic and African Americans (Merck Institute of Aging & Health and the Gerontological Society of America, 2002).

(8) Positive self-perceptions of aging are associated with longer life expectancy (F. M. Yang & Levkoff, 2005); those with positive self perceptions are associated with lower systolic blood pressure, cholesterol, and body mass index (Levy, Slade, Kunkel, & Kasl, 2002).

(9) For more information see Table 5.8.

b. Financial issues

(1) Health disparities exist because of lower income levels, lack of insurance, limited preventive care, and lack of access to care.

(2) Older adults who experienced prejudice and poverty many decades ago may have an impact on current health (Moody, 2006).

(3) Social security, pension, and health care systems receive increased attention in the developed world; in other parts of the world these policy issues are limited (Bongaarts & Zimmer, 2002; OECD, 1998; World Bank, 1994).

(4) Developing countries have little or no government-funded institutional support for older adults and as a result, rely heavily on family for their well-being and survival (Bongaarts & Zimmer, 2002).

(5) Filial piety honors and respects elder parents by providing support and co-residence; many older minorities reciprocate by providing important services such as cooking, cleaning, and childcare (F. M. Yang & Levkoff, 2005).

c. Initial assessment and treatment

(1) Older adults are a heterogeneous group requiring different approaches to care, support, and assistance (Andrew & Boyle, 2008); overgeneralization may lead to inaccurate stereotyping (Congress, 1997); assess both cultural group patterns and individual variation within the older adult group (Lipson & Dibble, 2009).

(2) Decisions and actions that are culturally congruent consider beliefs, practices, and values of the person (Leininger & McFarland, 2006).

(3) Establishing partnerships based on trust, respect, and responsible relationships between the provider, patient, their family, and communities is vital (Lipson & Dibble, 2009); demonstrating respect in a culturally appropriate way to older adults establishes a trusting relationship (McBride, 2008).

(4) Be alert for issues that are crucial to the success of the health care encounter, including lack of trust in health care providers, discomfort with Western biomedical systems, and fear of medical research, experimentation, and medications (Ethnogeriatrics Committee of the American Geriatrics Society, 2004).

(5) Openness to other health practices begins with self-knowledge (Lipson & Dibble, 2009) ethnic elders' common first attempts at treatment includes traditional medications and practitioners (traditional and spiritual leaders, medicine men/women).

Table 5.8. Chronic Illness and the Older Adult

Chronic Illness	Ethnicity
Alzheimer's disease and multi-infarct dementia	African Americans are at high risk (Ethnogeriatrics Committee, 2004); dementia is considered a mental illness in some cultures (McBride, 2008)
Cancer of the cervix	Vietnamese and African American women are at high risk (Ethnogeriatrics Committee, 2004)
Cancer of the colorectal	Filipinos are more likely to be diagnosed with advance stages and have low survival rates (Lin et al., 2002); occurs more frequently in Japanese Americans compared with Caucasians (Miller et al., 1996); colon cancer is more prevalent among Jews of Eastern European descent (Patai & Patai, 1989; Schurtz, 2008)
Cancer of the nasopharynx, liver, and stomach	Vietnamese men have a higher occurrence of these cancers (Ethnogeriatrics Committee, 2004); Chinese have a higher rate of nasopharyngeal cancer; men of Asian origin have a much higher than the overall rate in the United States of liver cancer (associated with chronic hepatitis B; Ethnogeriatrics Committee, 2004); liver and stomach cancer occur more frequently in Japanese Americans compared with Caucasians (Miller et al., 1996); stomach cancer is more prevalent among Jews from Europe and the United States and prostate cancer is higher in Jews of Eastern European descent (Patai & Patai, 1989; Schurtz, 2008); Vietnamese women are at high risk for stomach cancer (Ethnogeriatrics Committee, 2004)
Cancer of the prostate, lung, cervix, and esophagus	African Americans are at high risk (Ethnogeriatrics Committee, 2004)
Cancer of the thyroid	Vietnamese women are at high risk (Ethnogeriatrics Committee, 2004)
Cardiovascular disease	Higher in African American and Hispanic (American Heart Association, 2010); Vietnamese have a high rate of smoking (35% to 54%) resulting in an increased risk of heart disease; Asian Indians have a high risk for coronary artery disease (Ethnogeriatrics Committee, 2004); is the number one cause of death in African Americans (American Heart Association, 2010); Russia's cardiovascular deaths are 994 per 100,000 population (Marquez, 2005); the leading cause of death for Filipino Americans is heart disease (Hoyert & Kung, 1997)
Cerebrovascular disease	Occur at a younger age for African Americans, American Indians/Alaska Natives, and Asian/Pacific Islanders than non-Hispanic Caucasians (U.S. Department of Health and Human Services, 2005); the third leading cause of death for Filipino Americans (Hoyert & Kung, 1997)
Congestive heart failure	Higher in African Americans, Hispanic, and American Indian/Alaska Natives than in non-Hispanic Caucasians (American Heart Association, 2010)
Diabetes mellitus (type II)	Diabetes is the sixth leading cause of death for all older adults, but is the fourth for African American women and Hispanic men and women and fifth for African American men; African Americans have a 27% higher mortality rate, and American Indian and Hispanic women experience higher mortality rates than non-Hispanic Caucasians (American Heart Association, 2010); affects 18.3% in the United States with variance in prevalence by ethnic group and region; affects 27.8% of Native Americans living in the southeastern United States and 16.8% Mexican Americans (NIDDK, 2003); epidemic proportions in the Native American population resulting in a high incidence of end-organ injury with increased rates of coronary artery disease, blindness, renal failure, and limb amputation (Ethnogeriatrics Committee, 2004); Asian Indians have a high risk (Ethnogeriatrics Committee, 2004); Hispanics are more likely to require insulin to control, have more limb amputations and eye disease, have a six times higher incidence of kidney failure, and die at a rate of two to four times higher than non-Hispanic Caucasians (Gonzalez, Owen, Esperat, 2008; Otiniano, Black, Ray, Du, & Markides, 2002); Alaska Natives have seen an increase of 89% in the past 20 years, with the largest increase among Eskimos (Hall, Sberna & Utermohle, 2001)
Depression	Chinese women have seven times the suicide rate of Caucasian women in the United States (Ethnogeriatrics Committee, 2004); depression is stigmatized in many cultures
Glaucoma	More common in African American (19%; Higginbotham et al., 2004)
Hepatitis C	Occurs at higher rates among Mexican Americans than among non-Hispanic Caucasians (Gonzalez, Owen, Esperat, 2008)
Hepatitis B	Asian and Pacific Islander have a higher prevalence (Ethnogeriatrics Committee, 2004); high levels in Korean Americans (McBride, 2008); is endemic in South Asian populations, including the Vietnamese (Stauffer 2008; Hoang & Erickson, 1982); more than 80% of Vietnamese men have been exposed to hepatitis B with 14% being chronic carriers (Ethnogeriatrics Committee, 2004)

(continued)

Table 5.8. (continued)

Chronic Illness	Ethnicity
Hypertension	African Americans are at high risk (Ethnogeriatrics Committee, 2004); prevalence mortality due to myocardial infarction and stroke are greater among African Americans in the Southeast United States (Yusuf et al., 2001); Filipino Americans have one of the highest prevalence rates of hypertension, second only to African Americans (Requiro, 1988; Vance, 2008); compared with other Asians, Filipinos have highest prevalence characterized by sodium sensitivity (Garde, Spangler, & Miranda, 1994)
Osteoporosis	Varies with gender, race, and ethnicity; eight million women versus two million men; affects 20% Asian women and 10% Hispanic women (NIH, 2004; Ebersole et al., 2005); high levels in Japanese, African American, Puerto Rican, and Euro-European (McBride, 2008)
Submucosal fibrosis	Because of a habit of chewing *paan* (betel leaf, often chewed with tobacco and spices). Asian Indians have an increase rate of oral submucosal fibrosis (Ethnogeriatrics Committee, 2004)
Tuberculosis (active)	Asians and Pacific Islanders have a higher prevalence (Ethnogeriatrics Committee of the American Geriatrics Society, 2004); high levels in American Indian and immigrants from Africa, Asia, and Latin American (McBride, 2008); there is a high incidence in American Indians and varies among tribes (Hanley, 2008); exposure is common in Russia and multidrug-resistant TB is reaching unprecedented levels
Vascular dementia	Japanese have a higher rate; Chinese have increase prevalence (associated with hypertension, thalassemia, glucose-6-dehydrogenase deficiency; Ethnogeriatrics Committee, 2004); African Americans have a higher prevalence compared with non-Hispanic Caucasians (Miles, Froehlich, Bogardus, & Inouye, 2001)

(6) Assess the need for an interpreter early in the health care encounter; use trained interpreters or on-site interpreter services; be aware that using an interpreter may insult some minority older adults who may think you consider them intellectually limited (McBride, 2008).

(7) Increased response is seen in ethnic older adults when a calmer slower pace and speech is used (McBride, 2008); touch has substantial variations in meaning among cultures; personal space needs to be respected and understanding of distancing characteristics may enhance communication; eye contact must be interpreted within its cultural context; gestures and facial expressions vary among cultures; preferred greetings and acceptable body language also vary (Purnell, 2008); medical jargon is confusing and unclear.

(8) Formality of a health care encounters differ between cultural groups; a formal approach is likely the most appropriate initially; early in the relationship the health care provider should adopt conservative body language (Ethnogeriatrics Committee of the American Geriatrics Society, 2004); initially address an older person using a formal title, ask preference when appropriate (McBride, 2008).

(9) Some ethnic older adults, such as the Japanese and Filipinos, may laugh or smile to mask emotions; whereas other Asians tend to respond in accordance to social desirability (McBride, 2008)

(10) Assessing cultural history is essential; take into account the degree of acculturation and assimilation, age, gender, and individual variables; include enquiry about where the older adult grew up as well as the decade of their arrival to their new country (Lipson & Dibble, 2009); evaluating the level of acculturation assists with avoidance of mistaken assumptions in older minority adults (McBride, 2008).

(11) A mediator is a voluntary, nonbinding process in which parties reach an agreement; mediation is used among older adults in conflicts related to housing, consumer and neighbor disputes (Cox & Parsons, 1992; Persson & Castro, 2008); consider the use of a mediator in situations in which family members or friends petition for guardianship of an older adult (National Care Planning Council, 2008).

(12) See Table 5.9 for provider guidance in caring for the older adult.

d. Assessment tools

(1) Research-based, valid, and reliable, culturally and age appropriate assessment mechanisms are limited; trained administrators are needed; culturally valid definitions are important (Kobylarz, Health, & Spike, 2005).

(2) Use cultural interview tools such as the mnemonic ETHNICS (explanation, treatment, healers, negotiate, intervention, collaborate, and spirituality; Kobylarz, Health, & Like, 2002).

(3) Consider the level of education and literacy, vision and hearing deficits, nonverbal communication, and language during the interview and administration of assessment tools (Kobylarz, Health, & Like, 2002).

Table 5.9. Provider Guidance in Caring for the Older Adult

Ethnicity	Provider Guidance
Afghan	Older women avoid being touched by male providers and wear a head scarf and pants under their dresses; elders may prefer to wash the genital area by pouring water from a pitcher and expect assistance from hospital staff and children with care of their bodies; may see pain as punishment or as a part of life; vomiting is not embarrassing and may be described with a numerical scale and reported as "my food is coming up"; diarrhea is embarrassing; complaints of fatigue are common; reading of the Koran assists with symptom control, such as pain and fatigue; may use herbal/home remedies (Lipson & Askaryar, 2006)
African American	Respect is appreciated; independent self-care; a common skin problem in older women is melasma (patchy tan to dark discoloration of the face); a daily bowel movement is expected; may use herbal/home remedies (Waters & Locks, 2006); suspicious of health care providers; seeks assistance with family prior to medical care, delays early treatment of symptoms; perceives pain as a sign of disease; has stigma against mental illness; religion plays an important role in coping with illness and death; may consult a clergy or folk healer and use home remedies (Campinha-Bacote, 2008); illness is perceived as a collective event that disrupts the entire family system and is a natural occurrence resulting from disharmony in the individuals life; pain and illness is God's will (Cherry & Giger, 2008)
American Indian/ Alaskan Natives	A medicine bag or special items such as feathers or herb bundles may be worn; depression, which is prevalent, may be intergenerational resulting from memories of colonization and family stories about sexual and physical abuse at boarding schools earlier in life (Palacios, Butterfly, & Strickland, 2006)
Arab	Elders may prefer to wash their genital area by pouring water from a pitcher and believe that complete rest during illness is necessary; they expect to be cared for by family and providers; reading and placing the Koran or Bible (Ingeel) next to the bed may be important (Meleis, 2006); Islamic followers abstain from pork, alcohol, and illicit drugs, they practice moderation, and are conscious of hygiene; Muslims combine spiritual medicine, daily prayers, and reading of the Koran with medical treatment; Muslims believe that illness is considered punishment for sins; they acknowledge ailments when ill; women are reluctant to seek care, because of modesty; preventive care is not common; mental illness is stigmatized; family members care for and indulge the ill (Kulwicki, 2008); reactions to minor illness may be exaggerated; grave and terminal illness is fought relentlessly to prolong life to satisfy family or tribal members (Attia, 2003)
Cambodian	Older Khmer who are accustomed to squatting on the toilet may be uncomfortable with bedpans or urinals; string/ chain around the waist or neck with an amulet containing Buddha or inscription are worn to protect against evil spirits; Khmer elders will need direct questions about symptoms and prefer traditional practices before seeking pharmacological treatment; Khmer have died from unexplained sudden nocturnal death syndrome; older Khmer women attribute memory loss and posttraumatic stress disorder to the experiences of the Khmer Rouge War; older adults believe that Western medicine is "too strong" and may reduce dosages or not take medications; they often use herbal/home remedies and alternative healers (shaman, kru khmer, Buddhist monk) and practices (cupping [circular burning], coining [coin rubbing], acupuncture, and acupressure; Kulig & Prak, 2006); yin (cold) and yang (hot) concepts[a] utilized; illness caused by imbalance (chi) and restoring equilibrium cures illness; denies mental health issues; family expected to provide care (Touch, 2003)
Chinese	Some older women prefer to wash their genital area rather than using toilet paper; some older men expect family or providers to care for them; wearing jade or rope around the waist ensures good health; uses acupressure or acupuncture to treat illness; may ignore major illness until it is in an advance state (Chin, 2005); balance between the yin (cold) and yang (hot)[a] is important for health and imbalance between the two results in illness; illness is part of the life cycle and expected; they like treatments that do not harm and are noninvasive; family and friends take care of the sick person; traditional Chinese medicine is used and they may mistrust Western providers; older male providers are given more respect than younger and female providers (Wang & Purnell, 2008)
Dominican	Older women are expected to dress and behave conservatively; grandparents uphold modesty as the standard of behavior; charms, amulets, and healing pouches are common and charms or statues of Catholic saints are kept at the beside of the ill; folk remedies are usually the first line of treatment; older adults may suggest treating fatigue with beer to increase strength; they are passive recipients of care (Serra & Martinez, 2006); may believe the "evil eye" can cause symptoms; may seek healers (curanderos, santeras); "hot–cold" theory[a] considered (Lynch & Lynch, 2003)
East Indian	Traditional Sikh males do not cut or shave their hair; uses a water pitcher to wash their genital area; expects caregiver or family member to assist with personal hygiene and meals; uses herbal/home remedies prior to seeking medical advice; accustomed to care from family, friends, and community when sick (Zachariah, 2006); illness believed to be caused by upset of body balance; yoga is practiced to maintain a healthy body and mind (Chatterjee, 2003)
Ethiopian and Eritrean	Elder women wear a traditional cotton shawl at all times; may not want to shower daily but, if asked, may like assistance from a family member; hygiene is valued and some older women douche with warm water twice daily; may object to cutting nails at night; older women moan and appear helpless; older adults like to take daily naps after lunch; uses herbal/home remedies as a first line treatment; delays medical care until pain is severe and are not good at taking medications as prescribed (Beyene, 2005); uses traditional (magical–religious) healers and they believe in the "hot–cold" theory[a] (Kater, 2003a)

(continued)

Table 5.9. (continued)

Ethnicity	Provider Guidance
German/Amish	Older adults are very modest; they do not wash their hair daily, before sleeping, or going outdoors for fear of catching cold; Amish and Baptist men do not cut their beards; regular bowel movements are important and are described in detail; may not want to sleep without a window being opened; participates in self-care, advice from family and friends is considered, uses herbal/home remedies prior to medical care (Dodd & Eggert, 2006); health care providers are considered "outsiders", but hold them in high regard; Amish religion and cultural values are important believing that the body is the temple of God; involved in preventive care; uses folk medicine and alternative care (Wenger & Wenger, 2008)
Greek	Modest and prefer provider of same gender; may prefer sponge baths to showers; old-world ties result in older men preferring to leave nails on the little finger of right hand one inch-long; wears Greek Orthodox cross and/or pendant of the Virgin Mary at all times; family member may assist with personal hygiene; views rest and sleep as important to recovery and depression as disharmony with one's spirit and God; prefers prayer, over-the-counter medication, folk healing practices, and home remedies before seeking medical care (Genet, 2006); focuses on acute versus preventive care; religious belief that illness can be cured by atonement and forgiveness; wear amulets to protect from "evil eye" (Patiraki-Kourbani, 2003)
Hawaiian	Modest and prefer provider of same gender; traditionally baths two to three times a day; believes that hair and nails possess power, take great care when disposing of them; prefers independent self-care; may not trust Western biomedical care due to their history related to death from foreign born illnesses; traditionally believe that depression is a result of spiritual imbalance and needs to be treated by healers; incorporates massage, relaxation, prayer, and meditation in treatment of illness; uses herbal/home remedies; when hospitalized may expect family members to spend the night (Palakiko, 2006)
Israel	Preservation of life is the greatest priority and all people have a duty to maintain health; verbalization of pain is acceptable; family is central and assist with responsibilities during illness; regardless of age and level of disability the Torah teachings are expected (Purnell & Selekman, 2008); they believe in the value of health prevention and promotion, use complimentary and alternative care (Naturopathy, Feldenkrais, acupuncture, and homeopathy); have a stigma against mental illness with fear that it may decrease their children's marriage prospects; pray, wear religious objects, and carry religious pictures and booklets when ill; before signing consent forms they consult with a religious leader (rabbi; Kater, 2003b)
Iranian	Modest and prefer provider of same gender; if ill, may refrain from daily shower due to the belief that dampness accentuating weakness; may prefer to wash their genital area by pouring water from a pitcher; wears wrist chains and gold charm on their neck; prays with prayer beads; expects family and friends to assist with care; older adults are likely to manifest a somber mood due to a deeper understanding of human mortality; uses herbal/home remedies (Hafizi, 2006); balance is important to health; expressive about pain believing that suffering in this world assures a place in heaven; mental illness is stigmatized (Hafizi, Sayyedi, & Lipson, 2008); traditional healers may be consulted (Sadeghi, 2003)
Irish	Modest, wears black clothing to funerals and may wear an armband; may carry rosary beads or wear a crucifix or saint medal as a necklace, a scapular (two small pieces of cloth or laminated paper with religious images or text) may be worn around the neck or pinned to clothing; prefers to be independent in self-care; ignores symptoms as long as possible; reluctant to report symptoms or ask for pain relief; little understanding of mental illness; uses herbal/home remedies (Barnard, 2005)
Italian	Modest; when ill may avoid bath or shower and prefer a warm water sponge bathe; some wear horn or an amulet to protect against the evil eye; may carry rosary beads and wear religious medals or a card with a saint; women may wear black or navy when mourning the loss of child or husband; fears pain and expresses it by chanting "poor me, poor me"; overly concerned with digestive issues, when fatigued will rest or reduce activity; not inclined to seek mental health counseling or support groups; uses herbal/home remedies from different areas of Italy (Miceli, Breda, & Frank, 2006)
Japanese	Very modest, even with family and those of opposite gender; cleanliness and hygiene are important and are linked to restoring health; older women have their hair professionally cared for weekly; may use prayer beads if Buddhist; if ill, dependent on family members for personal care; describes symptoms in words instead of numerical scales (i.e., 1-5); especially concerned about becoming addicted to medications; mental illness is considered shameful; delays response to illness until advanced; relies on spouse or female family member to assist with illness; uses herbal/home remedies (Shiba, Leong, & Oka, 2006); less likely to express feelings verbally and bearing pain is considered a virtue; addiction is taboo; assuming the sick role is highly tolerated and recuperation periods are lengthy (Turale & Ito, 2008)
Korean	Very modest; tends to be very clean; older women may shampoo their hair once a week; Christians wear crucifix and Buddhist prayer beads around their neck; expect care from female children; fear addiction or complications to medication; stigma is attached to mental illness; symptoms ignored until severe; uses herbal/home remedies (Im, 2006); uses a holistic approach to health care; a balance of emotional and physical health is viewed as important; acupuncture and acupressure are used in conjunction to medical care; family care for the ill (Im, 2008); North Korean elders use traditional care (holistic, acupuncture, acupressure, herbal medicine, and cupping [circular burning]); illness considered a disturbance in "ki" (body's vital energy); malnutrition and lack of medical care common in North Korea (Chang, 2003a); South Korea elders consider mind-body interactions essential for health and believe in "ki" (Chang, 2003b)

(continued)

Table 5.9. (continued)

Ethnicity	Provider Guidance
Laos, Hmong	Older Hmong women are modest about their genitals, but not their breasts as a result of breastfeeding; in Laos bathing was infrequent due to lack of water; may were amulets, gold necklaces or bracelets to hold the soul in and keep evil spirits away; prefer to perform self-care but may expect family member to care for them; accepts analgesic medication (traditionally grew and used opium as an analgesic); posttraumatic stress disorder is common; uses herbal/home remedies extensively; alternative practices include cupping (circular burning) and coining (coin rubbing; Johnson & Hang, 2006); lack of health care and prevention programs in Laos is prominent; unhealthy and bad wind cause illness; pinching and scratching area of problem is done to release the "bad" wind; strings around the neck, ankles, or waist prevent the loss of the soul, which is believed to cause illness; loss of blood is considered irreplaceable; mental illness is stigmatized (D'Avanzo & Geissler, 2003)
Mexican	Modesty and cleanliness valued; wears crucifixes, scapulars, and religious medals; expects providers to assist with self-care; may interpret oxygen as a negative sign; uses herbal/home remedies, and spiritual healers or prayer (Guarnero, 2005); engage in folk medicine practices and use folk practitioners, including curandero(a); family is foremost; Catholicism is dominant (89%) and influences their health practices; health is considered a gift from God; they do not seek medical care until incapacitated; over-the-counter use of prescription medications purchased in Mexico is common (Zoucha & Zamarripa, 2008); diseases believed to be influence by "hot" (generated from within the body) and "cold" (invasion by outside sources)[a] imbalance (Dumonteil & Leon, 2003)
Nigerian	May refuse narcotics for moderate pain, as Islam forbids narcotics; complains of being tired due to aging, making it difficult to distinguish illness-related fatigue; views depression as spiritual unhappiness; prompt to respond to symptoms of discomfort; family recite the Koran or prayers and the older adult may pray or meditate when ill, uses herbal/home remedies (Hashwani, 2006)
Pakistani	Prefer provider of same gender; water is a symbol of purity; uses a water pitcher to wash their genital area; very religious older women reveal only their face and hands, may wear gold or silver charm with name of Allah on neck chain or Koranic verses in small cloth for protection against illness; assumes the dependent role (Hashwani, 2006); believe that health and sickness is provided by God; illness is a result of an evil dead or sorcery; mental illness is stigmatized and thought to be caused by evil spirits; prefer not being told about a grave diagnosis; uses allopathic, homeopathic, and indigenous methods (Parviz, 2003)
Philippines	Believe that cutting hair or nails on Friday is bad luck; uses a water pitcher to wash their genital area; wears religious medallions or keeps rosary beads or saint images by the bed while ill; may take an afternoon nap; fatalistic views may delay medical care; uses herbal/home remedies prior to seeking medical care (Rodriguez, de Guzman, & Cantos, 2006); predominantly Roman Catholic (80.9%); novenas and prayers for the sick are utilized; religion is an important component of health; decisions about care is influenced by the circle of family and they may consult the network of friends for advise; balance and moderation are important for health and illness is a result of imbalance; views pain as part of living an honorable life (Pacquiao, 2008); mental illness is stigmatized and believe it is rooted in witchcraft or demonic possession; they believe the "evil eye" can cause illness; if treatment is unsuccessful may attribute it to forces of nature, spells, or sins (D'Avanzo, 2003)
Polish	Modesty and privacy valued; they trim their nails short; they may wear crucifixes, religious medals, and scapular (two small pieces of cloth or laminated paper with religious images or text) around their neck; women care for self when ill, if possible, but men may expect more assistance; they are stoic with symptoms; believe suffering assists with personal salvation; recognizes mental illness; neglects self-care for sake of family; seeks medical help only when herbal/folk remedies ineffective (Carol, 2006); Catholicism is dominant with prayer used to ward off danger and illness; they fear being dependent on others; seek mental health care as a last resort; refrains from using extraordinary means for prolonging life (Plawecki, Plawecki, Plawecki, & Plawecki, 2008)
Russian	Values modesty; prefers a sponge bath when ill; women wear warm clothing for fear of becoming ill; family will assist with care; some Jewish families keep kosher; tend to be stoic; regular bowel movements are important; sleeping through the night is essential to recovery; they do not acknowledge mental illness; describes depression in terms of somatic symptoms; self-care prior to seeking medical care (del Puerto & Sigal, 2006); seriously ill who are religious consider prayer as a healing tool (Russian Orthodox, Russian Jew); alternative (cupping) and homeopathic remedies utilized; seek warmth when ill (Smith, 2008); oriental traditional medicine is popular; superstitions about magical healing powers of some drugs and objects is common; magical–religious practices may be followed (Knyazev & Slobodskaya, 2003)
Yugoslavian (former)	Uses baby soap, lotion, and facial cream feeling it is good for the skin; washes hair once or twice a week, believing wet hair may cause illness; women may wear a scarf if they lost a family in war; may wear thermal underwear in cold climates; wears religious amulets; family are caregivers, believing God will reward them for the deed; tolerates pain, thinking it is a inevitable result of aging; naps after lunch; mental illness is taboo; may delay medical care to avoid fear of illness; family assist with care (Alikadic, 2006)

a. According to the hot–cold theory, health is dependent on the proper distribution of the body's four humors: blood, phlegm, yellow bile, and black bile, which are classified based on their physical properties as hot or cold. The theory is based on the concept that an illness is hot or cold (e.g., arthritis is cold and an ulcer is hot) and that the medications, remedies, and foods that are used to treat is usually the opposite classification or property (Harwood, 1971; Kay & Yoder, 1987).

(4) Decision-making capacity relate directly to functional impairment in activities of daily living (ADLs; Spike, 2004).

e. Psychosocial Factors

   (1) When stressed and anxious, in an unfamiliar environment, and unable to communicate, it is common to feel isolated and misunderstood

   (2) Fears related to illness include unmanaged pain, emotional suffering, family burden, unwanted treatments, and wishes being ignored

   (3) Response to pain reflects cultural expectations and acceptable behavior based on years of social modeling (Jeffrey & Lubkin, 2002)

   (4) Religion and spiritual belief is a source of emotional and psychosocial support (McKenna, 2008); spiritual issues become more important with age (Koenig, Kvale, & Ferrell, 1988); religion is vital in the process of dealing with stressful life events or transition (Krause, 1998); health care providers need to assist with access to religion and spiritual beliefs (Ethnogeriatrics Committee of the American Geriatrics Society, 2009); many cultures rely on spirituality to assist with healing

   (5) Understanding patterns of decision making (designation to the firstborn son or extended family) increase communication (McBride, 2008); determining the person's decision-making preferences early promote better communication (Ethnogeriatrics Committee of the American Geriatrics Society, 2004)

   (6) Talking about death and disability is inappropriate in some cultures and should be approached after initial assessment and trusting relationships are developed

   (7) Knowledge and understanding of advance directives vary among ethnic elders, with some older adults believing that diminished care may result (Hopp, 2000; McBride, 2008); use of advance directives and health care proxies are less common in minority cultural groups; be sensitive to the possibility that some prefer alternative approaches, such as verbal directives or family dictated directive, whereas others need to avoid any discussion (Ethnogeriatrics Committee of the American Geriatrics Society, 2004)

   (8) See Table 5.9 for provider guidance in caring for the older adult

f. Health risks

   (1) Epidemiological and medical research has identified differences among ethnic and cultural populations related to health risks (Ethnogeriatrics Committee of the American Geriatrics Society, 2004)

   (2) Failure to prepare health care providers for this population's health care delivery will have a major impact on the health care of the older adult; cultural competence is a strategy to combat health disparities (Brach & Fraser, 2000)

   (3) The ethnic elder is less likely to be referred for screening procedures or to receive advanced surgical procedures (Ethnogeriatrics Committee of the American Geriatrics Society, 2004)

   (4) Current immunization rates for older adults is 23% to 49% with great ethnic disparities; the U.S. Public Health Service national goal is 90% by 2010 for pneumonia and influenza vaccines (Holtz, 2008; Weber, 2004)

   (5) Five out of six elders take at least one medication and nearly half take three or more (U.S. Department of Health and Human Services, 2004a); use of over-the-counter medications, sharing of medications, purchasing of medications out of the country, and home remedies must be considered in older ethnic adults

   (6) Depression is associated with the increased dependence of older immigrants; stigmas exist in many cultures against mental illness (Andrews & Boyle, 2008)

   (7) In 2002, there were 14.9 million refugees and 22 million displaced persons in the world; a large number suffer from PTSD resulting from traumatic events (Bolton, 2009; Porter & Haslam, 2001)

   (8) Oral health care is not covered by Medicare and there are not enough trained dentists to meet the needs (Lamster, 2004; U.S. Department of Health and Human Services, 2004b)

g. Elder abuse

   (1) Between one to two million older adults in the United States have been abused (Bonnie & Wallace, 2003); 1 in every 14 are abused in domestic settings (Pillemer & Finkelhor, 1988); financial exploitation is reported in 1 in 15 cases; every year there is one reported case of abuse for every five that go unreported (National Center on Elder Abuse, 1998)

   (2) Human rights of the older adult includes: protection (securing physical, psychological, and emotional safety; Human Rights Education Associates, 2003)

(3) Elder abuse includes physical abuse, neglect (including self neglect), emotional or psychological abuse, verbal abuse and threats, financial abuse and exploitation, sexual abuse, and abandonment (National Center on Elder Abuse, 2005)

(4) It occurs in the home, nursing homes, and institutions; affects older adults across all socio-economic groups, cultures, and races (National Center on Elder Abuse, 2005)

(5) The oldest old and women are more likely victimized; dementia is a risk factor; mental health and substance abuse (abuser and victim) is a risk factor; isolation may contribute (National Center on Elder Abuse, 2005)

(6) Warning signs include the following: marks, bruises, burns, blisters, pressure ulcers, hygiene issues, lack of medical care, malnutrition, dehydration, withdrawal from normal activities, changes in alertness or behavior, unexplained sexually transmitted diseases, sudden change in finances, altered wills and trusts, unusual bank withdrawals, and loss of property. (National Center on Elder Abuse, 2005)

(7) Risk factors include caregiver stress; childhood trauma; cultural sanctions against seeking help to care for older adult; delirium; dependency of abuser on victim for housing and finances; dependence of elder on caregiver for assistance with activities; family history of violence, financial strain, increased age, isolation of the caregiver or victim, lack of close family ties, mental illness in family members/caretakers; new, worsening, or prolonged depression or physical impairment; poverty/lack of financial resources; progressing dementia, shared living arrangement, substance abuse in family members/caretakers; and unsafe living situation (Fulmer, 2008; Wagner, Greenberg, & Capezuti, 2002)

(8) Decreased decision-making ability results in spouses, partners, and family members becoming involved in managing the older adult's assets potentially resulting in unintentional or intentional financial abuse (Wilson, Tilse, & Setterlund, 2009)

(9) Older homeless or imprisoned elders share environments with younger, frequently violent, persons who present increased risk and challenges (Dawes, 2009; Lipmann, 2009)

(10) An interdisciplinary assessment and intervention plan is essential to ensure the safety and health of older adults; assessment and intervention should be directed toward both the victim and the alleged perpetrator (Fulmer, 2008); the *Elder Mistreatment Assessment Tool* is a 41-item tool used to assess older adult abuse (Fulmer, 2008; Fulmer, Street, & Carr, 1984)

(11) The *Culturagram* is an assessment tool that incorporates cultural values, beliefs, and experiences into the assessment process (Brownell, 1998; Congress, 1994)

(12) Financial exploitation in minority communities is often unrecognized or inappropriately indentified; cultural considerations when assessing financial exploitation in minority families include: cultural differences in relation to living arrangements, financial status, family dynamics, systems of social support, and emotional/psychological stress; multigenerational households cannot be ignored (Sanchez, 1997)

h. Spiritual issues

(1) Sensitivity to spiritual needs (not simply those with religious beliefs) include acknowledgement of culture, language, customs, dietary needs, isolation, anxiety, fear, and so on; during times of crisis people may consciously or unconsciously experience spiritual needs (Bennion, 2000)

(2) Major religions of the world include Christianity (33%), Islam (21%), atheist, agnostic or nonreligious (16%); Hinduism (14%), Chinese Traditional (6.4), Buddhism (6%), Sikhism (0.4%), and Judaism (0.2%; Major Religions, 2007)

(3) Awareness of spiritual needs and practices promotes culturally competent care (Purnell, 2008)

(4) Older adults may find comfort in speaking to a religious leader during crisis, serious illness or eminent death; special arrangements for prayers or spiritual leader may be needed; comfort can be found in religious items (medals, books, statues) and removal avoided; family can help meet spiritual needs (Purnell, 2008)

(5) Some ethnic older adults may request body parts removed during surgery to be returned (McBride, 2008)

(6) "Grieving and death rituals vary across cultures and are often heavily influenced by religion" (Chachkes & Jennings, 1994; Lobar, Youngblut, & Brooten, 2006, p. 44; Younoszai, 1993); providers should be "aware of cultural perceptions and religious beliefs in order to assist families in their

preparations for death and to recognize the need for families to complete ceremonies and rituals surrounding the death of a family member" (Lobar, Youngblut, & Brooten, 2006, p. 50)

    (7) For more information see Table 5.9

i. Elder care

    (1) Informal caregiver role: *spouse, family, friends*

        (a) Informal caregivers are defined as people who, without payment, provide assistance to an older adult family member or friend who needs help because of frailty, illness, or disability

        (b) Ethnic minority caregivers have a lower socioeconomic status, are younger and less likely to be spouse; Asian American caregivers, but not African American and Hispanic caregivers, use less formal support than non-Hispanic Caucasian caregivers; African American caregivers have lower levels of caregiver burden and depression than Caucasian caregivers, Hispanic and Asian American caregivers are more depressed than their Caucasian non-Hispanic peers; all groups of ethnic minority caregivers reported worse physical health than non-Hispanic Caucasians (Pinquart & Sorensen, 2005)

        (c) Filial piety, a culturally defined set of respect norms with regard to age, influences the role that the family member will take in the care of the older adult (Harwood, 2007)

        (d) Recent immigrants and refugees have stronger family ties and expect caregiving by their adult relatives (Andrews & Boyle, 2008)

        (e) In many cultures, the eldest son has the responsibility for his aging parents, but the wife of the son provides the care; in developing countries the older adult lives with an adult child (Bongaarts & Zimmers, 2002); some cultures legally require the care for one's parent (Liu & Tinker, 2001); Muslim religious teachings encourages taking care of elders and nursing home placement is rare (Leininger, 1997)

        (f) There are more female caregivers (59% to 75%; Health and Human Services, 1998; The Henry J. Kaiser Family Foundation, 2002)

        (g) One in 10 older adults lives alone (greater for women than for men) and women are less likely to live with a spouse or the head of the household (Bongaarts & Zimmers, 2002)

        (h) Worldwide, as education increases, older adults are more likely to live alone or in smaller house-holds, with few children and other adults (Bongaarts & Zimmers, 2002)

        (i) In the United States, 34 million people aged 50 years and older live with an informal care giver (National Alliance for Caregivers and AARP, 2004); of those aged 70 years and older, 44% are Latino, 34% are African American, and 25% are non-Hispanic Caucasian (C. O. Weiss, Gonzalez, Kabeto, & Langa, 2005); 5.8 to 7.0 million people (family, friends, and neighbors) provide care to persons 65 years of age and older who need assistance with ADLs; National Long-Term Care Survey, 1994; W. D. Spector, Fleishman, Pezzin, & Spillman, 2000; U.S. Department of Health and Human Services, 1998); unpaid family caregivers is the largest source of long-term care services in the United States and the number is estimated to increase to 37 million by 2050 (U.S. Department of Health and Human Services, 2003)

        (j) Of those providing informal care in the United States, 21% are Caucasian and African American, 18% are Asian American, and 16% are Hispanic Americans (National Alliance of Caregivers and AARP, 2004); ethnic minority caregivers provide more care and report worse physical health than Non-Hispanic Caucasian caregivers (McCann et al., 2000; Pinquart & Morenson, 2005)

        (k) Of those 70 years of age and older who require care, Caucasians are most likely to receive help from their spouse, Hispanics are most likely to receive help from their adult children, and African Americans are more likely to receive help from a non-family member (National Academy on an Aging Society, 2000)

    (2) Informal caregiver burden

        (a) Caregivers feel marginalized and often overlook their own health and social needs (Arskey et al., 2003)

        (b) Participation of women in the workforce and the decrease in the number of adult children has resulted in families being unable to assist in care (Andrews & Boyle, 2008)

        (c) particularly women, provide most of the care with little support from formal caregivers (Navaie-Waliser, Spriggs, & Feldman, 2002)

- (d) A balance is needed between the care of the older adult and the active participation of their family and/or support system with consideration given to issues of dignity, safety, and security (Andrews & Boyle, 2008)
- (e) There are high disability rates among caregivers (Li & Fries, 2005)
- (f) Informal caregivers have increased blood pressure and insulin levels, may have impaired immune systems, have increased risk for cardiovascular disease, and, if older (66-69 years of age), have a 63% higher mortality rate (Cannuscio et al., 2002; Family Caregiver Alliance, n.d.; Kiecolt Glaser & Glaser, 2003; Lee, Colditz, Berkman, & Kawachi, 2003; Schulz & Beach, 1999)

(3) Informal caregiver barriers
- (a) Barriers to accessing support include lack of culturally sensitive services (for example, reluctance to access Meals-on-Wheels if no appropriate food) and services providing a range of languages (Department of Health, Social Services and Public Safety, Government of Ireland, 2004)
- (b) Changes in Social Security, Medicaid and Medicare will affect all, especially the ethnic elderly, and will determine quality of care
- (c) Many informal caregivers are unaware of availability of support services (Family Caregiver Alliance, n.d.)

(4) Formal care descriptions: *Board and care, assisted living, nursing home*
- (a) Formal care is defined as a caregiver who is paid and associated with a service system (Fradkin & Heath, 1992; McConnell & Riggs, 1994)
- (b) Board and care homes (residential care facilities), licensed by the U.S. Department of Social Services, provide care for seniors in residential private homes
- (c) Assisted living facilities offer housing alternatives for those who may need help with activities of daily living, but do not require medical and nursing care provided in a nursing home; licensing requirements vary by state; these facilities can be known by other names, including residential care, board and care, congregate care, and personal care (U.S. Department of Health and Human Services, 2005)
- (d) Nursing homes are long-term care facilities; the Nursing Home Reform Act, passed in 1987, established quality standards for nursing homes nationwide, emphasized the importance of quality of life, and preserved residents' rights (Turnham, n.d.)

(5) Formal care placement
- (a) The most consistent factor in determining placement outside of the home is the lack of informal support (Andrews & Boyle, 2008)
- (b) Assess family/support system for capacities of self-care with consideration given to culture, family size, location of residence, and socioeconomic factors (McKenna, 2008)
- (c) Most older adults report they would prefer to remain in their homes and community
- (d) Nursing homes are associated with stigma and utilized rarely in some cultures
- (e) Nursing home environments with schedules, order, daily care, and food selections may not be valued by other cultures (Andrews & Boyle, 2008)
- (f) Ethnic elders expect their preadmission folk care practices to be practiced, respected, and maintained (McFarland, 1997)
- (g) Disability rates are likely to affect the long-term care system; African Americans have higher disability rates than non-Hispanic Caucasians and other ethnic groups (Pandya, 2005)
- (h) Use of formal long-term care services by African Americans, Hispanics (non-Caucasian), and Asians have traditionally been substantially lower than that of non-Hispanic Caucasians most likely due to cultural preferences, language issues, and lower income (Dilworth-Anderson, Williams, & Gibson, 2002; Pandya, 2005; Wallace, Levy-Storms, Kingston, & Anderson, 1998)
- (i) Lower rates of formal care for Asians, Hispanics, and Native Americans may reflect preference for family caregiving (Pandya, 2005)
- (j) Older ethnic adults with special needs are aging; those with intellectual disabilities represent a challenge to families, care and service providers; persons with intellectual disabilities were not expected to outlive their caregivers consequently few services were developed (McCallion & McCarron, 2004)

    (6) Cultural sensitivity in formal care

        (a) It is necessary to support culturally competent policy development and education for the health care team; include healers from nonbiomedical traditions (McBride, 2008)

        (b) Build ethnic community partnerships to assist with coordinating health care interventions and traditional therapies (McBride, 2008)

        (c) Long-term care facilities reflect the awareness of cultural sensitivity through food service, environment, and activity policies (Gorek, 2002; Thomas, 1996); culture clusters (grouping of ethnic elders) can be used to provide traditional foods, language, and activities (Orlovsky, 2008)

        (d) Matching residents with staff members of their own culture, providing an area for residents of the same culture to socialize, involving family members, and reaching out to ethnic communities for resources may provide comfort (Lourde, 2007)

        (e) Be aware of comfort or discomfort related to cultural symbols, that is, images, color, and so on (McBride, 2008)

        (f) It is important to build patient–provider trust relationships by understanding the cultural contexts of health behaviors, and increasing one's sensitivity to the cultural relationship with decision making and health care preferences (McBride, 2008; McBride & Lewis, 2004)

        (g) Governments will be faced with funding challenges for health care programs for the aging (Flesner, 2008); exchange programs with other nations can lead to increased knowledge of the global issue

        (h) Alternative delivery models such as home-like environments need to be considered (Flesner, 2004)

        (i) Mediation can open doors to new ways of thinking about how to make long-term care facilities more cooperative places (Persson & Castro, 2008)

F. End-of Life Decisions and Practices

1. *Beliefs About Death*

    a. Culturally defined as a social transition; relating a change in the life cycle to changes in the social position within a society by linking the physiological and social aspects of an individual's life (Helman, 2007).

    b. Biological death is the end of the physiological organism, the end of the individual's lifespan; social death is the end of the person's social identity (Hertz, 1960).

      (1) The time between the two is variable, from days, months, to even years.

        (a) In many cultures a widow is prohibited from marrying for a specific period of time after her husband's death, sometimes forever.

        (b) For Orthodox Jews, the *shiv'ah* has a specific structure of 7 days of mourning after the funeral, mourning dress is worn until the 13th day, and recreation and amusement are forbidden for 1 year.

      (2) During this period, the deceased's soul is often considered to be in limbo, between the two worlds and thus dangerous to others

    c. Culturally defined rituals are performed at each stage in this process, with prescribed acts, dress and forbidden activities.

    d. Religious beliefs play a role in bereavement and rituals and overlap with cultural beliefs and rituals (Evers, Lewis, & Schaeffer, 1999. See Table 5.10).

2. *Role of the Family*

    a. Cultural differences in the role of the family are often cited as a major distinguishing factor among racial and ethnic groups (Lyke & Colon, 2004). Family member involvement in decision-making process is important across all racial and ethnic groups although preferences for how family members are involved differ across racial and ethnic groups

    b. Decision making (Kwak & Haley, 2005)

      (1) Decisions regarding end-of-life treatment preferences are often made by surrogates, because patients are too ill to participate in the process (Braun, Beyth, Ford, McCullough, 2008).

      (2) Across ethnic groups, medical decision making is likely to be viewed as a burden, but

        (a) Responses to the burden may vary across groups (Braun et al., 2008)

        (b) Some believe that it is the family's role to remove the burden of making treatment decisions from the patient (Born, Greiner, Sylvia, Butler, & Ahluwalia, 2004; R. S. Morrison, Zayas, Mulvihill, Baskin, & Meier, 1998)

Table 5.10. Beliefs and Values Regarding Organ Donation and Transplantation of Some Common Religions and Selected Cultures

Religion	Beliefs
African American	African Americans are half as likely to have signed a donor card and less likely to be willing to donate their own or a loved one's organs than Whites. African Americans express greater concerns about the trustworthiness of the health care system, both in general and in terms of the donation system specifically, and were more likely to want to see the organs that they give go to other African Americans (Cort & Cort, 2008; Dodd-McCue & Tartaglia, 2007; Siminoff, Burant & Ibrahim, 2006)
Amish	The Amish consent to transplantation if it is for the health and welfare of the transplant recipient
Asian Americans (from >20 countries)	Asian Americans are the least likely to donate organs among the major ethnic groups in the United States, comprising only 1.8% of deceased donors (OPTN, 2010). Beliefs range from a reluctance to talk about death or organ donation within the family to the importance of leaving the body whole at the time of death. Ancient Confusian philosophy taught that the body was not to be altered during life or death, and remnants of these beliefs remain in modern society (A. H. Cheung, Alden, & Wheeler, 1998; Kim, 2004; Wong et al., 2009)
Buddhism	Buddhists believe organ donation is viewed as a selfless act of charity, a dedicated act to one in need. It is even encouraged in some populations in Sri Lanka (Helman, 2007)
Catholicism	Catholics view organ donation as an act of charity, fraternal love, and self-sacrifice. Transplants are ethically and morally acceptable to the Vatican (Breitkopf, 2009)
The Church of Christ, Scientist	Christian Scientists do not take a specific position on transplants or organ donation. Christian Scientists rely on spiritual rather than medical means for healing, and the question of whether to donate is left to the individual church member
Hinduism	Hindus are not prohibited by religious law from donating their organs. Donation is an act of individual decision
Hispanic Americans	Hispanic Americans are less likely to consent to organ donation than non-Hispanic Whites. Barriers to consent include a reluctance to "plan for death," concern over body disfigurement, doubts that doctors do all they can to preserve life before pursuing organ donation, concerns about religious acceptance of donation, perceptions of inequity in the distribution of donated organs, and suspicion of a black market for organs, particularly in Mexico. Women are more likely to consent than men (Breitkopf, 2009)
Islam	In 1983, the Moslem Religious Council initially rejected organ donation by followers of Islam, but it has reversed its position, provided donors consent in writing before their death. The organs of Moslem donors must be transplanted immediately
Hmong culture	Historically, the Hmong have been opposed to organ donation, citing their belief bodies that are missing their organs consequently will lack those organs when they are reincarnated (Neidich et al., 2009)
Japanese Shinto	In Japan, brain death is still not widely accepted as human death (Japan Organ Transplant Homepage, 2010). It was not until 1997 that transplanation became legal, but with many restrictions (Kita, 2000). According to Shinto beliefs, the concept of personhood is communal and death is mot complete until a series of rituals is perfomed (Nudeshima, 1991). And if the body is incomplete, the soul will be sad and this sadness will affect the family members (Morioka, 1995)
Jehovah's Witnesses	According to the Watch Tower Society, the legal corporation for the religion, Jehovah's Witnesses do not encourage organ donation but believe it is a matter best left to an individual's conscience. With the advent of "bloodless" surgeries, Jehovah's Witnesses are charged with accepting these interventions according to their own conscience (Whyte, 2008). All organs and tissues, however, must be completely drained of blood before transplantation
Judaism	Judaism teaches that saving a human life takes precedence over maintaining the sanctity of the human body. In general, the Jewish faith condones organ donation and transplantation in order to preserve life. However, the Orthodox and Hassidic sects see harvesting of organs as mutilation of the deceased and forbid organ donation (Weber, 1996)
Mormonism	The Church of Jesus Christ of Latter Day Saints considers the decision to donate organs a personal one. Mormons must weigh the advantages and disadvantages of transplants individually and choose the decision that will bring them peace and comfort. The church does not interpose any objection to an individual decision in favor of organ and tissue donation
Protestantism	Protestants encourage and endorse organ donation. The Protestant faith respects an individual's conscience and a person's right to make decisions about his or her own body
Roma	Roma, disparagingly named "Gypsies", on the whole, are against organ donation. Although they have no formal resolution, their opposition is associated with their belief in the afterlife. Roma believe that for 1 year after death, the soul retraces its steps. All the body parts must be intact because the soul maintains a physical shape.

Source: Adapted from Evers et al. (1999). Reprinted with permission.

       i.   India, where filial ties are strong, relatives are often reluctant to leave the patient alone with the doctor and they may give strict instructions to the doctor not to reveal the diagnosis (Chaturvedi, Loiselle, & Chandra, 2009)

      ii.   In many Asian cultures, it is perceived as unnecessarily cruel to directly inform a patient of a terminal diagnosis (Holland, Geary, Marchini, & Tross, 1987; Matsumura et al., 2002)

      iii.   Even among people of European background, Bosnian Americans and Italian Americans perceive direct disclosure of illness as, at minimum, disrespectful, and more significantly, inhumane (Searight, 2005)

(3) Health care provider communication (Braun et al., 2008):

    (a) Is an important resource for coping with decision-making burden

    (b) Should be clear and sensitive

    (c) Should communicate condition and prognosis, if culturally appropriate. Suggested questions (Searight & Gafford, 2005)

      i.   "Some people want to know everything about their medical condition, and others do not. What is your preference?"

      ii.   "Is there anything that would be helpful for me to know about how your family, or comminuty or your faith views serious illness and treatment?"

c. Caregiving

  (1) Pain and other symptoms

  (2) Gender roles (Blackhall et al., 1999)

    (a) Across ethnic groups, is associated with both general attitudes about and personal desires for life support

    (b) Women less likely to want or view the use of life support favorably than men

d. Grief and bereavement:

  (1) Grief is a universal phenomenon, but it is shaped by cultural and religious factors and the following vary widely (Mantala-Bozos, 2003):

    (a) Expectations

    (b) Practices

    (c) Beliefs

    (d) Etiquette

    (e) Rituals

  (2) Cultures develop rituals to direct (Shuchter & Zisook, 1988; Zisook, Chentsova-Dutton, & Shuchter, 1998):

    (a) Care and disposal of the body, for example,

      i.   Burial

      ii.   Cremation

      iii.   "Sky funerals" of Tibet, wherein the body is placed on a high mountain ridge and left for the birds and the elements (Helman, 2007)

    (b) Incorporation of death into religious ceremony

    (c) Prescribed actions of mourning and memorials, for example,

      i.   Irish *wake* involves sitting with corpse for several dyas and nights, and sometimes includes feasting and drinking

      ii.   In Latin America, celebration of *El Día de los Muertos* (Day of the Dead) on November 2nd when the family spends the night at the gravesite of their deceased members, shares a meal, tells stories of the loved one, and attends to the gravesite (Sayer, 1990)

    (d) Some normative dimensions of cultural responses to grief may impact outcomes of grieving (Mantala-Bozos, 2003)

  (3) The majority of bereavement research is focused on

    (a) Heterosexual couples

    (b) Primarily married

    (c) Often in later years of life

  (4) Gay, lesbian, bisexual, or transgender (GLBT) culture may be hidden within mainstream societies, thus

    (a) Little is known about mortality, bereavement, and interventional support in GLBT communities

    (b) Research on loss of same-sex partner includes several studies of gay men who have lost partners or good friends from HIV-related illness

(5) Bereavement within GLBT communities
  (a) Kinship networks will determine who is bereaved by a death (Bent, & Magilvy, 2006)
  (b) May differ from those in traditional nuclear families and are often determined by:
      i.   Symbolic or practical ties
      ii. Choices
      iii. Love

3. ***Advance Care Planning (Advance Directives):*** Despite skepticism about the ability of advance directives to influence clinical decision making, they remain the primary means of guiding medical care for patients unable to make their own care decisions (Teno et al., 1997).
  a. Race and ethnicity appear to be independent of income and education in predicting possession of advance directives (Murphy et al., 1996; Hopp & Duffy, 2000).
  b. Discussion and preparation of *Advance Directives*
      (1) The preponderance of evidence is that African Americans are less likely than Whites to have some sort of advance directive.
      (2) There are fewer studies of frail older adults of other races and ethnicities.
      (3) Those studies also show that Whites are more likely than others to have completed advance directives, except where they are enrolled in special services targeted to reducing this disparity (Kwak & Haley, 2005).
  c. Disparate rates of advance directive completion are the source of much speculation
      (1) Reasons for disparities remain unclear.
          (a) The reluctance of Blacks to formally address end-of-life care may stem from a history of health care discrimination. Although individual studies vary, the preponderance of evidence indicates that non-Whites, even after controlling for income, insurance status, and age, are less likely to receive a range of common medical interventions such as cardiac catheterization, immunizations, and analgesics for acute pain (Steinbrook, 2004). Their nonacceptance of advance directives may be viewed as a way of limiting expensive health care costs (Searight, 2005).
          (b) Carrese and Rhodes (1995) noted that Navajo informants place a particularly prominent value on thinking and speaking in a "positive way." About one half of their Navajo informants would not even discuss advance directives, believing that these discussions could be injurious.
          (c) Similarly, the reluctance of Chinese patients and their families to discuss possible death is based on the belief that direct acknowledgement of mortality may be self-fulfilling (Liu et al., 1999).
      (2) Studies and articles may offer cultural explanations for end-of-life preferences, yet research has not examined
          (a) How aspects of culture influence decisions
          (b) How they affect and are affected by family processes (Kwak & Salmon, 2007)
  d. Areas that have been investigated include (Kwak & Haley, 2005):
      (1) Knowledge: Whites may be more knowledgeable about advance directives
      (2) Attitudes:
          (a) African Americans may be more likely to have negative attitudes toward advance directives than Whites
          (b) Culture-specific attitudes are important in other racial and ethnic groups
          (c) Studies generally suggest that the concept of advance directives may be problematic, particularly for less acculturated individuals
      (3) Access:
          (a) Lower completion rates among patients with access to health care may be due in part to barriers that can be addressed, such as knowledge
          (b) This effect has not been studied in individuals who do not have adequate access to health care (R. S. Morrison et al., 1998)
  e. The paradigm of advance directives
      (1) Best fits prevailing beliefs of a White, European American population, because they emphasize
          (a) Autonomy
          (b) Individuality
          (c) Legal factors

(2) Presents a paradox for patients who are

    (a) from non-Western cultures, which de-emphasize autonomy, perceiving it to be isolating rather than empowering. Cultures valuing nonmaleficense (doing no harm) protect patients from the emotional stress of addressing death and end-of-life decisions (Searight, 2005)

    (b) not oriented toward an internal locus of control

    (c) want or need family involvement in decision making

(3) These patients' choices may appear contradictory to a health care provider (Blackhall et al., 1999)

4. *Health Care Delivery*

a. Life support

    (1) Practices around forgoing life support under certain circumstances with permission of the patient or surrogate vary

        (a) over time

        (b) by country (Blackhall et al., 1999)

    (2) Some research has shown a strong relationship between ethnicity and *personal* wishes for the use of life sustaining technology, but this relationship is complex and contextual (Blackhall et al., 1999).

    (3) Use of life support technology at the end of life

        (a) African American and Hispanic adults seem to prefer the use of technology in interviews, in advance directives, and in real clinical situations.

        (b) There is no discernable pattern in findings about other groups, though directed service programs may have an effect (Kwak & Haley, 2005).

    (4) Attitudes may reflect

        (a) Reliance on the "doctor's judgment"

        (b) An expectation that technology will only be suggested or used if there is hope, thus favoring continuation. Professionals should not assume that information they present is being interpreted as mere information (Blackhall et al., 1999)

b. Hospice and palliative care

    (1) Older adults account for the majority of hospice patients. Minority older adults are the fastest growing segment of the elderly population (U.S. Census Bureau, 2002).

    (2) Racial and ethnic minorities use less hospice and palliative care than do non-Hispanic Whites.

        (a) Palliative and hospice care utilization by racial and ethnic minorities is nonproportional to both

            i. relative population size and

            ii. incidence of top hospice diagnoses and terminal illnesses in minorities (Hill, 2005).

        (b) This disparity is increasing over time (Lyke & Colon, 2004).

    (3) There has been much speculation about causes and factors of this disparity. Nevertheless, there are few data to support possible explanations (Colon, 2005; Crawley et al., 2000; Haber, 1999; Hill, 2005). Factors investigated for an effect on hospice use include

        (a) Beliefs about health care, death, and end-of-life care

        (b) Language difficulties

        (c) Lack of insurance

        (d) Lower referral rates

        (e) Home caregiver requirements

        (f) Acculturation

        (g) Poverty

        (h) Low levels of education

        (i) Lack of knowledge about hospice

    (4) Hospices lack (Gordon, 1996):

        (a) Involvement of minority health care professionals and

        (b) Clinical referral sources for minorities

        (c) However, there is no evidence that hospices with minority staff and volunteers are better able to attract and serve minority hospice patients (Haber, 1999).

    (5) There is no evidence to indicate that minority hospice patients want services but cannot obtain them; nor is there any evidence to indicate that they are dissatisfied with services once they receive them. For-profit hospice programs care for more non-White patients than do not-for-profits (Lorenz et al., 2002).

(6) All racial and ethnic groups have been found to lack information about the kind of care offered through palliative care or hospice programs (Reese, Ahern, Nair, O'Faire, & Warren, 1999).

(7) Issues of trust are often raised, yet conclusions about a "culture of mistrust," particularly among African Americans, remain largely unsubstantiated for lack of systematic measurement (Crawley et al., 2000).

(8) Hospices offer spiritual care to patients and families. Religious diversity may present a particular challenge for hospices because of the importance of religious beliefs and practices related to dimensions of death and dying such as (Lorenz et al., 2004):

    (a) Treatment of pain or suffering

    (b) Care of the body after death

    (c) Funeral rituals

    (d) Organ donation and autopsy

(9) Veteran culture

    (a) 54,000 American veterans die each month and account for one quarter of all U.S. deaths.

    (b) Military service can be a core experience in defining the way veterans live and the way they die.

    (c) Hospice care is now a covered benefit for all enrolled veterans and the Department of Veterans Affairs will purchase hospice services from local communities it serves (Hallerman & Kearns, 2006).

5. *Disclosure and Communication of Diagnosis, Prognosis, and Preferences* (Kwak & Haley, 2005)

  a. Some cultural differences exist in terms of preferences about disclosure of terminal illness among certain racial or ethnic groups

  b. Findings on each group have to be understood cautiously

    (1) Small number of studies

    (2) Important methodological differences between them

  c. Racial or ethnic differences in end-of-life communication may be associated with the individual's proximity to death

6. *Implications and Applications*

  a. Implications for education and practice: Reviews of research aimed at clinical audiences have provided concrete advice about how health care professionals can learn about and respect diverse cultures, values, health beliefs and practices and build trust as a foundation for culturally competent care.

    (1) As with other areas, better understanding of one's own culture is believed to be important for understanding culture and behavior without stereotyping.

    (2) Kagawa-Singer and Blackhall (2001) have adapted the ABCDE model (Attitudes, Beliefs, Context, Decision Making, and Environment) for assessing cultural influences at end-of-life to

      (a) reduce risk of miscommunication and

      (b) avoid dual pitfalls of

        i. cultural stereotyping or

        ii. ignoring the potential influence of culture.

      (c) In minority communities, death and dying may be associated with patterns of social and environmental disparities (Crawley et al., 2000). For example,

        i. Lorenz et al. (2004) reported that 26% of hospices are unwilling to admit a patient to hospice without a dedicated caregiver, which may disproportionately disadvantage racial and ethnic minority groups

        ii. African American patients have been found to receive less resource intensive care than do other hospitalized patients, despite preferences for more life-prolonging measures (Crawley et al, 2000)

      (d) *Patient Self-Determination Act*

        i. Reflects norms of Western culture

        ii. May ignore influence of family and larger social networks

        iii. Respecting and protecting rights of patients and their families require flexibility

      (e) Enquiring about military service has both practical and therapeutic benefits

        i. Hospice care is a covered benefit for all enrolled veterans

        ii. The Department of Veterans Affairs will purchase hospice services from local communities it serves (Hallerman & Kearns, 2006)

        iii. Knowing the components of a military history

aa.   can be a useful tool in bridging the silence that often surrounds the war experience

ab.   can act as a catalyst for discussions about end of life preferences

(f) The health care provider is

i.   critical to hospice and palliative care utilization and other care at the end of life

ii.   Many health care providers remain uncomfortable regarding care for the terminally ill, and

iii.   Associate this discomfort with lack of training and education (Hill, 2005).

(g) Advocacy needs

i.   Curricula and content that emphasize care at the end of life

ii.   Rigorously evaluations of the effectiveness of provider education for improving the actual, relevant patient and population outcomes

b. Implications for research: Research about culturally competent health care interventions, systems, and relationships has surged since the late 1990s, but the body of research has common and serious methodological limitations, including lack of theoretical framework, use of convenience samples, cross-sectional design, and self-developed measurement scales (Kwak & Haley, 2005)

(1) A growing body of research documents differences among major racial and ethnic groups in some important conceptual domains of end-of-life care

(2) Very little is known about (NHPCO, 2004):

(a) the unmet end-of-life care needs of racial, ethnic, and cultural minority populations

(b) the implications of those unmet needs for modifying or reorganizing the delivery of hospice, palliative care, or other end-of-life services

(c) creating a foundation of high quality, generalizable research about end-of-life care demands increased links between research and theory.

(d) Research is needed that will focus on

i.   identifying cultural factors that provide explanatory mechanisms for differences in end-of-life care practices and outcomes

ii.   identifying effects of culture apart from race or ethnicity

iii.   studying within group differences

iv.   improving measurement

v.   interventions to enhance culturally competent care

aa.   Designing these interventions

ab.   Evaluating the interventions

ac.   For example, in communities where political and spiritual perspectives privilege living over dying, quality of life may be seen existentially rather than functionally. Measurement tools need to be developed to account for these values (Doorenbos & Schim, 2004; Fowler, Coppola, Teno, 1999; Lynn, 1997)

7. Conclusions

a. Most studies of cultural diversity at the end-of-life only imprecisely imply cultural influence by measuring racial or ethnic group membership, while not fully examining within-group variations, such as social and acculturation differences, and personal values, and so on (Kwak & Haley, 2005).

b. Conceptual and methodological concerns and the small number of studies preclude making many definitive conclusions about how racial, ethnic, and cultural groups approach end-of-life decisions.

IV. CHAPTER SUMMARY

A. Continuing health disparities herald the call to extend efforts of health care clinicians and researchers to understand how people in diverse cultural groups understand and communicate their perspectives about health and illness.

B. Providers of health wellness education and illness care hold in their hands ethical and moral responsibility to learn the best ways to work effectively *with* as well as *for* the patients, families, and communities in their care.

C. While ethical and moral dimensions of care require the cultural dimension (Leininger, 1990), so also does culture care require the ethical and moral dimensions. Ethics, bioethics, and human rights are interrelated concepts that go hand in hand with cultural sensitivity and transcultural competence to assure protection of the rights and safety of patients and research participants in the health care arena (Buckster; 2009, Kutukdjian, 2009; Pavlish & Ho, 2009). Universal ethical decisions are likely to neglect the religious and cultural perspectives of individuals and small groups (Durante, 2009).

D. Cultural and linguistic competencies are critical components in the identification of perceptions of health and illness among people from diverse sociocultural groups and their resulting illness representations and explanatory models. Also required is a willingness to find ways to work effectively with patients in a partnership that addresses patients' explanations of their illness and their goals for seeking treatment.

NOTE: All references, additional resources, and important Internet sites relevant to this chapter can be found at the following website: http://tcn.sagepub.com/supplemental

Chapter 6
Culturally Based Healing and Care Modalities

Journal of Transcultural Nursing
21(Supplement 1) 236S–306S
© The Author(s) 2010
Reprints and permission:
sagepub.com/journalsPermissions.nav
DOI: 10.1177/1043659610382628
http://tcn.sagepub.com
$SAGE

Lauren Clark, PhD, RN, FAAN[1]
Alison Colbert, PhD, APRN-BC[2]
Jacquelyn H. Flaskerud, PhD, RN, FAAN[3]
Jody Glittenberg, PhD, RN, FAAN, TNS[4]
Patti Ludwig-Beymer, PhD, RN, CTN, NEA-BC, FAAN[5]
Akram Omeri, PhD, RN, CTN, FRCNA[6]
Aaron J. Strehlow, PhD, RN, FNP-BC, FNP-C, NPNP[7]
Kathryn Sucher, ScD, RD[8]
Sheryl Tyson, PhD, RN, PMHCNS-BC[9]
Rick Zoucha, PhD, PMHCNS-BC, CTN[10]

I. INTRODUCTION

   A. This chapter continues to address culture-based health and illness beliefs and care practices; however, these are not limited to specific periods of life but rather can be applied across the full spectrum of a lifetime.

   B. The topics in this chapter include mental health and illness, violence, care of refugees, pain management beliefs and practices, nutrition, complementary and alternative therapy, and pharmacogenetics.

   C. Each topic describes the cultural components of health and how the practice of ethical transcultural nursing and health care can be enhanced through application of the concepts presented.

II. MENTAL HEALTH AND ILLNESS

   A. **Cultural Definitions of Mental Health and Illness:** Cultural groups rarely define mental health and illness but instead make use of explanatory models in their understanding and labeling of behavior, thoughts, and emotions. They use these models to determine when the mental illness label is applied (Tyson & Flaskerud, 2009a).

   1. Definitions of mental illness remain subject to individual interpretation.

   2. Individual understanding evolves with age, increased exposure to life events, and differing explanatory models.

   3. There is no universal definition of mental health that represents all people within a cultural group.

   4. Many cultures have explanatory models of mental illness but not of mental health.

   a. Definitions of mental health are not distinguished from physical and spiritual well-being or illness, and day to day functioning.

   b. Mental health and illness are explained more than "defined."

   (1) Definitions and explanations occur within historic and contemporary social, cultural, political, migration, and religious contexts.

   (2) *Somatization*—manifestation of physical illness that cannot be explained in medical terms and may express psychological distress (U.S. Department of Health and Human Services [USDHHS], 2001).

Funding: The California Endowment (grant number 20082226) and Health Resources and Services Administration (grant number D11 HPO9759).
[1]University of Utah, Salt Lake City, UT, USA (Complementary & Alternative Therapy Modalities)
[2]DuquesneUniversity, Pittsburgh, PA, USA (Disaster Care: Care of Victims of Natural Disasters)
[3]University of California, Los Angeles, Los Angeles, CA, USA (Cultural Beliefs and Practices concerning Mental Health & Illness)
[4]University of Arizona, Tucson, AZ, USA (Intimate Partner Violence; Transcultural Nursing in War & Genocide)
[5]EdwardHospitaland Health Services, Naperville, IL, USA (Cultural Belief and Practices regarding Pain Management)
[6]Homebush, New South Wales, Australia (Care of Refugees and Asylees)
[7]University of California, Los Angeles, Los Angeles, CA, USA (Ethnopharmacology and Pharmacogenetics)
[8]San Jose State University, San Jose, CA, USA (Nutritional Practices: Diet and Culture)
[9]Azusa Pacific University, Azusa, CA, USA (Cultural Beliefs and Practices concerning Mental Health & Illness)
[10]Duquesne University, Pittsburgh, PA, USA (Disaster Care: Care of Victims of Natural Disasters)

Corresponding Author: Marilyn K. Douglas, Email: martydoug@comcast.net

Suggested Citation: Douglas, M. K. & Pacquiao, D. F. (Eds.). (2010). Core curriculum in transcultural nursing and health care [Supplement]. *Journal of Transcultural Nursing, 21*(Suppl. 1).

(3) Somatic symptoms are more acceptable than psychiatric symptoms, which are often stigmatized. *Stigma* is associated with mental illness in many cultures.

(4) Avoidance of stigma is influential in explanatory models (Kuo & Kavanagh, 1994; USDHHS, 2001; Waite, 2008)

5. Considerations related to worldview

   a. Explanatory models explain the origin and course of life, health, illness, treatment, and death (Kuo & Kavanagh, 1994)

   (1) Often not tested using comprehensive and objective methodology

   b. Health belief models are challenged and changed by traumatic experiences (e.g., war, victimization, forced migration)

   c. Contemporary Western Cartesian dualism separates mind and matter (body) into different but interacting substances (Blackburn, 2005)

   d. Holistic worldviews integrate physical, psychological, and spiritual dimensions that are integral to daily functioning (Kuo & Kavanagh, 1994)

6. Mental illness (Kleinman, 1988a)

   a. An interpretation of an experience

   b. Structural or functional abnormality does not indicate severity, functional impairment, or course/treatment response

7. The role of language (Kleinman, 1988)

   a. Cultures interpret the same words differently

   b. Illness beliefs are related to personal meanings of pain and suffering

   c. Practitioners use a taxonomic system to order and render experience understandable

   d. Medicalization is used to manage social problems (e.g., alcoholism, drug abuse, conduct-disordered children)

8. Mental health

   a. A state of well-being more than the absence of mental disorders (World Health Organization [WHO], 2007)

   (1) Individual realization of personal capacities

   (2) Coping capacity in response to normal life stresses

   (3) Work productivity

   (4) Contributions to one's community.

   b. The capacity to experience fulfilling relationships with other people (USDHHS, 2001)

9. Mental illnesses or disorders: Abnormal thoughts, emotions, behavior, and relationships, the majority of which can be successfully treated (WHO, 2007)

10. Mental health and mental disorders are determined by multiple and interacting biological, psychological, and social factors (WHO, 2007).

    a. Disadvantage, insecurity, rapid social change, and risk of violence and physical illness increase vulnerability

    b. Some disorders are recognized as occurring worldwide. These include schizophrenia, manic-depressive disorder, major depression, some anxiety disorders, various forms of substance abuse, and organic brain disorders.

    c. Higher rates for depression and anxiety occur among women than men.

11. Culture and urban mental health (Caracci, 2006)

    a. By the year 2030, the global urban population will reach 5.1 billion culturally diverse people

    b. Definitions of mental health affected by exposure to diverse cultural groups with explanatory models

12. Family/community responses to mental illness and patterns of care. Supportive nuclear and extended family, friends and communities facilitate effective coping with mental illness (USDHHS, 2001).

13. Guidelines for nursing care

    a. Educate the public to decrease stigma and increase help seeking

    b. Inform clients and encourage use of the many effective treatments that exist to assist them in living productive and fulfilling lives

    c. Involve communities in tailoring their own mental health care that will best meet their needs and conform to their explanatory models

B. **Traditional Views of Mental Health and Illness** (see Table 6.1)
   1. Introduction: Cultural groups accept and blend both modern and traditional explanations of mental illness into their understanding and approaches to treatment. Although Table 6.1 categorizes traditional views according to ethnicity and/or national origin, to avoid stereotyping, it is important to acknowledge that there is no universal explanation of mental illness that can be attributed to an entire cultural group. There is individual variation within any group when making the designation of mental illness and when determining who is mentally ill (Tyson & Flaskerud, 2009a).
   2. Cultural groups
       a. ***African Americans*** (Matthews, Corrigan, Smith, & Aranda, 2007; Waite & Killian, 2008)
           (1) Mental health is the individual's self will, capacity to maintain a strong mind, keep going, pray. Working and caring for others despite multiple psychological, economic, and social pressures (Matthews et al., 2007; Waite & Killian, 2008)
           (2) Depression is a "mind thing" that can be controlled (Waite & Killian, 2008)
               (a) Results from the inability to be strong
               (b) Perception of lack of self-control and decreased functional capacity
               (c) The greater the perceived lack of control and functioning capacity, the greater the experience of depression
           (3) Embarrassment about the need for mental illness treatment and socialization to be strong (Matthews et al., 2007)
           (4) Perception that mental illness is incurable (Matthews et al., 2007)
           (5) Family and/or community responses to mental illness and patterns of care
               (a) The family cues individuals to the need for support (Waite & Killian, 2008)
               (b) Friends and religious leaders cue women to seek treatment (Waite & Killian, 2008)
               (c) Social stigma, shame, embarrassment, and fear of rejection lead to denial of symptoms (Matthews et al., 2007)
               (d) Mistrust of health care services due to historical racism, for example, Tuskegee syphilis experiment (Matthews et al., 2007; Waite & Killian, 2008).
               (e) Professional services not sought because of the following: (Matthews et al., 2007)
                   i. Faith that God will heal
                   ii. Perception of being treated differently than Caucasian people
                   iii. Belief that once diagnosed, the label will remain for life
                   iv. Fear of dependence on psychotropic medication
       b. ***American Indians/Alaska Native Traditional Views of Mental Health and Illness***
           (1) A healthy self is inclusive and has permeable boundaries (Dana, 2000)
           (2) Includes nuclear family, extended family, tribe or community.
           (3) Healers may include animals, plants, and places as well as natural, supernatural, or spiritual forces
       c. ***Chinese Traditional Views of Mental Health and Illness***
           (1) Balance between two opposing forces of yin and yang (Kuo & Kavanagh, 1994)
               (a) Yin and yang forces are interdependent (Kuo & Kavanagh, 1994)
               (b) Form the basis of Chinese medicine (Wang, 2008)
               (c) Emphasizes the balance between organ systems (Wang, 2008)
               (d) Central to personal and social conditions and experiences (Wang, 2008)
               (e) Necessary for good physical and mental health (Kuo & Kavanagh, 1994)
               (f) Dependent on harmonious personal relationships (Kuo & Kavanagh, 1994)
           (2) Avoidance of emotional issues promotes stigmatization of mental illness (Kuo & Kavanagh, 1994)
           (3) Lack of Western psychiatric lexicon promotes somatization
           (4) Somatization is a source of explanation for mental disturbance (Kuo & Kavanagh, 1994)
               (a) Physical sickness is not a shortcoming
               (b) Maintains holistic rather than dualistic view of mind and body
               (c) Displaces mental illness and associated stigma
               (d) An immature defense against intrapsychic conflict in Western biomedical models (Cheung, 1995)
               (e) Fails to consider the role of somatic metaphor in Chinese culture

Table 6.1. Cultural Definitions of Mental Health and Illness

Group	Definition or Explanation of Mental Health	Mental Illness or Condition	Definition or Explanation of Mental Illness	Family and Community Responses to Mental Illness; Care Patterns; Additional Implications
African American women (Matthews, Corrigan, Smith & Arranda, 2007; Waite & Killian, 2008)	Staying strong Refusing to allow oneself to become "down" Going to work Taking care of others Coping with violence Focusing on gratitude	Depression Yelling Talking loud Acting crazy	Weak mind Poor health Troubled spirit Lack of self love Inability to resist stresses (e.g., job loss, crime, impoverishment) Trauma Oppression Racism Spiritual/demon possession	Stigma associated with depression and weakness Decreased treatment seeking Mistrust of health care system Decreased medication adherence Social isolation Empathy Illness is chronic, not treatable Cure comes through God
Chinese (Kuo & Kavanagh, 1994; Lin, 1983; Yamamoto, 1977)	Behaviors that reflect an internal state of well-being Ability to adjust to expectations. No display emotional expression or seek personal independence Each of five major emotions corresponds to a specific internal organ, i.e., Happiness/heart Anger/liver Worry/lung Desire/kidney Fear/spleen Optimal: Balanced emotions/ organs	Strong emotions (e.g., termed depression in Western medicine) Acknowledged psychiatric disorders	Feelings can cause someone to sicken and die: Anger Grief Sorrow Regret A dysfunctional organ explains an emotional state. For example, anxiety and sexual impotence is attributed to too much liver fire Heredity Punishment by the gods or ancestors for past behavior of the family Reflection of poor guidance and discipline of a family leader Responsibility ascribed to supernatural forces	Somatization allows displacement of mental illness symptoms onto biological conditions Avoidance of stigma Mental illness reflects poorly on the family Ill family members are kept at home Professional treatment sought only as a last resort Taiwanese traditional responses: Increase ancestral worship Seek advice from temple gods Answers received from gods decrease anxiety and reinforce adaptive behavior Patience, endurance, and maintenance of harmonious relationships encouraged Fortune tellers used by middle-class people
Chinese Americans (Loo, Tong, & True, 1989)	Mental disorders can be prevented by: Using relaxation Self-awareness Self-esteem Positive attitudes Positive emotions Clear thinking Not worrying Learning to be happy	Emotional tension Poor memory Nervousness Problems with: Appetite Sleep Headaches Worry Loneliness Psychological impairment	One or more of the following: Pressures Problems Personality Neglect Genetics Thinking too much Worrying too much Being overly sensitive Inability to use reason to calm the emotions	Mental health promotion practices may improve overall quality of health Belief that mental health problems cannot be prevented. Deter use of mental health services Less somatization than other Chinese subcultures Those who do seek mental health services may have more serious mental illness

(continued)

Table 6.1. (continued)

Group	Definition or Explanation of Mental Health	Mental Illness or Condition	Definition or Explanation of Mental Illness	Family and Community Responses to Mental Illness; Care Patterns; Additional Implications
	Mental health can be assisted by seeking professional Western-oriented help (e.g., counselor, physician) if needed		Psychological weakness Inability to deal with reality-based life stresses Some people feel that the causes of mental illness are unknown and that mental illness cannot be prevented	
Chinese Singaporeans (Lee & Bishop, 2001)	No information available	Psychological problems	Causes in Chinese medicine: Organ dysfunction Being easily disturbed by other people and things Abnormal weather Too much desire Not being easily satisfied Thinking too much Imbalance of yin/yang Having undesirable personalities and character *Dang-ki*: Doing something wrong in a previous life Being possessed by ghosts Black magic Neglecting ancestral worship Loss of soul after a shock Curse Not doing good in the world *Feng-shui*: Bad wind and water of ancestral graves The five elements (metal, wood, water, fire, earth) are not in harmony with the elements of other people Being born at an unlucky time (e.g. year, month, day, hour) Bad wind and water of one's home	Chinese Singaporens may hold multidimensional and overlapping beliefs regarding the etiology and manifestation of mental health problems and treatments
Filipino Americans (Sanchez & Gaw, 2007)	Balance (*timbang*) is central to health and is manifested in social relationships Demonstrated by Emotional restraint Self honesty Flexibility Inner strength (*lakas ng loob*)	Stress Illness Depression	A weak spirit A personal transgression Divine reckoning Ancestral spirits Excessive worry Overwork	Value coping mechanisms of patience and endurance Concern for family welfare and sensitivity to criticism are key factors for consideration when providing services to Filipino Americans

(continued)

Table 6.1. (continued)

Group	Definition or Explanation of Mental Health	Mental Illness or Condition	Definition or Explanation of Mental Illness	Family and Community Responses to Mental Illness; Care Patterns; Additional Implications
	Humor and the capacity to laugh at oneself during troubled times Sensitivity to shame and criticism Concessions to the collective Family and harmonious communal living are important			Willing interaction with mentally ill people Willingly care for ill family members Mentally ill people are not accepted as colleagues, partners Patient—family inclusion in collaborative treatment planning Discussion of physical ailments facilitates disclosure of psychiatric issues leads to underlying reason for visit
Haitians (Desrosiers & Fleurose, 2002)	Attributed to the positive relationship between an individual and the Loas The ability to forget about stresses is seen as strength Work is central to identity	Psychosis Inability to perform daily tasks Poor academic performance Depression Discouragement	A spell or curse sent by a jealous person through a *Bokor* (professional magician) More consistent with symptoms as described in the *Diagnostic and Statistical Manual of Mental Disorders*—Fourth Edition, Text Revision (APA, 2000)	Accepting of pharmacotherapy Targets of jealousy-based cursed have positive attributes (e.g., attractive, intelligent, successful) that contribute to healing. The spell must be lifted by a *Houngan* or *Mambo* Depression is not a mental illness but a weakness caused by malnutrition or anemia Excessive worry receives little sympathy because people are expected to exert control over such cognitive processes. People are expected to continue to fulfill their personal and social obligations Discouragement may manifest as somatization, which is socially acceptable
South Indians of Tamil Nadu (Joel et al. 2003; Saravanan et al., 2007; Saravanan et al., 2008)	Treatment and prevention focus on the quality of interpersonal interactions and relationships Moral living that is within social boundaries	Chronic psychosis/schizophrenia	Behavior definitions: Sitting alone Preoccupation and excessive thinking Does not talk to people Personality changes Angry Hits everyone Violent at times Runs like mad Removes clothes in public May beg Lazy	Psychotic behavior is not normal and is a problem Spiritual problems cause schizophrenia Result of bad karma, magic, family problems, unmarried men without a woman to provide care Response is to go to the temple to pray, seek treatment from traditional healers and shamans Religious treatment is essential Patients and relatives simultaneously pursue traditional and biomedical treatments

(continued)

Table 6.1. (continued)

Group	Definition or Explanation of Mental Health	Mental Illness or Condition	Definition or Explanation of Mental Illness	Family and Community Responses to Mental Illness; Care Patterns; Additional Implications
			Not inhibited Family members notice poor personal care, poor work functioning or scholastic performance, hearing voices, talking to oneself, distressed, suspicious Causes: Spiritual or mystical factors include: Encounters with black magic and evil spirits while alone in the forest at night Ancestors Punishment by God Punishment for previous ill deeds Psychological factors include interpersonal conflicts, problems with work, loss of a loved one, academic failure, mental tension, love, violence Biomedical factors include disease and heredity	Traditional beliefs regarding causes and treatment needs of psychosis may delay seeking treatment from biomedical health care resources Relatives stay with and help care for hospitalized family May not feel adequately informed
Italians (Magliano et al., 2004)	No information available	Schizophrenia	Mental disorders are very different from physical illnesses Prioritized causes: Heredity, alcohol, street drugs, psychological trauma, stress, family conflicts, problematic love relationships Illness makes people unpredictable	Partial belief in recovery Psychiatrist responsible for informing people of illness, drugs and side effects Community avoidance of ill people People with schizophrenia should not have children Recovered people can work as babysitters and in other jobs. Relatives are doubtful that recovering people can work Mental health reform Easier to seek professional treatment
Mexicans (Magana et al., 2007; Zacharias, 2006)	Balanced spirit (*espiritu*), soul (*alma*), body (*cuerpo*) Daily religious activities Dreams Altered states Positive self-identity	*Susto* *Mal de ojo* *Envidia* *Sentimientos Fuertes* *Brujeria* *Falta*	Magical fright Evil eye Envy of others Vehement feelings Illness caused by witchcraft Lack of faith	*Curanderismo*—treatment of mental illness is administered by a *curandero* or *curandera* Often the sole source of treatment

(continued)

Table 6.1. (continued)

Group	Definition or Explanation of Mental Health	Mental Illness or Condition	Definition or Explanation of Mental Illness	Family and Community Responses to Mental Illness; Care Patterns; Additional Implications
				Treatments include healing rituals, applications of states of altered consciousness, therapeutic talk, sweat lodges, cleansing rituals, psychospiritual healing rituals
Moroccans (Stein, 2000)	No information available	Hallucinations Chemical dependency Withdrawal behaviors Behaviors associated with schizophrenia The Western biomedical model Chronic pain, limb paralysis	Accidental ingestion of *SHour* *Tretat* (happens when someone throws *SHour* under a passerby's feet) *Djnoun* (take revenge when injured either by accident or intention) May be the result of jealousy, ill will, or the evil eye	Although a modern environment that embraces Western biomedical models of mental illness, many Moroccans also continue to believe in traditional explanatory models of mental illness Shrines (*Marabouts*) throughout rural and urban Morocco *Fquih* consulted by relatives to use his *Baraka* (divinity) to remove *SHour* or *Djnoun* via herbal remedies, amulets, Koranic readings, magical incantations Psychiatrists think *fquihs* are charlatans
Thais (Bernard et al., 2006; Rungreangklukij & Chesla, 2001)		Extreme illness or weakness Depression Schizophrenia Childhood schizophrenia	*Kwan* (life force or spirit) leaves the body *Kwan* does not go away *Kwan* goes away Caused by supernatural forces: Evil eye Ancient soul Spirit of the land Black magic Stresses Childhood preoccupations Genetics Drug and alcohol abuse *Karma* most common cause Escalating symptoms a sign of illness progression	People may be less likely to acknowledge symptoms of mental illness because mental illness may make *Kwan* go away. Families may be ashamed of and hide mentally ill members Mothers provide a calm environment *Thum-jai*: Meditative practice of smoothing a heart with water. Practice taught by priest, family, friends A skill that takes time to develop Practice with ill children, regardless of age Failure to practice thum-jai may increase child illness Mothers forfeit respect from child, which is a core cultural value

    (5) Family and/or community responses to mental illness and patterns of care (Shyu, 1989):

        (a) Family is greater than the individual

        (b) Mental illness attributed to ancestral spirits

        (c) Shamed by a mentally ill family

        (d) Family subject to social rejection (Kuo & Kavanagh, 1994)

        (e) Community isolation (Kuo & Kavanagh, 1994)

        (f) Increase in family worship of ancestral spirits

            i. Change location of ancestral burial sites

            ii. Divine instruction sought from temple gods

d. ***Chinese American and Singaporean Views of Mental Health and Illness***

    (1) Chinese Americans may adhere to explanatory models of mental illness and values of self-help espoused by other Chinese groups (Loo, Tong, & True, 1989)

    (2) Value mental illness preventive efforts and may use Western mental health resources if they are unable to independently resolve psychiatric issues

    (3) Dang-ki or Chinese shamanism contains elements of Buddhism, Taoism, and folk beliefs (Lee & Bishop, 2001)

    (4) Psychological problems attributed to external causes (e.g., fate, deities, demons, ancestral spirits) and astrological forces

    (5) *Feng-Shui*, translated as wind and water—human fate and fortune; directed by positive and negative cosmological forces inherent on the earth's surface (Lee & Bishop, 2001). Bad *feng-shui* causes psychological problems

e. ***Filipino American Views of Mental Health and Illness***

    (1) Perceptions of mental health and illness are influenced by regionalism (Sanchez & Gaw, 2007)

        (a) The Philippine islands consist of more than 7,000 islands

        (b) Sixty cultural minority groups speak more than 80 ethnic languages

        (c) Tagalog is spoken by approximately a third of the population

    (2) According to Sanchez and Gaw (2007), the following factors are associated with mental illness:

        (a) Mental illness is stigmatized and somatized

        (b) Depression manifests as sadness and other commonly recognized symptoms

        (c) Denial of depressive symptoms, for example, statement of feeling fine and simultaneously tearful.

        (d) Majority of Filipinos are Catholics

        (e) Faith healers (albularyos) are sought

        (f) Children with mental illness may bring good luck

        (g) Mentally ill adults are considered dangerous and unpredictable

    (3) Family and/or community responses to mental illness and patterns of care (Sanchez & Gaw, 2007)

        (a) Family, regional, and peer group affiliation over individualism

        (b) Individual illness is considered a family illness

        (c) Family shame and stigma

        (d) Family rather than professional assistance preferred

        (e) Family is decision maker regarding treatment

        (f) Treatment may involve rituals to reverse punishment administered through the spiritual world

f. ***Haitian Traditional Views of Mental Health and Illness***

    (1) Majority of Haitians are practicing Catholics and also practice Voodoo

    (2) Facts about Voodoo (Desrosiers & Fleurose, 2002; Morrison & Thornton, 1999):

        (a) A recognized religion

        (b) Arose out of a synthesis of African spiritual practice and Catholicism

            i. Families inherit ancestral spirits

            ii. Includes visible and an invisible (spiritual) forces that may be good or evil

            iii. Loas are the gods of Voodoo and are primarily spirits of African ancestors, deceased family members, and Biblical figures

            iv. Loas are channeled through a human being through a process of "possession" where the "self" of the person is inhabited by the spirit

          aa. Loas communicate through the possessed person
          ab. Loas possess the body of a Voodoo priest called a *Houngan* or a priestess called a *Mambo* who are respected community members
          ac. Do not engage in magic and curses. Loas are guardians and protect patrons from curses and stress
          ad. Loas are responsible for physical and mental health
          ae. Patrons care for the Loas through rituals
       v. Magicians, called bokors, buy spirits to send curses and achieve personal aims (Deren, 1983)

(3) Haitian explanations of mental health and illness (Desrosiers & Fleurose, 2002)
    (a) Western theories embraced by some middle and upper socioeconomic classes of Haitians
    (b) Most Haitians attribute some degree of mental illness to Voodoo
    (c) Mental illness is caused by a force that is external to the person
    (d) A curse sent on behalf of someone who is jealous of the victim who embodies positive attributes such as attractiveness and successfulness
    (e) The victim is not to blame for the externally caused illness—not burdened with guilt
    (f) Only a *Houngan* is able to intercede on the victim's behalf

g. ***Views of Psychosis and Schizophrenia in Vellore, India*** (Joel et al., 2003; Saravanan et al., 2007; Saravanan et al., 2008)
  (1) Vellore is located in Tamil Nadu, an industrialized state in southern India, with a population of approximately 100,000 residents who are predominantly practicing Hindus.
    (a) Most believe that schizophrenia must be treated by traditional healers or at temples (Joel et al., 2003).
    (b) Patient beliefs are similar to those of health care workers—black magic is the cause of schizophrenia (Saravanan et al., 2007).
    (c) High premorbid functional capacity increases confusion regarding illness symptoms (Saravanan et al., 2008).
      i. Black magic spirits reside in the forest and at night prey upon solitary individuals.
      ii. Schizophrenia may have a single or multiple causes (Saravanan et al., 2007).
      iii. Some patients believe in biomedical and heredity explanations of schizophrenia (Saravanan et al., 2007).
    (d) Family and/or community responses to mental illness and patterns of care (Saravanan et al., 2008)
      i. Relatives simultaneously believe traditional and biomedical explanations of mental illness (Saravanan et al., 2008).
      ii. Health care workers simultaneously maintain diverse and contradictory beliefs (Saravanan et al., 2008).
      iii. Psychosis is a biomedical disease and also caused by black magic (Saravanan et al., 2008).
      iv. Economic difficulties contribute to psychosis (Joel et al., 2003).
      v. Few Western trained health care workers believe that trained medical personnel can treat schizophrenia (Saravanan et al., 2007).
      vi. People may simultaneously use biomedical (e.g., medication) and traditional healing (e.g., temple prayer) methods.
      vii. Women are more likely to use traditional healing methods, whereas older patients and patients with severe symptoms prefer a Western psychosocial explanation and treatment mode (Saravanan et al., 2007).
      viii. Religious treatments are essential, even if Western treatment approaches are used (Saravanan et al., 2007).

h. ***Beliefs about schizophrenia among public, mental health professionals, and relatives of patients across Italy*** (Magliano, Fiorillo, De Rosa, Malangone, & Maj, 2004)
  (1) Causes of schizophrenia
    (a) Professionals prioritize causes as heredity, stress, family conflict, and street drugs.
    (b) General public prioritize causes as stress, heredity, psychological trauma, and family conflict.
    (c) Relatives prioritize causes as stress, psychological trauma, love problems, and family conflicts.
    (d) Stigma is not mentioned as a key factor in explanations or help seeking.

    (2) Family and/or community responses to mental illness and patterns of care (Magliano et al., 2004)
        (a) Community psychiatric treatment model used
        (b) Relatives should be informed by psychiatrist
        (c) General acceptance of biomedical explanations
        (d) Treated effectively with medication
            i. More relatives than professional and general public in favor of medication treatment
            ii. Relatives least likely to think psychosocial intervention useful
            iii. More relatives than general public or professionals believe that little can be done except to help ill people leave peacefully
            iv. Community-based care rather than institutionalization
            v. Psychiatric hospitals viewed as prisons
            vi. Relatives tend to believe that psychosocial factors are a greater cause of schizophrenia than is heredity
            vii. Almost a third of the sample of the general public and relatives, and almost 25% of the professional sample thought that disillusionment in love was a factor in the etiology of schizophrenia (Magliano et al., 2004).

i. ***Mexican Traditional Views of Mental Health and Illness***
    (1) Mental health is the product of balance between the spirit (*espiritu*), soul (*alma*), and body (*cuerpo*; Zacharias, 2006)
    (2) *Espiritu*—integration of spiritual practices into everyday life "Guardian" of mental and physical health
    (3) Mental illness results from imbalance between spirit, soul, and body
    (4) Treatment of mental illness (*curanderismo*) provided by curanderos (male) or *curanderas* (female) healers
        (a) Illnesses caused by relational conflicts or developmental crisis
        (b) Often referred to as culture-bound syndromes, for example, *susto* (fright)
        (c) Treatments involve spiritual, symbolic, and sensory interventions
    (5) Prevention of mental illness through maintenance of a balance of *espiritu*, *alma*, and *cuerpo*
    (6) Latino family and/or community responses to mental illness and patterns of care (Magaña, Ramíerez García, Hernández, & Cortez, 2007)
        (a) The term *Latino* includes people who identify as Mexican, Puerto Rican, Central American, South American, and Cuban
        (b) Profile of caregivers:
            i. Mothers as primary caregivers of the ill person
            ii. Fathers, siblings, or other relatives also assist
            iii. Caregivers range in age from 20 to 80 years
        (c) Caregiver depressive symptoms are related to stigma, young age, and low education levels
        (d) Avoidance of illness disclosure

j. ***Moroccan Traditional Views of Mental Health and Illness*** (Stein, 2000)
    (1) Explanations of mental illness originate with the Berbers
        (a) Animists who attributed magical or spiritual powers to natural surroundings
        (b) Supports concepts of sorcery—evil experienced through the senses, that is, sight, touch
    (2) Islamic (eighth century AD) and Koran influences on Moroccan views of mental health and illness
        (a) Allah populated the earth with four types of beings:
            i. Humans
            ii. Angels
            iii. Satan (*Iblis*)
            iv. Demons (*djnoun/jenoun* [*Djinn* is singular form])
        (b) Only humans are visible
        (c) Djnoun are invisible, nocturnal, and live in ways similar to humans, for example, eating, drinking, having children and families, forming communities, and dying
            i. Activities end at dawn with the morning call to prayer
            ii. Prefer to live close to water but may also live in the plumbing of a home

(3) Over time, Berber and Islamic beliefs synthesized and resulted in the following beliefs regarding mental illness:

    (a) SHour (seHour)—evil that can reside on, under, or within any surface, that is, ground, rocks, tables, creams, and food

        i. An inherent quality of the substances where it resides or it can be placed there by a person who seeks revenge

        ii. People may unwittingly walk next to or touch *seHour*, which can enter the person's body by some process of osmosis.

        iii. SHour may be ingested when eating or drinking food

        iv. It is not visible, has no odor or other property that would render it detectable to the average person

(4) Family and/or community responses to mental illness and patterns of care

    (a) Marabouts—originally holy men in the Sufi tradition

        i. Direct lineage from Mohammed

        ii. Imbued with divine blessing (*Baraka*)

    (b) Marabout is now the tomb and shrine of a holy man

        i. Pilgrimage site for those seeking *Baraka*

        ii. Marabout of Father (*Bouya*) Omar is the closest to Marrakesh and is most popular site for seeking help for mental illnesses

        iii. Wronged *djnoun* are compensated through ritual, prayer, and animal sacrifice

    (c) Religious scholar and holy man is the *Fquih*

        i. The living healer of mental illness

        ii. Well versed in the Koran

        iii. Most important attribute is his *Baraka* (divine blessing)

        iv. Navigates between human and spirit worlds

        v. Consulted by the family

k. ***Somali Traditional Views of Mental Illness***

(1) No continuum from mental health to illness. Someone is either "crazy" (*waali*) or not "crazy" (Perez, 2006; Schuchman & McDonald, 2004)

(2) Mentally ill people never return to their previous functioning and may never again be trusted (Perez, 2006)

(3) Caused by God or evil spirits (*jin*), another person or by oneself by bad behavior (Schuchman & McDonald, 2004)

(4) Spirits reside within the individual, and if angered, can cause fever, headache, and other illnesses (Lewis, 1996)

(5) *Evil eye* is caused when someone or their child is either intentionally or inadvertently praised or complemented (Lewis, 1996)

(6) Psychological problems are somaticized as headaches, chest pain, forgetfulness, sleep disturbance, and/or nightmares

(7) Depression is the feeling that a camel has when its mate dies (Schuchman & McDonald, 2004)

(8) The Koran teaches that suicide is a crime against God (Schuchman & McDonald, 2004)

(9) Refugee women identify mental health as being able to be strong and get on with life regardless of hardships endured (Whittaker, Hardy, Lewis, & Buchan, 2005)

(10) *Jinn* or *Zar* spirits—malevolent possession spirits (Morris, 2006)

    (a). Mentioned in the Koran, so they are under the control of God and therefore considered legitimate

    (b). *Jinn* or *Zar* spirits are not ancestors

    (c). May reside anywhere but prefer animals and dark places

(11) Family and/or community responses to mental illness and patterns of care (Stein, 2000)

    (a) Context of prolonged civil war resulted in repeated trauma

        i. Witnessed murder, torture of family/friends

        ii. Pervasive rape as a military tactic

    (b) Family and communal life is important to well-being. Not having family increases vulnerability to spirit position (Whitaker et al., 2005)

    (c) Community may conceal spirit possession from each other (Whittaker et al., 2005)

(d) Social isolation of mentally ill by community (Whittaker et al., 2005)
    i. Intensely felt by patient due to communal culture
    ii. May be self imposed to avoid stigma
    iii. Fear of stigma greater than fear of social isolation
    iv. Mental illness is hidden from family, friends, and health care providers
        aa. Families provide primary care for mental illness
            (i) Consult with elders, religious leaders, traditional healers
            (ii) Attributed to spiritual causes
        ab. Patient advocacy needed within the family and community to reduce stigma

l. ***Traditional Views of Mental Health and Illness in Thailand*** (Burnard, Naiyapatana, & Lloyd, 2006)
  (1) Thailand is predominantly Buddhist
  (2) Thai belief in spirits
  (3) Animism coexists with Buddhism and fosters beliefs in ghosts, poltergeists, gods, and goddesses among rural and some urban residents, which can promote psychological stability or instability
  (4) *Kwan* is life spirit, life force, and is also considered to be consciousness
  (5) Biomedical and traditional explanatory models of mental illness coincide
    (a) Caused by drug abuse, brain pathology, genetic factors, socioeconomic and environmental stresses, family breakdown, or by spirits
    (b) Simultaneous belief in both models
  (6) Mental illness is stigmatized, especially in rural areas
  (7) *Karma*—all actions in past lives or present life have consequences
    (a) Good actions result in good karma or positive experiences
    (b) Bad actions result in bad karma or negative experiences
    (c) Poor mental health may be attributed to bad Karma
  (8) Family and/or community responses to mental illness and patterns of care (Rungreangkulkij & Chesla, 2001)
    (a) Help sought from multiple traditional healers who use folk therapies
    (b) Famous spiritual healers (*Ajarns*) who bring holy water
    (c) After unsuccessful cures from healers, relatives seek help from hospitals
      i. Hospitalization and medication reasonably effective
      ii. Mothers must see symptom relief
      iii. Action of medication not understood
    (d) Mothers use *Thum-jai* to care for children with schizophrenia
      i. *Thum-jai* allows equanimity, acceptance, patience, understanding, reasonableness, sense of obligation, gentleness, nonconfrontational response to symptom escalation.
      ii. Used to face a situation that cannot be changed
      iii. Recognition that no one wants to be ill
      iv. Not responding to *Thum-jai* leads to negative social judgment
    (e) Maternal concerns that require *Thum-jai*
      i. Social expectation to care for ill children regardless of age, illness, or degree of disruptive behavior
      ii. Avoidance of escalation of symptoms that is believed to indicate worsening condition
      iii. Mothers "smooth their hearts with water" to gently manage symptomatic children (A meditative practice to replace fiery angry feelings with the peace of calm water)
    (f) Maternal intrapsychic conflict
      i. Cultural value of requiring maternal respect and practicing *thum-jai* for an ill but disrespectful child
      ii. To allow child disrespect is antithesis of core cultural value

m. ***Vietnamese Traditional Views of Mental Illness*** (LaBorde, 1996)
  (1) Mental illness is shameful and is stigmatized, denied, and feared
  (2) Caused by bad karma due to misdeeds in past lives
  (3) Mental health clinics are avoided and problems are somatized

3. Guidelines for the provision of culturally competent nursing care. The information below is in part included in the American Institute for Research 2004 report on cultural competence and nursing.

   a. Cultural competence improves nursing care to all people whether or not they are members of an identified minority group (Andrews & Boyle, 2003).

   b. Rather than focus on group-specific care, principles and strategies that apply across groups are recommended

   c. Culturally and linguistically appropriate services include

      (1) Self-awareness of difficulty with intercultural communication

         (a) Personal and professional biases (Van Ryn & Fu, 2003), institutional racism (Barbee, 1993), and White privilege

         (b) Assumed similarity, ethnocentrism, denial of difference, anxiety, or tension regarding anticipated conflict, comfort with what appears to be familiar

      (2) Individual recognition and acceptance of becoming rather than being culturally competent (Campinha-Bacote, Yahle, & Langenkamp, 1996)

      (3) Awareness of use of complementary and alternative medicines, for example, herbs, chiropractic, relaxation techniques, vitamins, massage, acupuncture, Chinese medicine, guided imagery, homeopathy

   d. Nursing guidelines for inclusion in the assessment of mental capacity include questions from Kleinman's (1980) Explanatory Belief Model. A determination of the following is required:

      (1) Whether the client believes there is an illness or if others (e.g., family) think there is an illness

      (2) How the client refers to the illness

      (3) If the illness is unique to the client or experienced by many

      (4) When the problem started

      (5) A precise behavioral description of the problem

      (6) Why the client thinks the problem started when it did

      (7) The seriousness of the problem

      (8) Beliefs regarding short- and/or long-term consequences

      (9) Fears and worries related to the problem

      (10) The main problems caused by the illness

      (11) Treatments the client believes work best for the illness

      (12) Styles of nonverbal communication may be related to culture and/or mental capacity

      (13) Culturally based values regarding modesty may influence appearance of apparent cooperation with the interview

4. Language access strategies

   a. Indicators of client lack of understanding

      (1) Nods or says "yes" to all questions

      (2) Brief residence in the United States or area where English is the primary language

      (3) Inability to explain key information

   b. Consider strengths and limitations of interpreters

      (1) Professional and trained staff interpreters

         (a) Consistent personnel, foster trust

         (b) May be costly

      (2) Untrained interpreters

         (a) May be more available than professional interpreters

         (b) Lack sufficient medical, mental health knowledge, terminology

      (3) On-call interpreters

         (a) Cover broader range of languages

         (b) May be trained on untrained in mental health

      (4) Bilingual staff

         (a) Available

         (b) Conflict of duties, usually untrained in mental health

      (5) Family members or friends

         (a) Available

         (b) Untrained, unfamiliar with specialized vocabulary, lack objectivity

      (6) Telephone interpretation services

         (a) Covers many languages, around the clock availability

         (b) Requires prior arrangement, telephone may decrease development of rapport, costly

5. Intervention
   a. Refrain from making ethnically or culturally based assumptions
   b. Present in a calm and unhurried manner
   c. Generally maintain physical space of 2 to 3 feet
   d. Be respectful in all situations, ask permission before touching
   e. Explain what is being written
   f. Determine if model should be client–nurse or client–family–nurse
   g. Determine gender role beliefs and importance to client
   h. Identify treatment goals of client (and family). Synthesize spiritual and/or religious beliefs and healing
   i. practices into treatment recommendations (e.g., praying with client/family)
   j. Negotiate treatment goals with client/family
   k. Learn biophysical vulnerabilities related to medication (e.g., more or less than usual dosages may be indicated given ethnic background—consult pharmacist to ensure optimal dosage
   l. Assist in connecting with cultural resources if desired
   m. Advocate and assist in negotiation of social service resources as indicated and desired

C. Dementia. This section focuses on the relationships among dementia, ethnicity and culture looking to epidemiologic studies, family studies, gene studies, cultural beliefs about dementia and caregiving, and studies of caregiver burden for evidence of consistency and differences (Flaskerud, 2009b).

1. There are various types of dementia, with Alzheimer's Disease (AD) being by far the most common, accounting for about 70% of cases of late-onset dementia.
   a. Other dementias include vascular dementia, HIV dementia, dementia due to head trauma, Parkinson's disease, Huntington's disease, Pick's disease, Creutzfeldt-Jakob disease, other medical conditions, multiple etiologies, and substance-induced persisting dementia (American Psychiatric Association [APA], 2000, p. 147; Edgar, White, & Cummings, 2002).
   b. Prevalence of different causes of dementia (infections, nutritional deficiencies, traumatic brain injury, endocrine conditions, cerebrovascular diseases, seizure disorders, brain tumors, substance abuse) varies substantially across cultural groups and geographic regions (APA, 2000, p. 151).
   c. African Americans and Hispanic Americans are more likely than Whites to have vascular dementia (Ethnic Elders Care Networks, n.d.).

2. Epidemiologic studies suggest that differences in prevalence of AD among population groups may be related more to geographic region rather than to genetic vulnerability (Malaspina, Corcoran, & Hamilton, 2002).
   a. Prevalence rates of AD in different ethnic groups who live in the same region are more similar than different.
   b. Groups with similar genetic backgrounds (ethnicity) who live in different parts of the world have a greater difference in prevalence rates.
   c. Non-Western countries have lower rates than Western countries.
   d. Differences in rates may be due to different etiologies, research methods, diet, life expectancy, educational levels, and other behavioral and lifestyle factors.
   e. African Americans (four times) and Hispanic Americans (two times) are more likely to develop AD by age 90 than White Americans (Ethnic Elders Care Network, n.d.).
   f. Limited studies of dementia in Asian Americans suggest prevalence rates similar to those of White Americans.

3. Family studies show an increased prevalence of dementia in the family members of AD patients (Malaspina et al., 2002).
   a. A total of 25% to 40% of patients with AD have at least one affected first-degree relative.
   b. Increased family prevalence occurs predominantly in those with early-onset disease.
   c. First degree relatives of African Americans with AD have a greater cumulative risk of dementia than do Whites (Ethnic Elders Care Network, n.d.) http://www.ethnicelderscare.net/ethnicity&dementiatitle.htm

4. Gene studies involve the possible genetic link of polipoprotein E4 (ApoE4) to development of AD, although other genetic factors also may be an influence (Reiman et al., 2007).
   a. The presence of ApoE4 as a determinant of risk for AD may differ between Whites and African Americans or Hispanic Americans (Ethnic Elders Care Care Network, n.d.).
   b. Genetic links would implicate family inheritance and the influence of ancestry/ethnicity on the occurrence of AD.

    c. Other factors may modify the effects of Apo E4 on disease risk within a group thought to be homogeneous genetically: culture and socioeconomic factors, early life experiences such as immigration, poverty and nutrition, and vascular process such as atherosclerosis, lipids, and metabolic, inflammatory and immune response, and other genetic factors.

    d. There may be interactions between genetic and cultural factors. In the ongoing, longitudinal Sacramento Area Latino Study on Aging (SALSA), 43% of AD was attributed to Type 2 diabetes mellitus, stroke, or both, far outdistancing the effect of the Apo E alleles.

    e. The relationship between hypertension, hypercholesteremia, and dementia is also a factor in the development of dementia in African Americans (Ethnic Elders Care Network, n.d.)

5. Beliefs about dementing illnesses differ among ethnic groups (Ethnic Elders Care Network, n.d.)

    a. Dementia is a form of normal aging (some Asian American groups, some African and White Americans)

    b. Dementia is a form of mental illness (Asian, Hispanic, and African Americans)

    c. Dementia as a culture specific syndrome—"worriation" and spells (southern state African Americans)

    d. Stigma and shame are associated with dementia; demented family members should be hidden from the community (some Asian American groups, Hispanic Americans)

    e. Caring for a relative with dementia is a family responsibility (some Asian American groups, African Americans, Hispanic Americans)

    f. Dementia is unavoidable, a result of fate, an imbalance in the body, a retribution for sins of family/ancestors (some Asian American groups)

6. Ethnic and cultural differences in care giving and caregiver burden occur with AD and other dementing illnesses (Janevic & Connell, 2001)

    a. More White Americans with AD are cared for in long-term care facilities than are African, Hispanic, or Asian Americans with AD (Daker-White, Beattie, Gilliard, & Means, 2002; Ethnic Elders Care Network, n.d.; Neary, 2005)

    b. Family caregiving is more common among minority groups and is related to cultural preference and tradition, lack of resources to place a relative in care, and lack of knowledge of available resources

    c. Evidence that the burden of care differs among ethnic groups is related often to which family member(s) provide the care—a spouse, multiple family members, or an adult child who is also caring for their own children (Wallace Williams, Dilworth-Anderson, & Goodwin, 2003)

7. Nursing guidelines for assessing mental capacity: Cultural and educational background and language should be taken into consideration in the assessment of an individual's mental capacity (APA, 2000, p. 151).

    a. Individuals from some backgrounds may not be familiar with the information used in certain tests of general knowledge

    b. Names of presidents, geographical knowledge, date of birth in cultures that do not routinely celebrate birthdays, and sense of place and location may be conceptualized differently in some cultures (APA, 2000, p. 151).

      (1) Translation of assessment instruments may be a problem

      (2) Concepts in one language may not translate accurately to another because they do not exist or have different meanings;

      (3) Inadequate translation methods may lead to erroneous conclusions/diagnosis (Flaskerud, 2000, 2007a)

8. Nursing/health care and social services for persons with AD and their caregivers should include

    a. Knowledge of language: Interpreters may bring added problems, distorting psychiatric interviews in three major ways:

      (1) Omitting, substituting, condensing, and changing the client's response to make sense of disorganized statements;

      (2) Normalizing thought processes and descriptions because of a lack of psychiatric knowledge;

      (3) Answering for the client to prevent stigma from being associated with their ethnic group (Flaskerud, 2007a)

    b. Knowledge of culture, including history of discrimination and institutional bias toward any racial or ethnic group

    c. Accurate assessments of clients' activities of daily living abilities

    d. Developing trust, communication, and collaboration with caregivers and designated family spokesperson

e. Knowledge of cultural explanation for etiology of disease and preferred treatment

f. Knowledge of community, social, cultural, economic, and health resources

g. Information about availability of long-term care, respite care, support groups, and individual and family counseling

h. Education and encouragement in the use of memory-enhancing drugs

D. Culture-Bound Syndromes (CBS)

1. This section focuses on information and resources that mental health nurses can use to educate themselves about the culture-bound syndromes, recognize these syndromes when they occur in the clinical practice settings, and provide culturally competent care that takes cultural behaviors and explanations into account when devising a treatment plan (Flaskerud, 2009a).

2. To facilitate this goal a table categorizing the CBS according to behavioral taxa is included (Table 6.2)

  a. The American Psychiatric Association has described the culture-bound syndromes as

  (1) "Recurrent, locality-specific patterns of aberrant behavior and troubling experience that may or may not be linked to a particular *DSM-IV* diagnostic category.

  (2) These patterns are indigenously considered to be 'illnesses,' or at least afflictions, and most have local names.

  (3) They are limited to specific societies or culture areas.

  (4) They are localized, folk, diagnostic categories that frame coherent meanings for certain repetitive, patterned, and troubling sets of experiences and observations." (APA, 2000, Appendix I, p. 898).

  b. Culture-bound syndromes have somatic, dissociative, anxiety, and/or depressive features (APA, 2000, pp. 353, 436, 487, 491, 524; Mezzich, Kleinman, Fabrega, & Parron, 2002, pp. 137-189). Categories can be distinguished among them as noted below:

  (1) An apparent psychiatric illness, locally recognized, does not correspond to a recognized Western disease category, no identifiable organic cause; may be stress related;

  (2) An apparent psychiatric illness, locally recognized, resembles a Western disease category, but has local features different from the Western disease, may be lacking symptoms seen as important in the West, no identifiable organic cause;

  (3) Culturally accepted explanatory mechanisms or idioms of distress, do not match Western mechanisms or idioms; in Western setting might indicate culturally inappropriate thinking and perhaps delusions or hallucinations;

  (4) A state or set of behaviors, often including trance or possession states; hearing, seeing, and/or communicating with the dead or spirits; or feeling that one has "lost one's soul" from grief or fright; may not be seen as pathologic within native cultural framework, could indicate psychosis, delusions, or hallucinations in a Western setting.

  c. Glossaries of the culture-bound disorders are available.

  (1) The most extensive was created by Simons and Hughes (1985) with more than 175 entries.

  (2) *DSM-IV* contains a glossary of common culture-bound syndromes in Appendix I (APA, 2000, pp. 899-903).

  (3) Glossaries and indexes plus extensive information on the culture-bound syndromes may be found also at Hall, T. McCajor: http://homepage.mac.com/mccajor/cbs.html.

  (4) These glossaries contain descriptions, symptoms, area(s) of the world in which the disorders are common and prominent features of the disorders. See Table 6.2 for a taxonomy of common culture-bound syndromes and culture-specific idioms of distress.

  d. A great deal of controversy surrounds the culture-bound syndromes because of the way in which they are portrayed and categorized and the implicit ethnocentric bias of the term itself (Mezzich et al., 2002, pp. 289-323; Simons, 2001).

  (1) Listing the culture-bound syndromes in the Appendix of *DSM* implies that the illness is not real or that it can be dismissed as merely exotic.

  (2) Disagreements about changing the *DSM*:

  (a) Since all psychiatric patterns are culturally constituted, perhaps a sixth cultural axis should be developed for use with the *DSM* diagnostic categories;

  (b) Modified forms of the culture-bound syndromes should be incorporated into existing *DSM* categories;

  (c) Create an additional Axis I diagnostic category in the anxiety disorders section and include the culture-bound syndromes there.

(3) Western psychiatry must acknowledge that all societies experience culture-bound syndromes.
    (a) Culture-bound illnesses occur in industrialized societies as well as nonindustrialized ones.
    (b) In the United States, "going postal," Type A pattern behavior and anorexia nervosa (prior to 1980) are examples (Mezzich et al., 2002, pp. 154, 183, 295-296).

  e. Guidelines for nursing care: Treatment for culture-bound syndromes and culture specific idioms of distress requires expanding the training of clinicians on basic concepts of cultural awareness and skills that encompass folk medical procedures (Simons, 2001).
    (1) Culturally competent care cannot be given without attention to racism at an individual, organizational, and societal level.
    (2) Incorporate acceptable traditional alternative treatments into psychiatric treatment.
    (3) Involve family, kin, friends, and clergy in treatment
    (4) Gather data by talking with the family and the patient. See above for additional information on language and for cautions about the use of translators and interpreters.
    (5) Observe patient's life situation including disturbances in interpersonal relations.
    (6) Name the cause of the disturbance using familiar words and terms consonant with the patient's own beliefs about forces in the world (natural and supernatural) that bring disturbance.
    (7) Prescribe a regimen of treatment appropriate to the cause attributed by the patient and family (includes pharmacologic, behavioral, interpersonal, and preventive, and involvement in ritual processes along with family; Mezzich et al., 2002, pp. 297-298).

E. Summary
1. The various explanations of mental illness that may be encountered by mental health nurses present a challenge. One challenge is to recognize these views when they are presented and incorporate acceptable traditional alternative treatments into psychiatric treatment.
2. Mental health nurses must establish trust, communication, and collaboration with traditional caregivers and family members to provide culturally competent care.
3. Knowledge of language and culture, including the life experience of different groups (e.g., a history of discrimination, war trauma) must be taken into account when making assessments and devising treatment plans.
4. A second challenge is to educate the public in order to decrease stigma and encourage help seeking.

III. CARING PRACTICES FOR PEOPLE AFFECTED BY VIOLENCE
  A. Intimate Partner Violence
    1. Introduction
      a. An overview of intimate partner violence (IPV)
        (1) Various terms used to describe the phenomenon
          (a) Domestic violence, family violence, spousal abuse, wife battering
          (b) IPV is the correct terminology
            i. Spousal abuse and wife battering are incorrect terms, as not all intimate partners are spouses or wives
            ii. Domestic violence includes other persons in a household, for example, elders, children, siblings, who are not intimate partners.
        (2) Culturally appropriate terms
          (a) Terms such as intimate partner and violence are culture-specific concepts, which occur within a cultural context (Heise, 1996; Macey, 1999; Nash, 2006)
          (b) Violence in some cultures is believed to be normal rather than a pathological behavior
          (c) Intimate behavior is culturally shaped between types of sexual partners, for example, heterosexual, homosexual, bisexual, and transgendered partners
          (d) Cultural norms are dynamic and shaped within a cultural context
            i. In Eurocentric cultures, victims are primarily female, but males are also abused (Finn & Clements 2006).
            ii. Females tend to use weapons in assaulting an intimate partner (Pearson, 1997).
            iii. Societal norms are more accepting of a battered wife than of a battered husband (Knauth 2003).
        (3) Types and process of violence eruptions
          (a) Categories of violence include physical, psychological, emotional, and financial.
          (b) Intensity and duration vary, but violent episodes usually occur in cycles.

Table 6.2. Mental Health and Illness: Taxonomy of Culture-Bound Syndromes (CBS) and Glossary of Culture-Specific Idioms of Distress

CBS Taxonomies or Classifications	Description/Symptoms	Syndrome Names and Culture/Country	Resemblance to DSM Diagnoses
Sudden mass assault taxon	A dissociative episode characterized by a period of brooding followed by an outburst of violent, aggressive, or homicidal behavior, often followed by a claim of amnesia The episode tends to be precipitated by a perceived insult or slight and seems to be prevalent among males	Amok or Mata elap (Malaysia) Cafard/Cathard (Polynesia, Laos, Philippines) Mal de pelea (Puerto Rico, Papua New Guinea) Iich'aa (Navajo) Going postal (United States)	Dissociative fugue Intermittent explosive disorders
Food restriction taxon	Severe restriction of food intake associated with morbid fear of obesity, may include excessive exercise Binge eating followed by purging through vomiting laxatives, diuretics, and morbid fear of obesity Severe restriction of food intake, associated with experience of religious devotion	Anorexia nervosa (North America, Europe, industrialized nations) Bulimia nervosa (North America, Europe, industrialized countries) Anorexia mirabilis	Eating disorders, anorexia nervosa Eating disorders, bulimia nervosa Historic term, not emic
Exhaustion taxon	Symptoms include unexplained physical and mental fatigue, difficulties in concentrating, remembering, thinking; dizziness, headaches and other pains; sleep disturbance May include gastrointestinal problems, dyspepsia, sexual dysfunction, irritability, and nervousness	Brain fag (West Africa) focus is on brain fatigue Shenjing shuairuo (China, Taiwan) Shinkeisui-jaku (Japan) Neurasthenia (19th century United States) Chronic fatigue syndrome, fibromyalgia, multiple chemical sensitivities (United States, Europe)	May resemble anxiety, depressive, or somatoform disorders Often attributed to somatic, biologic, and/or environmental causes or etiologies
Startle matching taxon	Hypersensitivity to fright often with echopraxia, echolalia, command obedience and dissociative trance-like behavior	Latah (Malaysia, Indonesia) Amurakh, Irkunii, Ikota, Olan myiachit, Menkeiti (Siberia) Bah-tschi, Bash-tsi, Baah-ji (Thailand) Imu (Japan) Mal-mali, Silok (Philippines)	Dissociative and anxiety features
Genital retraction taxon	Episode of sudden and intense anxiety that the penis will recede into the body and possibly cause death Occasionally occurs in local epidemics	Koro (Maylasia) Suo yang (China) Jinjinia bemar (Assam) Rok-joo (Thailand)	Anxiety and somatoform features
Running taxon	Characterized by a sudden onset of a high level of activity, a trance-like state, potentially dangerous or irrational behavior in the form of running, fleeing, breaking things, shouting, followed by amnesia May be accompanied by convulsive seizures, headaches, and anger	Pibloktoq or Arctic hysteria (Gtrrland Eskimos) Grisi sikni (Miskito Indians of Honduras and Nicaragua) "Frenzy" witchcraft (Navajo)	Dissociative fugue Dissociative trance disorder
Semen loss taxon	Severe anxiety and hypochondriasis associated with the discharge of semen, whitish discoloration of urine, and feelings of weakness and exhaustion Symptoms include dizziness, general weakness, insomnia, frequent dreams, sexual dysfunction, fears of loss of life	Dhat, Jiryan (India) Sukra prameha (Sri Lanka) Shenkui (China) Shen-k'uei (Taiwan)	Anxiety and panic features Somatization disorder

(continued)

Table 6.2. (continued)

CBS Taxonomies or Classifications	Syndrome Names and Culture/Country	Description/Symptoms	Resemblance to DSM Diagnoses
Spirit possession taxon	Spell (southern United States) Zar (Ethiopia, Somalia, Egypt, Sudan, Iran, North Africa, the Middle East) Not considered pathological locally	A trance-like state in which persons develop a relationship with deceased relatives or spirits May include apathy, withdrawal, not carrying out activities of daily living May also include laughing, weeping, or shouting	Dissociative features
Obsession with deceased taxa	Ghost sickness (American Indian groups) Hsieh-ping (Taiwan) Shin-byung (Korea)	Symptoms of insomnia, fatigue, panic, fear, anorexia, gastrointestinal symptoms, dizziness; may be associated with witchcraft or possession by ancestral spirits May include hallucinations, loss of consciousness	Dissociative, anxiety, somatoform features Sometimes psychotic features
Suppressed rage taxa	Hwa-bung or anger syndrome (Korea) Bilis and cholera (Latin America). See Idioms of Distress category below	Symptoms of insomnia, fatigue, panic, dysphoria, indigestion, anorexia, palpitations, aches, and pains In Korea includes a mass in the stomach Anger or suppressed anger believed to be the cause of illness	Anxiety, depressive, and somatoform features
Unclassified CBS	Boufée deliriante (West Africa and Haiti)	Sudden outburst of agitated and aggressive behavior, marked by confusion, psychomotor excitement, visual and auditory hallucinations	Brief psychotic disorder
Unclassified CBS	Qi-gong psychotic reaction (China)	Acute, time-limited episode characterized by dissociative, paranoid, or other psychotic or nonpsychotic symptoms after participating in the Chinese folk-healing practice of qi-gong	Brief psychotic disorder
Unclassified CBS	Locura (term used by Latinos in the United States and Latin America)	Severe form of psychosis attributed to familial vulnerability or a combination Symptoms of incoherence, agitation, auditory and visual hallucinations unpredictability and violence	Chronic psychotic disorder
Unclassified CBS	Tabanka (Trinidad) abandonment by wife Hi-Wa itck (Mohave American Indians) unwanted separation from loved one	Depression, insomnia, and sometimes suicide associated with the loss of a wife or other loved one	Major depressive disorder
Unclassified CBS	Taijin kyofusho (Japan)	Intense fear that a person's body parts are offensive to other people in appearance, odor or expression	Social phobia
Unclassified CBS	Falling-out (United States and Caribbean groups)	Sudden collapse, occurs without warning, dizziness, inability to see, powerless to move, no loss of consciousness	Conversion disorder Dissociative disorder

Culture-Specific Idioms or Expressions of Distress	Name of Idiom and Culture/Country	Description	Resemblance to DSM Diagnosis
Idiom	Ataque de nervios (Latinos–Caribbean, Latin America, Latin Mediterranean)	Occurs as a direct result of a stressful family event Expressions of distress include attacks of shouting, trembling, crying, heat in the chest rising to the head, verbal or physical aggression, seizure-like or fainting episodes and suicidal gestures	May range from normal expressions of distress to symptoms associated with anxiety, mood or somatoform disorders

(continued)

Table 6.2. (continued)

Culture-Specific Idioms or Expressions of Distress	Name of Idiom and Culture/Country	Description	Resemblance to DSM Diagnosis
Idioms	*Bilis* (Latin America) *Colera* or *Muina* (Latin America)	Expression of distress and explanation for physical and mental illness as a result of extreme emotions (in this case anger), which upset the hot and cold balance in the body	Anxiety, dissociative and somatic features ranging from normal distress to pathologic presentations
Idiom	*Mal de ojo* (evil eye) (Spain, Latin America, throughout the Mediterranean and Muslim worlds)	Common attribution of misfortune Social disruption and disease to the look of an envious or malevolent person Children are especially at risk Symptoms include fitful sleep, crying, diarrheas, vomiting, and fever	
Idioms	*Nervios* (Latin America) Case of nerves (Appalachian United States) *Nevra* (Greece)	Vulnerability to stressful life experiences and to a syndrome brought on by life stresses Nervousness, easy tearfulness, inability to concentrate, emotional distress	
Idioms	Rootwork (southern United States among African American and European populations and in Caribbean societies) *Mal puesto* (Latin American groups) *Brujeria* (Latino societies)	Explanation for illness as the result of hexing, witchcraft, voodoo, or the influence of an evil person Symptoms include gastrointestinal complaints, weakness, dizziness, fear of being poisoned and being killed	
Idiom	*Susto* (fright or soul loss) Other names: *espanto, pasmo, tripa ida perdida del alma, chibih* (Latinos in the United States and Latin America Similar beliefs and symptom constellations found in many parts of the world	Illness attributed to a frightening event that causes the soul to leave the body, leading to unhappiness and sickness. Symptoms include appetite disturbances, sleep problems, feelings of sadness, lack of motivation, low self-worth, muscle aches and pains, headache, stomach ache, diarrhea; in extreme cases death	Major depressive disorder Posttraumatic stress disorder Somatoform disorders

Note: Table constructed from material found in DSM-IV (APA, 2000, pp. 899-903), online glossary of Timothy McCajor Hall (2001), Simons and Hughes (1985, pp. 475-505), Flaskerud (2007b), Lin and Zheng (2001), and Shafer (2002). See reference list for full citations.

    i. A violent event is followed by regret, forgiveness, and then repeated violence

    ii. Triggers to a violent event are often unknown, examples include

        aa. alcohol or drug use can be a risk for both perpetrator and victim

        ab. financial downturns

        ac. pregnancy

        ad. mental or debilitating illness

    iii. IPV usually does not decrease with age, although the intensity may lessen. Older women share the same characteristics as younger women who are abused; the overall dynamics remain the same (Band-Winterstein & Eisikovits 2009). Victims feel trapped, uncertain, and fearful (Nagel 2003).

2. Societal Changes That Affected IPV

a. In the 19th century, industrialization and urbanization affected demographic transitions and role changes

    (1) Migration increased from rural to urban areas, lessening family ties and support (Brograd 2005; A. Raj & Silverman, 2003).

    (2) Fertility rates decreased as more infants survived, thus reducing the necessity for having a large number of children. With the increased infant survival rate over deaths, population exploded (Glittenberg, 1994; Korbin, 1981).

    (3) Lives became more public; IPV became more visible (Dobash & Dobash, 1992; Gelles, 2000).

b. Social awareness grew in the 20th century; structural and institutional protection and intervention began.

    (1) More than 2,000 years earlier, children (but not women) were protected in Greece and Rome (Gelles 2000).

    (2) For centuries women fought for equal rights with men (Dobash & Dobash 1992). English common law in 1768 used the "rule of thumb" that meant a husband could physically chastise his wife with a stick no thicker than his thumb (Gelles, 2000).

    (3) There were no advocates for abused women in the United States until the Civil Rights and Feminist Movements in the 1960s (Gelles, 2000).

c. Changes in sexual roles

    (1) In Western countries, women began working outside the home during and following World War II. They gained new roles and power (Dobash & Dobash, 1992).

    (2) Birth control gave women freedom and new choices.

    (3) In 1973, the *Roe v. Wade* Supreme Court decision prohibited outlawing abortion. It had the force of law in protecting a woman's right to choose to abort her pregnancy. This decision remains in dispute over the past 36 years, but it ushered changes in a female's power of decision making.

d. Research on IPV in the 1970s to 1990s shattered myths.

    (1) It was found that IPV exists in all sectors of society, classes, races, ethnicities, religions, and geographical locations (Dobash & Dobash, 1992; Gelles, 2000; Sachs, Kozial-McLain, Glass, Webster, & Campbell, 2002; Ventura & Miller, 2007).

        (a) Prevalence was highest among those who were on welfare assistance (Straus & Smith, 1990).

        (b) Rural women are at risk because they are isolated.

        (c) New immigrant women are victimized more often than the general population (A. Raj & Silverman, 2003).

    (2) During pregnancy, IPV rates rise and have implications for practice (Campbell & Lynch, 2006; Espinosa & Osborne, 2002).

    (3) A total of 20% to 50% of women coming to hospital emergency rooms are victims of violence, but all may not be IPV (Williams, 2005).

    (4) In the 1990s, violence was declared the number one public health problem in the United States, and it remains the same today (American Academy of Nursing, 1995; Glittenberg, 2008).

        (a) In 2000, the annual prevalence rate in the United States was found to be about 4 million women (Tjaden & Thoennes 2000).

        (b) World-wide lifetime estimate of IPV varies from 15% to 71% (WHO, 2008; Yick, 2008).

3. Institutional Interventions in IPV

a. Shelters for battered women and children were first established in England in 1974 and now exist in most developed countries. There are shelters for gay men, but not men in general (Bent-Goodley, 2001; Sullivan & Gillum, 2000).

   b. The first shelters were just havens with a good friend-in-need philosophy.
   c. Safe havens originally were not culturally sensitive to minorities or languages other than English and used Eurocentric norms and stereotypes for desired behavior (Bent-Goodley, 2001).
   d. Currently, shelters have competent professional, culturally aware staff (Wies, 2008).

4. *Legal Protection Acts to Guard Against IPV*
   a. The 1994 Violence Crime Control Bill and the Violence Against Women Act brought law enforcement, mandatory arrest, treatment for both the victim and the perpetrator.
   b. Zero tolerance laws aim to break the cycle of IPV and protect children (Gelles, 2000; Hawkins, 2002).
      (1) May not be culturally appropriate; need to understand local IP rules of behavior (Hurtado, 1999)
      (2) Glittenberg (2008) study of Mexican American/Mexican male perpetrators of IPV found no recidivism for 1 year when perpetrators were shamed by a culturally appropriate, Spanish-speaking judge.
   c. The Duluth Abuse Intervention Program deals with anger management with high success rates, but it is not necessarily culturally sensitive (Glittenberg, 2008; Yick, 2008).

5. *Cultural Awareness and Training in IPV Interventions*
   a. Ethnonursing defines behavior as relative to a specific culture (Leininger & McFarland, 2006).
   b. In the United States, there is a tendency to pathologize, stereotype, and stigmatize abused people and their perpetrators (Brograd, 2005; Winstok, 2007; Yick, 2008).
   c. Power and position of the husband vary according to cultural norms (Dobash & Dobash, 1992; Gelles, 2000; Hassouneh-Phillips, 2003).
   d. Even in the 21st century, wives' roles tend to be focused primarily on child-bearing, household economic production, and stability (Douai, Nacef, Belhadj, Bouasker, & Ghachem, 2003).
   e. Intergenerational learning perpetuates IPV.
   f. Children who witness IPV need support and opportunity to verbalize fear; they are often silent victims.
   g. Religious beliefs shape roles of interpersonal behavior, marriage, and reproduction (Ellison & Anderson, 2001; Ellison, Bartkowski, & Anderson, 1999; Foos & Warnke, 2003; Gelles, 2000; Kearney, 2001; Kwon, 2005; Nash, 2006; Nason-Clark, 2004; Pevey, Williams, & Ellison, 1996; Sherif, 1999).
      (1) Eurocentric religions favor patriarchal dominant male roles, for example, Catholic (Foos & Warnke, 2003; Neto, 2007; Yick, 2008).
      (2) Eastern religions: Hindu, Islamic, Buddhist, favor norms of equality and elder respect (Hassouneh-Phillips, 2001; Yick, 2007).
      (3) IPV prevalence rate is very low in Buddhist Thailand (Gelles, 2000). However, a study found 20% of Thai husbands surveyed reported abusing their wives.
   h. Global prevalence rates in 2000 were 15% to 71%, but statistics are questionable; suspect underreporting in many areas (WHO, 2008; Yick, 2008).
   i. A review by Campbell and Lynch (2006) of 35 developing countries describes from one quarter to one half of the surveyed women reported physical abuse by current or former male partner.

6. *Transcultural Nursing Education, Practice, and Research*
   a. Nursing curriculum
      (1) More attention is needed to prepare nurses for IPV prevention efforts (Bryant & Spence, 2002; Duma, 2007; Woodtli, 2001, 2002).
      (2) Teaching needs to be holist, including understanding cultural rules of the family system. Court systems and safe havens need to be understood (Duma, 2007; Glittenberg, 2008).
      (3) An increased comprehensive knowledge base of the physical, psychological, and spiritual signs of abuse is needed among nurses and other health care providers (Goodman, 2009).
      (4) A special awareness is needed about care for disabled persons' symptoms, including those with hearing and vision impairments, and those who are physically and mentally challenged (Moynihan, 2006).
   b. All clients need to be assessed for IPV, especially in emergency rooms and in primary care clinics; during in-home care visits, it is important to assess the environment and safety features (Moynihan, 2006).
      (1) Knowledge of intergenerational transmission of IPV is important to break the cycle of violence (Campbell, 1992; Campbell & Lewandowski, 1997; Magnussen et al., 2004).
      (2) Awareness of depression related to abuse is also needed.
   c. Use principles of transcultural nursing when evaluating, teaching, or researching IVP. See Table 6.3.
      (1) Use ethnonursing knowledge of intimate partner rules and norms, and norms of violent behavior in the cultural context of the community.

          (a) Respect of cultural taboos in questioning abuse; protect the victim by not questioning in front of perpetrator.

          (b) Be aware that in the United States, IPV is considered a crime (Hawkins, 2002).

          (c) Be sensitive for IPV when examining gay and lesbian clients.

    (2) Risk factors may include financial dependency, pregnancy, alcohol and/or drug use, failing health, and isolation, for example, for rural women (Campbell & Lynch, 2006).

    (3) Nurses are first responders in prevention and intervention.

    (4) Strive for early detection by nurse practitioners in primary care clinics and emergency rooms (B. R. Anderson, Marshak, & Hibbeler, 2002; Bryant & Spencer, 2002; Williams, 2005).

    (5) Nurses need to focus on family dynamics and the community context (Berry, 1995; Crenshaw, 1994; Day & Davy, 1998; Helton & Evan, 2001; Kakar, 1998; Knauth, 2003; Sumter, 2006).

    (6) Build recovery and resilience through spirituality, ethnonursing, and caring principles (Campesino & Swartz, 2006; R. E. Davis, 2002; Reed & Enrique, 2006; Sullivan & Gillum, 2001; J. Y. Taylor, 2004).

    (7) Be aware of and sensitive to emic views of violence of some Muslim, fundamentalist, and conservative subcultures (Ellison, Barkowski, & Anderson, 1999; Foss & Warnke, 2003; Giesbrecht & Sevick, 2000; Hassouneh-Phillips, 2003; Yicks, 2008).

    (8) Work within a multidisciplinary team and community partners. If possible intervene in the correctional systems to break a cycle of violence (Gelles, 2000; Glittenberg, 2008; Hayward & Weber, 2003).

    (9) Focus on developing social support networks and early teaching of survival techniques and alternative behaviors (Glittenberg, 2008; Watlington & Murphy, 2006).

  (10) Strengthen political awareness through testimony and social activism (American Academy of Nursing, 1995; Bent-Goodley, 2001; Brograd, 2005; Crenshaw, 1994).

B. War and Genocide

  1. War

    a. Types of war

      (1) Local wars are conflicts restricted in nature to small populations, such as tribes with opposing views of rights, privileges, or beliefs concerning ownership of land, food, and possessions (Ferguson 2004).

          (a) Such local wars may be confined to arguments, threats, restrictions on travel, access to goods, or they may be armed conflict with injuries and death.

          (b) Sometimes local wars are short-lived but at other times they continue over generations, such as family feuds.

          (c) Local conflicts may result in changes in cultural rules that influence laws on marriage, inheritance, or ownership of property, for example, minimum age for marriage, interracial, same-sex marriages, or distribution of land to new immigrants, such as in the Homestead Acts when indigenous lands were usurped.

          (d) Other conflicts may also arise when new immigrants, displaced persons, or refugees arrive or are forced to enter settled populations (Glittenberg, 1989).

      (2) Civil wars are conflicts within recognized national boundaries, between groups representing differences in ideologies, religions, political identities, or possessions, for example, Rwanda (Dallaire, 2003).

      (3) Revolutionary wars are conflicts between political powers within a country that result in an overthrow or an attempted overthrow of the political forces/party in power.

      (4) Global wars are conflicts between multiple nations on an international basis.

          (a) Societies have rules of engagement and forbidden use of certain forms of weaponry, such as gas or nuclear weapons.

          (b) Age of combatants has not been controlled by rules, but children under the age of consent are seldom used in direct combat.

          (c) The United Nations has a peace keeping armed force that is used when other negotiations fail. This force is controlled by the UN Security Council, representing the will of the whole UN.

          (d) In one sense, all wars are global, as energy and use of resources in conflicts/wars may threaten or deplete nonrenewable resources.

      (5) **Silent wars**, for example, withdrawal of support for the poor, homeless, and marginalized persons of minority status, have destructive effects on societies (Bourgois, 2004; Farmer, 2004; Glittenberg, 2008; Scheper-Hughes, 2004).

Table 6.3. Healing Pathways for Survivors of Violence

- Build upon emic cultural meanings of violence, partner, and intimate
- Use ethnonursing principles of holism, individual, family, and community
- Renewing self within cultural context

      (a) When such silent wars result in elimination of a population, the result is genocide (Palacio & Portillo, 2009; Peerwani & Lynch, 2006).

      (b) Examples of silent wars against a marginalized group include those against aboriginal populations in Australia, Native Americans, and First Nation peoples in North America.

b. Rules of War: In 1945 the United Nations ratified the Rules of War that apply to rights of prisoners, noncombatants, and refugees. Enculturation into a new society may be stressful and result in violent behavior (Lynch & Glittenberg, 2010).

c. Cultural aspects of war

    (1) War is dynamic and nonlinear. Cultural dimensions give it power and meaning. As nation states became organized units, war becomes more systematized and legalized (Glittenberg, 2008; Green, 2004; Scheper-Hughes, 2004; Velez-Ibanez, 2004).

    (2) Archaeological evidence illustrates that war and genocide have existed for thousands of years (Scheper-Hughes, 2004).

      (a) Accounts in the Bible refer to multiple wars and deadly battles in the region of modern Middle East for over 4,000 years.

      (b) Conquerors are often brutal to women and children, taking them as hostages or slaves, hence disrupting and changing two cultures, the conquering and the conquered (Castaneda, 1993; Dodgson & Struthers, 2005).

    (3) Colonization of less powerful nations results in enculturation of the conquered. Dynamic changes in cultural rules and norms redefine relationships, for example, former enemies may become allies.

    (4) Cultural rules of relationships toward "other" shape behavior in disagreement and conflict. For example, disrespect or "dissing" between gangs may be sufficient reason for armed conflict (Glittenberg, 2008). Cultural rules related to defined territory may lead to international disputes (Van Arsdale, 2006; Velez-Ibanez, 2004).

    (5) Cultural rules of some nations and local communities resist conflict.

      (a) For example, Sweden and Norway resist armed conflict.

      (b) Other nations have no standing armed forces, for example, Costa Rica.

      (c) Some local communities have "no gun" rules, for example, Oak Park, Illinois.

      (d) Some communities have rules of peaceful resolution in conflict, for example, Manitou Springs, Colorado.

      (e) Some elementary schools have educational programs that lead toward new cultural norms of resisting revenge and building respect (Glittenberg, 2008).

d. Role changes due to war

    (1) In the past, females and children tended to be more protected in war, seldom serving as combatants.

      (a) Archaeological evidence of the structure of houses was shaped by the status of females.

      (b) Those with higher status dwelled in houses with outside walls for protection from intruders (Voss, 2008).

      (c) Women from the Middle East may be covered from head to foot (a *burqa)* viewed emically by many as being protected from outside viewers.

    (2) Females in Western countries in the mid to late 20th century changed many behaviors during wartime.

      (a) Females served first in ammunition factories and military health care roles.

      (b) In the 21st century females now participate in as many combat roles as men.

      (c) If females in combat roles have children, they are left at home to be cared for by others, perhaps the father.

      (d) Male roles have changed as well, as they have taken on caregiver roles when the mother is on active duty.

      (e) Although these role changes are primarily found in the United States (because of the prolonged war in the Middle East), the principles may be found in other territories in conflict.

    e. Technological changes in weaponry

      (1) In the 21st century, changes have resulted in non-face-to-face conflict, for example, guns replaced swords and shields, and bow and arrows used in earlier times (Glittenberg, 2008). Advanced technology has resulted in larger numbers of casualties not defined as enemies but as "collateral damage."

      (2) Worldwide transcultural nurses need to be part of restitution in all disrupted areas. Awareness and participation in restoring fragmented cultures is part of the transcultural nurse's role (Glittenberg, 2008).

2. *Genocide* is defined as the purposeful, targeted elimination of a population or a subportion of a society (Hinton, 2002).

    a. Examples of well-known places and countries where genocide is documented: Bosnia (Van Arsdale, 2006), Chile, Darfur (Cheadle & Prendergast, 2007), Guatemala (Green, 2004); Jewish Holocaust (Arendt, 2004; Yahil, 1990), Jericho (the Bible), Native American Holocaust (Palacios & Portillo, 2009), Rwanda (Keane, 1995; Dallaire, 2003), and Turkey (Akcan, 2006).

    b. Racism, classism, and caste hierarchies target populations that are then dehumanized and marginalized to justify extermination of the population.

    c. Enemies are dehumanized, called rats, or savages, to justify internment or extermination, for example, Jewish Holocaust, Native American Holocaust, internment of Japanese Americans during World War II (Nagata & Cheng, 2003).

    d. Maltreatment and discrimination led to decimation of large populations of indigenous people, that is, the Native American Holocaust (Palacios & Portillo, 2009), First Nation populations of North America, and the aborigines in Australia (Arendt, 2004; Brimmer, 1994; Cheadle & Prendergast, 2007).

    e. Complicit, complacent, and broad constituencies of citizens too often become participant bystanders (Chester, 1992; Glittenberg, 2008; Scheper-Hughes & Bourgois, 2004).

    f. Silent genocides, like silent wars, may eliminate whole populations due to neglect, for example, in natural disasters a lack of timely response to save minorities, the elderly, and prisoners (Glittenberg, 1994).

    g. Another example is a criminal system where a disproportionate number of minority people or dissidents are imprisoned for long periods of time. Such incarceration interrupts family life (Glittenberg, 2008).

    h. Misdirected social laws may indirectly eliminate a culture, for example, forced adoption of indigenous children into the dominant culture to "save" the child from a life of poverty and lack of privilege. Also forced sterilization of targeted segments of the population (Palacios & Portillo, 2009; Springer, 2006).

    i. Genocide may result from an increase in mortality and morbidity of refugees or displaced persons (Palacios & Portillo, 2009; Palinkas et al., 2003).

    j. A type of genocide is the destruction of cultural symbols, for example, shrines, sacred places, flags, monuments, and language by the dominant culture thus disrupting a marginalized culture (Keane, 1995; Taussig, 2004; Velez-Ibanez, 2004).

    k. Torture is a specific, sadistic type of genocide (Chester, 1992). (Use caution when, from an etic perspective, something is labeled as "torture," as some coercive social customs may have different emic meanings.)

    l. United Nations definition of torture in the Convention Against Torture and Other Cruel, Inhuman, or Degrading Treatment or Punishment. Article 1 defines torture as "any act by which severe pain or suffering, whether physical or mental, is intentionally inflicted on a person . . . for reasons based on discrimination of any kind (Chester, 1992, p. 209).

    m. Torture, as defined by the UN, is used to instill fear, thus destroying cultural unity, and dissolving the will of survivors (Glittenberg, 2003; Springer, 2006; Van Arsdale, 2006).

    n. Rape is one form of torture used to demonstrate power, submission, and induce humiliation (Chester & Jaranson, 1994; Marcussen, 2001). Impregnation by the enemy is used as an ultimate destruction of family and may initiate a caste system (Voss, 2008).

3. *Human rights protection in war and genocide*

    a. Universality versus multiculturalism

      (1) United Nations Human Rights Declarations and Conventions (1948) are considered by some critics as being a Eurocentric, legalistic, top-down political decision-making process, and potentially coercive (Shell-Duncan, 2008).

      (2) Others believe there is a need to balance health human rights issues and multiculturalism. There is a need to respect culturally diverse solutions to human rights protection, for example, early indigenous populations had rules of war, care of victims, and prisoners (Ferguson, 2004).

b. Key events that organized universal protection of choice and freedom:
   (1) 1863: Henry Dunant organized protection of prisoners; organized International Red Cross;
   (2) 1867: National Aid Societies for the Nursing the War Wounded (Lynch, 2006)
c. Currently, a number of nongovernmental organizations (NGOs) and intergovernmental organizations (IGOs; see Resources for list) deal with casualties, food and water supplies, prisoners, displaced persons, and rebuilding community.

4. ***Principles of transcultural nursing care practices in war and genocide***
   a. Understand and use an ethnonursing perspective with survivors and perpetrators of war and genocide. Honor diversity in multicultural human rights agenda. Form interventions through a grassroots framework that includes emic definitions of conflict and resolution.
   b. Bear witness and give voice to those without advocates when issues of discrimination, scape-goating, or isolation prevents access to freedom and choice (Glittenberg, 1989).
   c. Include historical trauma, multigenerational transmission of marginalization, and accumulated trauma in addressing health disparities and ensuring healthy future generations (Kellerman, 2001; Lev-Wiesel & Amir, 2001; Nagata & Cheng, 2003; Palacio & Portillo, 2009; Steel, Silove, Phan, & Baumann, 2002; Struthers & Lowe, 2003; Wastell, 2002).
   d. Use ethical transcultural framework (Ray, 1994) to bring holistic healing to the wounded combatants, affected families and communities, including the grieving for the dead (Koff, 2004).
   e. In war, use the Nightingale code of ethics in treating both enemy and ally alike (Donahue, Russac & Christy, 1985). Maintain humanistic leadership in all military services. Teach and train cultural competence as a requirement for military, NGOs, and IGOs.
   f. Use theory of obligation and moral/ethical elements to guide humanitarian assistance and pragmatic approach with available resources (Van Arsdale, 2006).
   g. Reconciliation and forgiveness are positive healing modalities (Bhutto, 2008; Marcussen, 2001; Shell-Duncan, 2008).
   h. Bear witness to suffering, confinement, and lack of freedom through publications, hearings, social action, for example, Amnesty International (Chester, 1992; Glittenberg, 2003; Sheehan, 2006).
   i. When intervening with a victim of torture or severe trauma, use personal narratives to reconnect with meaning, especially with cultural symbols and artifacts (Ray, 1994, Rushton, Scott, & Callister 2008). Use narratives both with individuals and communities (Chester & Jaranson, 1994).
   j. Use informed inquiry and critical thinking with social activism when individual, family, or community rights are being abused (Glittenberg, 1998; Ray, 1994).
   k. Promote and participate in educational nursing exchanges that embrace multiculturalism and peace, for example, Fulbright Fellowships, Peace Corps.

5. ***Summary***
   a. Understanding the sociocultural forces of war and genocide is critical for transcultural nursing as this topic challenges nursing skills of the highest nature.
   b. Limiting knowledge to only Eurocentric viewpoints, cultural blinders, and narrow solutions adds pain and misery to those who are experiencing or have experienced these wounds.

C. **Care of Refugees and Asylees**
   1. *Introduction.* This section covers three subject areas:
      a. The first provides definitions for refugees, asylees and immigrants and other categories of people outside their homelands.
      b. The second area provides an overview of the evolution of the Geneva Convention introduced to protect the rights of asylees and refugees.
      c. The third part identifies health issues and models of health care to meet the health care needs of this group of people.
   2. *Definitions*
      a. The following definitions distinguish the circumstances of people displaced from their homelands for whatever reason.
      b. The bureaucratic responses in host nations vary according to the status of individuals defined by these terms. There are practical implications therefore conferred by the nomenclature.
         (1) ***Refugee:*** United Nations High Commission on Refugees' (UNHCR)'s founding mandate defines refugees as (UNHCR, 2009b):

(a) People outside their country of origin

(b) Persons who cannot return to their country of origin owing to a well-founded fear of persecution due to their:
 i. race,
 ii. religion,
 iii. nationality,
 iv. political opinion, or
 v. membership of a particular social group (UNHCR, 2009b; Universal Declaration of Human Rights [UDHR], 1948)

(2) **Asylum seeker**

(a) A person who has exercised the legal right under the Geneva Convention of 1951 to apply for personal and legal protection;

(b) Someone who has made a claim that he or she is a refugee; and

(c) is waiting for that claim to be accepted or rejected (UNHCR, 2006).

(d) Some asylum seekers will be judged to be refugees and others will not.

(3) **Stateless person**

(a) Definition:
 i. Someone who is not considered as a national by any state (de jure stateless);
 ii. or possibly someone who does not enjoy fundamental rights enjoyed by other nationals in their home state (de facto stateless);
 iii. Statelessness can be a personal disaster (Richter, 2005; UNHCR, 2009b)

(b) The Universal Declaration of Human Rights 1948–Article 15 states unequivocally that "everyone has the right to a nationality. No one shall be arbitrarily deprived of his nationality, nor denied the right to change his nationality."

(c) The UDHR, 1948 Article 14.1 states that "Everyone has the right to seek and to enjoy in other countries asylum from persecution." (UDHR, 1948)

(4) **Immigrant/migrant**

(a) A wide ranging term that covers most people who move to a foreign country for a variety of reasons, such as, financial, educational, and/or family reunion.

(b) Someone who takes up permanent residence in a country other than his or her original homeland.

(c) Migrants can be refugees as well (Richter, 2005; UNHCR, 2009b).

(5) **Internally displaced person (IDP):** Someone who has been forced to move from his or her home because of

(a) conflict,

(b) persecution,

(c) natural disaster, or

(d) some unusual circumstances,

(e) Unlike refugees, IDPs remain inside their country of birth (Darling, 2009; Richter, 2005) http://may.unricmagazine.org/fact-sheet.html

c. Immigrants and refugees differ fundamentally in one aspect: Immigrants have the freedom to choose when and where they go.

d. Additionally, immigrants are able to return to their home country if things do not work out for them in their adopted country.

e. Deciding to return to their homelands is not an easy option for refugees and may not ever be possible.

3. *Historical highlights*

a. Seeking asylum is an ancient act, dating back to ancient times when people sought help and protection from the divine by sheltering in sacred places. Today, the protection of sovereign states is sought by asylum seekers rather than divine the protection of the sacred.

b. In modern times, the League of Nations Health Commission for Refugees, in 1921, set up the first international effort to coordinate refugee affairs. A refugee at that time was defined as a person in a group for which the League of Nations had approved a mandate, as opposed to a person to whom a general definition applied.

c. The large numbers of refugees seeking to enter the United States caused Congress to pass the Emergency Quota Act of 1921, a precursor to the Immigration Act, which followed in 1924.

d. The Treaty of Lusanne in 1923 between Greece and Turkey denaturalized people who had crossed borders during their conflict and made them refugees.

e. In 1930, the Nansen International Office for Refugees created a passport for refugees.

f. So many people were fleeing Germany with the rise of Nazism that the League of Nations created a High Commission specifically for people coming out of Germany.

g. World War II conflict produced massive forced migrations.

h. Following World War II, refugees were defined as a legal group in response to large numbers of people fleeing Eastern Europe.

i. The Allies create the United Nations Relief and Rehabilitation Administration (UNRRA) to assist the millions of displaced people and to assist refugees (http://en.wikipedia.org/wiki/Refugee).

j. The League of Nations dissolved both the Nansen Office and the German High Commission and replaced them with the Office of the High Commissioner for Refugees, which remains the leading international agency coordinating refugee protection.

k. United Nations High Commissioner for Refugees (UNHCR) was established on December 14, 1951, to protect and support refugees and to assist in their return or resettlement.

   (1) Except for a few specific groups, all refugees in the world are under the UNHCR mandate.

   (2) UNHCR provides protection and assistance to

      (a) Asylum seekers

      (b) Refugees who have returned home but still need help in rebuilding their lives

      (c) Local civilian communities directly affected by the movements of refugees

      (d) Stateless people and IDPs.

   (3) The agency is mandated to

      (a) Safeguard the rights and well-being of refugees

      (b) Ensure that everyone can exercise the right to seek asylum and find safe refuge in another state, with the option to return home voluntarily

      (c) Lead and coordinate international action to protect refugees

      (d) To resolve refugee problems worldwide

      (e) Integrate asylum seekers locally or to resettle in a third country

   (4) Under the 1951 Refugee Convention and 1967 Protocol, UNHCR's mandate has expanded to include protecting and providing humanitarian assistance to other persons "of concern." (http://en.wikipedia.org/wiki/Refugee)

l. The concept of a refugee was expanded by the refugee convention 1976 Protocol and by regional conventions in Africa and Latin America to include persons who had fled war or other violence in their own home country.

4. **Global mandate for refugees:** *United Nations High Commission for Refugees–1951 Statute*

a. The Geneva Convention 1951 outlined the details of the rights of refugees, including the right to seek employment, freedom of movement, and access to national courts (UNHCR, 2009b).

b. Signatories to the UNHCR: A total of 146 countries have signed the 1951 UN Refugee Convention and /or its 1967 protocol and recognize people as refugees based on the definitions contained in these and regional instruments (UNHCR, 2009b).

c. Refugee population statistics, released by the UNHCR: http://www.unhcr.org/4c11f0be9.html.

   (1) In 2009, there were 43.3 million forcibly displaced people worldwide, the highest number since the mid-1990s. Of these, 15.2 million were refugees; 10.4 million who fell under UNHCR's responsibility, and 4.8 million Palestinian refugees under the mandate of United Nations Relief and Work Agency (UNRWA) for Palestinian refugees in the Near East.

   (2) The figure also includes 983,000 asylum seekers and 27.1 million internally displaced persons. This increase includes refugees and civilians who have returned home but still need help, people displaced internally within their own countries, asylum seekers, and stateless people.

   (3) Afghan and Iraqi refugees accounted for almost half of all refugees under UNHCR's responsibility worldwide; one out of four refugees in the world was from Afghanistan (2.9 million).

   (4) Afghans were located in 71 different asylum countries; however, 96% were located in Pakistan and Iran. Afghanistan has been the leading country of origin of refugees for the past three decades.

   (5) Iraqis were the second largest refugee group, with 1.8 million having sought refuge primarily in neighboring countries.

(6) The third largest group of refugees is from Somalia, with security conditions and severe drought being major factors for leaving their country of origin.

(7) Other main sources of refugees were Myanmar, Colombia, and Sudan.

d. Global trends in asylum applications (UNHCR, 2010) http://www.unhcr.org/4ba7341a9.html

(1) There was a 3% increase in asylum applications from 2008 for the 27 countries of the European Union.

(2) Among the European countries, the largest increase in asylum applications was reported by 11 Central European countries, followed by similar increases in the Nordic Region (13% increase).

(3) The only European region to experience a decrease in the asylum seeker applications was Southern Europe

(4) Asylum applications in North America were 5% less in 2009 than in 2008. Yet, for the fourth year in a row, the United States received the largest number of new applications for asylum, accounting for 13% of all claims of the 44 industrialized nations.

(5) The 2009 number of asylum seekers in Australia increased by 29% over the previous year.

(6) The 2009 UNHRC report indicates that sociopolitical influences have brought changes in policy direction, leading to a decline in asylum seekers in a number of countries (http://www.unhcr.org/4adebca49 .html)

5. *Changing political circumstances and the dynamics of displacement*
Evolution of UNHCR to fulfill its mandate

a. 1960s and 1970s: Shift from Europe to the global South.

b. 1980: Increased emphasis on humanitarian assistance over protection.

c. 1990s: Wider role in humanitarian assistance and repatriation

d. End of the 1990s/early 2000s: Greater responsibility for IDPs, returnees, stateless, and a number of other "persons of concern."

e. Call for UNHCR to be responsible for persons displaced by natural disasters, climate change and other migration (http://canada.metropolis.net/mediacentre/new_challenges_internat refugee_protection_e.ppt).

f. Example: The Australian experience:

(1) Although it is Australian government law to detain people until a determination is made, the right to seek asylum is an absolute right determined through international law (UNHCR, 2006).

(2) Temporary protection for 3 years was afforded asylees by way of a Temporary Protection Visa (TPV).

(3) TPV holders have limited access to social security and education services, but no access to family reunion programs.

(4) On expiration of the TPV—the end of 3 years—such visa holders could apply for refugee status.

(5) On May 13, 2008 the Rudd Government announced the abolishing of the TPV (http://news.in.msn .com/international/article.aspx?cp-documentid=1398286).

(6) On May 14, 2008 Human Rights and Equal Opportunities Commission Press Release, announced that "end of TPVs for refugees is a step forward for human rights" (http://www.hreoc.gov.au/ about/media/media_releases/2008/56_08.html).

(7) Although TPV was first introduced in Australia, other countries such as the United States allowed TPV for people from Bosnia, El Salvador, Lebanon, Liberia, Kuwait, Rwanda, and Somalia. A number of other European countries have also followed the same pattern.

(8) The uncertainty of such a temporary situation can create an enormous physical and psychological toll. For many TPV holders, suicide is considered a very real option (Procter, 2004a, 2004b; http:// www.refugeecouncil.org.au/docs/resources/ppapers/pp-tvp-qanda-sep03.pdf).

g. Detention of asylum seekers, within the countries in which they seek asylum, is a worldwide concern for health professionals because of the potential detrimental effects on the mental health of detainees (Steel et al., 2004; Steel et al., 2006; Sultan & O'Sullivan, 2001).

6. *Health issues of refugees and asylum seekers*

a. The mental and psychological impact of war, conflict, and the resultant dislocation and resettlement out of their country of origin has been well documented (Gessner, 1994; Halimi, 2002; Kalipeni & Oppong, 1998: Khamis, 1998; Lipson & Omidian, 1997; Lipson, Omidian, et al., 1995; Omeri, Lennings, & Raymond, 2004, 2006; Procter, 2005a, 2005b; Silove, et al., 1988; Silove & Steel,

1998; Silove, Steel, & Mollica, 2001; Silove, Steel, & Walters, 2000; Steel & Silove, 2001; Sultan & O'Sullivan, 2001).

    b. A range of physical and psychological reactions to this dislocation have been identified.

        (1) Emotional responses to trauma, immigration and resettlement (Omeri et al., 2006; Steel & Silove, 2006)

        (2) Loss and grief (Harris & Telfer, 2001; Keyes, 2000; Omeri et al., 2004, 2006; Proctor, 2005a, 2005b).

        (3) Feeling unsafe and living in limbo (Omeri et al., 2004, 2006)

        (4) Lack of trust (Omeri et al., 2004, 2006)

        (5) Mental illness, such as anxiety and depression (Lipson & Omidian, 1997: Omeri et al., 2004, 2006; Steel et al., 2006; Steel & Silove, 2001).

        (6) Posttraumatic stress disorder (PTSD; Cunningham & Cunningham, 1997; Silove et al., 2000; Procter, 2004a, 2005b).

        (7) Disempowerment and helplessness (De Santis, 1997; Omeri et al., 2006)

7. Health care and health services/models: *Caring for refugees and asylum seekers*

    a. Refugees represent persons from diverse cultural contexts across the globe. It is important therefore to use model of health care that integrates the unique perspective of each cultural group.

    b. Primary health care (PHC) model:

        (1) PHC delivers care to families and communities by means of encouraging their full participation in their own health care, self-reliance and self-determination.

        (2) PHC can form an integral part of the country's health system, which is a central function of overall social and economic development of the community (WHO, 1978, p. 3).

        (3) To achieve primary health care for all, the Alma-Ata conference (WHO, 1978) issued five calls to action:

            (a) A call for equity—universal health coverage with care provided according to need.

            (b) A call for self-reliance and self-determination with communities assuming more responsibility for their own health.

            (c) A call for effective and culturally acceptable, manageable, and affordable services. Cultural acceptability cannot be sacrificed for effectiveness.

            (d) A call for primary health care not to be limited to first contact with medical, health, or nursing care.

            (e) A call for primary health care not to be limited to health care interventions (WHO, 1978).

        (4) Australia example:

            (a) Community Health Centers provide primary health care to diverse communities, including refugees and asylum seekers in both urban and remote rural areas.

            (b) Community Controlled Primary Health Care has been adopted by Indigenous communities as the method of choice in health care delivery, as well as reaching and providing care for refugees who reside in remote rural areas (Couzos & Murray, 2008; McMurray, 2008; Omeri & Malcolm, 2004).

    c. Challenges for provision of mental health nursing services:

        (1) Nurses need knowledge of the stressors affecting TPV holders to avert mental health problems, suicide, and mental illness.

        (2) Nurses need to employ trusting, culturally appropriate interactions with groups and individuals.

        (3) Nurses need to develop, disseminate, and implement effective strategies that are culturally and linguistically appropriate (Omeri et al., 2004, 2006)

    d. Three-dimensional model

        (1) To take into account the complexities of the refugee experiences and circumstances, Watters (2001, p. 1609) suggests a "three-dimensional model" for mental health services to allow for analysis of institutional factors on the mental health of individuals, particularly PTSD.

        (2) Models that tend to homogenizes a diverse range of refugees and condense their cultures in ways that ignore the dynamic interaction between cultures of various groups are to be avoided.

        (3) Consideration of a three-dimensional model that includes the interaction between services and refugees may be helpful in the provision in mental health service (Watters, 2001, pp. 1709-1718).

(4) Without allowing refugees to voice their stories and needs, they may be the subjects to stereotypical institutional responses (Leininger, 2006; Muecke, 1982; Omeri et al., 2006).

   e. Transcultural nursing model

     (1) A number of terms have been used interchangeably to describe the core concept of this model: cultural congruence, cultural sensitivity, culturally appropriate, culturally competent, and cultural awareness, among others.

     (2) Leininger's Theory of Culture Care Diversity and Universality provides an appropriate and useful theoretical framework for the study and provision of culturally congruent and meaningful care to diverse populations of refugees and asylum seekers across the world. See Chapter 3 for discussion of this theory (Leininger & McFarland, 2006).

8. *Research studies on the care of refugees or immigrants*

   a. Leininger (2006) conducted an ethnonursing study with a Sudanese refugee family in Nebraska.

   b. Transcultural nursing care values, beliefs, and practices of Iranian immigrants/refugees in Australia (Omeri, 1996).

   c. Beyond asylum: Implications for nursing and health care delivery for Afghan refugees in Australia (Omeri et al., 2004, 2006).

   d. A study by DeSantis (1997) examined the impact of prolonged stays in refugee camps. She discovered that such experiences foster learned helplessness, fear of strangers, incapacity to make decisions for themselves and does not foster empowerment.

   e. A U.K. study highlights primary health care as a framework to meet the recognized health needs of refugees and asylum seekers that can be used in planning and evaluating services as model of care for refugees and asylum seekers (Feldman, 2006).

   f. A population-based study between 2003 and 2004 among refugees and asylum seekers from Afghanistan, Iran, and Somalia, in Netherlands, showed no differences between refugees and asylum seekers in the self-reported use of health care services. However, respondents from Somalia reported fewer contacts with general practitioners, less use of mental health services, and less medication use than respondents from Afghanistan and Iran (Gerritsen et al., 2006).

   g. Interviews with 34 primary health care nurses (PHCN) from two municipalities in Sweden revealed that PHC's can facilitate strengthening the identity of the families and reducing the effects of socioenvironmental stressors by adopting a family system perspective (Samarasinghe & Arvidsson, 2006).

9. *Global services for refugees and asylees*

   a. UNHCR provides protection and assistance not only to refugees but also to other categories of displaced or needy people. See section 3.k(2) above.

   b. In 2006, UNHCR was applying its long-time expertise in specific areas, such as protection, emergency shelter and camp management to help 6.6 million IDPs, working in close collaboration with other UN agencies and NGOs.

   c. Globalization means that local conflicts and disease outbreaks are no longer local but global with extensive consequences (Kalipeni & Oppong, 1998).

   d. Example: Services for refugees and asylum seekers in Australia:

     (1) Integrated Humanitarian Settlement Strategies (IHSS) are in place in Australia and include specialized services for the treatment and rehabilitation of torture and trauma survivors (STARTTS).

     (2) Services are comprehensive and cover major resettlement issues such as: employment, accommodation, health care, counseling among others. More detail can be obtained from the following website: http://www.racgp.org.au/refugeehealth

IV. DISASTER ASSISTANCE: CULTURALLY CONGRUENT CARE OF VICTIMS OF NATURAL DISASTERS

  A. Definition of Terms

    1. Disaster: "A serious disruption of the functioning of a community or a society causing widespread human, material, economic or environmental losses which exceed the ability of the affected community or society to cope using its own resources. A disaster is a function of the risk process. It results from the combination of hazards, conditions of vulnerability and insufficient capacity or measures to reduce the potential negative consequences of risk" (United Nations, International Strategy for Disaster Reduction, 2004).

2. *Natural disaster*: Consequence of a natural hazard that affects human activities. Human vulnerability, exacerbated by the lack of planning or appropriate emergency management, leads to financial, environmental or human losses (Bankoff, Frerks, & Hilhorst, 2004).

3. *Disaster risk management*: Systematic process of using administrative decisions, organization, operational skills and capacities to implement policies, strategies and coping capacities of the society and communities to lessen the impacts of natural hazards (United Nations, International Strategy for Disaster Reduction, 2004).

4. *Vulnerable populations:* Social groups that may experience health disparities as a result of lack of resources and/or exposure to risks (Flaskerud et al., 2002).

5. *Transcultural nursing:* "A formal area of study and practice focused on comparative human-care (caring) differences and similarities of the beliefs, values, and patterned lifeways of cultures to provide culturally congruent, meaningful and beneficial health care to people" (Leininger & McFarland, 2002, pp. 5-6).

B. Scope of the Problem

1. Over the past 20 years, the number of recorded disasters has increased 100%, from approximately 200 to 400 per year.

2. Nine out of 10 recorded disasters have been climate related; current data suggest this will continue with the potential for increasing frequency and intensity.

3. Various issues contribute to increased vulnerability worldwide, including
   a. poverty;
   b. increasing urbanization in potentially unsafe and unplanned urban areas;
   c. disease patterns (HIV, infectious disease); and
   d. disparities, including health and access to services (United Nations Secretariat of the International Strategy for Disaster Reduction [UN/ISDR] and the United Nations Office for Coordination of Humanitarian Affairs [UN/OCHA], 2008).

C. Types of Natural Disasters

1. Hurricanes
   a. Often accompanied by widespread, torrential rains, causing deadly and devastating flooding, some persisting days after storm.
   b. May also trigger landslides or mud slides.

2. Tornadoes

3. Tsunamis/seismic (tidal) waves
   a. Most often instigated by earthquake or landslide; if those happen close to shore, a tsunami can reach the coastline very quickly.
   b. Most vulnerable are those less than 25 feet above sea level and within a mile of shoreline.
   c. Other natural hazards include resultant flooding and fires.

4. Monsoons

5. Earthquakes: Includes the initial quake and aftershocks or subsequent vibrations.

6. Volcanic eruptions: Often accompanied by other natural hazards such as earthquakes, flash floods, landslides, fire, and (under very particular circumstances) tsunamis.

7. Floods
   a. Includes flash floods and slow developing floods, some without sign of rain.
   b. Danger areas in low-lying, near water, or downstream from a dam.

8. Landslides and debris flows
   a. Can be of any magnitude, slow or fast.
   b. Often activated by other natural disasters (storm, fire, earthquakes, etc) or human modification of land.

9. Drought

10. Winter storms and extreme colds/heat: Extreme heat exacerbated by poor air quality and stagnant atmospheric conditions, making urban dwellers more vulnerable.

11. Wildfires (Federal Emergency Management Agency, n.d.).

D. Theoretical Underpinning of Culture for Pre- and Post-Disaster Management

1. *Leininger's Sunrise Model:* Cultural care worldview refers to the way in which people of particular cultures understand the world around them (Leininger & McFarland, 2006). See Chapter 3 for more extensive description.

  a. Cultural and social structure dimensions (found in most cultures)
   (1) Technological factors
   (2) Religious and philosophical factors
   (3) Family and kinship factors
   (4) Cultural values and lifeways
   (5) Political and legal factors
   (6) Economic factors
   (7) Educational factors
  b. Diverse health systems
   (1) Generic or folk health systems: culturally learned and transmitted folk knowledge and skills to promote health and treat illness from the people
   (2) Nursing care system (see definition of Transcultural Nursing)
   (3) Professional health systems: formal and cognitively learned knowledge and practice skills learned at institutions promoting a particular system of care and cure
  c. Nursing care decisions and actions
   (1) Cultural care preservation/maintenance: nursing actions that are assistive, supportive to help people retain or maintain cultural practices that promote heath and well-being.
   (2) Cultural care accommodation/negotiation: nursing actions that are assistive, supportive in negotiating care that may use both professional and folk beliefs for meaningful health outcomes.
   (3) Cultural care repatterning/restructuring: nursing actions that are assistive, supportive for people to reorder, change or modify their current lifeway to promote health and well-being.
  d. Culturally congruent nursing care: The goal of nursing in promoting care that is culturally meaningful and beneficial for health, well being, or to face death and disability (Leininger & McFarland, 2006).

 2. *Vulnerable Populations Model* (Aday, 1994)
  a. Vulnerability refers to social groups who have an increased susceptibility to adverse health outcomes, in this case, victims of natural disaster.
  b. This model posits that there are interrelationships between health status (morbidity), resource availability (social and environmental resources), and relative risk (increased risk factors, health promoting behaviors).
  c. "Resource availability" is the optimal place for intervention by the transcultural nurse. By increasing resources available to the individual, the nurse seeks to reduce risk, and therefore maintain (or improve) health status.

E. Critical Issues in Disaster Preparedness Related to Culture and Culturally Congruent Care
 1. *Dislocation*
  a. Dislocation from home environment for some period of time is inevitable in most natural disasters, ranging from hours to years (including permanent dislocation).
  b. Loss of home can also mean loss of culture and day-to-day life.
 2. *Identity*
  a. Identity related to home, job, or role functioning may be disrupted.
  b. Disaster may result in "identity crisis," secondary to significant disturbance to the understanding of self (Dugan, 2007).
 3. *Sources of information and method of delivery*
  a. Includes questions regarding who is presenting information, who should be told how the community leaders are used in communication, establishing credible sources.
  b. Traditional methods may be compromised or unavailable after a disaster.
  c. Response to methods (television, community leaders, police) may differ within communities.
 4. *Gender*
  a. Internationally, gender is an organizing principle in societies.
  b. Interventions must incorporate gender differentiation, so that strategies can be effectively implemented (United Nations Secretariat of the International Strategy for Disaster Reduction [UN/ISDR] and the United Nations Office for Coordination of Humanitarian Affairs [UN/OCHA], 2008).
 5. *Priorities* and priority setting will vary between and among cultures.
 6. *Language difference* between disaster workers and victims.

7. *Cultural definitions of grief, mourning, and loss.*
    a. Disaster workers must be diligent to ensure that they do not use their own definitions of grief, mourning, and loss to develop plans of care and nursing diagnoses.
    b. Special consideration should be given to language and culturally specific psychological factors when planning intervention for those suffering great loss (Gilbert, 2005).

F. Examples of Lessons Learned From Domestic and Global Disasters
    1. U.S. disasters
        a. Rural North Carolina, post Hurricane Floyd (Aderibigbe, Bloch, & Pandurangi, 2003)
            (1) African Americans are more likely to seek assistance from clergy, increased use of support group.
            (2) Culturally congruent intervention: Identify health seeking behaviors.
        b. Alaskan Natives, post Exxon Valdez oil spill (Palinkas, Petterson, Russell, & Downs, 2004)
            (1) Social disorder triggered posttraumatic stress disorder (PTSD), prevalence associated with decreased social support.
            (2) Culturally congruent intervention: Define "disaster" and assess for culturally patterns of PTSD symptoms.
        c. Impact of 9/11 on elderly in NYC Chinatown (Chung, 2003)
            (1) Very limited resource availability related to language, as well as physical and socioeconomic barriers to seeking assistance.
            (2) Feelings of loss associated with personal history of immigration, war, famine
            (3) Culturally congruent intervention: Identify barriers, including cultural history and previous experiences of disaster
        d. Latino disaster vulnerability: Hurricane mitigation information (Peguero, 2006)
            (1) Latinos prefer family and friends as sources
            (2) Culturally congruent intervention: Identify effective sources of information and support

    2. Global disasters
        a. Meta-analysis of psychological response of Japanese disaster victims (Goto & Wilson, 2003)
            (1) Suggests that Japanese disaster victims tend to express psychological distress somatically, allowing them to ask for help from health/medical resources.
            (2) There is no clear understanding of PTSD in this population and culture, creating confusion about treatment and a degree of stigma for those who may manifest those symptoms.
            (3) Culturally congruent intervention: Include psychological assessment with all medical interventions. Educate individuals, families, and communities about PTSD.
        b. Cultural considerations for treatment when a tsunami hit the Indian shore (Ranjan & Saraswat, 2005)
            (1) Comparing tribal and nontribal relief camps, researchers found that tribal families were composed of 15 to 100 members, each of whom could function in various community roles. Each family functioned as an individual societal unit, with many of the units displaying homogenous characteristics related to religion (almost all followed Christianity), family structure, decision making, and child rearing.
            (2) Conversely, the nontribal population was more heterogeneous, with various religious and cultural backgrounds, within the nuclear family structure.
            (3) Culturally congruent intervention: Identify familial and societal constructs when planning interventions. Use the infrastructure created by the community to implement interventions.
        c. Experience of nurses from Western countries volunteering for humanitarian aid work, including disasters (Zinsli & Smythe, 2009)
            (1) Qualitative study finding that nurses in this work should embrace difference, while honoring sameness and shared experience
            (2) Challenges encountered when nurses may need to persuade individuals that their "way" is not safe
            (3) Issues of "differences" may be most obvious when the nurses' life or safety is in danger
        d. Cultural consideration for assessing needs of people in developing countries (Africa, South America, and Asia; Wright & Walley, 1998; Zwim, Gee, Meece-Hinh, & Meuhlenkord, 2006)
            (1) Emergency health needs related to disasters may be the same regardless of the disaster.
            (2) Nurses and other health care providers need to assess the needs of large groups of people based on mass casualty.

(3) Community involvement predisaster is imperative. Community appraisal can provide valuable insight and empower the community for postdisaster and future planning. Therefore seek predisaster appraisal on arrival at disaster site.

(4) Consider the health systems and beliefs of the community and understanding of illness, health, and meaning of disasters.

(5) Appraise the health status of the community especially those most vulnerable such as children and elders.

(6) Consider the culture and cultural needs of the community.

(7) Promote self-care after the period of assistance is over.

G. Role of the Transcultural Nurse

  1. Member of an Interdisciplinary Team

   a. Coordinated and timely response by all individuals and entities is a critical component of an effective response.

   b. Teams may include military, police, health care providers, emergency personnel, lay persons, social service providers, and government employees.

   c. Efforts led by trained response teams from governmental agencies, NGOs, volunteer agencies, and affected and neighboring communities.

   d. There is no unique role for the nurse or any responding professional immediately after a disaster. This requires nurses have a broad perspective, and to take a more holistic approach that incorporates the unique needs and circumstances of the individuals (Clive, Davis, Kushma, & Mincin, 2007).

   e. The unique contribution of the transcultural nurse may be most clearly seen in coordination of efforts and communication between responders, victims, and communities; this includes before, immediately after, and well after the event.

  2. Preparation and Planning

   a. Assess services and community

   (1) Consider and assess current level of vulnerability and health care services.

   (2) Consider and assess current cultural practices of determining services needed.

   b. Involve appropriate community members in planning

   (1) Develop relationships with leaders and stakeholders in the communities for full participation in all aspects of planning. Identifying those individuals is a critical step, and will vary considerably across communities.

   (2) "Informed engagement" may mean avoiding problems when hazard events occur. Participatory activities can maximize capacities of communities, as they may be more sensitive to gender, cultural, and other issues that can undermine or empower particular groups.

   (3) Incorporating the perspective of locals may also ensure recognition of changes in vulnerability and perception of risk (United Nations Secretariat of the International Strategy for Disaster Reduction [UN/ISDR] and the United Nations Office for Coordination of Humanitarian Affairs [UN/OCHA], 2008).

   c. Assist in the development of a Disaster Plan

   (1) Developing a disaster plan may increase access and services and decrease vulnerability in the process.

   (2) Plan for disaster and potential dislocation, including things such as meeting place, medication and health care needs.

   (3) Use current research and literature to develop plans that are culturally appropriate and congruent for disaster preparedness plan sanctioned by the community.

   (4) The humanitarian values of neutrality and impartiality must be incorporated into all planning and response. Nondiscriminatory response is provided according to the needs of the individual (Ferris & Paul, 2009; United Nations Secretariat of the International Strategy for Disaster Reduction [UN/ISDR] and the United Nations Office for Coordination of Humanitarian Affairs [UN/OCHA], 2008).

  3. Immediate Response to Disaster

   a. First and foremost, all responding personnel must focus on the preservation of life and ongoing safety for communities and first responders.

   b. Attention must also be paid to protecting people from discrimination, exploitation, and other human rights violations (Ferris & Paul, 2009).

    c. Consider and promote culturally congruent nursing care actions postdisaster with individuals and communities.

    d. Intent for providing services should be on working *with* the community (as opposed to providing services *to*), and endorsing inclusiveness in all stages (Clive et al., 2007).

    e. Many humanitarians see the event as a natural phenomenon, whereas a "disaster" is a combination of that phenomenon and the human action or response, for example, Hurricane Katrina and the now widely acknowledged poorly executed immediate disaster response (Ferris & Paul, 2009).

  4. *Long-Term Issues*

    a. The transcultural nurse works in tandem with the community and community leaders to reduce vulnerability and increase access to health care during contemporary event; this will reduce the effects of disaster.

    b. If dislocation is a significant issue, special attention must be paid to helping individuals maintain their own cultural identity.

    c. Long-term relocation may involve some degree of adaptation to a new culture. The transcultural nurse can help individuals deal with loss concerning their culture and potential loss of identity.

    d. The longer the displacement, the greater the risk for human rights violations. These can range from violations of basic necessities, that is, food, shelter, and separation from family, to personal rights violations, for example, sexual assault, human trafficking (Ferris & Paul, 2009).

    e. Engagement in the process of advocacy with the community to have basic and long-term health care services in place that is culturally congruent and appropriate.

V. PAIN MANAGEMENT BELIEFS AND PRACTICES

A. Historical Perspectives

  1. Early societies considered pain to be a result of magic and treated pain using ritual activities to ward off demons (Warfield, 1988).

  2. Early Hebrews considered pain and suffering a punishment form God, based on biblical interpretations (P. P. Raj, 1995).

  3. Ancient Egyptians thought pain resulted from spirits entering living bodies by way of the ears and nose (Bonica, 1990).

  4. Ancient Buddhists believed pain resulted from frustration of desires (Keele, 1957).

  5. Ancient Hindus thought pain originated from and was experienced in the heart (Warfield, 1988).

  6. Ancient Greek philosophers held that pain originated in the heart and began with increased sensitivity to touch (Warfield, 1988) or that pain resulted from a disequilibrium of the humors (Bonica, 1990).

  7. The Chinese believe that yin and yang forces maintain balance and vital energy (chi) in the body (Bonica, 1990).

    a. Within the beliefs of Taoism, pain occurs if Qi, or blood circulation, is blocked. Pain is relieved through removal of blockage removal and living in harmony with the universe.

    b. Within the beliefs of Buddhism, pain is a power that may only be removed by following the eight right ways.

    c. Within Confucian beliefs, pain is an essential element of life, a trial, and a sacrifice. A person will endure pain until it is intolerable (Chen, Miaskowski, Dodd, & Pantilat, 2008).

  8. Pain in ancient Mesoamerica was viewed as accepted, anticipated and a necessary part of life (Villarruel & Ortix de Montellano, 1991).

    a. The ability to endure pain and suffer stoically was valued.

    b. Pain and suffering were viewed as a consequence of immoral behavior.

    c. Pain management was aimed at maintaining balance within the person and the environment.

B. Definitions and Frequency

  1. The term *pain* is derived from the Latin word *poena* for penalty or punishment.

  2. Pain is subjective and "is whatever the experiencing person says it is, occurring whenever the experiencing person says it does" (McCaffery & Pasero, 1999).

    a. Pain perception cannot be defined simply in terms of a particular type of stimuli.

    b. Pain is a personal experience that depends on cultural learning, the meaning of the situation, and other factors unique to the individual.

  3. Pain is a private experience that is influenced by a variety of factors, as identified in Table 6.4 (Ludwig-Beymer, 2008).

  4. Melzack, a pioneer in pain research, states that "The neuromatrix theory of pain proposes that pain is a multidimensional experience produced by characteristic 'neurosignature' patterns of nerve impulses

Table 6.4. Factors That Affect the Expression of Pain

Factor	Explanation
Age	Biological and psychosocial factors influence elderly people's perceptions and experience of pain. Elderly people may believe that pain is a normal part of aging and should be tolerated, staff members are too busy to hear complaints of their pain, and telling nurses about pain may result in further testing and expenses. The elderly may also be resigned to pain, ambivalent about the benefits of pain relief, and reluctant to express pain (for further information, see Herr & Mobily, 1991; Hofland, 1992; Melding, 1991; Witte, 1989; Yates, Dewar, & Fentiman, 1995)
Cultural group	Patterned attitudes toward pain behavior exist in every culture, and appropriate and inappropriate expressions of pain are culturally prescribed. Cultural responses to pain can be divided into two categories: stoic and emotive. Patients who are stoic are less likely to express their pain, whereas emotive patients are more likely to verbalize the expressions of pain
Emotional factors	The perceived significance of pain affects response to pain
Family	Experiences and attitudes of one's family affect response to painful situation
Gender	Studies suggest that women tend to express distress and strain related to pain more openly and more often than men (Kleinman, 1988; Encandela, 1993; Lawlis, Achterberg, Kenner, & Kopetz, 1984)
Spirituality and religious heritage	Studies suggest that spiritually focused or strongly religious people find meaning and expression for their pain through religious doctrines (Encandela, 1993; Kotarba, 1983; Ohnuki-Tierney, 1984)

generated by a widely distributed neural network." The "output pattern is determined by multiple influences, of which the somatic sensory input is only a part . . ." (Melzack, 2005, p. 85).

5. Pain as an unpleasant sensory and emotional experience arising from actual or potential tissue damage or described in terms of such damage (U.S. Department of Health and Human Services, 1992).

6. The definition of pain is culturally influenced. Expectations about pain and its manifestations and management are embedded in a cultural context (Ludwig-Beymer, 2008).

7. Regardless of its definition, pain is a universal human experience (Villarruel, 1995).

8. Pain is one of the top three reasons for seeking health care (Chang, 2009).

   a. Using data from the United States National Health and Nutrition Examination Survey, Hardt, Jacobsen, Goldberg, Nickel, and Buchwald (2008) found that

      (1) Women had higher odds than men to report headache, abdominal pain, and chronic widespread pain

      (2) Mexican Americans had lower odds compared with non-Hispanic Whites and Blacks for chronic back pain, legs/feet pain, arms/hand pain, and regional and widespread pain

   b. According to a survey of adults in the United States, reported by Meghani and Cho (2009):

      (1) 75% reported experiencing "any type of pain"

      (2) 17% reported being diagnosed with chronic pain

      (3) Minorities reported a higher average amount of daily pain than Whites

   c. According to research conducted by Gureje, Von Korff, Simon, and Gater (1998) in 15 centers in Asia, Africa, Europe, and the Americas,

      (1) 22% of primary care patients reported persistent pain (range 5.5% to 33%)

      (2) Persistent pain was consistently associated with psychological illness across centers

   d. Pain management has been identified as a significant issue by regulatory and professional groups

      (1) The Joint Commission (The Joint Commission, 2009b)

         (a) Speak Up campaign

            i. Addresses what patients need to know about pain management

            ii. Includes sections on talking about pain and managing pain

         (b) Comprehensive Accreditation Manual for Hospitals (The Joint Commission, 2009a)

            i. Addresses pain management

            ii. Addresses patient education related to pain

      (2) The Anesthesia-Analgesia Organization recognizes pain management as a human right (Fishman, 2007)

      (3) Pain is considered the fifth vital sign (Quan, 2006)

C. Expressions of Pain

   1. The information below references research that has been conducted on pain expression and meaning. The list is not exhaustive and is not meant to stereotype groups. The information serves as a starting point; the clinician must take into account other key variables, such as age, gender, language, degree of acculturation, and other individual differences when planning and providing care (see Table 6.4)

2. Early research on pain (Zborowski, 1952 & 1969) suggested patterned responses to pain based on ethnicity and religion:
   a. Irish Americans—little emotion to pain, difficulty describing and talking about pain, deemphasis of pain, social withdrawal.
   b. Italian Americans—expressive when in pain, preferred company of others while in pain, requested relief of pain, generally satisfied when pain relieved.
   c. Jewish Americans—freely expressed pain, preferred company while in pain, sought relief from pain, skeptical and suspicious of pain, concerned about implications of pain.
   d. "Old Americans" (defined as third-generation Americans)—displayed little emotion, precise when defining pain, preferred to withdraw socially when in pain.
3. Neill (1993) found similar pain styles in men experiencing an acute myocardial infarction, with expressive pain responses demonstrated by Jewish and Italian men and stoic behaviors found in "Yankee" (American) and Irish men.
4. Responses to pain have been divided into two categories: stoic and emotive (Llewellyn, 2003).
   a. Stoic patients are less expressive about their pain and tend to withdraw socially. Stoic patients often have Northern European and Asian backgrounds.
   b. Emotive patients tend to verbalize expressions of pain and prefer people to be present to react to their pain and assist then through their suffering. Expressive patients often have Hispanic, Middle Eastern, and Mediterranean backgrounds.
5. Pain is often perceived by African Americans as a sign of illness or disease (Campinha-Bacote, 1998).
   a. Some African Americans believe that suffering and pain are inevitable and must be endured.
   b. Prayers are thought to free the person from suffering and pain.
6. For many Appalachians, pain is something to be endured and accepted stoically (Miles, 1975).
   a. During illness or pain, an individual expects to be cared for by others.
   b. Some believe that a knife or ax placed under the bed or mattress will help cut the pain (Purnell & Counts, 1998).
7. Research with Arab Americans suggests that the group views pain as unwelcome and unpleasant (Reizian & Meleis, 1986).
   a. Responses are aimed at avoiding painful situation and attending to pain immediately.
   b. Verbal expression of pain is appropriate, particularly with family members.
8. The Bariba of the Republic of Benin in Africa idealize stoicism in response to pain (Sargent, 1984).
9. Cardoso and Faleiros Sousa (2009) found that the words used to describe chronic pain by patients and health care providers in Brazil vary significantly.
10. Chinese tend to describe pain in terms of diverse body symptoms and use explanations of pain from the traditional Chinese perspective of imbalances in yin and yang (Moore, 1990).
11. For Cuban Americans, pain is a signal of a physical disturbance (Grossman, 1998).
    a. Pain requires consultation with a traditional or biomedical healer.
    b. Tend to be expressive in their pain, with verbal complaints, moaning, crying, and groaning as appropriate ways of dealing with pain.
12. Egyptians avoid pain and seek prompt relief and tend to be verbally and nonverbally expressive about pain.
    a. Pain is described in general terms, using metaphors such as earth, rocks, fire, heat, and cold (Reizian & Meleis, 1986).
    b. Children are expressive about pain (Meleis & Meleis, 1998).
    c. Childbirth pain is intense and having a female family member present provides care and comfort (Meleis & Sorrell, 1981).
13. Filipinos may appear stoic toward pain (Miranda, McBride, & Spangler, 1998).
    a. They view pain as part of living an honorable life
    b. Some view pain as a way to atone for past transgressions or reach a fuller spiritual life
14. Conflicting research exists with French Canadians.
    a. Choinière and Melzack (1987) found that French-speaking Canadians described pain as more intense and more affective than English-speaking Canadians.

b. Rukholm, Bailey, and Coutu-Wakulczyk (1991) found that English-speakers rated their distress at seeing a relative in pain higher than did French-speakers.

15. For Greek Americans, pain is the chief symptom of ill health (Tripp-Reimer & Sorofman, 1998).
    a. It needs to be immediately treated rather than endured.
    b. Family members are expected to find resources to relieve the pain or share the experience of suffering

16. Iranians are typically expressive of their pain, with men more stoic than women. Some use future rewards to justify their suffering (Lipson & Hafizi, 1998).

17. Research findings hold that Japanese Americans (Nissei):
    a. Often appear stoic in situations that are likely to cause pain due to cultural norms.
    b. Their norms suggest that one should have the ability to withstand discomfort and that expressions of pain indicate a weak character (Kagawa-Sincer, 1987).

18. For Jewish Americans, the verbalization of pain is acceptable and common (Fischel & Pinsker, 1992). Knowing the reason for the pain is as important as obtaining pain relief (Zborowski, 1969).

19. To many Mexican-Americans, good health is being pain free and bearing pain stoically because it is God's will (Condon, 1985). Research conducted by Villarruel and Ortix de Montellano (1991) suggests that Mexican Americans:
    a. experience more pain than other ethnic groups
    b. report pain less frequently
    c. endure it for longer periods
    d. tend to accept and anticipate pain as a necessary part of life
    e. endure pain
    f. suffer stoically
    g. seek methods to alleviate pain while maintaining balance within the person and environment
    h. pain and suffering are viewed as a consequence of immoral behavior
    i. pain is divinely predetermined

20. Navajo Indians view pain as something to endure. They may not request analgesics, using herbal medicine without the knowledge of the health care provider (Still & Hodgins, 1998).

21. Somali women express pain both verbally and nonverbally (Ness, 2009).

22. Vietnamese Americans view pain fatalistically, as a punishment.
    a. Pain is accepted as a part of life, and is managed with self-control and little expression of pain.
    b. The use of pain medication may be viewed as a sign of weakness and thus may be limited (Nguyen, 1985).
    c. The person in pain relies on family for care and attention (Calhoun, 1985).

23. Additional cross-cultural studies suggest:
    a. Research conducted by Sanders et al. (1992) found that among patients with chronic low back pain from 11 countries:
       (1) Mexican and New Zealander patients had fewer physical findings to explain the pain.
       (2) U.S., New Zealander, and Italian patients reported more impairment in psychsocial, recreational and work areas, with the U.S. patients most dysfunctional.
    b. Palmer et al. (2007) compared South Asians and Whites in the United Kingdom and found that
       (1) South Asians more commonly reported widespread pain and consultation rates for pain.
       (2) Increased acculturation was associated with decreased reporting of widespread pain.
    c. Hobara (2005) researched verbal and behavioral expressions of pain and found:
       (1) Japanese men and women considered pain expressive behavior less acceptable than did Euro Americans.
       (2) Both males and females were more accepting of pain expressions in females than in males.

D. **Pain Assessment**
   1. Pain assessment has three major objectives:
      a. Allow the clinician to understand what the patient is experiencing.
      b. Evaluate the effect the pain is having on the client.
      c. Determine the cause of the pain (Ludwig-Beymer, 2008).
   2. The emic (insider) perspective presents a true knowledge base for providing culturally congruent care (Leininger, 1991).
   3. Self-report is the single most reliable indicator of the existence and intensity of pain (National Institutes of Health, 1987).

4. Clinicians tend to use other, less reliable measures for assessing pain. McCaffery, Ferrell, and Pasero (2000) found that five of the six top factors identified by nurses as helpful in assessing pain were influenced by the patient's culture. The factors include
   a. facial expression
   b. position and movement
   c. vocalization
   d. request for relieve
   e. verbalization
5. Neither vital signs nor behavior can substitute for self-report of pain.
6. Clinicians must approach pain assessment as an important interaction with the client.
7. Davidhizar and Giger (2004) suggest the following strategies to assist in culturally appropriate assessment and management of pain:
   a. Use assessment tools to measure pain.
   b. Appreciate variations in affective response to pain.
   c. Be sensitive to variations in communication styles.
   d. Recognize that communication of pain may not be acceptable within a particular culture.
   e. Appreciate that the meaning of pain varies between cultures.
   f. Use knowledge of biological variations.
   g. Develop personal awareness of values and beliefs that may affect responses to pain.
8. The following questions may guide the nurse to discover individual and group perspectives on pain (Villarruel, 1995):
   a. What do you think caused the pain?
   b. What have others told you about the pain (what caused it, how it should be cared for, who can provide care)?
   c. How do you let others know you are in pain?
   d. What words do you use to describe your pain?
   e. How do you manage your pain at home? In the hospital? In other settings?
   f. Who do you turn to for help when you are in pain?
   g. What do you think should be done for you, by you and by others when you are in pain?
   h. When you experience pain, when do you ask for help? How do you ask for help?
   i. How do you think you should act when you are in pain? Is it the same for men, women and children?
9. A variety of pain assessment tools exist, as identified in Table 6.5.
10. While the tools are helpful, the most important aspect of pain assessment is to facilitate communication about what is being experienced.

E. Identifying Personal Attitudes Toward Pain
1. Crowley-Matoka, Saha, Dobscha, and Burgess (2009) suggest three key features of the biomedical culture that strongly affect pain management:
   a. Mind–body dualism
   b. A focus on disease versus illness
   c. A bias toward cure rather than care
2. Clinicians bring their own attitudes toward pain to each client interaction.
3. Research suggests that as a subculture, nurses have been socialized to certain pain expectations.
4. In research conducted by Im (2006), White women with cancer indicted that their pain was not taken seriously by health care providers and wanted to have control of their pain management process.
5. Clinicians must identify their personal beliefs about pain and suffering (Ludwig-Beymer, 2008). The questions below ask that the clinician think about the last time she or he experienced pain and may be helpful in identifying personal values and beliefs:
   a. Describe the pain.
   b. Did you want others to know about it?
   c. How did you respond to the pain?
   d. Did you want to be with others or alone?
   e. What treatments did you use for the pain?
   f. Did you worry about the pain?

Table 6.5. Pain Assessment Tools

Tool	Description
The Adolescent Pediatric Assessment Tool	The Adolescent Pediatric Assessment Tool, which takes about 20 minutes to complete, is a multidimensional self-reported pain assessment tool that includes a body outline, a word graphic rating scale, and a qualitative descriptive word list of 67 words representing sensory, affective, evaluative, and temporal dimensions of pain. It has been used effectively to assess complex pain such as sickle cell disease in children and adolescents (Crandell & Savedra, 2005)
The Brief Pain Inventory (BPI) tool	The Brief Pain Inventory (BPI) tool takes about 15 minutes to complete and is helpful when behavioral expressions for pain vary. It has been found to be reliable and valid in the United States (Zelman, Gore, Dukes, Tai & Brandenburg, 2005), Singapore (Cleeland & Ryan, 1994), France, the Philippines, and China (Cleeland et al., 1996)
Face Rating Scales	A number of face rating scales have been developed. The Oucher Scale (Villarruel & Denyes, 1991) allows children in pain to compare their pain intensity with pictures of children in pain. It is available in Caucasian, African American, and Hispanic versions (Beyer & Kuott, 1998). The Wong–Baker faces scale is available in Chinese, English, French, Italian, Portuguese, Romanian, Spanish, and Vietnamese. It has been used in children aged 3 years and older (Wong & Baker, 1988). One study suggests that African American children prefer the Faces Scale to the Oucher Scale (Luffy & Grove, 2003)
Numerical Rating Scale	This scale asks individuals to rate their pain on a scale of 0-5 or 0-10. The numerical rating scale correlates well with the visual analog scale (Cork, 2004; Ohnhaus & Adler, 1975) and the 0-10 scale is more precise than the 0-5 scale (Carpenter & Brockopp, 1995). The scale is widely used in clinical practice and can be easily administered to critically ill patients. It is available in Chinese, English, French, German, Greek, Hawaiian, Hebrew, Italian, Japanese, Korean, Pakistan, Polish, Russian, Samoan, Spanish, Tagalog, Tongan, and Vietnamese (McCaffery & Pasero, 1999). The scale may not be reliable when used with cognitively-impaired individuals (Kaasalainen & Crook, 2003)
The Visual Analog Scale (VAS)	This is a vertical or horizontal line with the words "no pain" on one end and "pain as bad as it can be" on the other end (Scott, 1976). Cultures that read from top to bottom or right to left will understand the vertical presentation, whereas those that read from left to right will be comfortable with the horizontal display

F. Pain Management

1. *Under treatment of pain* has been identified as a problem for many years (U.S. Department of Health and Human Services, 1992).

2. A 17-nation survey found that the majority of participants were dissatisfied with acute pain service for hospitalized surgical patients (Rawal, Allvin, and EuroPain Acute Pain Group, 1998).

3. There is still a tendency to under medicate for pain, even within hospice programs, both in the United States and in other countries.

   a. Studies show that 75% to 90% of cancer pain in terminally ill patients can be well controlled when the WHO approach is used: mean medication doses are as high as 30 milligrams of morphine every 4 hours.

   b. Appropriate doses are often not used.

4. *Barriers* to effective palliative care appear to be similar worldwide (Rhymes, 1996).

   a. A German-language study of treatment of cancer pain (cited in Rhymes, 1996) found that

      (1) Only 322 of 16,630 cancer patients received strong opiates.

      (2) Adjuvant therapy was rarely used.

      (3) Treatment for breakthrough pain was rarely given.

      (4) Health care professionals may be concerned about addiction and respiratory depression or may think that morphine is a drug only for those actively dying.

   b. Similar beliefs exist among patients and family members. A study conducted in Poland (cited in Rhymes, 1996) identified common lay myths, including the following beliefs:

      (1) Morphine is to be given only in the very last stages of disease

      (2) Morphine will cause addiction

      (3) If morphine is used too early there will be nothing stronger to use for pain relief later.

5. *Management of pain* needs to take into account the strategies the patient finds helpful.

   a. Im et al. (2009) found the following in patients with cancer:

Table 6.6. Pain Expectations in the Nursing Subculture

Expectations	Description
Ability to describe pain	Nurses expect people to be objective about the very subjective experience of pain. In clinical practice, nurses may expect a person experiencing pain to report it and give a detailed description of it, but to display few emotional responses to the pain
Pain minimization	Individuals who are in frequent contact with people in pain may minimize pain. Nurses may deny or downplay the pain they observe in others. Research suggests that the ethnic background of both the client and the nurses is an important determinant for inference of suffering caused by both physical and psychological distress. One study asked nurses from 13 countries to infer physical and psychologic pain for clients described in brief case studies. Nurses from these cultures differed markedly. Korean nurses inferred the highest level of psychologic distress, followed by Puerto Rican and Ugandan nurses. Nepalese, Taiwanese, and Belgian nurses inferred the least amount of psychological distress. Korean nurses also inferred the greatest amount of physical pain, followed by Japanese and Indian nurses. Nurses from Belgium, the United States, and England inferred the least amount of physical pain (for further information, see Acheson, 1988; E. Baer, Davitz, & Lieb, 1970; L. J. Davitz & Davitz, 1975; J. R. Davitz & Davitz, 1981; L. J. Davitz, Sameshima, & Davitz, 1976)
Silent suffering	Social customs and practices in society at large, particularly in health care, have been dominated by White Anglo-Saxon Protestants. Regardless of their ethnic backgrounds, most nurses have been somewhat influenced by these dominant values and beliefs. The majority of nurses in the United States and Canada are White, middle-class women who have been socialized to believe that self-control is better than open displays of strong feelings. Nurses may be socialized to place a high value on self-control in response to pain (for further information, see Acheson, 1988; Benoliel & Crowley, 1974; Howell, Butler, Vincent, Watt-Watson, & Stearns, 2000)

         (1) White patients were highly individualistic and focused on how to control their pain and the treatment selection process; they used diverse strategies for pain management.

         (2) Ethnic minority patients were family oriented and controlled pain by minimizing and normalizing it; they tried to maintain normal lives and used natural techniques for pain.

    b. Anie, Dasgupta, Ezenduka, Anarado, and Emodi (2007) found the following in patients with sickle cell disease:

         (1) Compared with Nigerians with sickle cell disease, patients in the United Kingdom experienced more pain episodes of longer duration and had more frequent visits to the emergency department.

         (2) Nigerian patients used psychologically active coping strategies such as distraction to deal with their pain.

    c. Kvarén and Johansson (2004) found the following in patients requiring physiotherapy:

         (1) Patients from Iran and Iraq reported higher levels of sensory and affective pain and pain intensity when compared with Swedish patients.

         (2) Swedish patients had stronger confidence that the physiotherapy was an effective treatment.

    d. Fenwick and Stevens (2004) found that Aboriginal women expect nurses to "see within" and "just know" about their pain and to provide care similar to that provided by their own traditional tribal healers

6. Several studies (Carpenter & Brockopp, 1995; Cohen, 1980; Rankin & Snider, 1984; Teske, Daut, & Cleeland, 1983) suggest that the nurses' perception of pain is not consistent with the patients' perspective. See Table 6.6.

7. Dudley and Holme (1984) found that nurses tended to infer more psychological than physical distress from pain, which may result in inappropriate interventions.

8. Griffin, Polit, and Byrne (2008) found that nurses perceived high levels of pain in pediatric research vignettes and indicated they would administer appropriate doses of analgesia and use other strategies to manage the pain in children, regardless of race/ethnicity, age, education, and experience.

9. Several research studies suggest that analgesia administration varies by race and ethnicity, that pain medications may be withheld from less vocal clients, and that interventions are affected by race and gender.

    a. Nurses limited analgesia for Whites, Hawaiians, and Asians, and gave significantly fewer analgesics to Japanese, Filipino, and Chinese patients who were the least vocal about pain (Streltzer & Wade, 1981).

    b. Nampiaparampil, Nampiaparampil, and Harden (2009) found that physician specialty, gender, ethnicity, and professional status significantly affected treatment plans, including analgesic prescriptions and referrals for invasive therapy.

10. *The race or ethnicity of patients affects pain management* in a variety of settings (Bonham, 2001; Cleeland, Gonin, Baez, Loehrer, & Pandya, 1997; Todd, Samaroo, & Hoffman, 1993).
   a. White males receive more interventions than women and minorities (Ang, Ibraham, Burant, & Kwoh, 2003; B. A. Taylor et al., 2005).
   b. Hispanic ethnicity and Medicaid insurance is strongly associated with nonuse of epidural analgesia in laboring women (Athertoon, Feeg, & El-Adham, 2004).
11. Some conflicting research exists.
   a. When responding to clinical vignettes, emergency department physicians developed similar treatment plans for pain management regardless of the race or ethnicity mentioned in the vignette (Tamayo-Sarver et al., 2003).
   b. A large survey of emergency department physicians found that opioids are less likely to be prescribed for Blacks when compared with Hispanics and Whites, particularly for migraines and back pain (Tamayo-Sarver, Hinze, Cydulka, & Baker, 2003).
   c. Type of analgesic received for pain from long-bone fractures was not associated with patient race or ethnicity in two academic urban emergency departments (Bijur, Bérard, Esses, Calderon, & Gallacher, 2008).
   d. Research suggests that the use of opioids to manage pain in the emergency department has increased, but differences in opioid prescribing by race/ethnicity have not diminished (Pletcher, Kertesz, Kohn, & Gonzales, 2008).
12. *Family presence*
   a. Clinicians often make assumptions about what patients and family members prefer.
   b. Jones, Qazi, & Young (2005) examined ethnic differences in parents' desire to remain present for venipuncture, laceration repair, lumbar puncture, fracture reduction, and critical resuscitation.
      (1) Overall, White, Black, and Hispanic parents (both English and Spanish speaking) wished to remain with their child.
      (2) English-speaking Hispanic parents were statistically significantly less likely to wish to remain during critical resuscitation and more likely to want physicians to decide whether they should be present.
      (3) Black parents were less likely to want physicians to decide whether they should be present.
      (4) Parents generally preferred to actively participate through coaching and soothing rather than simply observing.
   c. It is important to have this dialogue with patients and their family members.
13. *Ethnopharmacologic research* has identified significant differences in how people in diverse ethnic groups metabolize drugs (Munoz & Hilgenberg, 2005).
   a. Genetic variations may cause differing drug response.
   b. Considerable research has been conducted on psychotropic agents and antihypertensive agents.
   c. Additional discussion is found later in this chapter.
14. Evidence suggests that disparities in pain care continue to exist. Resources identified by Fan, Thomas, Deitrick, and Polomano (2008) and the author are summarized in Table 6.7.
G. **Complementary and Alternative Medicine (CAM) Practices for Pain Management**
   1. This section is designed to sensitize the clinician to the many options available to clients, as listed in Table 6.8, and to foster dialogue between the health care professional and the client.
   2. In CAM therapies, the connection between mind, body, and spirit is emphasized
      a. Many practices have been used for centuries in the management of pain, but the predominant biomedical system has adapted very few of these techniques.
      b. This has resulted in the growth of CAM.
   3. Research indicates that alternative therapies are being used.
      a. CAM use was reported by 42% of persons in both the United States and Canada in 1997 (Eisenberg et al., 2000; National Council for Reliable Health Information, 1998).
      b. Nearly 48% of Hispanic and Vietnamese elderly report using CAM over the past year, with most not informing their physicians of the use. Pain was the most common indicator for use of CAM in Hispanics (Najm, Reinsch, Hoehler, & Tobis, 2003).
      c. A total of 68.1% of Midwestern urban adolescents reported using one or more CAM therapies.
         (1) Most commonly, CAM was used by adolescents for alleviation of physical pain.
         (2) Very few adolescents disclosed their use to health care providers (Braun, Bearinger, Halcón, & Pettingell, 2005).

Table 6.7. Web-Based Resources to Assist Health Care Providers in Overcoming Pain Disparities

Site	Content
Agency for Healthcare Research and Quality: http://www.ahrq.gov	Sections of the website are devoted to specific populations Supports Excellence Centers to Eliminate Ethnic/Racial Disparities (EXCEED) Houses National Healthcare Disparity Report
Alliance of State Pain Initiatives: http://aspi.wisc.edu	Provides support for clinician education, patient education, outreach, and advocacy to address undertreatment of pain
American Academy of Pain Medicine: http://www.painmed.org	Demonstrates strong advocacy for pain treatment, including appropriate use of opioids for chronic pain Annual meeting topics include access to care, racial and ethnic disparities, and care of vulnerable populations
American Cancer Society: http://www.cancer.org	Provides pain information to health care providers and consumers Addresses existing disparities in pain management
American Medical Association: http://www.ama-assn.org	Houses continuing medical education on pain management, including a section "Racial and Ethnic Considerations in Pain Management"
American Pain Foundation: http://www.painfoundation.org	Provides information, advocacy, and support to people in pain and strives to remove barriers and increase access to effective pain management
American Pain Society: http://www.ampainsoc.org	Provides advocacy through the Pain Care Coalition Has a pain advocacy position statement: "Racial and Ethnic Identifiers in Pain Management: The Importance to Research, Clinical Practice, and Public Health Policy" Includes a special interest group on pain and disparities
American Society for Pain Management Nursing: http://www.aspmn.org	Has developed multiple position papers on pain management Developed Core Curriculum for pain management nursing, which includes content on culture and pain
California Health Care Foundation: California Healthline: http://www.californiahealthline.org	Mission of California Health Care Foundation is to "expand access to affordable, quality health care for underserved individuals and communities and to promote fundamental improvements" Website provides information on health disparities and disparities related to pain management
CultureMed: http://cuituremed.binghamton.edu; https://culturedmed.binghamton.edu/index.php/bibliographies-by-cultural-aspect/ethnopharmacology	Mission is to facilitate the provision of culturally competent health care to refugees and immigrants worldwide Extensive bibliography on culture and ethnopharmacology
Institute of Medicine: http://www.iom.edu	Although not specific to pain, has strong commitment to addressing racial and ethnic disparities and care for the underserved and uninsured Committee of volunteer scientists conducted the study "Unequal Treatment: Confronting Racial and Ethnic Disparities in Health Care," which found that U.S. racial and ethnic minorities are less likely to receive routine medical procedures
International Association for the Study of Pain: http://www.iasp-pain.org	Founded in 1973, has more than 6,500 members from 123 countries Brings together scientists, health care providers, and policy makers to support the study of pain and translate that knowledge into improved pain relief worldwide November 2009 focus was on opioid use
Intercultural Cancer Council: http://iccnetwork.org	Provides information for both health care providers and consumers, focused on pain, clinical assessment, disparities, and communication
National Guideline Clearinghouse: http://www.guideline.gov	Sponsored by Agency for Healthcare Research and Quality Provides guidelines that include recommendations and evidence
National Pain Foundation: http://www.painconnection.org	Advocates for people with pain Provides knowledge and education Raises awareness of disparities through brief reports on pain and race/ethnicity, pain and socioeconomic status, and disparities in pain Provides monitored online support groups for people experiencing pain

Table 6.8. Complementary and Alternative Methods of Pain Control

Modality	Description
Acupressure	Acupressure involves a deep-pressure massage of the appropriate acupoints. Shiatsu is the most widely known form of acupressure, used in Japan for more than 1,000 years to treat pain and illness and maintain general health (for more information, see Novey, 2000)
Acupuncture	Acupuncture, practiced for at least 3,000 years, is a method of preventing, diagnosing, and treating pain and disease by the skilled insertion of special needles into the body at designated locations and at various depths and angles. According to Chinese thought, life energy, or *ch'i*, constantly flows and energizes humans through a pattern known as meridians. *Ch'i* may be intercepted at various acupoints throughout the body. Acupuncture has been used as an alternative to other forms of analgesia for many minor surgical procedures in China. It has also been used in the treatment of pain in a variety of other countries. There are no simple explanations for the mechanisms that underlie the analgesia-producing effects of acupuncture. However, research has documented the release of endorphins into the vascular system during acupuncture, contributing to pain relief (Novey, 2000)
Alexander technique	This is based on the belief that tension restricts movement and tightens the body. An Alexander technique teacher works to restore freedom of movement and enhance body awareness by applying subtle adjustments in posture and alignment (see Novey, 2000)
Aromatherapy	Aromatherapy may take a variety of forms, including aesthetic (aromas used for pleasure), holistic (aromatherapy used for general stress), environmental fragrancing (aromas used to manipulate mood), and clinical (essential oils used for specific measurable outcomes). Aromatherapy has been used in pain management to enhance strong analgesics. The specific essential oils used are based on the type of pain (see Novey, 2000)
Autogenic training	This emphasizes passive attention to the body. The training, which was first recognized within the biomedical model in 1910, incorporates elements of hypnotism, spiritualism, and various yogic disciplines (see Luthe & Schultz, 1969, for specific meditative exercises)
Benson's relaxation response	Relaxation is achieved through six basic steps: sit quietly, close eyes, deeply relax all muscles, breathe through nose, continue for 20 minutes, allow relaxation to occur at its own pace (for further information, see Benson, 1976)
Biofeedback	Biofeedback techniques use instrumentation to provide a client with information about changes in bodily functions of which the person is usually unaware. Clients are taught to manipulate and control their degree of relaxation and tension by way of biofeedback training using electroencephalography (EEG) or electromyogram (EMG) muscle potential
Craniosacral therapy	This manual procedure is used to remedy distortions in the structure and function of the brain, spinal cord, skull, and sacrum. It is used to treat chronic pain and migraine headaches (see Novey, 2000)
Cutaneous stimulation	This reduces the intensity of pain or makes the pain more bearable. Types of cutaneous stimulation for pain relief include massage/pressure, vibration, heat or cold application, topical application, and transcutaneous electrical nerve stimulation (TENS). Stimulation need not be applied directly to the painful site to be effective (McCaffery, 1990)
Distraction	Distraction from pain is a kind of sensory shielding in which one is protected from the pain sensation by focusing on and increasing the clarity of sensations unrelated to the pain. Research suggests that distraction techniques, like pain, may be a cultural phenomenon. Clinical and research findings suggest that distraction may be a potent method of pain relief, usually by increasing the client's tolerance for pain by placing pain at the periphery of awareness. Distraction techniques include watching television, listening to music, reading, telling jokes, walking, playing with pets, crocheting, doing housework, interacting with children, animal-assisted therapy, and getting out of the house. Distraction appears to place the pain at the periphery of awareness (for further information, see Kaplan & Ludwig-Beymer, 2005; McCaffery, 1990; Miller, Hickman, & Lemasters, 1992; Zadinsky & Boyle, 1996)
Herbal remedies	Herbal treatments have been used in many cultures for centuries. Although adherence to herbalism diminished in the West, interest is currently increasing, as exemplified by the popularity of herbal teas. Many of the herbs used have a physiologic effect and must be understood by the health care professional (for additional details, see Novey, 2000)
Hypnosis	This technique was introduced into Western medical practice in the 18th century by Franz Anton Mesmer. A hypnotic state may be induced either by a hypnotist or by the client (autohypnosis). Hypnosis is based on the power of suggestion and the process of focusing attention. It has been used as an adjunct to other pain-relieving therapies and has been found to be helpful in dentistry, surgery, and childbirth as well as malignancies
Imagery	Imagery techniques for physical healing date back hundreds of years. Guided imagery involves using one's imagination to develop sensory images that decrease the intensity of pain or that become a nonpainful or pleasant substitute for pain. During guided imagery the client is alert, concentrating intensely and imagining sensory images. Research suggests that pleasant imagery can effectively reduce the perception of postsurgical pain. Music therapy is being used with increased frequency to augment imagery and other relaxation techniques (for further information, see McCaffery & Pasero, 1999; Novey 2000)
Progressive relaxation	Originated by Jacobson (1964), this is probably the most widely used relaxation technique today. The method teaches the client to concentrate on various gross muscle groups in the body by first tensing and then relaxing each group

(continued)

Table 6.8. (continued)

Modality	Description
Reiki therapy	"Reiki" is a Japanese word meaning life energy. In this therapy, a Reiki master or Reiki practitioner uses hands to effect healing (see http://www.holistic-online.com/Reiki/hol_Reiki_home.htm)
Relaxation techniques	Many relaxation techniques result in physiologic changes that reduce the damaging effects of stress and promote a sense of physical, mental, and spiritual well-being. All these techniques result in an altered state of consciousness and produce a decrease in sympathetic nervous system activity. Each technique requires a calm and quiet environment, a comfortable position, a mental device or image, and a willingness to let relaxation happen
Religious rituals	Prayer is more often reported as coping mechanisms in African American and Hispanics (Ang, Ibrahim, Burant, Siminoff, & Kwoh, 2002; Edwards, Moric, Husfeldt, Buvanendran, & Ivankovish, 2005; Hastie, Riley & Fillingim, 2004); prayer/hoping and diverting attention is used as a coping technique more often with Blacks than with Whites (Jordan, Lumley, & Leisen, 1998); and religion is a major source of coping for those with sickle cell disease (Harrison, Edwards, Koenig, Bosworth, Decastro & Wood, 2005; Strickland, Jackson, Gilead, McGuire, & Quarles, 2001). This finding holds true in Muslim as well as Christian patients. Voigtman (2002) found that religious precepts derived from Islamic teaching support tolerance for pain and suffering, and seeking cure. Clients should be encouraged to use their religious practices as they desire, to help in pain management. Privacy should be provided as needed. Prayer, chanting, songs, amulets, and charms should be respected and incorporated into the care provided. Christianity has included the notion of healing through divine intervention since its inception. Roman Catholic clients in pain may wish to pray the rosary or attend mass. Clients of many Christian denominations may actively seek healing through prayer and other rituals. Jewish clients experiencing pain may ask to speak to a rabbi. In other faith traditions, a shaman may conduct a religious ritual for the purpose of healing or pain relief. In this context, the illness or pain is viewed as a disorder of the total person, involving all parts of the individual as well as relationships to others. Working with client, family members, and others, the shaman focuses on strengthening or stimulating the client's own natural healing powers
Trager	Practitioners move the client's trunk and limbs in a gently rhythmic way. These noninvasive movements help to release physical and mental patterns, allowing the recipient to experience new sensations of freedom and lightness (see Novey, 2000)
Transcendental meditation	This type of meditation is taught individually, involves the use of a specific mantra during the meditation, and was originally developed by the Maharishi Mahesh Yogi, an Indian scholar and teacher
Yoga	Yoga techniques have been used within the Hindu culture for thousands of years. Yoga involves the practice of both physical exercise (hatha yoga) and meditation (raja yoga). The correct performance of yoga results in deep relaxation without drowsiness or sleep

    d. According to data derived from the United States National Health Interview Survey, 80.9% of women with female-specific cancer used CAM therapies (Eschiti, 2007)

4. Patients are turning to CAM for several reasons, which include the following:
    a. Frustration with conventional medicine
    b. Increasing evidence of the influence of lifestyle, nutrition, and emotions on disease
    c. Expectations of wellness rather than just the absence of symptoms
    d. The desire to take less medication and decrease health costs
    e. Increasing awareness of other cultures and their practices

5. A Health Forum survey suggests that 37% of acute care hospitals offer one or more CAM therapy. The primary rationale for offering CAM services was patient demand (84%) followed by clinical effectiveness (67%; Allen & Fenwick, 2008). Many of these hospitals use relaxation, hypnosis, acupuncture, and acupressure to help patients reduce their need for pain medication.

6. Clinicians are being encouraged to consider CAM therapies as they manage care (Ang-Lee, Moss, & Yuan, 2001; Novey, 2000).

7. The culturally competent nurse talks with patients about their use of CAM therapies.
    a. To begin dialogue, the nurse might simply ask what the patient is doing to reduce pain or improve health.
    b. As the patient identifies the use of CAM therapies, the nurse can explore areas such as the following:
        (1) The safety and effectiveness of the therapy
        (2) The experience of the practitioner
        (3) The cost of therapy (most patients must pay for CAM therapies themselves because they are typically not covered by insurance)
        (4) The benefits and risks of therapy
        (5) Other activities, therapies, or medications to be avoided during the CAM therapy

H. Summary
1. Pain has been experienced throughout the ages.
    a. People define, express, cope with, and manage pain in a variety of ways.
    b. Sophisticated pharmacologic interventions do not necessarily relieve pain,
2. Culture is a major influence in this process.
    a. Culture helps determine the innermost feelings of the individual.
    b. According to Mead (1934), the behavior of an individual may be understood only in terms of the behavior of the whole social group of which he or she is a member.
    c. Nurses encounter clients experiencing pain in virtually every clinical setting and provide care for people from a variety of cultural backgrounds.
    d. Recognizing cultural differences in beliefs about pain and suffering, and cultural views about appropriate responses to pain, can prevent misunderstanding and lead to the delivery of culturally competent care.
    e. Evidence-based practice is defined as the integration of best research evidence with clinical expertise and patient values (Sackett, Straus, Richardson, Rosenberg, & Haynes, 2000).
    f. Only through the use of evidence-based practice will nurses provide culturally congruent or culturally competent care.
    g. Understanding cultural similarities and differences will prevent problems with stereotyping, miscommunication, and interpersonal stress; and will result in adequate pain control (Al-Atiyyat, 2009).

VI. NUTRITIONAL PRACTICES
A. Introduction
1. *What do Americans eat?*
    a. Eggs/cereal for breakfast, sandwiches/salads for lunch, and meat and potatoes for dinner is what many would say.
    b. But in reality, our food habits are as diverse as our population and demand for ethnic foods is growing.
    c. Today a fast food restaurant is just as likely to offer pizza, egg rolls, and tacos as hamburgers and French fries.
    d. The American food fare is a mix of old and new, traditional and innovative foods.
2. *Definition*
    a. Food is defined as any substance that provides the nutrients necessary for growth and maintenance of life when usually ingested (Kittler & Sucher, 2007).
    b. However, we do not eat nutrients.
    c. We eat food/ingredients transformed by cooking.
    d. Health professionals must be aware how culture influences what we eat.

B. Diet and the Food Culture
1. Food culture, or cultural food habits, is the term used to describe the nonnutritive significance of food, such as
    a. When food is eaten
    b. Who grows, purchases, prepares, and serves food
    c. Who eats the food (Kittler & Sucher, 2007)
2. Food culture also includes
    a. The way foods are flavored
    b. Which foods are considered edible or inedible
    c. How often certain food items are eaten
    d. Pairing of foods (like French fries and ketchup)
    e. Additional factors that affect a client's food choices, such as cost, availability, personal preference, and so on.
3. Manifestations of food culture are reflected in the composition of the meal and the meal cycle (daily, weekly, and yearly).

C. Core/Complementary Foods (Passim & Bennett, 1943).
1. *Foods can be grouped by frequency of consumption.*
    a. Food eaten everyday are "core foods" and are commonly complex carbohydrates, such as rice for many Asian cultures and rice, beans and tortillas for Mexicans.
    b. Secondary foods are eaten several times a week
    c. Peripheral foods are eaten just occasionally, such as tamales for Mexicans.

2. *Nutrition therapy*
   a. It is difficult for individuals to eliminate core foods from their diet but the *quantity* can be modified.
   b. Modifying serving sizes of carbohydrate core foods are especially important for clients with Type 2 diabetes. For Asians this would be rice and noodles; for Mexicans—rice, beans, and tortillas; and for South Asians—rice and bread products, such as chapattis.

3. *Flavor principles* (E. Rozin, 2005)
   a. Food flavor has significant impact on how foods are prepared and seasoned and are usually associated with cultural core foods. Salt is one of the most widely used seasoning. Examples of three cultural flavor principles are
      (1) South Asians: *garam masala* (curry blend of spices, for example, coriander, cumin, fenugreek, turmeric, black pepper, cayenne, cloves, cardamom, cinnamon, chili peppers)
      (2) Chinese: soy sauce, rice wine, and ginger root
      (3) Vietnamese: *nuoc mam* (fermented fish sauce common throughout Southeast Asia countries)
   b. As with core foods, it is difficult to eliminate an ingredient that is culturally important for flavoring the dish/meal, such as soy sauce but it can be modified by decreasing the quantity or using the low sodium variety. This would be important for an Asian American with hypertension.

D. **Edible/Inedible Foods** (Lowenberg, 1970).
   1. *Early food habit model*, which classifies foods and food appropriateness in a culture by:
      a. *Inedible foods*—food are poisonous or not eaten because of strong beliefs or taboos (e.g., poison mushrooms, worldwide or in the United States; dogs and rats, both of which are eaten in several Asian countries)
      b. *Edible by animals*, but not by humans (e.g., horse meat in the United States)
      c. *Edible by humans*, but not one's own cultural group, for example,
         (1) blood sausage is eaten in Europe and Mexico but not common in the United States
         (2) liver is a good examples of food that is eaten by Americans but not by everyone
      d. *Edible by one's own cultural group*—Dietary recommendation should be modified for an individual's food choices and not based on ethnic stereotypes
   2. *Nutrition therapy*
      a. Do not assume an ethnic client does or does not eat certain culturally based foods. It is important to assess dietary habits before recommending modifications.
      b. Only modify diet components that can affect the client's health/treatment. If unfamiliar with a food item, research it before making a recommendation.
      c. Ethnic clients may be curious about "American" foods. Do not assume they may or may not want to try them.

E. **Manifestation of Food Culture**
   1. *Meal and meal cycle* (Douglas, 1972).
      a. *Meals*—the elements that make up the meal; food appropriateness, serving order, portion size.
         (1) Typically, Americans eat three meals a day plus one snack, the elements for dinner/supper are usually meat, starch, and vegetable, with the soup and/or salad served before the entrée.
         (2) A tuna fish sandwich would not usually be an appropriate item for an American breakfast.
         (3) One cup of rice would be an acceptable portion size in the United States, for many Asians this would not be considered enough.
      b. *Meal cycle*—each culture has a daily cycle (e.g., breakfast, lunch, and dinner), a weekly cycle (weekday and weekend), and yearly cycle which include holidays/religious days that include a feast or a fast.
         (1) Some cultures have a small breakfast, large mid-day meals, and a small evening meal.
         (2) Other cultures encourage a large breakfast, small lunch, and large evening meal.
         (3) One of the first changes seen with acculturation is adoption of the daily meal cycle, probably since employment dictates when you eat (Kittler & Sucher, 2007).
         (4) *Feasting*: secular (Christmas, Passover, etc.) and nonsecular (Thanksgiving, New Year, birthdays, etc.)
            (a) Typically, the elements of the normal meal are multiplied for a feast and special dishes with expensive ingredients are prepared.
            (b) It has been observed that traditional foods are also served at Thanksgiving along with the turkey, stuffing and other side dishes.

(5) *Fasting:* partial or total.
  (a) In some cases, it is the elimination of one item from the diet, such as meat on Fridays during Lent for Roman Catholics.
  (b) Moslems will not eat or drink from dawn to sunset during the month of Ramadan.
  (c). On Yom Kippur, observant Jews will not eat or drink for the entire day (sunset to sunset).

(6) *Social aspects of eating*—who eats the meal is important since it defines the boundaries of interpersonal relationships.
  (a) At one time it was common that doctors had their own dining room in hospitals.
  (b) Many cultures (Middle Eastern, Native Americans, and Mexican) will not refuse food or not finish all the food, even if they know they shouldn't eat it, since it would be disrespectful to the host.

2. *Consumer food choices:* The consumer food model explains factors influencing individual decisions about dietary choices, especially with acculturation (Drewnowski, 2002). Food selection is motivated by
  a. *Taste*—There is a physiological preference for salt, sweets, and fats. Although the desire for sweets diminishes with age, bitter/sour foods increases (coffee, citrus fruits, etc.; C. H. Anderson, 1995).
  b. *Cost* (Jetter & Cassady, 2005)—Many convenience foods are inexpensive, salty and fatty, which makes them very attractive to new immigrants as well as most Americans. Healthy foods, such as fruit and vegetables may be more expensive than convenience foods.
  c. *Convenience*—Not only obtaining food but also in the preparation of food. Takeout food is on the increase, especially for working couples with children.
  d. *Self-expression.* This reflects
   (1) cultural identity, often noticeable in recent immigrants, with acculturation usually occurring in subsequent generations;
   (2) adherence to religious-related food rules. Example of medically related religious food recommendations:
     (a) hypertensive observant Jews may need to reduce the use of some koshered meat since it is salted to remove remnants of blood and
     (b) Moslems with Type 2 diabetes may fast from sunrise to sunset during the month of Ramadan requiring adjustment of medications and carbohydrate intake.
   (3) regional food habits, such as grits in southern United States
   (4) self-identity
     (a) Many African Americans, even if not living the in the South have remnants of southern food habits—sweetened ice tea, ribs, ham hocks, greens, and sweet potato pie or peach cobbler.
     (b) Since they identify with Southern soul food, it is important to modify recipes to decrease calories and fat without changing its flavor (modified recipes can be found online at the Office of Minority Health Resource Center website).
   (5) Advertising—self-expression may be influenced by creating the desire for specific foods/restaurants (Lannon, 1986).
  e. *Variety*
   (1) The Omnivore's Paradox
     (a) Humans can consume a wide variety of plants and animals and we must be flexible to obtain necessary nutrients but cautious enough to prevent poisoning.
     (b) This leads to two contradictory impulses related to food choices: We are attracted to new foods but we have a preference for familiar foods (Fischler, 1998; P. Rozin, 1976).
   (2) Desire to try new foods but a preference for familiar foods.
     (a) One will try new foods that are similar to foods already known and liked.
     (b) Thus, for a new immigrant, many of the U.S. foods they might be willing to try are not necessarily that nutritious, such as sugary soda or fast food (both being tasty, convenient, and inexpensive).
     (c) Acculturation to the Western diet is thought to have increased the incidence of several chronic diseases (e.g., Type 2 diabetes, cardiovascular disease, hypertension) in the United Staes and the rest of the world.

3. *Food as a manifestation of physical and spiritual well-being*
  a. Physiological characteristics such as: age—culturally acceptable food items/physiology/preferences change through the lifespan as the ability to eat and digest foods changes (Birch, 1999).
  b. In many cultures, many elders prefer being overweight and is a visible sign of wealth (Crawford et al., 2001; Grivetti, 2001; Renzaho, 2004).

    c. Gender: In the United States, salads and yogurt are considered women's food, whereas steak and beer are for men. Interestingly, men are more likely to cook food outside (barbecue) the house whereas women primarily cook inside the house. Therefore, it may not be appropriate to ask a man to eat a salad for lunch.

    d. State of health

        (1) In many cultures, certain foods or combinations of food are eaten to prevent illness and treat disease, such as the balancing of yin/yang foods in many Asian cultures and hot/cold in Hispanic cultures (Chau, Lee, Tseng, & Downes, 1990; Kittler & Sucher, 2007).

            (a) Yin foods are considered cool, whereas Yang food are hot.

            (b) Dietary recommendations should not conflict with cultural food combination.

            (c) For example, in China, as the body "cools" with age, one needs to consume hot/yang foods, which tend to be high in calories, often fried in oil.

            (d) Therefore, reducing the serving size of fried foods and substituting lower caloric "hot" foods is recommended for weight loss.

        (2) Specific diets are recommended for pathophysiological conditions, such as, lactose intolerance, Type 2 diabetes mellitus, and so on (Nelms, Sucher, Lacey, & Roth, 2010).

            (a) People of color have a higher incidence of lactose intolerance and, of more concern, the growing rate of Type 2 diabetes (National Institute of Diabetes, Digestive, and Kidney Diseases, 2010).

            (b) For lactose intolerance, nondiary sources of calcium should be recommended if traditional food sources of calcium are no longer prepared (e.g., bones soaked in vinegar to make a sauce) or use of *lactase* products if dairy products are consumed.

            (c) Dietary recommendation for Type 2 diabetes can include traditional food but serving sizes usually need to be modified. In addition, educational material should be provided on the carbohydrate content of traditional foods.

            (d) Foods used during an illness may include chicken soup, used by many cultural groups, and congee (rice porridge) used by the Chinese.

  4. *Nutrition therapy*

    a. Dietary modifications should recognize the above influences on choice and that they may change as a person matures.

    b. Food selection in infants is based on taste factors while, children become more interested in self expression and peer pressure. (Appleton, Gentry, & Shepherd, 2006).

    c. Young adults continue to be concerned with taste and self expression but cost and convenience is added, especially in families with children.

    d. In most cultures, as individuals' age, well-being becomes more important and leads to healthier food choices.

  F. Summary. Recommended changes to the diet must be individualized, culturally appropriate and conform to traditional health beliefs as well.

VII. COMPLEMENTARY AND ALTERNATIVE THERAPIES

  A. Introduction

    1. *Complementary and alternative modalities* for preventing illness and treating disease are only "complementary" when we consider biomedicine as the "benchmark" or dominant form of medical care in the Western world (Loustaunau & Sobo, 1997).

    2. *Biomedicine*, also called conventional medicine in the United States, is practiced by biomedical providers, such as those with an MD (medical doctor) or DO (doctor of osteopathy) degree, as well as registered nurses, psychologists, and physical therapists, among others.

    3. *Complementary and alternative medicine* (CAM) is "a group of diverse medical and health care systems, practices, and products that are not presently considered to be part of conventional medicine" (National Center for Complementary and Alternative Medicine [NCCAM], NIH, 2010; http://nccam.nih.gov/health/whatiscam/).

  B. Definitions

    1. *Complementary therapy:* used *together with* biomedicine. For example, using hand massage to treat anxiety is a complement to pharmaceutical agents or psychotherapy (National Institutes of Health, n.d.)

    2. *Alternative therapy:* used *in place of* biomedical care. For example, using a special diet to treat cancer instead of radiation or chemotherapy (National Institutes of Health, n.d.).

    a. *CAM* is an acronym that means complementary and alternative medicine and is often used as a shorthand way of referring to both of these practices.

    b. A therapy may be used as a complementary therapy in one situation or for one person; the same therapy may be used as an alternative therapy for person or situation. The words are not interchangeable, but may be used interchangeably given the variability with which people employ CAM.

3. *Traditional healing systems*:

    a. Sometimes called "folk healing systems" (Chrisman, 1977) or

    b. "indigenous healing systems" (Freund & McGuire, 1999)

    c. A vast array of these systems have been documented around the globe, including in modern industrialized countries.

    d. Traditional healing practices are widespread, even among educated, fully acculturated, and economically secure persons.

    e. These include

        (1) Traditional Chinese medicine

        (2) Christian faith healing

        (3) Ayurveda is practiced in India

        (4) Santeria from the Caribbean

        (5) Mexican *curanderismo*

    f. Integrated traditional healing systems are often systematized and practiced by an eclectic group of practitioners (Freund & McGuire, 1999).

C. Prevalence and Place of Complementary/Alternative Healing Practices

1. Approximately 38% of adult Americans and 12% of children used some kind of alternative therapy in 2007, according to the National Health Survey (Barnes, Bloom, & Nahin, 2008).

2. CAM use may vary with illness condition, geography of residence, language use, and acculturation status

    a. Among patients with chronic pain in one clinical setting, 81% reporting current or previous use of CAM.

        (1) Most commonly, CAM treatments were massage therapy, spiritual healing, and vitamin and mineral supplements (Ho, Jones, & Gan, 2009).

        (2) There was no difference in CAM use by ethnic group

    b. *Curanderismo* is the predominant traditional healing system in the greater southwestern United States and parts of Latin America.

        (1) Approximately 5% of respondents in both convenience and population-based samples of Mexican Americans reported consulting a traditional healer or *curandero/a* in the previous year (Feldman, 2006).

        (2) Lifetime use of a *curandero* varies in published reports, ranging from 13% of adults to approximately 1/3 of Latinos in Texas

        (3) Spanish-language preference and less than 5 years residence in the United States were predictive of seeking care from *curanderos*.

3. CAM use across the life span

    a. CAM is used in childhood

        (1) In a small survey of Latinas in Houston, Texas, 20% of mothers had taken their children to a *curandero*.

        (2) A total of 39% believed a medical practitioner's medicine was more reliable and effective for most illnesses, and 31% believed that *curanderos*' medicine was more effective for treatment of folk illnesses (Risser & Mazur, 1995).

    b. CAM is used by older adults

        (1) In assisted living centers, 5% to 9% of older adult residents report ingesting some kind of herbal remedy (Moquin, Blackman, Mitty, & Flores, 2009).

        (2) Sometimes older adults select these themselves, or they are encouraged by family members who believe certain herbal preparations may prevent dementia or other conditions.

        (3) Older adults may hide "stashes" of herbal preparations in their rooms at an assisted living facility, unable to gain assistance in preparation or dosing by nurses, who cannot administer medications without a physician order.

D. What Are the Overall Safety Concerns About CAM? (see Table 6.9)

1. Delayed entry into treatment: by using an "alternative" to evidence-based biomedical care, delayed health care seeking may prove dangerous.

Table 6.9. Examples of Potentially Serious, Direct Adverse Effects Associated With Complementary and Alternative Medicine (CAM)

Therapy	Definition	Effectiveness	Adverse Effects (Examples)	Comment
Acupuncture	Insertion of a needle into special sites of the skin for therapeutic or preventative purposes	Positive evidence from systematic reviews of back pain, dental pain, idiopathic headache, nausea, and vomiting	Puncture of vital organs; infections	Adverse effects are rare with adequately trained therapists; deaths have been reported
Aromatherapy	Use of plant essences for therapeutic purposes	Probably reduces anxiety	Allergic reactions	Frequency of adverse effects depends on the nature of the oil used
Chelation therapy	Intravenous injection of EDTA	No evidence of effectiveness as used in CAM	Depletion of calcium and other minerals	Deaths have been reported
Chiropractic	Drug-free treatment with spinal manipulation to realign vertebral subluxations	Might be helpful for lower back pain but the evidence is unconvincing. For all other indications, the evidence is even less compelling	50% of patients experience minor adverse effects. Serious complications, such as vertebral arterial dissections occur in an unknown number of cases	Numerous cases of adverse effects have been reported; deaths have been reported
Traditional herbalism (including traditional Chinese medicine, Ayurveda)	Use of botanical preparations according to the individual characteristics of a patient	Only scant evidence exists for all types of traditional (individualized) herbalism	Intrinsic toxicity (e.g., liver damage), drug interactions, contamination with heavy metals	Nature of adverse effect caused by contaminants depends on contaminant
Herbalism and phytotherapy	The medical use of preparations that contain exclusively plant material	Some herbal medicines are supported by strong evidence (e.g., *Hypericum perforatum* for depression)	Intrinsic toxicity (e.g., liver damage), drug interactions	Frequency of adverse effect depends on remedy; deaths have been reported

Note: Data from Ernst, Pittler, and Wider, 2006. Adapted from Ernst (2007). "First, do no harm" with complementary and alternative medicine. *Trends in Pharmacological Sciences, 28*(2), 48-50. Reprinted with permission of Edzard Ernst, Complementary Medicine, Peninsula Medical School, Universities of Exeter and Plymouth, 25 Victoria Park Road, Exeter EX2 4NT, UK.

    a. Twenty cases of delayed or missed diagnoses in children occurred through consulting a chiropractor (Ernst, 2007).

    b. In cancer treatment, reported use of alternative medicine was associated with a significant delay in biomedical treatment (G. E. Davis et al., 2006).

  2. Vulnerable populations

    a. Remedies taken by women who are pregnant may have unknown consequences for fetal growth and development (Murphy, Kronenberg, & Wade, 1999).

    b. Remedies taken by children may have unanticipated toxic effects because of the immaturity of the liver in metabolizing these substances, and due to a potential for overdose due to the smaller body weight of children that may not be accounted for in certain kinds of remedy administration practices.

  3. Toxicities, substitutions, and wrong kinds of treatment (see section on plant-based medicine for more specifics).

  4. Advice against immunizations

    a. The majority of U.S. homeopaths do not recommend immunization and 9% openly oppose it (Ernst, 2007).

    b. Recent outbreaks of measles, pertussis, and other preventable communicable diseases can be linked to parental refusal of childhood immunizations.

  5. Lack of coordination among medical systems: In one study, three quarters of those who used an alternative therapy did not tell their primary care providers they were using complementary or alternative treatments (Eisenberg et al., 1993; Murphy et al., 1999).

E. History of Food and Fluids and Complementary Therapies

  1. Galen, an early Greek who followed Hippocrates' approach to humoral pathology, described food and fluid as two of the extrinsic factors that determine health and disease and to which human beings are exposed on a daily basis (Kay, 1982).

2. When ill or well, we must answer questions such as "What can she have? What must he have? What must he avoid?" What one eats from infancy through old age is to some degree culturally regulated and monitored (L. Clark, 2003).

3. In some cultures, food is sparingly administered in times of illness or pregnancy.
   a. American Indian women are urged to eat sparingly during pregnancy, and Mexican women are urged to avoid milk to prevent a large baby (Kay, 1982).
   b. In other societies, "eating for two" by consuming extra calories is encouraged (as in Egypt and Japan; Kay, 1982).

4. Across generations, cultural views of health and therapy guide the selection of complementary and alternative practices.

F. **Food and Fluids for Health Promotion, Disease Prevention, and Therapy**
   1. *Healing foods*
      a. What characterizes a "food" in times of sickness and health is culturally determined.
      b. What is considered a healing food may be determined by considering the nature of the disease in a biomedical, folk, or traditional system of disease classification, and then identifying the corresponding types of foods that can counteract the illness or restore balance to the ill person.
      c. Another way to determine a healing food is to consider what brings comfort or familiarity to the sick person, or what food will nourish (mentally, spiritually and/or physically) the person who is ill.
   2. *What is food?*
      a. What is considered "edible" varies among cultural groups, with some prizing horse flesh, others insects, and still others who are repulsed by foods like pork.
      b. Pica is the eating of nonfood substances (like dirt), and is common in various cultural groups, particularly among pregnant women (Kay, 1982).
   3. *Fasting*
      a. Cultural groups, particularly religious groups, may prescribe periods of fasting on a weekly, monthly, or annual basis.
      b. Fasting may be considered a healing intervention or a form of religious observance in the absence of illness (Andrews & Hanson, 2003; Lipson, Omidian, & Paul, 1997).
      c. For some groups, fasting is abstinence from both food and water.
      d. Others consider fasting to consist of refraining from certain kinds of foods, or from food eaten during certain times of the day.
      e. Assessing what fasting means and how it is implemented as a complementary healing strategy informs care planning related to nutritional intake.
   4. *Foods for daily consumption and health promotion*
      a. For certain cultural groups, a meal is not a meal unless it contains certain foods.
      b. For some families living in the rural Midwestern United States, dinner contains meat and potatoes.
      c. Chinese families may prepare rice for every meal.
      d. In addition to *kinds* of food, "cultural preferences [also] determine the style of food preparation and consumption, the frequency of eating, the time of eating, and eating utensils" (Boyle, 2003, p. 345).
   5. *Food avoidances*
      a. In contract to daily food preferences, food avoidances can be a daily pattern of learned behavior shared within an ethnic or cultural group.
      b. Lactose intolerance among some populations is linked to avoidance of milk products as a health promotion strategy (Boyle, 2003).
      c. Other groups may avoid protein sources (like insects or horse flesh) that may be preferred in other societies
   6. *Humoral systems* organize illnesses and prescribe certain kinds of food
      a. Minor health deviations, as well as major illnesses, are identified and treated with home-based remedies, including special foods and beverages.
      b. Cultural systems for classifying and understanding illness provide a framework for determining when and how to modify an ill person's diet.
         (1) *Hot and cold systems.*
            (a) A long-standing system in many parts of Latin America and derived from Greco-Roman concepts of humoral qualities.
            (b) Suggests that there are inherently "hot" diseases that should be treated with "cold" remedies, and inherently "cold" diseases that should be treated with "hot" remedies.

      (c) Asian, Middle Eastern, Caribbean, and Hispanic patients may be familiar with hot/cold balance (Galanti, 1997; Loustaunau & Sobo, 1997).

      (d) In some contexts, rather than counterbalancing the hot disease with cold or vice versa, the goal of treatment is to accentuate the hot or cold state.

      (e) For example, if the body is heating up to expel some toxin, further heating might help the body accomplish this task, further aiding recovery (Loustaunau & Sobo, 1997).

    (2) Examples of hot and cold states

      (a) Menstruation and childbirth are both considered hot states in many Latin American and Caribbean groups (Loustaunau & Sobo, 1997).

      (b) Diseases that include inflammation are often classified as "hot," and include sore throats and skin eruptions.

    (3) Foods to treat hot/cold imbalance

      (a) The qualities of the foods that treat these diseases are not based on temperature of the food, and their designation as "hot" or "cold" may appear arbitrary in different classification systems.

      (b) Honey, for example, is almost always "hot," whereas pork is by nature "cold" (Foster, 1994).

    (4) Evolution of hot/cold systems of classification

      (a) Anthropologic fieldwork suggests that hot/cold balance and the classification of diseases and foods in this system is no longer as common as it once was, and that the systems of different cultural groups classify the same items into "hot" or "cold" categories differently (Shutler, 1977; Urdaneta, Aguilar, Livingston, Gonzales-Bogran, & Kaye, 2001).

      (b) Assessing the classification scheme being used and the related treatment in a hot/cold system is important for caregivers who seek to provide the food and drink that is believed to aid, rather than forestall, healing.

      (c) Providing adequate nutrition within a hot/cold system of belief is possible with consultation by the patient and family.

7. *Sickness foods* or *comfort foods* culturally identified in times of illness and may have pathways of action amenable to scientific discovery

  a. Chicken soup as a prototypical sickness food

    (1) Many Americans are familiar with the idea of chicken soup feeding the depleted spirit of the ill person as well as the sick body (M. J. Clark, 1996).

    (2) Healing or comfort foods may include special drinks (a fizzy soft drink or juice) to remediate dehydration or a sodium and protein-rich soup (like chicken soup) to replenish nutrients.

  b. Scientific basis for sickness foods as a complementary form of care.

    (1) Rennard, Ertl, Gossman, Robbins, & Rennard (2000) conducted laboratory tests of homemade and commercial chicken soups and detected inhibition of neturophils in a concentration-dependent manner.

    (2) Findings in this study suggested beneficial medicinal effects of the ingredients and/or a mild anti-inflammatory effect of the soup.

  c. Transmission of cultural knowledge about sickness foods

    (1) Comfort food for an ill person is determined by families over time and is based on lay understandings of disease and care.

    (2) Sayings like "feed a cold and starve a fever" encapsulate folk beliefs about the relationship between nutrition and healing.

  d. Incorporating cultural assessment into sickness food clinical care

    (1) Assessing preferred illness and comfort foods and providing those to achieve hydration and caloric needs may be challenging given dietary restrictions.

    (2) Helping the patient attain psychological comfort through sickness foods or comfort foods is also a consideration in providing culturally competent care.

8. *Food preparation*

  a. Preparing food may be guided by cultural and religious preferences and prohibitions.

    (1) The Hebrew word kosher means "proper," and refers to the way slaughter animals should be killed.

    (2) "Many people think that 'kosher' refers to a type of food. If a patient asks for kosher food, it is important to determine what he or she means" (Andrews & Hanson, 2003, p. 485).

   b. Other cultural groups, including vegetarians, may adhere to individual or shared food preferences and patterns of avoidance.

   9. *Caregiving and Cultural Relationships established through Food and Feeding*

   a. How a parent or grandparent shows he or she cares about his family can be demonstrated through the provision and preparation of food.

   b. Food "expresses affection or friendship in every society" (Lipson & Steiger, 1996, p. 131). Families may wish to provide particular foods to a patient as a way of demonstrating their concern and care.

   c. The urge to show love and concern toward a family member who is feeling ill may over-ride prescribed dietary restrictions.

   d. Examples of parents "sneaking" favorite family foods to their loved one on a restricted diet abound, a reminder of the power of culture to shape both ideas about therapeutics and the enactment of cultural role obligations.

G. Plant-Based Remedies

   1. For certain ailments, particularly self-limiting or common problems, such as gastrointestinal upset, herbal teas may be recommended by mothers, grandmothers, midwives, traditional healers, herbalists, and others.

   2. Teas may be considered strengthening, soothing, or calming.

   3. Chamomile tea, for example, is a herbal tea recommended for its soothing gastrointestinal properties in many European, American Indian, and Mexican households (L. Clark, 2003; Mendelson, 2003).

   4. Anecdotal evidence reminds health care providers of the need to assess safety of even the most benign and common herbal teas. An American infant died of botulism that he contracted through chamomile tea. This is an example of a rare but nonetheless fatal encounter with an herbal remedy (Kemper, 1996).

   5. Locating evidence of plant-based remedy safety: Evidence-based care of those who prefer herbal teas as a complement or alternative to biomedical care includes consulting with a poison-control hotline or pharmacy about the active ingredients in an herbal product and interactions of herbally derived active ingredients with pharmaceutical products.

   a. Misperception of safety of plant-based remedies: Even though some mothers and traditional healers commonly use herbal teas, to the extent that such plant-based remedies contain pharmacologically active ingredients, they are not "safe" or "safer" than pharmaceuticals (Kay, 1996). Types of dangers (see Table 6.9; Medicines and Healthcare Products Regulatory Agency, 2008) include

   (1) toxic plants used, for example, *Senecio* species used in traditional Chinese medicine may cause liver cancer or toxicity.

   (2) side effects, as with any other medicine.

   (3) interactions with other medicines (St. John's Wort can interact with contraceptive pills and immunosuppressant medicines)

   (4) wrong plants may be used due to lack of expertise or intentional substitution in preparation

   (5) addition of analogues of pharmaceutical substances (sometimes of unknown toxicity) into herbal products

   b. Other health risks encountered by patients using plant-based remedies (Medicines and Healthcare Products Regulatory Agency, 2008) may include:

   (1) Delay in effective treatment, such as in the case where a traditional practitioner advertises that an herbal remedy will obviate the need for surgery.

   (2) Addition of heavy metals/toxic elements as ingredients. Both traditional Chinese and Ayurveda use heavy medals and other toxic elements as ingredients. These include arsenic and mercury compounds (Medicines and Healthcare Products Regulatory Agency, 2008).

   (3) Contamination during manufacturing processes with pesticides or microbes because of poorly controlled and inadequately monitored conditions.

   (4) Inaccurate or missing information in plant-based product labeling.

   (5) Communicative lapses in practitioner–patient interchanges because of language discordance and inability to determine patient's comorbidities or conditions, such as pregnancy or lactation, that might limit safety of herbal remedy prescription

H. Spiritual and Religious Care

   1. *Religious rituals* and personal religious observance can be viewed as promoting health, preventing disease, and aiming to heal those who are ill mentally, physically, or spiritually.

2. Care arising from religious or spiritual traditions is part of treatment for many patients as a complement or alternative to biomedical care.

3. Health promotion and prevention practices
   a. *Prayer*
      (1) Offering prayers, attending a religious service, displaying a shrine in one's home, or wearing a particular symbolic piece of clothing or jewelry are all examples of religious practice that may reaffirm a sense of religious belonging and harmony with the cosmos.
      (2) These daily or routine practices may be emphasized in response to illness or upheaval (Andrews & Hanson, 2003).
      (3) Prayer is the most commonly employed complementary and alternative healing strategy used in the United States, with 43% of adults reporting use of prayer in the past year for their own health and 24% reporting praying on behalf of others.
      (4) These two uses of prayer surpassed the use of all other complementary and alternative treatments, including natural products (18.9%), deep breathing exercises (11.6%), prayer groups (9.6%), meditation (7.6%), chiropractic care (7.5%), yoga (5.1%), massage (5.0%), and diet-based therapies (3.5%; Barnes, Powell-Griner, McFann, & Nahin, 2004).
   b. *Healing ceremonies for illness*
      (1) Ritual or folk healers across cultures tend to blur the distinctions biomedical providers make between physical and mental affliction. Healing ceremonies similarly seek to remedy illness and suffering with different etiologies and culturally specific nosologies or classifications (Csordas, Storck, & Strauss, 2008).
      (2) Healing ceremonies may include using a broom or egg to sweep away or draw away the evil causing disease, as in the case of *curanderismo* as practiced among Mexicans (Ceja-Zamarripa, 2007; Trotter & Chavira, 1997; Urdaneta et al., 2001).
      (3) Religiously based Christian healing ceremonies may involve the administration of rites or healing ceremonies by a priest or pastor. These may include the laying on of hands, anointing with holy oil, and the use of prayer clothes and aprons (Andrews & Hanson, 2003; H. Baer, 2001).
      (4) Navajo tribal practices may include a singer, who is able to cure through the power of song in a ceremony that may last from one to many days and nights (H. Baer, 2001; Still & Hodgins, 1998).
   c. *Biomedical inclusion of complementary healing ceremonies*
      (1) Research to evaluate the efficacy of complementary and alternative healing ceremonies is lacking. Despite this lack of evidence, biomedical health care systems have incorporated aspects of traditional healing ceremonies in care.
      (2) Burning sage, providing space for sand painting, or offering consultation from a medicine man are ways some facilities seek to provide a culturally competent integration of biomedical care with traditional healing ceremonies on the Navajo reservation.
      (3) A pilot study of sweat lodges used by American Indians indicated that participation resulted in improved well-being of participants in both spiritual and emotional domains (Schiff & Moore, 2006).

I. Energy Therapies

1. Foundations
   a. Energy field therapies are based on the "concept that human beings are infused with a subtle form of energy. This vital energy or life force is known under different names in different cultures" (National Institutes of Health, n.d.).
   b. Chinese medicine, with a history of more than 2,000 years, postulates that the flow and balance of life energies (or *qi*) are necessary for maintaining health. *Qi gong*, a Chinese practice, combines movement, meditation, and controlled breathing to improve blood flow and the flow of *qi* (National Institutes of Health, n.d.).

2. Disturbances in the energy field necessitate intervention
   a. Acupuncture, moxibustion, cupping, and coining, among other energy field treatments, all act by changing the energy flow within the individual (Spector, 2008).
   b. Acupuncture is described here as an exemplar of an energy field therapy.
      (1) *Acupuncture* is a traditional Chinese medicine technique in which thin needles are inserted into the skin then are manipulated by the hands of the practitioner or by electrical stimulation.

(2) Placement of the needles is guided by "meridians" and the assumption that certain meridians extend internally throughout the body in a fixed network.

(3) The way to treat internal problems is to puncture the meridians to restore a balance of yin and yang (Spector, 2008).

3. The scientific evidence for the efficacy of energy field treatments is not yet definitive for most forms of this therapy. However, a few limited studies have been conducted.

a. One recent study found that in the case of osteoarthritis of the knee, acupuncture, in addition to regular medical care, reduced the pain and functional impairment experienced by research subjects, in comparison to a sham acupuncture treatment and a treatment of self-help.

b. This study showed that acupuncture was an effective complement to conventional arthritis treatment (Berman et al., 2004).

J. Manipulative and Body-Based Practices

1. Foundations: The underlying focus of body-based practices is on the structures and systems of the body, including bones, joints, soft tissue, and the circulatory and lymphatic systems.

2. The body-based practices focus on self-regulation.

a. These different practices share the commonality that the body is self-regulating and that it has the ability to heal itself (National Institutes of Health, n.d.).

b. This category of alternative and complementary practices includes chiropractic and osteopathic manipulation, massage therapy, reflexology, and other types of therapies.

c. *Massage*, as one example, is the manipulation of soft tissue with some degree of friction, tension, motion, or vibration using the hands, arms, elbows, or a device.

3. The scientific evidence for the efficacy of manipulative and body-based practices is not yet definitive.

a. A recent study found that patients with advanced cancer who experienced massage over six weeks had lower pain intensity ratings immediately after the massage and improved mood compared to those who received only simple touch.

b. There is evidence that massage may have immediate beneficial effects in this circumstance (Kutner et al., 2008).

K. Mind–Body Medicine

1. Foundations

a. Mind–body medicine considers that interactions between the brain, mind, body, and behavior are powerful ways that health can be affected (National Institutes of Health, n.d.).

b. Enhancing the capacity for self-knowledge and self-care are techniques grounded in this approach.

2. Mind–body medicine focuses on interventions to promote health, such as yoga, relaxation, hypnosis, visual imagery, meditation, biofeedback, and other similar approaches.

3. The scientific evidence for mind–body medicine:

a. The effects of energy field treatments suggest that mechanisms in the brain and central nervous system influence immune, endocrine, and autonomic functioning.

b. Evidence suggests that multiple approaches to cancer, arthritis, and other chronic conditions may work together to decrease symptoms, speed recovery time, or decrease hospital days (National Institutes of Health, n.d.).

L. Cultural Preferences and Alternative Uses of Biomedical Therapies

1. Cultural preferences for different kinds of treatments shape the selection of particular therapeutic regimens (whether from a biomedical or alternative or complementary source)

2. Preferences for biomedical cures vary across cultures

a. *Injection versus oral delivery of medication*

(1) For some Mexican immigrants, selection of an injection over an oral form of a medication is preferred, as the "shot" is seen as more powerful and faster acting (L. Clark & Redman, 2007; Flaskerud & Nyamathi, 1999).

(2) What is believed to be the "best" or "strongest" medicine for a particular condition depends on the cultural evaluation of these treatments.

b. *Color and shape aspects of medications*

(1) Color of medication is important for people of many cultures, as color is associated with humoral properties.

(a) *Red*, for example, may be considered a *strong or "hot" medicine* in a humoral system, and not appropriate for children or women weakened by illness.

(b) Similarly, *blue* may be associated with *sleep*.

(c) *Yellow* may be associated with *malaria*. In Nigeria, malarial symptoms, including jaundiced sclera, are associated with a yellow-colored medication.

(2) A new program to administer age-appropriate dosing for adults and children was associated with yellow pills for adults and blue for children.

(3) This program was met with uncertain reactions from both medication vendors and community members, and education is needed to assure that symptoms and patient age, rather than pill color, are linked to the correct treatment (Brieger, Salami, & Oshiname, 2007).

3. Evolution and synthesis of complementary and alternative therapeutics

   a. Selection of complementary/alternative therapeutics is a matter of identity and social relations as well as treatment.

   As they [Kachitunos of Bolivia] discuss what they and their neighbors suffer from, and as they draw upon three medical traditions and resources, they are also saying something about themselves, the person they are talking to, and the person they are talking about. They are saying something as well about the social relationships between these individuals. (Crandon-Malamud, 1991, p. 31)

   b. There are indications that during the last half-century traditional complementary/alternative treatments are decreasing across the globe, from India to Latin America, as biomedical treatment is taking hold (Bentley, 1988; Browner, 1989; L. Clark, 1993; M. Clark, 1959).

   c. The ascendance of biomedical hegemony makes new combinations of therapeutic approaches possible.

      (1) Patients may combine a traditional therapeutic with a modern biomedical understanding of the body. For example, a woman described using a traditional plant-based purgative as "just like Draino," employing a mechanistic biomedical understanding of the body with traditional therapeutics.

      (2) Active resistance to the biomedical paradigm by patients who prefer a different, "more natural" approach to treatment. This may be an explanation for the increasing proportion of primarily affluent, White women who access CAM (Murphy et al., 1999).

      (3) The political and economic context of alternative therapies is an area still being explored, since culture is not the only factor in selecting a treatment for illness or misfortune.

      (4) Diabetes care, for example, is not rendered by traditional *curanderos* in barrios where popular discourses of "addiction" and "control" have replaced traditional cosmologies (L. Clark, Vincent, Zimmer, & Sanchez, 2009).

M. Economics of CAM

1. Economics for Practitioners of CAM

2. Economics for Patients who use CAM

   a. For patients with chronic pain, the amount of money spent on prescription medication was $114 ± 222 whereas the amount spent on CAM was $62 ± 96.

   b. CAM was less expensive if used alone, but patients who used both CAM and prescription medication paid more than those who used only one or the other (Ho et al., 2009).

N. Current Recommendations for CAM Use

1. Assess safety

2. Assess efficacy

3. Translation into practice

   a. Biomedical providers, including nurses, may lack familiarity with scientific research about effective CAM therapies. Even if they are familiar with the outcomes of such studies, they may not apply findings to their practice (Tilburt et al., 2009).

   b. Less than half of the providers in a national survey were aware of two well-publicized and successful randomized controlled trials of CAM therapies for osteoarthritis of the knee. One study was an acupuncture trial, the other a glucosamine trial.

   c. The nature of the evidence—a randomized clinical trial, one's personal clinical experience, or patient preference—was viewed differentially by CAM and biomedical providers, signaling different values and familiarity with interpreting research literature.

   d. CAM may be translated into practice if clinicians become more aware of CAM scientific evidence and have opportunity to apply findings in their own practice.

VIII. ETHNOPHARMACOLOGY AND PHARMOCOGENETICS

A. **Definitions** (Kalow, 2006; Lesher, 2005; National Center for Biotechnology Information [NCBI], 2004; Nebert, 1999)

  1. Ethnopharmacology: Study of ethnic or raciogeographic origin effects on drug response

  2. Pharmacogenetics

   a. Study or clinical testing of genetic variation involved in drug metabolism

   b. Gives rise to differing response to drugs

   c. Considers one or at most a few genes of interest

   d. How inherited differences affect drug metabolism and response

  3. Pharmacogenomics

   a. Broader application of genomic technologies to new drug discovery

   b. Further characterization of older drugs

   c. Considers the entire genome

   d. How a person's genetic makeup affects drug behavior

   e. Study of the relationship between specific deoxyribonucleic acid (DNA) sequence variation and drug effect

  4. Difference between pharmacogenetics and pharmcogenomics, although distinct areas of study, is sometimes considered minor and the terms are often used interchangeably in the literature (Kalow, 2006; Lesher, 2005; Nebert, 1999; Sheffield & Phillimore, 2009).

B. **Adverse Drug Reactions:** Clinical drug trials are aimed at evaluating

  1. Safety (Phase I trials)

  2. Efficacy and toxicity (Phase II trials)

  3. Decreasing serious events caused by adverse drug reactions based on an individual's genetic profile.

C. **History of the Discipline** (Cavallari & Lam, 2008; Relling & Giacomini, 2006; Weber, 2008)

  1. Ethnic specificity

   a. During World War I, Marshall, Lynch, and Smith (1918) found that Blacks were more resistant than Whites to the blistering of skin by mustard gas.

   b. During the 1930s, ethnic studies of phenylthicarbamide taste sensitivity found a hereditary deficit in sensory perception.

   c. Showed the prevalence of nontasters in European populations (35% to 40%) was higher than in African subpopulations, Chinese, Japanese, South Amerinds, and Lapps (<10%; Weber, 1999).

   d. During the 1930s and 1940s, it was recognized that sudden hemolytic anemia induced by sulfanilamide and primaquine:

     (1) Occurred preferentially in Black males and other dark-skinned people.

     (2) Cause of this trait, G6PD (glucose-6-phosphate dehydrogenase) deficiency, was discovered in World War II.

  2. Pharmacogenetic history

   a. First observation of genetic variation in drug response occurred in the 1950s,

   b. Involved the muscle relaxant suxamethonium chloride [Anectine®, Quelicin®], and

   c. Drugs metabolized by *N*-acetyltransferase.

     (1) One in 3,500 Caucasians has less efficient variant of the enzyme butyrylcholinesterase, which metabolizes suxamethonium chloride.

     (2) As a result, drug's effect is prolonged with slow recovery from surgical paralysis.

  3. In 1959, Fredrich Vogel introduced the term *pharmacogenetics* (Vogel, 1959).

  4. In 1962, Kalow published a monograph revealing the potential significance of genetic variations to responses of a host of organisms (Kalow, 1962).

  5. In 1988, the U.S. Congress commissioned the Department of Energy and the National Institutes of Health to plan and implement the *Human Genome Project* (NCBI, 2004; National Human Genome Research Institute [NHGRI], 2009).

   a. Goal of the Human Genome Project:

     (1) To determine the entire sequence of the human genome.

     (2) The aim was to better understand the genetic contributions to disease susceptibility.

   b. Data from this project are in a freely accessible database operated by the National Center for Biotechnology Information [NCBI] (http://www.ncbi.nlm.nih.gov).

    c. Following completion of this project in 2003, the NHGRI announced its goal to develop genome-based approaches in predicting drug responses (Collins, Green, Guttmacher, & Guyer, 2003).

6. In 2005, the U.S. Food and Drug Association [FDA] approved the AmpliChip CYP450 test (http://www.roche.com).

    a. First pharmacogenetic test that determines a patient's ability to metabolize about 25% of all drugs, including many antidepressants and antipsychotics, specifically, genetic variations in the CYP2D6 and CYP2C19 enzymes (Medical Letter, 2005).

    b. Several other companies have developed similar tests.

      (1) Genelex (http://www.healthanddna.com/)

      (2) Luminex (http://www.luminexcorp.com; Cavallari, Ellingrod, & Kolesar, 2005; Cupp & Lesher, 2008).

7. *Current recommendations for genetic testing prior to prescribing* certain drugs in the United States, for example,

    a. Warfarin (Coumadin®),

    b. Carbamazepine (Tegretol®),

    c. Human immunodeficiency virus (HIV) treatment guidelines for the drug abacavir (Ziagen®; Cupp & Lesher, 2008; Sheffield & Phillimore, 2009; U.S. Department of Health and Human Services, 2008)

    d. In some countries, such as those in Europe, screening is mandatory before prescribing (Pirmohamed, 2009)

D. Genetic Definitions and Concepts (Cavallari & Lam, 2008; Jorde, 2006)

  1. Genes are composed of deoxyribonucleic acid (DNA), which has three components:

    a. A pentose sugar molecule, deoxyribose;

    b. A phosphate molecule; and

    c. Four type of nitrogenous bases.

  2. Two of the bases, cytosine and thymine are single carbon–nitrogen rings called pyrimidines;

  3. The other two bases, adenine and guanine are double carbon–nitrogen rings called purines

  4. The human genome contains approximately three billion purine and pyrimidine nucleotide bases that code for thousands of protein-coding genes. These bases are

    a. Adenine (A)

    b. Guanine (G)

    c. Cytosine (C)

    d. Thymidine (T)

  5. Nucleotide bases make up the structure of the DNA

  6. Pyrimidines and purines always pair together as

    a. Cytosine–guanine, and

    b. Adenine–thymidine in the two strands that make up the DNA structure

  7. Most nucleotide pairs are identical from person to person. *Only 0.1% contribute to individual differences* (Cavallari & Lam, 2008; Jorde, 2006; Kalow, 1999).

  8. When a strand of DNA is transcribed into ribonucleic acid (RNA) and translated to make proteins, three consecutive nucleotides form a *codon.*

    a. Each codon specifies an amino acid.

    b. *Amino acids* are the basic units for all proteins found in the human body.

  9. *A gene is a series of codons that specifies a particular protein.*

  10. In most cases, individuals carry one *allele* from each parent, at each gene locus.

  11. An *allele is the sequence of nucleic acid bases at a given gene chromosomal locus.*

  12. Two identical alleles make up a homozygous genotype.

  13. Two different alleles make up a heterozygous genotype.

  14. The outward expression of the genotype is referred to as the phenotype.

E. Types of Genetic Variation (Cavallari & Lam, 2008; Relling & Giacomini, 2006)

  1. *Genetic variation* occurs either as a

    a. rare defect or

    b. polymorphism

      (1) A locus that has two or more alleles that occur with an appreciable frequency in a population (Jorde, 2006) or

        (2) The existence of two or more variants, such as, alleles, sequence variants, chromosomal variants, that are nonpathogenic (Firth, Hurst, & Hall, 2005)
           (a) for example, common blood types such as the ABO system
           (b) sickle cell anemia

  2. Polymorphisms: Genetic variations occurring at a frequency of at least 1% in humans (Cavallari & Lam, 2006; Weber, 2008).

  3. Rare mutations occur in <1% of the population and are thought to cause inherited diseases, such as
    a. Huntington's disease,
    b. hemophilia, and
    c. cystic fibrosis.

  4. Snips, or *single nucleotide polymorphisms* (SNPs) are the most common genetic variations in human DNA.

  5. SNPs may change the codon, resulting in amino acid substitution that may or may not change the function or amount of the encoded protein.

F. Underlying Pharmacokinetic Principles (Gutierrez, 2008; Lehne, 2010; Weber, 2008)

  1. Definition and processes of pharmacokinetics
    a. Study of drug movement throughout the body
    b. Based on four major processes:
      (1) absorption,
      (2) distribution,
      (3) metabolism, and
      (4) excretion.

  2. These four processes, acting in concert, determine the concentration of a drug at its site of action.

  3. At each process, drugs pass across cell membranes by
    a. Passing through ion channels or pores,
    b. Passage with the aid of transport systems such as P-glycoprotein, and
    c. Direct penetration of the membrane itself.

  4. Pharmacogenetics may affect the response rate for each of the above four pharmacokinetic processes, whereby the processes may be
    a. accelerated,
    b. decreased, or
    c. inhibited—with the strongest evidence to date on the process of metabolism.

  5. Absorption
    a. Movement of a drug from its site of administration into the blood
    b. How a pill taken orally gets absorbed through the gastrointestinal tract and into the blood stream where the drug is carried to its site of action

  6. Distribution:
    a. Drug movement from the blood to the interstitial space of tissues and from there into the cells
    b. How the drug gets from the blood stream and penetrates the phospholipid layer of cells

  7. Metabolism
    a. Enzymatically mediated alteration of drug structure
    b. How the drug is broken down by metabolic enzymes into its active state
    c. Commonly takes place in the liver
      (1) Common metabolic enzymes are the hepatic microsomal enzyme system
      (2) Also known as the cytochrome P450 system
      (3) Active state stimulates drug receptors
      (4) Stimulation of receptor causes the anticipated drug response
    d. Drug metabolism results in six possible consequences of therapeutic significance, that is,
      (1) promotes drug elimination,
      (2) converts pharmacologically active compounds into inactive forms,
      (3) increases the effectiveness of some drugs,
      (4) converts products into active forms,
      (5) decreases drug toxicity, or
      (6) increases toxicity.
    e. Pharmacogenetics plays a major role in this pharmacokinetic process (Table 6.10).

8. *Excretion*
   a. Movement of drugs and their metabolites out of the body
   b. How the drug is eliminated by the kidneys into the urine
9. In contrast to the above pharmacokinetic interactions, *pharmacodynamic interactions* also occur.
   a. Most interactions are not clearly understood.
   b. Even though there is limited data available about specific ethnic group variations in pharmacodynamic interactions as there is in pharmacokinetic interactions, knowledge of pharmacodynamic interactions is still clinically significant (Lesher, 2005; Sheffield & Phillimore, 2009; Wilkinson, 2005; see Table 6.11)
      (1) For example, some women (not specifically from a distinct ethnic group) with metastatic breast cancer and a specific oncogene appear to derive the greatest benefit from trastuzumab (Herceptin®).
      (2) As a result, these women have a better clinical response to treatment, which includes disease-free and overall survival, than those without the oncogene.
10. However, genetic polymorphisms do occur in drug transporter genes such as in
    a. P-glycoprotein
    b. Drug target proteins, including
       (1) receptors,
       (2) enzymes,
       (3) ion channels and
       (4) intracellular signaling proteins.
          (a) For example, beta-1 (β_1) and beta-2 (β_2) adrenergic receptor genes have been shown to have polymorphisms in some individuals,
          (b) It is possible that certain persons who appear to be unresponsive to use of beta adrenergic medications (e.g., metoprolol [Lopressor®, Toprol-XL®]) in the treatment of their hypertension or asthma may actually have genetic polymorphic differences (Cavallari et al., 2005; Cavallari & Lam, 2008; Johnson & Terra, 2002; Litonjua, 2006).

G. Many genes have been associated with disease pathways and outcomes, and have been found to influence response to pharmacologic disease management (Table 6.12).
   1. This mechanism is the least understood.
   2. Mechanism is complicated by the fact that for many diseases, multiple genes affect the disease pathway.
      a. Limited data available about specific ethnic group variations in pharmacodynamic interactions (Lesher, 2005; Sheffield & Phillimore, 2009; Wilkinson, 2005)
      b. For example, oral contraceptive use in some women (not specifically associated with an ethnic group) is associated with an increased risk for the development of thromboembolic disorders, including
         (1) thrombotic stroke,
         (2) deep vein thrombosis, and
         (3) pulmonary embolism.
      c. Individuals who have been shown to have genetic variation with coagulation factors prothrombin and factor-V Leiden have been identified as being at an increased risk for the development of thromboembolic disorders and should use alternate forms of contraceptive measures (Cavallari & Lam, 2008; Martinelli, Battaglioli, & Mannucci, 2003).

H. **Polymorphisms in Drug-Metabolizing Enzymes** (Cavallari et al., 2005; Cavallari & Lam, 2008; Gonzalez & Tukey, 2006, Ingelman-Sundberg, Sim, Gomez, & Rodriguez-Antona, 2007; Lehne, 2010; Relling & Giacomini, 2006; Wilkinson, 2005; Zhou, 2009; see also Table 6.10)
   1. The first recognized and most documented examples of polymorphisms are in the cytochrome P450 (CYP450) superfamily of isoenzymes (also known as isozymes) that are responsible for the metabolism of drugs.
   2. *CYP450 enzymes reduce or alter the pharmacologic activity of many drugs* and facilitate their elimination.
   3. Individual cytochrome CYP450 enzymes are classified by their amino acid similarities, and are designated by
      a. a family number,
      b. a subfamily letter,
      c. a number for an individual enzyme within the subfamily, and
      d. an asterisks followed by a

Table 6.10. Examples of Genetic Polymorphisms (Pharmacokinetic Interactions) That Influence Drug Effects in Humans With Known Ethnopharmacologic Variability

Drug and/or Drug Class Affected	Specific Gene/Protein Involved	Observed Clinical Effect by Type of Drug Metabolizer		Frequency of Observed Clinical Effect Among Ethnic Groups	
		Poor Drug Metabolizers	Ultra-Rapid Drug Metabolizers	Poor Drug Metabolizers	Ultra-Rapid Drug Metabolizers
Antidepressants Antipsychotics Antiarrhythmics Atomoxetine (*Strattera*®)	CYP2D6	Greater likelihood of observing drug's known adverse reactions	Greater likelihood of treatment failure	Caucasians: 5%-10% Southeast Asians (Chinese, Japanese, Koreans): 1%-2% Kung San Bushmen: (Indigenous Black Africans from Southern Africa): 18.8%	Scandinavians: 1% Germans: 3.6% Spaniards: 10% Saudi Arabians: 20% Ethiopians: 39%
Codeine	CYP2D6	Greater likelihood of treatment failure	Greater likelihood of observing drug's known adverse reactions		
Beta-blockers	CYP2D6	Marked differences in plasma levels reported; clinical significance not currently known			
Tamoxifen (*Nolvadex*®)	CYP2D6	May have reduced response. If appropriate, consider an aromatase inhibitor (e.g., anastrozole [*Arimidex*]) instead			
Warfarin (*Coumadin*®) Tolbutamide (*Orinase*®) Glipizide (*Glucotrol*®) Phenytoin (*Dilantin*®)	CYP2C9	May exhibit toxic drug effects; testing recommended in U.S. product labeling for warfarin (*Coumadin*®)		"Ultra"-poor metabolizers Europeans: 0.2% to 1% Southeast Asians: relatively uncommon, close to 0%	
Proton pump inhibitors	CYP2C19	Marked differences in plasma levels reported Increased gastric and duodenal ulcer healing rates documented	Decreased gastric and duodenal ulcer healing rates documented	Caucasians: 2%-3% Blacks: 4% Southeast Asians: 10%-25%	

Note: Adapted from "Pharmacogenomic Examples" by Cupp and Lesher (2008), Pharmacogenomics. *Pharmacist's Letter/Prescriber's Letter*, 24(2): 240211. Copyright 2008 by Therapeutic Research Center. Reprinted with permission. Table is meant to be representative and not comprehensive. Ansell, Ackerman, Black, Roberts, and Tefferi (2003); Belle and Singh (2008); Bertilsson, Dahl, and Tybring (1997); Dervieux, Meshkin, and Neri (2005); Evans and Relling (2004); Goetz, Ames, and Weinshilboum (2004); Garber et al. (2005); Litman and Rosenberg (2005); Masimirembwa, Persson, Bertilsson, Hasler, and Ingelman-Sundberg (1996); Maitland-van der Zee, Klungel, and de Boer (2004); Wilkinson (2005).

Table 6.11. Pharmacogenetic Examples That May Affect Clinical Outcomes Either Pharmacokinetically or Pharmacodynamicaly, but Limited Ethnic Variation May Be Known

Drug and/or Drug Class Affected	Specific Gene/Protein Involved	Observed Clinical Effect	Frequency of Observed Clinical Effect
Mercaptopurine (*Purinethol®*) Thioguanine (*Tabloid*) Azathioprine (*Imuran®*)	Thiopurine methyltransferase (TPMT)	Patients with TPMT deficiency experience profound myelosuppression with normal doses	10% of population is heterozygous for polymorphism requiring dosage reduction of 10%-50% but can also be at risk for severe toxicity
Irinotecan (*Camptosar®*)	Uridine diphosphate glucuronosyl-transferase 1A1 (UGT1A1)	Patients with UGT1A1 deficiency are at an increased risk of developing severe toxicities, including gastrointestinal toxicities and neutropenia	Chinese: 16% Europeans: 40% East Indians: 40%
Imatinib (*Gleevec®*)	ber-abl tyrosine kinase	Administration to patients with chronic myeloid leukemia results in decreased proliferation and survival of leukemia cells	
Trastuzumab (*Herceptin®*)	HER2/neu oncogene	Administration to patients with tumor cells that overexpress HER2/neu results in decreased tumor cell proliferation	HER2/neu overexpressed in 25%-30% of primary breast cancers
Warfarin (*Coumadin®*)	VKORC1	Patients with variation in VKORC1 are relatively warfarin resistant; testing recommended in U.S. product labeling	Caucasians: 14% African Americans: 37% Asian: 89%
Fluorouracil Capecitabine (*Xeloda®*)	Dihydropyridine dehydrogenase (DPD)	Patients with DPD deficiency experience profound toxicity effects including life-threatening gastrointestinal toxicity, myelosuppression, and neurological toxicities	Caucasians: 0.9% Japanese, Taiwanese, African Americans with deficiency have not shown toxicities

Note: Adapted from "Pharmacogenomic Examples" by Cupp and Lesher (2008). Pharmacogenomics. *Pharmacist's Letter/Prescriber's Letter*, 24(2): 240211. Copyright 2008 by Therapeutic Research Center. Reprinted with permission. Table is meant to be representative and not comprehensive. Ansell, Ackerman, Black, Roberts, and Tefferi (2003); Belle and Singh (2008); Dervieux, Meshkin, and Neri (2005); Evans and Relling (2004); Goetz, Ames, and Weinshilboum (2004); Garber et al. (2005); Litman and Rosenberg (2005); Maitland-van der Zee, Klungel, and de Boer (2004); Wilkinson (2005).

  (1) number and
  (2) letter for each genetic (allelic) variant.
e. For example, CYP1A2*1K is
  (1) family 1;
  (2) subfamily A;
  (3) gene number 2 and
  (4) allelic (*) variation 1K (Gonzalez & Tukey, 2006; Zhou, 2009)
4. A total of 57 different CYP450 genes have been identified in humans
  a. Fifteen are known to be involved in the metabolism of drugs.
  b. Three of the encoded proteins dominate the metabolism of therapeutic drugs and toxicants:
    (1) CYP1,
    (2) CYP2, and
    (3) CYP3
5. The liver is the major site of cytochrome P450 mediated metabolism, but the enterocytes in the epithelium of the small intestine are also a potentially important site.
6. The variability in genes encoding drug metabolizing enzymes often affects outcome in drug treatment to a very high extent and the polymorphism of the cytochrome P450 enzymes plays a major role in this respect.

Table 6.12. Examples of Genetic Polymorphisms in Disease Treatment Modifying Genes That Alter Drug Response in Humans, However Specific Ethnic Variation May or May Not Be Known

Drug and/or Drug Class Affected	Disease Modifying Genes	Observed Clinical Effect	Frequency of Observed Effect
Abacavir (e.g., *Ziagen*®)	HLA-B*5701	Increased risk of hypersensitivity reactions; U.S. HIV guidelines recommend not prescribing for patients with this variant	Hypersensitivity reactions 114 times more common in patients with HLA-B*5701 allele
Allopurinol (*Zyloprim*®)	HLA-B*5801	Increased risk of hypersensitivity reactions	
Carbamazepine (e.g., *Tegretol*®)	HLA-B*1502	Increased risk of hypersensitivity reactions; testing recommended in U.S. labeling ("black box" warning for patients of Asian (e.g., Chinese, South Asian Indian) ancestry	Risk for serous dermatologic reaction to carbamazepine is 5% in patients with HLA-B* 1502 allele
Oral contraceptives	Factor-V Leiden	Increased incidence of deep vein and cerebral vein thrombosis	5% White North Americans
General anesthetics	Ryanodine receptor (RYR1)	Increased incidence of malignant hyperthermia in patients with a mutation in the gene for RYR1	Maturations found in 25% of individuals susceptible to malignant hyperthermia

Note: Adapted from "Pharmacogenomic Examples" by Cupp and Lesher (2008). Pharmacogenomics. *Pharmacist's Letter/Prescriber's Letter*, 24(2): 240211. Copyright 2008 by Therapeutic Research Center. Reprinted with permission. Table is meant to be representative and not comprehensive. Ansell, Ackerman, Black, Roberts, and Tefferi (2003); Belle and Singh (2008); Dervieux, Meshkin, and Neri (2005); Evans and Relling (2004); Goetz, Ames, and Weinshilboum (2004); Garber et al. (2005); Litman and Rosenberg (2005); Maitland-van der Zee, Klungel, and de Boer (2004); Wilkinson (2005).

7. Because of this variability, populations are classified into the following *phenotypes* (outward expression of genotypes)
   a. *Poor metabolizers* (PMs)
      (1) have a defective mutant gene for the isoenzyme,
      (2) cannot manufacture a fully functional isoenzyme,
      (3) cannot metabolize the drug substrate very well, and
      (4) may achieve toxic concentrations of the drug with usual doses or may fail to have any pharmacologic effect from the drug.
   b. *Extensive metabolizers* (EMs),
      (1) have the standard gene for the isoenzyme and
      (2) metabolize the drugs normally.
   c. *Ultra metabolizers* (UMs)
      (1) metabolize too quickly and
      (2) may not exhibit a drug response.
   d. *Intermediate metabolizers* (IMs)
      (1) metabolize too slowly and
      (2) may have an adverse effect
8. Poor metabolizers are usually a minority of the general population.
9. *Ethnic background can affect the likelihood that the individual will be a poor metabolizer* (Table 6.10).
   a. Examples
      (1) Incidence of poor metabolizers for CYP2D6 is approximately 5% to 10% for Whites, and approximately 0% to 1% for Asians (Cavallari et al., 2005; Cavallari & Lam, 2008; Marez et al., 1997).
      (2) Incidence of poor metabolizers for CYP2C19 make up approximately 3% to 6% of White population and pproximately 20% of the Asian population (Cavallari & Lam, 2008; Ghoneim et al., 1981).
      (3) Approximately 7% of the White population are poor metabolizers for CYP2C9 substrates.
      (4) CYP3A5 is reported to be polymorphic in approximately 60% of African Americans and 33% of Whites.
10. *Functional genetic polymorphisms* (fully operational/"causative" vs. reduced function or null [nonfunctional]) have been discovered for
    a. CYP2A6

    b. CYP2C9
    c. CYP2C19
    d. CYP2D6
    e. CYP3A4
    f. CYP3A5 (Cavallari & Lam, 2008; Zhou, 2009)
    g. A polymorphism in the regulatory encoding for CYP1A2 has been identified but its importance remains to be determined (Cavallari & Lam, 2008; Sachse, Brockmöller, Bauer, & Roots, 1999).
  11. *Changes in drug metabolizing enzymes are subjected to selection pressure*
    a. They may adapt to a changing dietary environment (Ingelman-Sundberg, 2005; Ingelman-Sundberg et al., 2007)
    b. Dietary habits are important factors among differing ethnic groups and cultures.

I. **Enzyme Genes and Drug Response** (see Table 6.11)
  1. Some enzymes involved in drug responses are known to be under the influence of genetic polymorphisms.
  2. Examples:
    a. *Vitamin K epoxide reductase* (VKOR) is involved in warfarin's (Coumadin®) anticoagulant effect. Individuals who have VKOR mutations and are given warfarin may fail to achieve effective anticoagulation or fail to respond to any dose of warfarin administered (Cavallari & Lam 2008; Medical Letter, 2008; Rost et al., 2004).
    b. Evidence exists that there are *racial differences in response to angiotensin converting enzyme (ACE) inhibitors* (captopril [Capoten®], benazepril [Lotensin®]). African Americans in general are believed to have diminished antihypertensive responses to angiotensin-converting enzyme (ACE) inhibitors compared with Whites (Belle & Singh, 2008; Brugts et al., 2008; Materson, Reda, & Cushman, 1995).
  3. *Human leukocyte antigens* (HLAs) are proteins found on all cells, but particularly on white blood cells, where they help the immune system distinguish between self and non-self (see Table 6.12).
    a. Knowledge of these protein variations is clinically significant, but there is limited data available on its presence among specific ethnic groups
    b. Certain *variants of the HLA gene* put individuals at risk for *hypersensitivity reactions* to certain drugs (Cupp & Lesher, 2008). For example, about 1 in 20 patients with HLA-B*1502 will have a serious dermatologic reactions, such as
      (1) Toxic epidermal necrolysis
      (2) Stevens–Johnson syndrome due to carbamazepine
      (3) Approximately 10% to 15% of people of China, Malaysia, the Philippines, Taiwan, and Indonesia may carry this gene.
      (4) Incidence is lower in South Asian Indians, averaging about 2% to 4% but may be higher in some groups
      (5) Incidence is <1% in Japan and Korea
    c. Newest U.S. HIV guidelines recommend testing for HLA-B*5701 before starting patients on abacavir (Ziagen®; Trizivir® [abacavir, lamivudin, zidovudine]; DHHS, 2008).
    d. Severe hypersensitivity reactions to abacavir are more common in patients with the HLA-B*5701 variant.

J. **Pharmacogenetics of Mind-Altering Substances**
  1. After a person's first exposure to a drug, genes exert a major influence on whether he or she will go on to become dependent.
  2. Approximately 89 genes have been linked to drug abuse and dependence (National Institute on Drug Abuse [NIDA], 2008).
    a. Most of these genes were associated with substance dependence among
      (1) European Americans
      (2) African Americans
      (3) Although some appeared to affect risk in only one ethnic group.
    b. Findings support the idea that many of the variants that predispose to addiction first occurred relatively early in human evolution, before humankind's diaspora out of Africa led to the formation of separate Asian, African, and European ethnicities.
    c. Because an individual has one or more of the predisposing gene variants does not mean they are bound to abuse drugs or develop addiction.
    d. Pharmacogenetic studies in alcohol-dependent individuals have shown that optimal therapeutic response to the drug naltrexone [ReVia®] may be dependent on genetic polymorphism in the

(1) opioid mu receptor gene, and

(2) A118G SNP (Haile, 2008)

e. Data exist that highlights genetically determined individual variability in response to opioids

(1) not only for analgesia

(2) but also to the analgesic effects of opioids in prescription opioid abuse.

(3) May be relevant in the pharmacologic treatment of opioid abuse (Haile, 2008).

(4) Poor metabolizers (see Table 6.10) of CYP2D6, the enzyme used to convert codeine and tramadol (Ultram®) to morphine may be protected from abusing opiates such as

(a) Codeine,

(b) Oxycodone, and

(c) Hydrocodone.

(5) Investigators have used such drugs as fluoxetine (Prozac®), a CYP2D6 inhibitor, as adjunctive therapy in the management of opiate abuse to metabolically convert drug abusers who are extensive metabolizers (EMs) to poor metabolizers (PMs; Cavallari & Lam, 2008; Romach, Otton, Somer, Tyndale, & Sellers, 2000).

K. Genetic Testing

1. Several companies offer testing for HLA variants such as

a. Kashi Clinical Laboratories,

b. Laboratory Corporation of America Holdings (http://www.labcorp.com),

c. Speciality Laboratories (http://www.specialtylabs.com), and

d. Quest Diagnostics Nichols Institute (http://www.questdiagnostics.com).

2. Several companies offer tests that determine a patient's ability to metabolize drugs, such as Roche (e.g., AmpliChip; See Types of Genetic Variation above)

3. Depending on health insurance coverage

a. These tests may cost upward of $1,000

b. May not be covered by third-party payers.

4. Ethnopharmacologic responses: Some ethnic groups appear to have more pharmacogenomic responses to drugs than other groups. Table 6.13 highlights some of the reported responses in three groups.

M. Ethical Issues

1. Despite theoretical advantages of knowing a patient's CYP450 metabolizing profile, whether CYP450 genotyping improves outcomes or reduces costs is still unknown (Maitland-van der Zee, Klungel, & de Boer, 2004; Sheffield & Phillimore, 2009; Wilkinson, 2005).

2. Pharmacogenetic testing may generate complex risk information that would

a. Require detailed pretest counseling to assure informed consent.

b. Make genetic counseling mandatory (Haga & Burke, 2008).

c. Affect eligibility for health care and life insurance (Maitland-van der Zee et al., 2004).

d. Affect patient/clinician interactions because of the lack of regulated oversight systems for direct-to-consumer advertising of genetic testing (Ameer & Krivoy, 2009)

3. Pharmacogenetic profiling of infants and children raises particular ethical concerns regarding

a. Benefit of early testing in the absence of an immediate benefit,

b. Potential for ancillary information (Freund & Clayton, 2003), or

c. Correlations of neonatal ontogeny (genotype–phenotype) where apparent gene interest is not yet expressed (Leeder, 2009).

4. Genetic differences between racial groups may result in

a. Preferential drug development

b. Could favor one ethnic group over another (Evans & Relling, 2004)

N. Areas for Future Research

1. Discovery of genes that confer disease has led to

a. An improved understanding of the molecular mechanisms involved in disease pathophysiology.

b. Raises the possibility of examining these genes as targets for drug therapy (Cavallari & Lam, 2008).

2. Gene therapy has emerged as a possibility to

a. Treat and cure diseases

b. Study the role of pharmacologic therapy.

c. Gain information on gene therapy trials. Current information may be found from the U.S. FDA's clinical trials website (http://www.clinicatrials.gov)

Table 6.13. Ethnopharmacologic Responses Reported in Three Ethnic Groups

Ethnic Group		
Blacks	European Population	Southeast Asian
More resistant to blistering of skin by mustard gas	Deficiency in taste sensitivity to phenylthicarbamide (35%-40%)	Marked differences in plasma levels of proton pump inhibitors with increased gastric and duodenal ulcer healing rates [CYP2C19] (10%-25%)
Deficiency in taste sensitivity to phenylthicarbamide (<10%)	Toxic effects to drugs such as warfarin, phenytoin [CYP2C9] (0.2%-3%)	Deficiency in taste sensitivity to phenylthicarbamide (<10%)
Increased frequency of G6PD deficiency	Greater likelihood of adverse events with codeine use (1%-10%)	Marked differences in beta-blocker plasma levels [CYP2D6] (1%-2%)
Codeine treatment failure/adverse drug reactions	Marked differences in beta-blocker plasma levels	Risk of developing toxicity with Irinotecan [UGT1A1] (16%)
Marked differences in beta-blocker and proton pump inhibitor plasma levels [CYP2C19, CYP2D6] (4%-18%)	Risk of developing toxicity with Irinotecan (40%)	Toxic effects to drugs such as warfarin [VKORC1] (89%)
Toxic effects to drugs such as Warfarin [VKORC1] (37%)	Greater likelihood of treatment failures to antidepressants, antipsychotics, antiarrhythmics, and atomoxetine [CYP2D6] (1%-10%)	Increased risk of severe immune-mediated adverse effects caused by Carbamazepine (10%-15%)
CYP3A5 polymorphism (60%)		Greater likelihood of adverse reactions to antidepressants, antipsychotics, antiarrhythmics, and atomoxetine. [CYP2D6] (1%-2%)
Decreased response to angiotensin-converting enzyme (ACE) inhibitors		
Greater likelihood of adverse reactions to antidepressants, antipsychotics, antiarrhythmics, and atomoxetine [CYP2D6] (18%)		

Note: Adapted from "Pharmacogenomic Examples" by Cupp and Lesher (2008). Pharmacogenomics. *Pharmacist's Letter/Prescriber's Letter*, 24(2): 240211. Copyright 2008 by Therapeutic Research Center. Reprinted with permission. Table is meant to be representative and not comprehensive. Ansell, Ackerman, Black, Roberts, and Tefferi (2003); Belle and Singh (2008); Dervieux, Meshkin, and Neri (2005); Evans and Relling (2004); Goetz, Ames, and Weinshilboum (2004); Garber et al. (2005); Litman and Rosenberg (2005); Maitland-van der Zee, Klungel, and de Boer (2004); Pirmohamed (2009); Wilkinson (2005).

3. Genetic testing, even though it usually refers to screening individuals for genetic material in order to identify genotypes associated with disease susceptibility or carrier status, also may have a role in the search for variations that are linked to drug efficacy or toxicity.

4. More affordable, rapid genetic testing may improve the clinical utility of pharmcogenonic testing (Sheffield & Phillimore, 2009).

5. Knowledge of the
   a. Ontogeny (genotype-phenotype) of processes involved in
      (1) drug disposition
      (2) drug targets, and
   b. Role of genetic variations: could improve the value of the information on which therapeutic decisions in children are based (Leeder, 2009).

6. Lack of oversight "regulatory" controls over direct-to-consumer/patient advertising of genetic testing can have both immediate and long-term effects on public health and the future adoption of pharmacogentic/genomic testing (Ameer & Krivoy, 2009).

O. **Summary of Key Points**
   1. Many factors must be taken into consideration when prescribing the best drug for an individual patient. Pharmacogenetics and ethnopharmacology are just two important concepts.

2. A drug may be metabolized by more than one cytochrome P450 isoenzyme.
   a. Generic blanket statements about ethnic drug metabolism are intended as guidelines only.
   b. Standard pharmacology texts and references often contain specific cytochrome P450 enzyme substrate, and inhibitor and inducer information that is useful to the prescriber in avoiding drug–drug interactions.
3. Significant interindividual variability in enzyme activity exist as a result of
   a. induction
   b. inhibition
   c. genetic inheritance
4. Genetic variations occur for
   a. drug target proteins
   b. drug transporter systems
   c. drug metabolism
   d. disease-associated genes
5. Genetic polymorphisms may be linked to
   a. drug efficacy
   b. drug–drug interactions
   c. adverse drug events
   d. toxicity
6. Understanding which cytochrome P450 isozyme is responsible for the metabolism of a drug is useful in
   a. understanding drug interactions and
   b. predicting drug interactions
7. The cost of genotyping can be considerably less than that incurred in a patient with a serious adverse drug reaction. However, standard of practice does not specifically recommend genotyping individuals initially (Pirmohamed, 2009).
8. Broad public initiatives, such as the NIH-funded Pharmacogenetics and Pharmacogenomics Knowledge Base (http://www.pharmGKB.org), provide useful resources to permit clinicians to access information on pharmacogenetics.
9. Pharmacogenetics has the possibility of eliminating trial-and-error approaches to drug prescribing for many diseases and racial and ethnic groups.
10. Pharmacogenetic studies need to be interpreted carefully.
    a. Often studies are relatively small and the populations studied are not always well characterized.
    b. Ethnic categories often include persons from widely diverse geographic and sociocultural backgrounds with varying genetic composition.
    c. Results might not apply to all members of each ethnic population.
11. The critical determinant is the genotype of the particular enzyme involved in drug metabolism
    a. Not race or
    b. Ethnic group
    c. Both of which are assigned by subjective criteria.
12. Even though ethnicity/racial difference may not be known for a particular polymorphism, environmental, dietary, and cultural practices may still alter genetic polymorphisms affecting drug metabolism.
13. Because of possible ethnic and pharmacogentic differences, nurses and other health care providers need to perform comprehensive health history assessments, including
    a. family history,
    b. social history,
    c. ethnic and racial background,
    d. cultural practices,
    e. dietary habits,
    f. medication and food allergies,
    g. previous reactions to medications,
    h. past medical history, and
    i. values and beliefs
14. A drug response has inter-individual variability and is mutifactorial, influenced by
    a. environment,
    b. genetics, and
    c. disease determinants.

15. Currently, there are no treatment guidelines taking pharmacogenetic data into account (Klotz, 2007).

16. There have been no prospective clinical trials showing that knowledge of a patient's genotypic profile before prescribing drugs
    a. increases drug efficacy,
    b. prevents adverse drug reactions,
    c. reduces adverse drug reactions, and
    d. lowers overall costs of therapy and associated sequelae.

17. When providing quality care to multicultural and ethnically diverse individuals and groups, health care providers who use or recommend pharmaceuticals should consider a multidisciplinary team approach, which includes, but is not limited to,
    a. primary care clinicians,
    b. pharmacists,
    c. physicians,
    d. pharmacologists,
    e. nurses, and
    f. geneticists

IX. SUMMARY

A. In this chapter, culturally based health and illness beliefs and practices were presented as complementary content that round out the cultural and ethical basis for transcultural care, which begun in the previous chapter.

B. This content prepares the base for and leads to the next step in the process, which is cultural health assessment that is presented in the next chapter.

NOTE: All references, additional resources, and important Internet sites relevant to this chapter can be found at the following website: http://tcn.sagepub.com/supplemental

Chapter 7
Cultural Health Assessment

Journal of Transcultural Nursing
21(Supplement 1) 307S–336S
© The Author(s) 2010
Reprints and permission:
sagepub.com/journalsPermissions.nav
DOI: 10.1177/1043659610377208
http://tcn.sagepub.com
⑤SAGE

Nancy L. R. Anderson, PhD, RN, FAAN[1]
Joyceen S. Boyle, PhD, RN, CTN, FAAN[2]
Ruth E. Davidhizar, DNSc, RN, APRN, BC, FAAN (deceased)[3]
Joyce Newman Giger, EdD, APRN, BC, FAAN[4]
Marilyn R. McFarland, PhD, RN, FNP-BC, CTN-A[5]
Irena Papadopoulos, PhD, MA, RN, RM, FHEA[6]
Larry Purnell, PhD, RN, FAAN[7]
Rachel Spector, PhD, RN, CTN-A, FAAN[8]
Mary Tilki, PhD, MSc, RN[9]
Hiba Wehbe-Alamah, PhD, RN, FNP-BC, CTN-A[10]

I. INTRODUCTION

A. This chapter provides the cultural assessment that complements the content in the previous two chapters (5 and 6).

B. The conduct of a thorough assessment blends physical, psychosocial, and cultural foci as the basis for planning quality care.

C. Chapter 7 outlines several approaches to the conduct of a holistic health assessment.

II. GUIDELINES FOR ASSESSMENT OF PERSONS FROM DIFFERENT CULTURES

A. Assessment begins with ethical, cultural, and social justice considerations by clinicians.

  1. Engage in self-reflection regarding personal beliefs, life experiences, explanatory models, and potential personal biased attitudes

   a. Learn how to tap those beliefs in ways that help you to be open to the belief systems of patients and families

   b. Monitor your reactions to people and settings

  2. Preserve personal and professional integrity which is essential for establishing trust, demonstrating respect and sincerity of purpose (Winslow & Wehthe-Winslow, 2007).

  3. Determine ethnolinguistic orientation of patient in advance of encounter

   a. If barriers to effective communication are anticipated, seek best available translation/interpretation options.

   b. Review available records/charts for relevant cultural and linguistic information, prior to initiating establishing contact.

  4. Ethical approaches to clinical assessment require equitable management of the power differential between provider and patient/family.

   a. Vulnerable populations (such as underrepresented minorities, persons with disabilities, those who are homeless, and/or living in poverty) may find it difficult to communicate with providers if the providers' power status and prestige make them potentially unapproachable or disinterested

Funding: The California Endowment (grant number 20082226) and Health Resources and Services Administration (grant number D11 HPO9759).

[1]University of California -Los Angeles, Los Angeles, CA, USA (Guidelines for Assessment; Interviewing Techniques, Community Assessment)
[2]University of Arizona, Tucson, AZ, USA (Andrews & Boyle Transcultural Nursing Assessment Guide)
[3]Bethel College, Mishawaka, IN, USA (Cultural Health Assessment: Physical Assessment)
[4]University of California -Los Angeles, Los Angeles, CA, USA (Cultural Health Assessment: Physical Assessment)
[5]University of Michigan -Flint, Flint, MI, USA (Leininger's Cultural Assessment Tools, Instruments and Guidelines)
[6]Middlesex University, London, UK (Papadopoulos, Tilki & Lees Cultural Assessment Tool (CCA Tool)
[7]University of Delaware, Newark, DE, USA (Assessment of the Domains of the Purnell Model of Cultural Competence)
[8]Cultural Care Consultant, Needham, MA, USA (The Heritage Assessment Tool)
[9]Middlesex University, London, UK (Papadopoulos, Tilki & Lees Cultural Assessment Tool (CCA Tool)
[10]University of Michigan -Flint, Flint, MI, USA (Leininger's Cultural Assessment Tools, Instruments and Guidelines; Case Study)

Corresponding Author: Marilyn K. Douglas, Email: martydoug@comcast.net

Suggested Citation: Douglas, M. K. & Pacquiao, D. F. (Eds.). (2010). Core curriculum in transcultural nursing and health care [Supplement]. *Journal of Transcultural Nursing, 21*(Suppl. 1).

b. Some patients are reluctant to disclose personal information if they anticipate receiving discriminatory treatment.

c. These patient concerns often result in miscommunication and misdiagnosis, particularly among those with mental health problems (Kendrick, Anderson, & Moore, 2007).

5. Demonstrate respect
   a. Introduce self by name and clinical role
   b. Greet by using patients' and/or family members' surname(s)
   c. Observe for signs of comfort levels with (Hall, 1984)
      1) Space between self and patient/family member
      2) Eye contact
      3) Touch (ask permission prior to any touch, including hand shake)

6. Establish mutual trust
   a. Employ active listening techniques
   b. Show interest
   c. Assure safety
   d. Assure confidentiality
   e. Consider the possibility that patient may have experienced stigma, discrimination, and/or racism

B. Conducting the interview
   1. When asking questions:
      a. First determine the appropriate person with whom to initiate the interview
         1) Usually this is the patient
         2) In some ethnic and cultural groups a man or elder of either gender is designated to serve as the authority for all communications
      b. Start with general questions
      c. Avoid intrusive questions (if they must be asked, first establish rapport with less intrusive questions)
      d. Avoid coercion (Kallert, 2008)
      e. Use patient verbal and behavioral cues as signals for more personal questions
      f. Offer opportunity but avoid directive style for seeking personal disclosures
   2. Types of general information to seek:
      a. Patient and family explanatory models (see Chapter 5)
      b. Endeavor to learn patient and family strengths before seeking weaknesses
      c. When asking about cultural and ethnic orientations, consider the possible interconnections with religion and spirituality.
   3. Ethical considerations during assessment blend well with the concept of a working partnership between clinician and patient/family (Anderson, Calvillo, & Fongwa, 2007).
   4. The environmental context, including socioeconomic and political factors significantly influences patients' and families' response to illness as well as their dynamic interactions with health care providers in institutional settings that have implications for health disparities.
   5. Provider behaviors that may account for disparities in health outcomes (Gaston-Johansson, Hill-Briggs, Oguntomilade, Bradley, & Mason, 2007) include
      a. Ineffective communication
      b. Poor service delivery
      c. Inefficiency
      d. Cultural incompetence
   6. Patient recommendations (Anderson et al., 2007; Gaston-Johansson et al., 2007)
      a. Provide ways to empower patients throughout the care process
      b. Provider and staff training in effective communication
      c. Consider alternative models for patient care
      d. Explore accessible mechanisms for monitoring care quality
      e. Establish partnerships with patients and their families
   7. See culturally relevant assessment tools and strategies below.

III. METHODS FOR CONDUCTING ASSESSMENT (Gathering Data)
   A. Interview Techniques
      1. Interviews in the health care arena often occur at stressful times when:

    a. Patients may be in pain or anticipating the pain of unknown procedures, or are experiencing other forms of life stress,

    b. Family members may be experiencing varying degrees of concern and fear for or with the patient, and/or other stressors,

    c. Clinicians may be stressed by staff shortages, system or personal issues, or multiple emergent situations.

2. Clinical interview formats

    a. Patient and clinician

    b. Patient and clinician with one or more family members present

        1) Some cultural and ethnic groups prefer to have the family spokesperson involved

        2) Among some groups the family spokesperson speaks for the patient.

    c. Clinician and family members, for example, especially if the patient is a woman and the clinician is male, the female patient may not be present

3. Employing strategies and techniques from ethnography during interactions with patients and their families

    a. Definitions of Ethnography

        1) The study of ". . . human behavior and attitudes . . . in the natural setting" where they occur (Ragucci, 1990, p. 164)

        2) A ". . . process of learning *about* people by learning *from* them" (Roper & Shapria, 2000, p. 1)

        3) Focus on how people interpret experience and shape their behavior within the context of their culturally constructed environments (Aamodt, 1991)

        4) ". . . neither subjective nor objective. It is interpretive . . ." (Agar, 1986)

    b. Ethnographic components include

        1) Participant observation—watching behavior and interaction dynamics (Shatzman & Strauss, 1973)

        2) Informal interviews and conversations

        3) Listening to patient/family stories—these stories often include important revelations not obtainable by direct questioning (Mason, 2002)

        4) Review of relevant documents

    c. Ethnographic participant observation blends a combination of:

        1) Various degrees of participation in dynamic interaction with the patient/family—a reciprocal process (Byerly, 1990; Pearsall, 1965)

        2) Observation of verbal and nonverbal behavior, and interactive dynamics

        3) Observation of clinical signs

        4) Informal discussion and/or interviews for the purpose of clarification and verification of observed behaviors and clinical signs

        5) Reflection with the patient/family regarding observed behaviors and/or informal disclosures

    d. Ethnographic interviewing

        1) More formal semistructured or structured interviews for the purpose of assessment should be based on:

            a) Issues identified during participant observation (Pelto & Pelto, 1978)

            b) Review of relevant documents (e.g. patient chart)

            c) Patient and family questions, stated concerns

            d) Patient's expressed cultural and ethnic identity

            e) Respectful and ethical considerations relevant to the patient/family culture and ethnicity

        2) A speech event based on cultural rules for initiation, turn taking, asking, listening, and closure (Mason, 2002; Spradley 1979)

        3) General types of questions (Spradley, 1979)

            a) *Descriptive questions:* Ask for a description that provides insights about the patient, for example, "Please tell me about your pain."

            b) *Structural questions:* Seek information about how patients organize their perceptions about their health or health problem, for example, "What kinds of pain are you having?"

            c) *Contrast questions:* Determine how patients distinguish the meaning of two or more kinds of phenomena, for example, "What is the difference between your nighttime and daytime pain?"

        4) The clinical assessment focus for questioning

            a) Patient/family explanatory models regarding causation, course of the illness, and expected/desired outcomes (see Explanatory Models in Chapter 5)

b) Symptom relevant questions

c) Questions that clarify observed clinical signs

d) Questions relevant for planning evidence based care derived from expert sources and relevant literature

4. Ethnographic and community-based participatory action strategies relevant to working with groups for assessment/identification of population-based health disparities and policy establishment purposes

a. Establish collaborative partnerships

b. Respond to community, neighborhood, or social group requests

c. Determine need to address health disparity

d. Participation and partnership with community members give them the opportunity to

1) Have a voice in decisions that affect their communities (Glasson, Chang, & Bidewell, 2008)

2) Assist in the creation of programs that assist them to change health behaviors (Wagemakers et al., 2008)

3) Learn new skills (Horn, McCracken, Dino, & Brayboy, 2008)

4) Participate in the implementation of programs intended to reduce health disparities in their neighborhoods (Anderson et al., 2007; Gaston-Johansson et al., 2007)

5. Community assessment

a. Participant as observer and observer as participant

1) Attend community meetings

2) Observe the dynamic interactive process

3) Talk with community members and leaders

4) Listen to community concerns

5) Seek to learn community assets and strengths

b. Collaborative examples of work with community members and leaders to:

1) Conduct a Rapid Assessment Response and Evaluation (RARE) of the neighborhood (Brown et al., 2008)

a) Form an interdisciplinary team that includes community membership

b) Develop training materials appropriate for team members

c) Use more than one method to collect data

d) Collect and analyze data simultaneously

e) Complete the process expeditiously

2) Blend a cultural systems paradigm with an ethnographically informed evaluation to assess community strengths (Aronson, Wallis, O'Campo, Whitehead, & Schafer, 2007)

3) Use strategies to assess and map community strengths and needs:

a) Members of the community participate with clinicians and researchers in community assessment and mapping procedures by creating maps that show community assets (i.e. location of schools, clinics, public service facilities) and community deficits (i.e. absence of accessible transportation (Aronson, Wallis, O'Campo, & Schafer, 2007)

(1) Windshield surveys—A team of two or more people including community members and researchers drive through a rural area to locate and map sources of health services and distance from homes to these services.

(2) Walk-through surveys—The team walk through an urban neighborhood to collect information for their map locating youth recreation resources and safety issues for adolescents seeking to participate in sports activities.

b) Geographic information system (GIS) mapping using electronic and technological resources for census, epidemiological and geographic location sources to conduct assessments of community health status, issues, and resources (Chong & Mitchell, 2008; Graves, 2008; Sowmyanarayanan, Mukhopadhya, Gladstone, Sarkar, & Gagandeep, 2008)

4) Examine the context within which community and neighborhood health status issues emerge and where care is provided (Anderson et al., 2007; Townley, Kloos, & Wright, 2008)

5) Analyze and synthesize information gathered for the purpose of collaborative development of culturally and ethnically relevant community-based interventions

B. Physical Assessment

1. Bio-cultural ecology

a. The purpose of biocultural ecology is to transcend the fragmentation inherent in the separation of culture, human biology, and ecology and the environment.

    b. Biocultural ecology is an examination of diverse human populations by means of this three-way interaction system and focuses on specific, localized individuals and populations within a given environment (Giger & Davidhizar, 2008).

    c. Data relative to all the variables significant to people within a racial group are essential for complete understanding of the people.

    d. No two persons or two cultural or racial groups are alike, and all phenomena relative to both individuals and cultural or racial groups must be understood (Giger & Davidhizar, 2008).

2. ***Disease incidence and prevalence among culturally diverse populations***

    a. Diabetes among culturally diverse populations

      1) There is a high incidence of diabetes mellitus in certain American Indian tribes, including the Seminole, Pima, and Papago (Giger & Davidhizar, 2008).

      2) However, until very recently diabetes was thought to be quite rare among Alaskan Eskimos.

      3) Diabetes mellitus is a major health problem in the in the United States with 11.1 million diagnosed cases and more than 5.9 million undiagnosed cases, accounting for 6.2% of the total population in the United States (American Diabetes Association, 2006; Centers for Disease Control and Prevention [CDC], 2005; National Center for Health Statistics, 2007).

      4) More than 800,000 new cases of diabetes are reported in the United States each year (American Diabetes Association, 2006; CDC, 2005; National Center for Health Statistics, 2007).

      5) The prevalence of diabetes is so widespread in the United States making it the seventh leading cause of death in the United States in 2001 (American Diabetes Association, 2006; CDC, 2005; National Center for Health Statistics, 2007; U.S. Department of Health and Human Services, 2005).

      6) In 2006, diabetes was reported as the underlying cause for more than 40,000 deaths and a contributory factor in approximately 160,000 other deaths (National Center for Health Statistics, 2007).

      7) It is estimated that some 7.8% (11.4 million) of all non-Hispanic Whites have diabetes, as well as 13.0% (2.8) million of Blacks and 10.2% (2 million) of Hispanics (National Center for Health Statistics, 2007).

      8) American Indians have a disproportionately high incidence of diabetes than other racial/ethnic groups totaling 15.1% of their population (105,000), and Alaska Natives have the lowest percentage of diabetes (5.3%; National Center for Health Statistics, 2007).

      9) By geographical region, American Indians residing in the Southeastern United States have the greatest incidence of diabetes at 25.7% (American Diabetes Association, 2006).

      10) By race, diabetes is ranked as the seventh leading cause of death in the United States among Whites, Blacks, Chinese, and Filipinos (American Diabetes Association, 2006; National Center for Health Statistics, 2007).

      11) Women in the general U.S. population have a higher mortality associated with diabetes than their male counterparts (Giger & Davidhizar, 2008).

      12) In 2004, the age-adjusted death rate for diabetes by race was Whites, 22.8; Blacks, 50.1; American Indian or Alaska Natives, 50.3; Asian or Pacific Islanders, 18.4; and Hispanics, 33.6 (National Center for Health Statistics, 2007).

      13) The prevalence of diabetes varies according to race and gender and increases with age; at all ages, is highest among African American women.

      14) In 1999, the prevalence rate of diabetes for African American women (50.9 per 1,000) was twice the rate for their White counterparts (23.4 per 1,000; Mirsa, 2001).

      15) The Institute of Medicine's report *Unequal Treatment* (Smedley, Stith, & Nelson, 2003) suggests that ethnic minorities sometimes receive unequal treatment in regard to health care; it is further illuminating in regard to care for diabetes.

      16) Although Blacks, Hispanics, and American Indians experience a 50% to 100% higher burden of illness and mortality due to diabetes than their White counterparts, the disease appears to be more profoundly under-managed among these vulnerable populations (National Center for Health Statistics, 2007).

      17) Chin, Zhang, and Merrell (1998) noted that even when gender, education, and age were controlled, African Americans were still less likely to undergo measurements of glycosylated hemoglobin, lipid testing, ophthalmologic visits, and influenza vaccinations than their White counterparts.

      18) Blacks and Latinos with type 2 diabetes are more likely to be treated with insulin as opposed to an oral anti-hyperglycemic agent than their White or Mexican counterparts (Cowie & Harris, 1997).

      19) When conducting a physical assessment consider the race of the client and the family medical history.

b. Hypertension among Blacks
  1) The incidence of hypertension has been reported to be significantly higher in African Americans than in White Americans (Giger & Davidhizar, 2008).
  2) The onset by age of hypertension is earlier in African Americans, and the hypertension is more severe and associated with a higher mortality in African Americans (Giger & Davidhizar, 2008).
  3) Equal prevalence of hypertension among both sexes in the Black race and incidence increases with advancing age (Giger & Davidhizar, 2008).
  4) However, contrasting opinions indicate that hypertension may occur slightly more often in men than in women (Joint National Committee, 2003).
  5) A total of 35% to 40% of African Americans have hypertension, which accounts for 20% of African American deaths in the United States (Giger & Davidizar, 2008).
  6) African Americans with hypertension have an 80% higher chance of dying from a stroke and 20% higher chance of developing heart disease than in the general population (Joint National Committee, 2003).
  7) Africans Americans have four times greater risk of developing hypertension related end-stage kidney disease than the general population (Joint National Committee, 2003).
c. Metabolic syndrome is a well-defined constellation of symptoms that eventually leads to the development of cardiovascular disease; to date, race has not been established as a clear correlate for causation, but the condition bears watching for this relationship (Appel et al., 2005).
  1) The essential components of the metabolic syndrome are
    a) Abdominal adiposity
    b) Hypertriglyceridemia
    c) Low high-density lipoprotein (HDL) cholesterol
    d) Hypertension
    e) Impaired fasting glucose
  2) Although the metabolic syndrome is a disease of lifestyle, it does seem to have greater propensity in some racial/ethnic groups as opposed to others (i.e., African Americans and Mexican Americans).
  3) The metabolic syndrome is characterized by a pro-inflammatory state.
  4) Other names for the metabolic syndrome included:
    a) Syndrome X
    b) Insulin resistance syndrome (IRS)
    c) Multiple-metabolic syndrome
    d) Deadly quartet
    e) Dysmetabolic syndrome ICD-9 code: 277.7
  5) Markers for insulin resistance or hyperinsulinemia (indices for metabolic syndrome)
    a) Acanthosis Nigricans (more common in African Americans and Latinos)
    b) Skin tags (more common in Whites)
    c) Hirsutism
    d) Acne
    e) Menstrual irregularities
    f) Android appearance in women
    g) Virilization
    h) Male pattern vertex balding
  6) Look for markers for hyperinsulinemia by race/ethnicity. For example, acanthosis nigricans (darkly pigmented areas behind the neck maybe more commonly found among African Americans and Latinos and may be a precursor for the metabolic syndrome.
  7) Genetic risk factors, including but not limited to:
    a) Sickle-cell anemia
    b) African American population
d. Cancer and Asian Americans and Pacific Islanders
  1) The burden of cancer for Asians Americans and Pacific Islanders (AAPIs) is *unusual*, *unequal*, and *unnecessary* (Chen, 2000).
  2) The burden of cancer is *unusual* in that cancer is and has been the leading cause of death for AAPI females as early as 1980, when these statistics were first collected.

3) No other racial/ethnic/gender group has experienced this unequal burden for cancer.

4) Cancer is also the leading cause of death for AAPIs between 25 and 64 years of age; by comparison, cancer does not become the leading cause of death for Whites until they reach the 45- to 64-year age bracket (Chen, 2000).

5) The burden of cancer for AAPIs is also *unequal* because cancer death rates for AAPIs have increased at higher rates than any other racial/ethnic group in the United States.

6) For example, cancer of the stomach, colon, rectum, and liver occurs more frequently among Japanese Americans than among their White counterparts (Miller et al., 1996).

7) A possible cause of stomach cancer is thought to be chronic gastritis. Yet, Among Asian Americans, it is believed that eating dried salted fish is a predisposing factor for gastric cancer (Nomoura, et al., 2002; National Cancer Center, 2006).

8) Diets high in salt-cured foods and nitrites and poor in vitamin C intake have been commonly associated with greater incidence of stomach cancer.

e. Glucose-6-phosphate dehydrogenase (G-6-PD; Giger & Davidhizar, 2008)

1) G-6-PD deficiency is a red blood cell defect causing fragility of the red blood cells.

2) G-6-PD is an enzyme constituent of the red blood cells and is involved in the hexose monophosphate pathway, which actually accounts for 10% of glucose metabolism of the red blood cells.

3) Under normal circumstances, it is expected that the proportion of glucose metabolized through this pathway might increase greatly if the cells are subjected to oxidation.

4) Chinese and Mediterranean people have relatively high incidences of thalassemia and G-6-PD deficiency.

5) Persons with G-6-PD deficiency are prone to anemia when exposed to certain drugs, such as analgesics (aspirin, phenacetin), sulfonamides and sulfones, antimalarials (primaquine, quinacrine), antibacterials (nitrofurantoin, chloramphenicol, *para*-aminosalicylic acid), vitamin K, probenecid, and quinidine.

f. Thalassemia (Giger & Davidhizar, 2008)

1) Thalassemia is an autosomal recessive blood disorder inherited from both parents.

2) This genetic defect actually causes a reduced rate of synthesis of one of the globin chains that make up hemoglobin.

3) Reduced synthesis of one of the globin chains causes the formation of abnormal hemoglobin molecules, which in turn causes anemia.

4) Thalassemia differs from sickle cell anemia in that thalassemia is a quantitative problem of too few globins synthesized, unlike sickle cell anemia, which is thought to be a qualitative problem of synthesis of an incorrectly functioning globin.

5) Thalassemia is particularly prevalent among Mediterranean people where it gets its name from the Greek words for sea, which is *Thalassa (θάλασσα)*, and blood, which is *Haema (αίμα)*.

6) The Greeks once were thought to have a higher prevalence of thalassemia; Asia now has even greater prevalence, with the highest concentration of carriers (18% of the population) in the Maldives.

g. Sickle cell anemia

1) Sickle cell anemia is the most common genetic disorder in the United States.

2) It has been projected that 50,000 African Americans have sickle cell anemia (Wyngaarden & Smith, 1985).

3) Sickle cell anemia or the trait also occurs in people from Asia Minor, India, the Mediterranean, and Caribbean areas but to a lesser extent than what has been reported in African Americans (Giger & Davidhizar, 2008).

4) Sickle cell anemia is characterized by chronic hemolytic anemia and is a homozygous recessive disorder.

5) The basic disorder lies within the globin of the hemoglobin (Hb), where a single amino acid (valine) is substituted for another (glutamic acid) in the sixth position of the beta chain (Giger & Davidhizar, 2008).

6) A single amino acid substitution profoundly alters the properties of the Hb molecule; Hb S is formed instead of normal Hb A as a result of the intermolecular rearrangement (Giger & Davidhizar, 2008).

7) The normal oxygen-carrying capacity of the blood is found in Hb A but as a result of deoxygenation, there is a change in the solubility of protein, which makes the Hb molecules lump together, causing the cell membrane to contract, with the resultant sickle cell shape (Giger & Davidhizar, 2008).

8) Affected cells have a shortened life span of 7 to 20 days, which is profoundly different from the life span of normal cells, which is 105 to 120 days.

9) Hb SA is the heterozygous state and is often an asymptomatic condition referred to as sickle cell trait.

10) Sickle cell anemia is believed to have occurred for many years in Africa along the Nile River valley as an adaptive disease. In Africa, this disorder was believed to produce resistance to malarial transmission by the anopheles mosquito (Williams, 1975).

11) In Africa, sickle cell anemia or the trait affects approximately 10% of the Black population, and the death rate before 21 years of age has been 100% in those affected with the disease.

12) Before full recognition of the clinical significance of sickle cell anemia in the United States, the death rate was almost of the same magnitude as that in Africa.

13) Today in the United States, as a result of improved and comprehensive care, as well as early recognition of the crisis of the disease, persons with sickle cell anemia may live through their third and fourth decades of life (Giger & Davidhizar, 2008).

3. **Skin color and skin assessment**

a. When working with people from diverse cultural backgrounds it is important to understand how different races evolved in relation to the environment.

b. Biological differences noted in skin color may be attributable to the biological adjustments a person's ancestors made in the environment in which they lived (Giger & Davidhizar, 2008).

c. Scientists have postulated that the original skin color of humans was black (Overfield, 1977, 1995) and that white skin may be result of mutation and environmental pressures exerted on persons living in cold, cloudy northern Europe (Giger & Davidhizar, 2008).

1) Skin color is probably the most significant biological variation in terms of culturally appropriate care.

2) Appropriate health care delivery is based on accurate client assessment, and the darker the client's skin, the more difficult it becomes to assess changes in color (Giger & Davidhizar, 2008).

3) When caring for clients with highly pigmented skin, first establish the baseline skin color, and daylight is the best light source for doing so (Giger & Davidhizar, 2008).

4) If possible, dark-skinned clients should always be given a bed by a window to provide access to sunlight.

5) When daylight is not available to assess skin color, a lamp with at least a 60-watt bulb should be used.

d. To establish the baseline skin color observe those skin surfaces that have the least amount of pigmentation, which include the volar surfaces of the forearms, the palms of the hands, the soles of the feet, the abdomen, and the buttocks (Giger & Davidhizar, 2008).

1) When observing these areas, the nurse should look for an underlying red tone, which is typical of all skin, regardless of how dark its color.

2) Absence of this red tone in a client may be indicative of pallor.

3) Additional areas that are important to assess in dark-skinned clients include the mouth, the conjunctivae, and the nail beds.

4) The darkness of the oral mucosa correlates with the client's skin color.

5) The darker the skin, the darker the mucosa; nonetheless, the mucosa is lighter than the skin.

6) Oral hyperpigmentation can occur on the tongue and the mucosa and can alter the value of the oral mucosa as a site for observation.

7) In many cases, the occurrence of oral hyperpigmentation is directly related to the darkness of a person's skin.

8) Oral hyperpigmentation appears in 50% to 90% of African Americans, compared with 10% to 50% of Whites (Giger & Davidhizar, 2008).

9) Look at the hard palate because it takes on a yellow discoloration, particularly in the presence of jaundice as it is frequently affected by hyperpigmentation in a manner similar to that of the oral mucosa and the tongue.

10) Assess the lips because they may be helpful in assessing skin-color changes (such as jaundice or cyanosis).

11) In assessing the lips of some Black people, it is important to remember that there may be a natural bluish hue (Rouch, 1977).

12) Establish the baseline color of the lips, particularly if they are to be of value in detecting cyanosis (Branch & Paxton, 1976).

13) Establish the normal color of the conjunctivae when working with persons from transcultural populations.

14) In some diverse populations, the conjunctivae often will reflect the color changes of cyanosis or pallor and is a good site for observing petechiae.

15) Be sure to assess for the presence of jaundice in the sclera.

16) Establish a baseline color for the sclerae as first priority because the sclerae of dark-skinned persons often have a yellow coloration caused by subconjunctival fatty deposits.

17) One common finding in persons with highly pigmented skin is the presence of melanin deposits or "freckles" on the sclerae.

18) Lastly, assess the nail beds as they are useful to detect cyanosis or pallor.
    a) It is difficult to assess the nail beds in dark-skinned persons because they are often highly pigmented, may be thick, or lined or contain melanin deposits.
    b) Notice how quickly the color returns to the nail bed after pressure has been released from the free edge of the nail (Rouch, 1977).
    c) A slower return of color to the nail bed may be indicative of cyanosis or pallor.

19) It is also difficult to detect rashes, inflammations, and ecchymoses in dark-skinned persons.
    a) It may be necessary to palpate rashes in dark-skinned persons because rashes may not be readily visible to the eye.
    b) When palpating the skin for rashes, the nurse should notice induration and warmth of the area.

20) Other visible physical characteristics
    a) Note other aberrations in the skin such as Mongolian spots on the skin of African American, Asian American, American Indians, or Mexican American newborns.
    b) Mongolian spots are bluish discolorations that vary tremendously in size and color and are often mistaken for bruises.
    c) Another aberration that is more common in African Americans than in other racial groups is keloids.
    d) These ropelike scars represent an exaggeration of the wound-healing process and may occur as a result of any type of trauma, such as surgical incisions, ear piercing, or insertion of an intravenous catheter (Giger & Davidhizar, 2008).

IV. CULTURAL ASSESSMENT TOOLS, INSTRUMENTS, GUIDELINES

A. The Transcultural Nursing Assessment Guide (Andrews & Boyle, 2008)

1. *Biocultural Variations and Cultural Aspects of the Incidence of Disease*
   a. Some common diseases, such as diabetes, cardiovascular diseases and sickle cell anemia are more prevalent in specific cultural groups.
   b. Socioeconomic conditions may contribute to the incidence of disease conditions.
   c. There is increased resistance to certain diseases in specific cultural/ethnic groups.

2. *Communication*
   a. Language
      1) Language spoken at home
      2) Preferred language with health care provider
      3) Other languages spoken by client and family members
      4) Fluency level of client's and family members' English
   b. Choosing an interpreter
      1) Consider the preferences of family and client
      2) Culturally inappropriate interpreters may be:
         a) Members of the opposite sex
         b) Person older or younger than client
         c) Member of a rival tribe, ethnic group, or nationality
   c. Rules and style of client's communication

    d. Vary the techniques and style of communication to accommodate cultural background of the client
       1) Tempo and intensity of conversation
       2) Eye contact can be culturally important or taboo
       3) Sensitivity to certain taboos subjects
       4) Norms regarding confidentially
       5) Styles of nonverbal communication
       6) The client's and the family's feelings and views about health care providers who are not of the same cultural or religious background

3. Cultural Affiliations
    a. The client's cultural affiliation
    b. Differences and similarities with other family members
    c. Country of origin

4. Cultural Sanctions and Restrictions
    a. Expressions of emotion, feelings, spirituality, religious beliefs
    b. Culturally defined expressions of modesty, male–female relationships
    c. Restrictions related to sexuality, exposure of various parts of the body, or of certain types of surgery

5. Developmental Considerations
    a. Distinct growth patterns and characteristics vary with cultural background
    b. Factors such as circumcision, growth rates, culturally acceptable ages for toilet training, length of breast-feeding, gender differences, discipline, and socialization to adult roles
    c. Beliefs and practices associated with developmental events such as pregnancy, birth, and death
    d. Cultural perceptions of aging as well as practices associated with care of elders

6. Economics
    a. Primary wage earner and income level; other sources of income
    b. Insurance coverage
    c. Impact of economic status on lifestyle and living conditions
    d. Experiences of client and family with the health care system in terms of reimbursement, costs and insurance coverage

7. Educational Background
    a. Client's highest educational level
    b. Value of education achievements
    c. Effect of educational level on health literacy and health behavior of client
    d. Client's preferred learning style; written materials, oral explanations, videos, and/or demonstrations
    e. Preferences of client and family for intervention settings
       1) Community sites such as churches and schools are conducive to open discussions, demonstrations, and reinforcement
       2) Home settings provide privacy, convenience, and one-on-one learning

8. Health-Related Beliefs and Practices
    a. Beliefs about causation of illness and disease
       1) Divine wrath
       2) Hot–cold imbalance
       3) Yin–yang
       4) Punishment for moral transgressions, past behaviors
       5) Soul loss, hexes
       6) Pathogenic organisms
    b. Beliefs about ideal body size and shape; concept of body image in relation to the ideal
    c. Terms used by client to express health conditions such as ways of expressing of pain and discomfort
    d. Client's and family members' beliefs about health promotion
       1) Eating or avoiding certain foods
       2) Wearing amulets for good luck or to keep away the evil eye (red earrings, bracelets, hats, etc.)
       3) Sleep, resting, or napping for children
       4) Stress reduction techniques such as exercise, yoga, meditation, prayer, rituals to ancestors
    e. Client's religious affiliation and involvement in religious practices and activities; similarities and differences in religious beliefs and practices between client and family members

       f. Reliance on cultural healers such as curanderos, shamans, spiritual advisors

          1)   Types of cultural healing of healing practices engaged in by the client

          2)   Perceptions of client and family members about biomedical or scientific health care providers

       g. Provisions made by family to care for client at home

       h. Client's and family's view of mental disorders

9. *Kinship and Social Networks*

       a. Client's social network such as family, friends, peers, neighbors

       b. Composition of a "typical" family versus composition of the client's family

       c. Roles of family members and social networks during health and illness episodes

       d. Decision makers in the family who make decisions about health and health care

       e. Participation by family members in promotion of health such as lifestyle changes in diet and/or activity levels

       f. Participation by family members in nursing care procedures such as bathing, feeding, touching, being present when client is ill

       g. Influence of cultural, ethnic or religious organizations on the lifestyle and quality of life of the client

       h. Gender issues within the cultural group such as conformity to traditional gender roles wherein women are the caretakers of the home and children while men work outside of the home and have primary decision-making responsibilities

10. *Nutrition*

       a. Cultural influences on nutrition; *meaning* associated with food or meal sharing for the client and his or her family

       b. Nutritional disorders such as obesity, bulimia, anorexia or lactose intolerance

          1)   Nutritional disorders of family members

          2)   How client and family members view nutritional disorders

       c. Overview of eating patterns of client and family

          1)   What the client defines as "food"

          2)   What is considered a "healthy" diet

          3)   Congruency of beliefs with what the client actually eats

       d. Family member who shops for food and/or prepares meals

       e. How family members are involved in nutritional choices, values, and choices about food

       f. How foods are prepared at home

       g. Nutritional practices of client and family members such as vegetarianism and abstinence from red meat or alcoholic beverages

       h. Influence of religious beliefs on client's and family's diet

          1)   Observance of religious prescriptions or holidays that require abstinence or avoidance of certain foods such as kosher diets, observance of Ramadan, fasting on certain occasions

          2)   How fasting practices are observed within the family, periods of fasts, and exceptions to fasting

       i. Home remedies or special foods used to treat illnesses

11. *Religious Affiliation*

       a. Ways in which the client's religious affiliation and views influence health and illness

       b. Special rites or ceremonies associated with healing, recovery, illness, and/or death

          1)   Who performs the special religious ceremonies

          2)   Preparations that are necessary for the nurse to make prior to the practice of these rituals

       c. Role of religious representatives during health and illness.

12. Value orientation

       a. Client's and family members' attitudes, values and beliefs about health and illness

       b. How attitudes, values and beliefs influence health and illness behavior

       c. Stigmas associated with client's illness

       d. Reactions of client and family to changes that occur with illness or surgery

       e. Client's and family's views about biomedical health care

       f. Other cultural views that may influence health and illness behaviors

B. Leininger's Assessment Guides

  1. *Definition, Goal, Focus, Purpose, and Principles of Effective Cultural Assessments*

a. *Culture care assessments* refer to the systematic identification and documentation of culture care beliefs, meanings, values, symbols, and practices of individuals or groups within a holistic perspective, which includes worldview, life experiences, environmental context, ethnohistory, language, and diverse social structure influences (Leininger, 2002c, p. 117). [See also Leininger, 1995, p. 115; refer also to Sunrise Enabler #3 below and Section 2, Chapter 3, III B-2, V-4.]

b. *Goal of assessment*: To obtain a full and accurate account of the client so appropriate nursing care decisions can be made with the client for beneficial client health outcomes (Leininger, 2002c, p. 117).

c. *Major focus of assessment:* To identify culture care beliefs, values, patterns, expressions, and meanings related to the client's needs for obtaining or maintaining health or to face acute or chronic illness, disabilities, or death; include but go beyond traditional psychophysiological and medical foci (Leininger, 2002c, pp. 118-119).

d. *Purposes of assessment*: (Leininger, 2002c, p. 119)
   1) To discover the client's culture care and health patterns and meanings in relation to the client's worldview, lifeways, cultural values, beliefs, practices, context, and social structure factors;
   2) To obtain holistic culture care information as a sound basis for nursing care decisions and actions;
   3) To discover specific culture care patterns, meanings, and values that can be used to make differential nursing decisions that fit the client's values and lifeways, and to discover what professional knowledge can be helpful to the client;
   4) To identify potential areas of cultural conflicts, clashes, and neglected areas resulting from emic and etic value differences between clients and professional health personnel;
   5) To identify general and specific dominant themes and patterns that need to be known in context for culturally congruent care practices;
   6) To identify comparative cultural care information among clients of different or similar cultures, which can be shared and used in clinical teaching, and research practices; and
   7) To use theoretical ideas and research approaches to interpret and explain practices for congruent care and new ideas of transcultural nursing knowledge for discipline users.

e. *Principles of culturalogical assessment* (Leininger, 1995, pp. 121-129) [See also Leininger, 2002c, p. 121.]
   1) First Principle: Give attention to gender differences, communication modes, special language terms, interpersonal relationships, use of space and foods, and other additional aspects which the client may share [with you]; attention to attitudes and physical and dress appearance are important throughout the assessment.
   2) Second Principle: Show a genuine interest in the client and learn from and maintain respect for the client.
   3) Third Principle: Study the Sunrise Enabler before doing the assessment in order to draw upon these factors.
   4) Fourth Principle: Discover and remain aware of one's cultural biases and prejudices; learn to be aware of cultural blindness.
   5) Fifth Principle: Be aware that clients may belong to subcultures or special groups/situations such as homeless, person living with AIDS/HIV, drug abuse/recreational use, gay/lesbian, deafness, persons with mental retardation; be aware of stereotyping.
   6) Sixth Principle: Know one's own culture with its variabilities, strengths, and assets.
   7) Seventh Principle: Clarify and explain to the client (individual, family, or group) at the onset of assessment that the focus of a culturalogical or lifeway assessment is to help the client.
   8) Eighth Principle: Maintain a holistic or total view of the informant's world and environmental context by focusing on the multiple components depicted in the Sunrise Enabler.
   9) Ninth Principle: Remain an active listener to discover the client's emic lifeways, beliefs, and values, as well as etic professional ways, to fit client expectations and create a climate that is trusting, so client feels it is safe and beneficial to share his or her beliefs and lifeways.
   10) Tenth Principle: Reflect on learned "transcultural holding knowledge" about the client's culture and research-based care and health knowledge currently available.

2. ***Culturalogical Care Assessment***
   a. Long Guide [Refer to #7 below]
   b. Short Culturalogical Assessment Guide Enabler (Leininger, 2002c, p. 129) [See also Leininger, 1995, p. 142.] This is an alternative brief and general cultural assessment guide for use by nurses in short-term emergency and acute-care centers.
      1) Phase I: Record observations of what is seen, heard, or experienced; focus on dress and appearance, body condition features, language, mannerisms, and general behavior, attitudes, and cultural features.

    2) <u>Phase II</u>: Listen to and learn from client about cultural values, beliefs, and daily/nightly practices related to care and health in the client's environment.

    3) <u>Phase III</u>: Identify and record recurrent client patterns and narratives with client meanings of what has been seen, heard, or experienced;

    4) <u>Phase IV</u>: Synthesize themes and patterns of care derived from Phases I to III above;

    5) <u>Phase V</u>: Develop a culturally based client–nurse care plan as coparticipants for actions and decisions for culturally congruent care.

3. ***Sunrise Enabler*** (Leininger, 1997, pp. 37, 40) [See also Leininger, 1991a, p. 49; 2002b, pp. 80-81; 2006a, p. 25.]

    a. *Let the sun rise* figuratively means to have nurses open their minds in order to discover many different factors influencing care and ultimately the health and wellbeing of clients.

    b. Developed as a conceptual holistic research and assessment guide and enabler to help nurses and researchers discover multiple dimensions related to the theoretical tenets of the Theory of Culture Care.

    c. Enabler:

      1) Comprehensive and yet specific tool to depict different components that need to be studied systematically for the theory;

      2) Serves as a cognitive guide to tease out culture care phenomena from a holistic set of factors influencing care in cultures under study;

      3) Not the theory per se but depicts areas that need to be examined in relation to the theory tenets and the specific domain of inquiry under study;

      4) Differs from other nurse theorists' concepts or models as it serves different purposes within the qualitative paradigm and the Culture Care Theory;

      5) Focuses on multiple care influencers (not causes) that can explain emic and etic phenomena in different historical, cultural, and environmental contexts;

      6) Important to note that certain social structure factors: gender, class, race, historical and contextual factors, kinship, politics, cultural norms, legal factors, religion/spirituality, ethnohistory, biophysical, emotional, genetic, professional and generic health care are included;

      7) Extremely helpful in guiding nurses in thinking about these multiple factors and their influences on care meanings, patterns, symbols, and expression of care in different cultures; and,

      8) Has opened the minds of nurses to look for new and embedded knowledge areas related to human care and health.

4. ***Inquiry Guide for Use with the Sunrise Enabler to Assess Culture and Health*** (Leininger, 1995, pp. 145-148; 2002c, p. 137) [See also color insert #5, Leininger & McFarland, 2002.]

    a. Holding Knowledge

      1) Definition: Substantive background knowledge about a culture that serves as known knowledge on which to reflect on ideas and experiences (Leininger, 2002a, p. 10).

      2) Value: The constructs of *culture* and *care* are two domains that require in-depth study of people to have holding knowledge to guide nurses' thinking, actions, and decision; without such knowledge, nurses can be ineffective and even dangerous; it takes time to gain understanding of clients (Leininger, 2002a, p. 6).

    b. Purpose of the Guide: To enter into the world of the client and discover information to provide holistic, culture-specific care through the use of broad and open inquiry modes rather than direct confrontational questions (Leininger, 1995, pp. 145-148; Leininger, 2002c, pp. 137-138]

      1) Move with the client to make inquiry natural and familiar;

      2) Identify at outset if client is individual, family, group institution, or community; and

      3) Identify self and purpose of inquiry to the client (to learn from client their lifeway to provide nursing care that will be helpful or meaningful).

        a) Worldview

          (1) "I would like to know how you see the world around you."

          (2) "Please share with me your views of how you see things are for you."

        b) Ethnohistory

          (1) "Tell me something about your cultural background." "Where were you/your parents born? Where have you/your parents lived?"

          (2) "Tell me any stories you may have about how you were treated in a discriminatory way because of your cultural background."

      (3)   "Tell me about any special events in your life/your parents' lives."

  c) Kinship/social structure factors

      (1)   "I would like to hear about your family and/or close friends and what they mean to you."

      (2)   "Who are the caring or non-caring persons in your life?"

  d) Cultural values, beliefs, and lifeways

      (1)   "Please share with me what values and beliefs you would like nurses to know to help you regain or maintain your health."

      (2)   "What specific beliefs or practices do you find most important for others to know to care for you?"

  e) Religious/spiritual/philosophical factors

      (1)   "How do you think your beliefs and practices have helped you to care for yourself and others in keeping well or to regain health?"

      (2)   "How does religion help you to heal or to face crisis, disabilities, or even death?"

  f) Technological factors

      (1)   "In your daily life what 'high-tech' modern appliances or equipment are you greatly dependent upon?"

      (2)   "In what ways do you think technological factors help or hinder keeping you well?"

  g) Economic factors

      (1)   "In what ways do you believe money influences your health and access to care or to obtain professional services?"

      (2)   "How is money necessary to keep you well?"

  h) Political and legal factors

      (1)   "What are some of your views about politics and how you and others maintain your well-being?"

      (2)   "In your community or home, what political or legal problems tend to influence your well-being or handicap your lifeways in being cared for by others?"

  i) Educational factors

      (1)   "I would like to hear in what ways you believe education contributes to your staying well or becoming ill."

      (2)   "What educational information, values, or practices do you believe are important for nurses or others to care for you?"

  j) Language and communication factors

      (1)   "How would you like to communicate your needs to nurses?"

      (2)   "What languages do you speak or understand?"

  k) Professional and generic care beliefs and practices

      (1)   "What professional nursing care practices or attitudes do you believe have been or would be most helpful to your wellbeing within the hospital or at home?"

      (2)   "What does health, illness, or wellness mean to you and your family or culture?"

  l) General and specific nursing care

      (1)   "In what way would you like to be cared for in the hospital or at home by nurses?"

      (2)   "What is the meaning of care to you or in your culture?"

5. **Stranger to Trusted Friend Enabler** (Leininger, 1991b, 1995, 2002b, 2006b)

  a. This enabler is helpful as the nurse/HCP (health care provider) cares for the client(s) who may consider him or her to be a stranger.

  b. With this enabler, the nurse/HCP can learn much about herself or himself and the people he or she cares for.

  c. The goal is to move from a stranger and become a trusted friend. It is essential for the nurse/HCP to be trusted so the cultural assessment will reveal honest, in-depth, and credible data from clients.

  d. The following are indicators of being a *stranger* (largely etic or outsider's view):

    1) Actively protects self and others; acts as gatekeeper and guards against outside intrusions; suspicious and questioning.

    2) Actively watching and attentive to what the nurse/HCP says and does; limited signs of trusting the nurse/HCP or stranger

    3) Skeptical about the nurse/HCP's motives and work; may question how findings will be used by the nurse/HCP or stranger.

4) Reluctant to share cultural secrets and views as private knowledge; protective of local lifeways, values, and beliefs; dislikes probing by the nurse/HCP or stranger.

5) Uncomfortable in becoming a friend or confide in stranger; may come late, be absent, and withdraw at times from nurse/HCP.

6) Tends to offer inaccurate data; modifies truths to protect self, family, community, and cultural lifeways. Emic values, beliefs, and practices are not shared spontaneously.

e. Some indicators that the nurse/HCP is becoming a *trusted friend* (largely emic or insider's view):

1) Less active in protecting self; more trusting of nurse/HCP (less gate keeping); less suspicious and less questioning of nurse/HCP.

2) Less watching of nurse/HCP's words and actions; more signs of trusting and accepting new friend.

3) Less questioning of nurse/HCP's motives, work, and behavior; signs of working with and helping the nurse/HCP as a friend.

4) Willing to share cultural secrets and private world information and experiences; offers mostly local views, values, and interpretations spontaneously or without probes.

5) Signs of being comfortable and enjoying friendship—a sharing relationship; gives presence, is on time, and gives evidence of being a genuine "true" friend.

6) Wants assessment truths to be accurate regarding beliefs, people, values, and lifeways; explains and interprets emic ideas to nurse/HCP; nurse/HCP has accurate data of the client and his or her culture.

6. *Observation–Participation–Reflection Enabler*

a. Guides the nurse/HCP to move slowly and politely in conducting a cultural assessment after seeking permission to be with the client (Leininger, 2002b, p. 90) [See also Leininger, 1991b, p. 83; 2006b, p. 60]

b. Phase I focus: Primarily observation and active listening (no active participation);

c. Phase II focus: Primarily observation with limited participation;

d. Phase III focus: Primarily participation with continued observations; and

e. Phase IV focus: Primarily reflection with reconfirmation of findings with clients.

7. *Acculturation Health Care Assessment Enabler* (Leininger, 2002c, 139) [See also Leininger, 1991b, p. 93; 1995, p. 139; 2006b, p. 60].

a. Provides a qualitative assessment of traditional and nontraditional lifeways of clients.

b. Part I: A rating scale is used to assess traditionally and nontraditionally patterned cultural lifeways or orientations (1, mainly traditional; 2, moderate; 3, average; 4, moderate; 5, mainly nontraditional)

1) Criteria to be rated:

a) Language, communication, gestures (narrative and nonnarrative)

b) General environmental living conditions (symbols, material, and nonmaterial signs)

c) Wearing apparel and physical appearance

d) Technology used in the living environment

e) Worldview (how person looks out on the world)

f) Family lifeways (values, beliefs, norms)

g) General social interactions and kinship ties

h) Patterned daily activities

i) Religious or spiritual beliefs and values

j) Economic factors (approximate cost of living estimates and income)

k) Educational values or belief factors

l) Political or legal influencers

m) Food uses and nutritional values, beliefs, and taboos; specify

n) Folk (generic, lay, or indigenous) health care-cure values, beliefs, and practices; specify

o) Professional health care-cure values, beliefs, and practices; specify

p) Care concepts or patterns that guide actions, that is, concern for, support, presence, and so on.

q) Caring patterns or expressions

r) Client's ways to prevent illness, preserve or maintain wellness or health, and care for self or others.

s) Other indicators to support more traditional or nontraditional lifeways, including ethnohistorical and other factors.

t) Other notations

c. Part II: Acculturation profile form assessment factors using a numerical rating (1, mainly traditional; 2, moderate; 3, average; 4, moderate; 5, mainly nontraditional) for each of the following (see Leininger, 2002c, p.141):

1) Language and communication modes
2) Physical–social environment and ecology
3) Physical–apparel appearance
4) Technological factors
5) Worldview
6) Family lifeways
7) Social ties and kinship
8) Daily/nightly lifeways
9) Religious or spiritual orientation
10) Economic factors
11) Educational factors
12) Political or legal factors
13) Food uses/abuses
14) Folk (generic) care-cure
15) Professional care-cure expressions
16) Caring patterns
17) Curing patterns
18) Prevention/maintenance factors
19) Other indicators, that is, ethnohistorical

C. Purnell Model for Cultural Competence (Purnell, 2002)

1. *Metaparadigm Concepts: Global Society, Community, Family, Person, and Health*
2. *Domains*
   a. Overview, inhabited localities, topography
      1) Origins/ethnicity/ancestry
      2) Residence past and present
      3) Topography of current and past residence
      4) Economics
      5) Politics
      6) Educational level
      7) Occupation present and past
   b. Communication
      1) Dominant language and dialects
      2) Contextual use of the language
      3) Voice volume and tone
      4) Spatial distancing practices
      5) Use of eye contact and facial expressions
      6) Acceptable greetings
      7) Temporality
      8) Time social and work
      9) Name format
      10) Use of touch
   c. Family roles and organization
      1) Head of household and decision making
      2) Gender roles
      3) Family goals and priorities
      4) Developmental tasks
      5) Roles of older people
      6) Extended family
      7) Social status
      8) Alternative lifestyles
   d. Workforce issues
      1) Acculturation and work
      2) Autonomy in the workforce
      3) Language barriers

    e. Biocultural ecology
      1) Biological variations
      2) Skin color
      3) Hereditary and genetic diseases
      4) Drug metabolism
      5) Ecology and diseases/illnesses/injuries
    f. High-risk behaviors
      1) Tobacco and recreational substance use
      2) Alcohol
      3) Physical activity
      4) Safety measures
    g. Nutrition
      1) Meaning of food
      2) Common foods and limitations
      3) Food rituals
      4) Nutritional deficiencies
      5) Food and health promotion
    h. Pregnancy and childbearing practices
      1) Fertility practices
      2) Views toward pregnancy
      3) Prescriptive, restrictive, and taboo practices during pregnancy
      4) Prescriptive, restrictive, and taboo practices during labor and delivery
      5) Prescriptive, restrictive, and taboo practices during postpartum
    i. Death rituals
      1) Rituals during the dying process
      2) Meaning of death
      3) Bereavement practices
    j. Spirituality
      1) Religious practices
      2) Use of prayer
      3) Meaning of life
      4) Individual sources of strength
      5) Spirituality and health
    k. Health care practices
      1) Focus of health care
      2) Traditional and folk practices
      3) Magicoreligious beliefs and health care practices
      4) Responsibility for health and health care
      5) Views toward organ donation and transplantation
      6) Acceptance of blood and blood products
      7) Views toward chronicity and rehabilitation
      8) Self-medication practices
      9) Pain and the sick role
      10) Mental health views
      11) Barriers to health care
    l. Health care practitioners
      1) Perceptions of allopathic practitioners
      2) Folk practitioners
      3) Gender and health care
3. ***Primary and Secondary Characteristics of Culture: Not Categorically Imperative***
    a. Primary characteristics
      1) Nationality
      2) Age
      3) Race

    4) Color
    5) Gender
    6) Religion
  b. Secondary characteristics
    1) Educational status
    2) Socioeconomic status
    3) Occupation
    4) Military experience
    5) Political beliefs
    6) Urban versus rural residence
    7) Enclave identity
    8) Marital status
    9) Parental status
    10) Physical characteristics
    11) Sexual orientation
    12) Gender issues
    13) Length of time away from country of origin
    14) Immigration status (sojourner, immigrant, undocumented)

D. The Papadopoulos, Tilki, and Lees CCATool

1. *Background*
  a. The self-assessment Cultural Competence Assessment Tool (CCATool; Papadopoulos, Tilki & Lees, 2004; Table 1) was originally designed for mental health practitioners).
  b. Modified versions were subsequently developed for public health nurses and for practitioners working in the area of child and adolescent mental health.
  c. The rationale for this assessment approach is based on the principles of:
    1) Context specificity
    2) Client group specificity
    3) Culture-generic and culture-specific competencies
  d. The self-assessment CCATool is based on the Papadopoulos, Tilki, and Taylor (1998) model for developing cultural competence. The model consists of four constructs:
    1) Cultural awareness
    2) Cultural knowledge
    3) Cultural sensitivity
    4) Cultural competence

2. *Definitions and Concepts* (Papadopoulos, 2006)
  a. *Cultural competence* is the process one goes through to continuously develop and refine one's capacity to provide effective health and social care, taking into consideration people's cultural beliefs, behaviors and needs, as well as the effects that societal and organizational structures may have on them.
  b. Cultural competence requires the synthesis and application of previously gained awareness, knowledge and sensitivity into practice.
  c. A most important component of cultural competence is the ability to recognize and challenge racism and other forms of discrimination and oppressive practice.
  d. Throughout one's professional life, an individual develops a set of culture-generic competencies that are applicable across cultural groups (Gerrish & Papadopoulos, 1999).
  e. Using culture-generic competencies, enables the practitioner to develop culture-specific competencies according to their practice needs as it is impossible to have culture-specific competencies for an infinite number of cultures.

3. *Development of the CCATool* (Figure 1)
  a. The CCATool is divided into the following 4 sections each containing 10 statements:
    1) cultural awareness
    2) cultural knowledge
    3) cultural sensitivity
    4) cultural practice

Table 1. Cultural Competence Assessment Tool (CCATool)

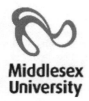

Middlesex University

RESEARCH CENTRE FOR
TRANSCULTURAL
STUDIES IN HEALTH

The RCTSH Cultural Competence Assessment Tool (CCATool)

(Mental Health Service Staff Specific)

Thank you for agreeing to complete this questionnaire. The data gathered from this will be used to help assess your cultural competence. The questionnaire is completely confidential. Any reporting of data will be done in such a way that none can be assigned to a particular individual.

The questionnaire is a self-assessment exercise. In the *tables* of statements please tick the response that seems most appropriate. Do not spend much time thinking about your answer. Please tick all the boxes. Leaving unticked boxes or responding 'not applicable' will negatively affect your total score. Please use the *box* to elaborate on any of your responses, noting the statement number. On the *lines* please circle the number that is nearest to where you feel you are regarding the statements.

Please send to Research Centre for Transcultural Studies in Health, Middlesex University, 2-10 Highgate Hill, London N19 5LW or contact Shelley Lees on 020 8411 5283, s.lees@mdx.ac.uk.

Thank-you very much

For Office Use Only

Id	
Site	
Score		

(continued)

Table 1. (continued)

A) Assessing Cultural Awareness   For office use only   ☐

	Statements	Strongly agree	Agree	Disagree	Strongly disagree
1	Cultural upbringing impacts on the way in which individuals view other people				
2	People from different ethnic groups share many of the same values and beliefs as people from the host community				
3	There are many differences in values and beliefs within any single ethnic group				
4	Gender, age, class and generation are as important as ethnicity in forming a person's identity				
5	Ethnic identity changes with time and the influence of wider social factors				
6	Some aspects of culture are more important to a person than others				
7	People select the most relevant aspects of their culture in different situations				
8	People from different ethnic groups may have the same needs but they may be expressed in different ways				
9	To avoid imposing values on a client practitioners should be aware of their own value and belief systems				
10	Ethnic identity is influenced by personal, social and psychological factors				

Please elaborate on any statement/s

Please circle the number you feel nearest to

I am not at all aware of my own ethnic and cultural identity	I am highly aware of my own ethnic and cultural identity

   1   2   3   4   5   6   7   8   9   10

(continued)

Table 1. (continued)

B) Assessing Cultural Knowledge   For office use only   ☐

	Statements	Strongly agree	Agree	Disagree	Strongly disagree
1	Monitoring the ethnicity of all clients can help identify the effectiveness of service access and delivery				
2	Effective care requires an adequate knowledge of the client's culture				
3	It is not possible to have full knowledge of all cultures				
4	There is much to be learned from the folk systems of the client				
5	People from minority ethnic groups have particular difficulty accessing day care services				
6	Discrimination and harassment in everyday life leads people to engage in behaviours which may be damaging to mental health				
7	Compulsory admission/ detention rates are higher for black people				
8	Black people with mental health problems are more likely to have contact with the criminal justice system				
9	It is important to acknowledge particular cultural beliefs and practices in relation to mental health of minority ethnic groups				
10	Clients who perceive themselves to be possessed by spirits are invariably mentally disturbed				

Please elaborate on any statement/s

Please circle the number you feel nearest to

I am not at all informed about the culture and social situation of the majority of my clients	I am very well informed about the culture and social situation of the majority of my clients

          1   2   3   4   5   6   7   8   9   10

(continued)

Table 1. (continued)

C) Assessing Cultural Sensitivity   For office use only   ☐

	Statements	Strongly agree	Agree	Disagree	Strongly disagree
1	It is almost impossible to communicate with a client whose first language is not English				
2	Greeting family members before the client may be appropriate in some minority ethnic groups				
3	Clients who avoid eye contact are always suspicious or withdrawn				
4	Practitioners need to be trained in the use of interpreters and advocates				
5	Interpreters and advocates need to be trained in order to effectively represent the best interests of the client				
6	People from some minority ethnic groups can be very demanding				
7	It is important to discuss the impact of ethnicity on the therapeutic relationship where the client and practitioner are from different cultures				
8	Religion can be a source of comfort and reassurance for some clients				
9	People from minority ethnic groups get little benefit from psychological therapies				
10	The stigma of mental illness is greater in some minority ethnic groups than in the host community				

Please elaborate on any statement/s

Please circle the number you feel nearest to

I am very uncomfortable working with people whose beliefs, values and practices are different from my own	I am very comfortable working with people whose beliefs, values and practices are different from my own

1   2   3   4   5   6   7   8   9   10

I am not at all confident of my ability to establish trust, show respect and empathy to all people whatever their culture	I am very confident of my ability to establish trust, show respect and empathy to all people whatever their culture

1   2   3   4   5   6   7   8   9   10

(continued)

Table 1. (continued)

D) Assessing Cultural Practice　　　For office use only　　□

	Statements	Strongly agree	Agree	Disagree	Strongly disagree
1	Subtle forms of racism are as damaging as overt forms				
2	Institutional racism is seen in unwitting prejudice, ignorance and thoughtlessness				
3	Recognising and challenging institutional racism is the responsibility of each individual health practitioner				
4	User participation is a critical component of good practice and should be encouraged at all levels of service provision				
5	Professionals and clients need training in user participation				
6	Best practice can be achieved by joint partnership between statutory and voluntary sectors				
7	The expertise of the minority ethnic voluntary sector should be used more effectively to obtain advice on good practice				
8	Stereotypes have an impact on how clients are assessed				
9	Stereotypes may account for the high level of compulsory detention and treatment of people from minority ethnic groups				
10	The type and route of medication should be based on sound clinical judgement of client need and the degree of danger to self and others				

Please elaborate on any statement/s

Please circle the number you feel nearest to

I am not at all able to incorporate the clients cultural beliefs into the care and treatment I provide	I am very able to incorporate the clients cultural beliefs into the care and treatment I provide

1　2　3　4　5　6　7　8　9　10

I am not at all confident to challenge racism and discrimination towards clients, carers and staff	I am very confident to challenge racism and discrimination towards clients, carers and staff

1　2　3　4　5　6　7　8　9　10

(continued)

Table 1. (continued)

About You

Please tick the relevant box

1. **Name** _____ (this will be kept confidential)

2. **Gender**   Male   Female   3. **Age** _____   years

4. **Ethnic Group (2001 UK Census Categories)**

White   *Mixed*

☐ British   ☐ White and Black Carib
                                                     ☐ White and Black African
☐ Irish   ☐ White and Asian
☐ Any other white background   ☐ Any other mixed background

Asian or Asian British   *Black or Black British*

☐ Indian   ☐ Caribbean
☐ Pakistani   ☐ African
☐ Bangladeshi   ☐ Any other Black Background
☐ Any other Asian background

Other Ethnic groups

☐ Chinese
☐ Any other ethnic group

5. **Country of birth** _____

6. **If you were born outside the UK, how many years have you lived in the UK?** _____ years

7. **What religion are you?**

☐ Buddhist   ☐ Jewish   ☐ Other (please state) _____
☐ Christian   ☐ Muslim   ☐ Atheist
☐ Hindu   ☐ Sikh   ☐ None

8. **Languages**

What is your first language? _____ Other Languages spoken _____

9. **Work Experience**

(a)   *Role*

☐ Social Worker   ☐ Community Psychiatric Nurse
☐ Occupational therapist   ☐ Counsellor
☐ Doctor   ☐ Psychologist
☐ Psychiatric Nurse   ☐ Unqualified Mental Health Worker
☐ Other (Specify) _____

    (b) How many years have you worked in your profession? _____ Years

    (c) How many years have you worked in your current location? (site) _____ Years

---

Table 1. CCATool. The Papadopoulos, Tilki and Taylor Model for developing Cultural Competence. Source: Papadopoulos, Tilki & Lees (2004). Promoting cultural competence in health care through a research based intervention. *Journal of Diversity in Health and Social Care*, 1(2), 107-115). Permission to reprint from Radcliffe Publishing

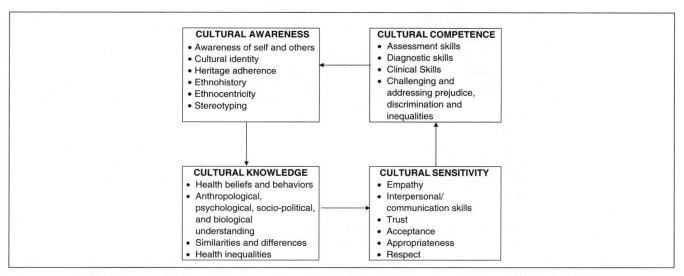

Figure 1. The Papadopoulos, Tilki and Taylor Model for developing Cultural Competence. Source: Papadopoulos, Tilki & Lees (2004). Promoting cultural competence in health care through a research based intervention. *Journal of Diversity in Health and Social Care*, 1(2), 107-115). Permission to reprint from Radcliffe Publishing

    b. The Delphi approach was used to develop the statements of the CCATool and assure content validity.
       1) A panel of experts was established.
       2) A data collection document was developed in order to collect the panel's opinions on the relevance and importance of an initial list of statements.
       3) The panel could suggest alternative statements which were included in the next round of the Delphi process.
       4) The Delphi process was repeated until consensus was achieved on which statements to include in the tool.
    c. Characteristics of the CCATool
       1) All statements in the "cultural awareness" area are culture generic.
       2) Four statements in each of the other areas are culture generic.
       3) Six statements in each of the other areas are culture specific.
       4) Piloting of the tool was conducted to ascertain the reliability of the tool.
       5) Each statement correctly answered receives one point, whereas incorrectly answered statements receive zero points.
       6) The maximum points that can be awarded are 40.
    d. The CCATool has four levels of cultural competence. These are determined by the scores on the tool which are interpreted as:
       1) *Cultural Incompetence* (CI). A person is culturally incompetent if he or she receives a score of less than 5 in cultural awareness, whatever his or her score is in the other three areas included in the tool.
       2) *Cultural Awareness* (CA) A person is culturally aware if he or she achieves a score of 5 or more in cultural awareness, without necessarily having all the generic statements in the other areas correct.
       3) *Cultural Safety* (CS). A person is culturally safe if he or she achieves a score of 5 or more in cultural awareness, and all the generic statements in the other stages correct.
       4) *Cultural Competence* (CC). A person is culturally competent if he or she achieves a score of 10 in all of the four stages (a perfect score).
    e. The CCATool contains a subjective measurement of cultural competence using the Visual Analogue Scale (VAS).
       1) Each area of self-assessment contains a continuum of competence, for example:
"I am not at all aware . . .   I am highly aware . . ."

---

1   2   3   4   5   6   7   8   9   10
       2) Assessees are asked to indicate their level on a scale of 1 to 10.
       3) Assessees can compare their perception of their scores in each area with their score achieved by their responses to the statements included in each area.

4. ***Principles of CCATool Development*** that guide the adaptation of the tool to suit health professionals working in other areas of practice.
    a. Context specificity: The CCATool is based on the principle that tools derived within and for a particular country or health care system are largely inappropriate in another country or health care system.
    b. Client group: The CCATool is also based on the principle that tools developed to assess the cultural competence of practitioners working with a specific group of clients are largely inappropriate for use with other client groups and must be adapted before use.
    c. Culture-generic and culture-specific statements:
        1) Culture-generic statements of the original CCATool are broadly applicable to all contexts and clients groups. They remain constant in all versions of the CCATool but may require some amendment of the terminology.
        2) Culture-specific statements of the original CCATool must be amended to the specific context and client group.

5. ***Modified Versions of the CCATool***
    a. The CCATool is now available for public health nurses (Knight-Jackson, 2008)
    b. The CCATool is also available for practitioners working in the area of child and adolescent mental health (Papadopoulos, Tilki, & Ayling, 2008)
    c. The CCATool is currently being adapted for practitioners working with older adults in Denmark.

6. ***Adaptation of the CCATool***
    a. The tool offers a basic framework for assessing cultural competence.
    b. The value of adapting it lies in the exploration and the inclusion of elements pertinent to a specific national and professional context.
    c. Adapting the tool using the Delphi method affords many opportunities to debate widely held or common-sense assumptions.
    d. It provides for the exploration of issues related to particular ethnic groups and to national issues.
    e. It can encourage discussion of organizational customs and practices which may not be a problem for the majority but which may inadvertently discriminate against some groups.
    f. Working with a group of colleagues, clients and possibly community leaders is more time consuming but the added value of the debate and dialogue involved is immeasurable.
    g. Drawing on the expert knowledge of the Delphi panel can make the tool more valid as well as give a team a sense of pride and ownership of the whole project.

E. Heritage Assessment Tool (Spector, 2008)

1. ***Purpose:*** *To assess the degree to which a given person/family/community adheres to traditional ethno-religious-cultural health and healing beliefs and practices.*

2. ***Designed to assess***
    a. Culture
    b. Ethnicity
    c. Religion
    d. Socialization
    e. Acculturation
    f. Assimilation

3. ***Interpretation of assessment***
    a. Heritage Consistent—Identification with a traditional heritage and family relations
    b. Heritage Inconsistent—Identification with modern, dominant culture than ethnic practices

4. ***Factors inherent in heritage*** (Table 1)
    a. Childhood development occurred in the person's country of origin or in an immigrant neighborhood in the United States of like ethnic group
    b. Extended family members encouraged participation in traditional religious and cultural activities.
    c. Frequent visits to country of origin or to the "old neighborhood" in the United States
    d. Family homes are within the community of heritage
    e. Participation in religious/ethnic cultural events, such as festivals
    f. Raised in an extended family setting
    g. Maintains regular contact with the extended family
    h. Name has not been Americanized
    i. Engages in social activities primarily with others of the same heritage
    j. Knowledge of the culture and language of origin
    k. Personal pride about heritage

Table 2. The Heritage Assessment Tool

This set of questions is to be used to describe a given person's—or your own—ethnic, cultural, and religious background. In performing a *heritage assessment* it is helpful to determine how deeply a given person identifies with his or her traditional heritage. This tool is most useful in setting the stage for assessing and understanding a person's traditional HEALTH and ILLNESS beliefs and practices and in helping to determine the community resources that will be appropriate to target for support when necessary. The greater the number of positive responses, the greater the degree to which the person may identify with his or her traditional heritage. The one exception to positive answers is the question about whether or not a person's name was changed.

1. Where was your mother born? _____
2. Where was your father born? _____
3. Where were your grandparents born?
   a. Your mother's mother? _____
   b. Your mother's father? _____
   c. Your father's mother?
   d. Your father's father? _____
4. How many brothers _____ and sisters _____ do you have?
5. What setting did you grow up in? Urban _____ Rural _____
6. What country did your parents grow up in?
   Father _____
   Mother _____
7. How old were you when you came to the United States?
8. How old were your parents when they came to the United States?
   Mother _____
   Father _____
9. When you were growing up, who lived with you? _____
10. Have you maintained contact with
    a. Aunts, uncles, cousins?   (1) Yes _____ (2) No _____
    b. Brothers and sisters?   (1) Yes _____ (2) No _____
    c. Parents?   (1) Yes _____ (2) No _____
    d. Your own children?   (1) Yes _____ (2) No _____
11. Did most of your aunts, uncles, cousins live near your home? 1) Yes ___ (2) No ___
12. Approximately how often did you visit family members who lived outside of your home?
    (1) Daily _____ (2) Weekly _____ (3) Monthly _____
    (4) Once a year or less _____ (5) Never _____
13. Was your original family name changed? 1) Yes _____ (2) No _____
14. What is your religious preference?
    (1) Catholic _____ (2) Jewish _____ (3) Protestant _____ Denomination _____
    (4) Other _____ (5) None _____
15. Is your spouse the same religion as you?
    (1) Yes _____ (2) No _____
16. Is your spouse the same ethnic background as you?
    (1) Yes _____ (2) No _____
17. What kind of school did you go to?
    (1) Public _____ (2) Private _____ (3) Parochial _____
18. As an adult, do you live in a neighborhood where the neighbors are the same religion and ethnic background as yourself?
    (1) Yes _____ (2) No _____
19. Do you belong to a religious institution? (1) Yes _____ (2) No _____
20. Would you describe yourself as an active member?
    1) Yes _____ (2) No _____
21. How often do you attend your religious institution?
    (1) More than once a week _____ (2) Weekly _____ (3) Monthly _____
    (4) Special holidays only _____ (5) Never _____
22. Do you practice your religion in your home?
    (1) Yes _____ (2) No _____ (if yes, please specify):
    (3) Praying _____ (4) Bible reading _____ (5) Diet _____
    (6) Celebrating religious holidays _____
23. Do you prepare foods special to your ethnic background?
    (1) Yes _____ (2) No _____
24. Do you participate in ethnic activities?
    (1) Yes _____ (2) No _____ (if yes, please specify)
    (3) Singing _____ (4) Holiday celebrations _____ (5) Dancing _____
    (6) Festivals _____ (7) Costumes _____ (8) Other _____

(continued)

Table 2. (continued)

25. Are your friends from the same religious background as you?
    (1) Yes _____ (2) No _____
26. Are your friends from the same ethnic background as you?
    (1) Yes _____ (2) No _____
27. What is your native language? _____
28. Do you speak this language?
    (1) Prefer _____ (2) Occasionally _____ (3) Rarely _____
29. Do you read your native language?
Yes _____ (2) No _____

Source: Spector, R. (2008). Cultural diversity in health and illness. Upper Saddle Rover, NJ: Pearson. Permission to reprint from Pearson Education Publications.

V. SUMMARY

A. This chapter focuses on cultural assessment that addresses cultural and religious beliefs and practices; includes both subjective (interview) and objective (physical) data; and provides guidance for how to integrate the assessment data into the overall plan for care.

B. Cultural assessment models in this chapter include those by Andrews and Boyle, Giger and Davidhizar, Leininger, Purnell, and Spector.

C. These models offer clinicians a range of interrelated concepts and guidelines for the conduct of cultural assessments.

D. Wehbe-Alamah and McFarland include a case example that demonstrates Leininger's culturalogical assessment.

E. The content in this chapter links with the life span content in Chapters 5 and 6 to provide an overview of cultural health beliefs and practices and related assessment approaches. Thus the three chapters in Section III are interrelated in addressing the objectives of this core curriculum text.

Case Study

Assessment of a Traditional Lebanese Muslim Patient

Objectives:

1. Apply Leininger's principles of culturalogical assessment and enablers to a traditional Lebanese Muslim patient.
2. Identify important cultural beliefs, expressions, and practices of a traditional Lebanese Muslim patient.
3. Determine nursing actions and decisions needed to provide culturally congruent care for a traditional Lebanese Muslim patient.

Mrs. Rana Salam is a 20-year-old Lebanese Muslim woman who has been experiencing labor pain for the past 4 hours. Her expected due date was 1 week ago. She immigrated to the United States 9 months ago. She is a student enrolled in the local university and speaks fluent English. This is her first pregnancy. The only family member she has with her in the United States is her husband. Mrs. Salam is wearing a head cover, a long skirt, and a shirt with long sleeves. She has a gold necklace with an emblem that has some writings and a blue stone on it. She reports a yellowish greenish nasal discharge for the last four days accompanied by a feeling of pressure over her sinuses and forehead. The physician on call today is Dr John Adams. You are a nursing student assigned to do her cultural assessment and to follow her through her delivery and discharge.

1. Applying Leininger's principles of culturalogical assessment and cultural assessment enablers to a traditional Lebanese Muslim patient

To get an accurate cultural assessment of your assigned patient and to prevent potential *cultural clashes*, *cultural pain*, or *cultural imposition practices*, you decide to apply Leininger's principles of culturalogical assessment in conjunction with Leininger's Sunrise Enabler, Observation–Participation–Reflection Enabler, Stranger to Trusted Friend Enabler, Acculturation Health Care Assessment Enabler, Inquiry Guide for Use with the Sunrise Enabler to Assess Culture and Health Enabler, and Short Culturalogical Assessment Guide Enabler.

As you have learned that an antecedent to conducting accurate cultural assessment is the discovery of one's own culture and areas of cultural competencies as well as deficits, you examine your own *cultural values*, *beliefs*, and *practices* as well as *biases, prejudices*, and *stereotypes* in relation to the Lebanese Muslim culture by relying on an adaptation of the Sunrise Enabler and the Inquiry Guide and your knowledge of the Culture Care Theory. Questions you may ask yourself include:

a. What are my important cultural values and beliefs?
b. Who or what has influenced the development of my cultural values and beliefs?
c. What important cultural traditions do I engage in?
d. What does family mean to me and what role do family members play in my health care?
e. What types of food are important in my culture and what is their significance to health care?
f. What are important verbal expressions and body language used in my culture and what is their meaning?
g. What do I know about Lebanese Muslims?
h. What stereotypes have I formulated about members of this culture?
i. What transcultural holding knowledge have I been exposed to in relation to the Lebanese Muslim culture?

Following your cultural self-assessment and reflection on *holding knowledge* in relation to the Lebanese Muslim culture, you decide to approach your client with an open mind and a genuine desire to learn about her culture in order to provide her with culturally congruent care. Your goal at this point is to remain fully aware of your own prejudices and biases and to obtain an individualized cultural assessment of your client. You need to be aware that *differences exist within and between cultures* and members of any culture may also belong to *subcultures* within their own culture. Discoveries from applications of Leininger's principles of culturalogical assessment and cultural assessment enablers will assist you in seeking a holistic view of your Lebanese Muslim patient's world by focusing on familiar and multiple factors depicted in the Sunrise Enabler that influence *health, care, illness*, or *well-being*.

As you enter Mrs. Salam's room, you begin by introducing yourself to her and inquire how she likes to be addressed. You explain the purpose of your presence and your interest in learning about her cultural values, beliefs, and lifeways so you can provide her with care that is meaningful to her. By doing so, you begin to establish trust with your client. Establishing trust will allow you to move from the role of a *Stranger* to that of a *Trusted Friend* and will assist you in obtaining *accurate, in-depth*, and *reliable* data as you proceed with the cultural assessment of your client. This process can further be facilitated by paying close attention to your client's *body language, gender issues, eye contact, communication modes*, and *interpersonal space*, as well as by *remaining an active listener* throughout the cultural assessment process.

Based on your knowledge of Leininger's Culture Care Theory and relevant enablers, you proceed with your cultural assessment. Questions you may ask Mrs. Salam based on all of the above include:

a. Which cultural group do you identify yourself with?
b. What cultural beliefs and practices are important for you to maintain in the health care setting?
c. What is your belief about the evil eye, what causes it, and how do you prevent it? In your culture, how do men, women, children, and nurses provide care?
d. Who is the health care decision maker in your family?
e. Who helps you when you are sick or need care?
f. What does religion mean to you?
g. How do you practice it and how does it help you?
h. What types of technology are forbidden or discouraged by your religion?
i. What are restrictions you may have in relation to diet?
j. What are areas I did not cover yet that I need to know about in order to provide you with care that fits with your cultural beliefs and practices?

2. Discovering important cultural beliefs, expressions, and practices of a traditional Lebanese Muslim patient

The cultural assessment you just engaged in revealed the following information: Mrs. Salam identifies herself as a traditional Lebanese Muslim. She values modesty and privacy from a cultural and religious perspective. She prefers to have same gender health care providers but will accept to have a male caregiver in the event of an emergency and in the absence of a female health care provider. She prefers to remove her head cover while in the hospital provided that measures are taken by the hospital staff to protect her from being exposed to male visitors and health care professionals. A respectable amount of personal space as well as fleeting, indirect nonprolonged eye contact are the norm in her culture in relation to interaction with males. She does not shake hands with men and prefers to have no physical contact with them unless absolutely necessary such as for medical procedures. She believes that effusive or passionate admiration may cause someone and especially newborns to be afflicted by the evil eye. She explains that the necklace she is wearing is supposed to protect her from the evil eye because it has writings from her holy book, the *Qur'an*. Similar emblems are pinned to the newborn's clothing to protect him or her from the evil eye. Expressions such as *Mashallah* are used to ward off the evil eye when admiring newborns. The father of the newborn is supposed to whisper the call of prayer in the newborn's right ear as soon as possible after birth. This is supposed to introduce the baby to Islam and to protect him or her from the devil.

You learn that in Mrs. Salam's culture, females provide emotional and physical care whereas men provide financial care but may also engage in physical or emotional care. It is customary for hospitalized individuals to receive many visitors since visiting the sick is considered a cultural and religious duty. Females from her community will stop by her house following her discharge from the hospital and will provide her with nutritious meals and assist with cleaning her if needed. According to Mrs. Salam, nurses are considered caring if they engage in the following activities: smiling, respecting, and accommodating the cultural needs of their patients, and responding promptly to their clients when called. While her husband consults with her in various matters, she considers him to be the ultimate decision maker in the family. Mrs. Salam is a devout Muslim and believes that her religion guides all aspects of her life. She finds solace and an inner sense of peace by reading her holy book and praying five times a day. She adheres to the Muslim food code (*halal*) which forbids the consumption of alcohol and pig products such as gelatin, ham, lard, pepperoni, etc. She explains that as non-halal gelatin is an ingredient of Jello and most gelatin-encapsulated medications, she is unable to consume any of these products. Mrs. Salam is interested in birth control following delivery. Her religion allows her to use reversible forms of birth control. Irreversible methods such as tubal ligation or vasectomy are considered unlawful in her religion.

3.   Nursing actions and decisions needed to provide culturally congruent care for a traditional Lebanese Muslim patient

Based on the information you discovered from conducting a cultural assessment using Leininger's cultural assessment enablers and principles for culturological assessment, you decide to devise a care plan that incorporates nursing actions and decisions needed to provide culturally congruent care for your traditional Lebanese Muslim patient. You start by reporting your findings to the registered nurse assigned for your patient and other staff in the OB and nursery units and proceed to attempt to locate a female physician because the OB-GYN physician on call was a male. Luckily for you, the physician who has been caring for Mrs. Salam, Dr. Sally Smith, had left a note in her chart requesting to be notified of Mrs. Salam's admission. Dr. Smith informs you that she will come to the hospital to deliver the patient's baby. In the meantime, you put a sign on Mrs. Salam's door that reads: "Request and wait for permission before entering room." This sign is designed to give your client time to cover her head before receiving male visitors or health care providers.

After four additional hours of labor, Mrs. Salam gives birth to a healthy baby boy. Having been briefed by you about the cultural practice of reciting the call of prayer in the newborn's right ear after birth, the nurse assisting with the delivery hands the baby to the father who proceeds with fulfilling this cultural practice. The mother pins a silver pendant with religious emblems to the hat covering the baby's head. You and the rest of the health care providers abstain from effusive expressions of admirations in relation to the newborn baby. The baby is sent to the nursery for additional follow-up. Having read your cultural assessment notes in the chart, Dr. Smith refrains from discussing tubal ligation with Mrs. Salam and discusses oral contraceptives for birth control instead. You notice that Dr. Smith has also ordered amoxicillin for the patient's sinusitis. You call the pharmacy and explain to them that the medication should not be sent in gelatin encapsulated form. Amoxicillin tablets are provided instead. In addition, you contact the hospital dietary department and explain the food restrictions of your patient. You arrange for *halal* gelatin to be provided to your patient and ensure that no pork derivatives will be served. Finally, in anticipation of a potentially large number of visitors, you arrange for a waiting room and negotiate with the client a predetermined number of visitors at a time.

Before her discharge, Mrs. Salam insists on taking a picture with you and shares with you that you made her stay memorable and very comfortable. She especially is thankful for the way you respected and accommodated her cultural beliefs and practices.

NOTE: All references, additional resources, and important Internet sites relevant to this chapter can be found at the following website: http://tcn.sagepub.com/supplemental

Section IV. Cultural Competence in Education, Organizations, Research and Professional Roles

Associate Editor: Stephen R. Marrone, EdD, RN-BC, CTN-A

Chapter 8
Educational Issues for Students, Organizational Staff, Patients, and Communities

Journal of Transcultural Nursing
21(Supplement 1) 338S–356S
© The Author(s) 2010
Reprints and permission:
sagepub.com/journalsPermissions.nav
DOI: 10.1177/1043659610364635
http://tcn.sagepub.com

Marianne R. Jeffreys, EdD, RN

I. **Theoretical Framework for Teaching Cultural Competence: Jeffreys's Cultural Competence and Confidence (CCC) Model (Jeffreys, 2006; see Chapter 3)**
   A. **Proposed as an organizing framework** for examining the multidimensional factors involved in the process of learning cultural competence (CC) to:
      1. Identify at-risk individuals
      2. Develop diagnostic-prescriptive strategies to facilitate learning
      3. Guide innovations in teaching and educational research
      4. Evaluate strategy effectiveness
   B. **Interrelates concepts** that explain, describe, influence, and/or predict the phenomenon of learning (developing) CC and incorporates the construct of transcultural self-efficacy (TSE; confidence) as a major influencing factor
   C. **Cultural competence** is defined as a multidimensional learning process* that integrates:
      1. Transcultural skills in all three learning dimensions
         a. Cognitive
         b. Practical
         c. Affective
      2. Involves transcultural self-efficacy (confidence) as a major factor
      3. Aims to achieve cultural congruent care
         Learning process emphasizes that the cognitive, practical, and affective dimensions of transcultural self-efficacy can change over time as a result of formalized education and other learning experiences.
   D. **Transcultural skills**
      1. Those skills necessary for assessing, planning, implementing, and evaluating culturally congruent care for diverse populations
      2. Incorporate cognitive, practical, and affective dimensions
   E. **Transcultural self-efficacy** is defined as:
      1. Perceived confidence for performing or learning transcultural skills
      2. Degree to which individuals perceive they have the ability to perform the specific transcultural nursing skills needed for culturally competent and congruent care despite obstacles and hardships
   F. **Cognitive learning dimension**
      1. General: focuses on knowledge outcomes, intellectual abilities, and skills
      2. Specific to transcultural learning: knowledge and comprehension about ways in which cultural factors may influence professional care among clients of different* cultural backgrounds and throughout the lifecycle
         *Different refers to clients representing various different racial, ethnic, gender, socioeconomic, and religious groups
   G. **Practical learning dimension**
      1. General: similar to psychomotor learning domain and focuses on motor skills or practical application of skills
      2. Specific to transcultural learning: refers to communication skills (verbal and nonverbal) needed to interview clients of different cultural backgrounds about their values and beliefs

Funding: The California Endowment (grant number 20082226) and Health Resources and Services Administration (grant number D11 HPO9759).
[1]The City University of New York (CUNY) Graduate College and CUNY College of Staten Island, Staten Island, NY

Corresponding Author: Marianne R. Jeffreys, Email: marianne.jeffreys@csi.cuny.edu

Suggested Citation: Douglas, M. K. & Pacquiao, D. F. (Eds.). (2010). Core curriculum in transcultural nursing and health care [Supplement]. *Journal of Transcultural Nursing, 21*(Suppl. 1).

H. **Affective learning dimension**
    1. General
        a. Concerned with attitudes, values, and beliefs
        b. Considered to be crucial for developing professional values and beliefs
    2. Specific to transcultural learning: Includes:
        a. Self-awareness
        b. Awareness of cultural gap (differences)
        c. Acceptance
        d. Appreciation
        e. Recognition
        f. Advocacy

I. **CC is influenced by**:
    1. TSE
    2. The learning of transcultural skills (cognitive, practical, affective)
    3. Formalized educational experiences
    4. Other learning experiences

J. **TSE pathway**
    1. *Traces the proposed influences of TSE on a learner's* actions, performance, and persistence for learning tasks associated with cultural competency development and culturally congruent care
    2. *First step is self-efficacy appraisal, an individualized* process influenced by four information sources: (Bandura, 1977, 1982, 1986, 1989, 1997)
        a. Actual performances
        b. Vicarious experiences (role models)
        c. Forms of persuasion (encouragement from others)
        d. Emotional arousal (physiological indices, such as sweating)
    3. *Resilient individuals* (realistically medium–high self-efficacy)
        a. Highly motivated and actively seek help to maximize their CC and transcultural skill development
        b. Most likely to persist in CC development
        c. Most likely to achieve cultural congruent care actions
        d. Following CC educational interventions, changes in TSE noted
    4. *Low self-efficacy (low confidence) individuals*
        a. Poorly motivated and reluctant to actively seek help in CC and transcultural skill development
        b. At risk for avoiding transcultural tasks
        c. Unlikely to persist in CC tasks
        d. Unlikely to achieve cultural congruent care actions
        e. Most improvement noted in TSE gains following CC educational interventions
    5. *Supremely efficacious (overly confident) individuals*
        a. May be totally unaware of their cultural incompetencies and weaknesses
        b. Likely to underestimate the transcultural task or its importance
        c. At risk for overestimating their abilities, overrating their strengths
        d. Unlikely to recognize the need for adequate preparation for CC
        e. Unlikely to recognize the need to restructure priorities or time management to accommodate transcultural tasks
        f. Unlikely to achieve cultural congruent care actions
        g. Following CC educational interventions, more likely to become more conservative (realistic) in TSE appraisals

K. **Components of comprehensive CC education**
    1. Weave together cognitive, practical, and affective learning
    2. Encompass assessment, planning, implementation, and evaluation
    3. Integrate self-efficacy appraisals and diagnostic-prescriptive interventions
    4. Coordinated program planning and updates

L. **Assumptions of CCC model** (Jeffreys, 2006, pp. 32-33)
    1. "*Cultural competence is an ongoing, multidimensional* learning process that integrates transcultural skills in all three dimensions (cognitive, affective, and practical), involves TSE (confidence) as a major influencing factor, and aims to achieve cultural congruent care.

2. **TSE is a dynamic construct** that changes over time and is influenced by formalized exposure to culture care concepts (transcultural nursing).

3. **The learning of transcultural nursing skills is influenced** by self-efficacy perceptions (confidence).

4. **The performance of transcultural nursing skill competencies** is directly influenced by the adequate learning of such skills and by TSE perceptions.

5. **The performance of culturally congruent nursing skills** is influenced by self-efficacy perceptions and by formalized educational exposure to transcultural nursing care concepts and skills throughout the educational experience.

6. **All students and nurses (regardless of age,** ethnicity, gender, sexual orientation, lifestyle, religion, socioeconomic status, geographic location, or race) require formalized educational experiences to meet culture care needs of diverse individuals.

7. **The most comprehensive learning involves** the integration of cognitive, practical, and affective dimensions.

8. **Learning in the cognitive, practical, and affective** dimensions is paradoxically distinct yet interrelated.

9. **Learners are most confident about their attitudes** (affective dimension) and least confident about their transcultural nursing knowledge (cognitive dimension).

10. **Novice learners will have lower self-efficacy** perceptions than advanced learners.

11. **Inefficacious individuals are at risk for decreased** motivation, lack of commitment, and/or avoidance of cultural considerations when planning and implementing nursing care.

12. **Supremely efficacious (overly confident)** individuals are at risk for inadequate preparation in learning the transcultural nursing skills necessary to provide culturally congruent care.

13. **Early intervention with at-risk individuals** will better prepare nurses to meet cultural competency.

14. **The greatest change in TSE** perceptions will be detected in individuals with low self-efficacy (low confidence) initially, who have then been exposed to formalized transcultural nursing concepts and experiences."

II. **Teaching Learners of Various Cultural and Educational Backgrounds (Jeffreys, 2004, 2006)**
   A. **Assessing diverse learner needs**
      1. *Nontraditional students in nursing (one or more of the following)*
         a. Age 25 or older
         b. Commuter
         c. Enrolled part-time
         d. Male
         e. Member of an ethnic and/or racial minority group
         f. Speaks dominant culture language as a second (other) language
         g. Has dependent children
         h. Has a general equivalency diploma for secondary school
         i. Required remedial classes
      2. *Cultural factors*
         a. Identity and background
            (1) Ethnicity
            (2) Race
            (3) Gender
            (4) Sexual orientation
            (5) Class (economic background)
            (6) Immigration history
            (7) Minority vs. nonminority group
            (8) Religion
         b. Pertinent role perceptions
            (1) Role of the teacher or nurse
            (2) Role of the learner or patient (sick role)
            (3) Role of family/group in learning process
            (4) Role in active help-seeking behaviors
      3. *Educational factors*
         a. Prior education
            (1) Highest level or degree
            (2) Place (location, e.g., geographic, public, private, at-risk school)
            (3) Language

          (4) Views on education
          (5) Type of secondary education (college prep, vocational, etc.)
          (6) Gaps in educational experience
          (7) Prior CC education
          (8) Prior educational experience with culturally diverse (CD) learners
          (9) Learning with technology
          (10)Prevalent teaching-learning strategies
     b. Family educational history (as above)
     c. Work experience
  4. ***Health literacy***
     a. Primary language
     b. Other spoken and written languages
     c. Preferred spoken language
          (1) Family
          (2) Friends
          (3) Work
          (4) Health issues
     d. Preferred written language
          (1) Family
          (2) Friends
          (3) Work
          (4) Health issues
     e. Reading level
          (1) Dominant language
          (2) Preferred language
          (3) Language of educational setting
     f. Level of consciousness and mental alertness
     g. Level of comfort
     h. Level of stress
  5. ***Psychological factors***
     a. Motivation
     b. Self-efficacy (confidence)
     c. Stress
     d. Presence or history of psychological disorders or illnesses
  6. ***Physical factors***
     a. Presence or history of underlying physical illnesses
     b. Comfort or pain level
     c. Rest or fatigue level
     d. Level of consciousness and mental alertness
     e. Influence of medications, alcohol, other drugs
     f. Age
B. **Teaching-learning principles for diverse populations**
  1. ***General considerations—Taxonomy of Learning*** (Bloom, 1956; Gronlund, 1985; Harrow, 1972; Krathwohl, Bloom, & Masia, 1964)
     a. Cognitive learning domain
          (1) Levels
             (a) Knowledge
             (b) Comprehension
             (c) Application
             (d) Analysis
             (e) Synthesis
             (f) Evaluation
          (2) Sample strategies
             (a) Lecture
             (b) Written paper

   (c) Reading cultural journal articles
   (d) Computer-assisted instruction (CAI)
   (e) Programmed instruction
 b. Psychomotor learning domain
  (1) Levels
   (a) Perception
   (b) Set
   (c) Guided response mechanism and complex overt response
   (d) Adaptation
   (e) Origination
  (2) Sample strategies
   (a) Demonstration and return demonstration
   (b) Positive reinforcement
   (c) Guided coaching
   (d) Culturally appropriate films
   (e) Interview with culturally different person
 c. Affective learning domain
  (1) Levels
   (a) Receiving
   (b) Responding
   (c) Valuing
   (d) Organization
   (e) Characterization
  (2) Sample strategies
   (a) Guided self-reflection—thinking, thinking and written)
    i. Guided questions or programmed instruction
    ii. Diary or journal
    iii. Paper component
   (b) Shared reflection—verbal or written with small or large group)
    i. Discussion board, blog, wiki
    ii. Conference style
    iii. Reading shared written drafts or final copies
   (c) Interview with culturally different person
   (d) Immersion experiences
   (e) Field trip experiences

2. ***Adapting educational strategies to specific cultural groups***
 a. Students
  (1) General considerations
   (a) Immediate relevance to course grade
   (b) Relevance to progression in the curriculum
   (c) Publicized relevance to future career goals
  (2) Specific considerations
   (a) Cultures with group orientation may perceive debate, gaming, and other competitive activities as stressful
   (b) Cultures educated outside the United States may prefer (be more familiar with) rote memorization, lecture, and essay tests
   (c) Cultures with group orientation may have difficulty selecting choices on multiple choice exams when family vs. individual needs are opposing choices
   (d) Cultures educated within U.S. at-risk school districts may find standardized testing and multiple choice exams more challenging because of lack of experience, preparation, and societal/community expectations
   (e) Economically disadvantaged groups may not be able to purchase required books and/or have easy access to computers
   (f) Students from groups with very high expectations for academic excellence may experience increased stress, dissatisfaction, and decreased confidence with less than perfect performances (faculty advisement essential)

   (g) Learner groups representing much cultural and academic diversity may need explanations about how and why specific teaching-learning strategies are chosen

   (h) All learners benefit from academic and social support services integrated proactively and ongoing throughout the curriculum (e.g., enrichment programs, peer mentor tutoring, nursing neighborhoods)

   (i) Learning about cultures within dominant and minority group designations is important

   (j) Help-seeking behaviors vary so faculty must reach out to diverse students in culturally congruent ways

   (k) Cultural groups that put family responsibilities first over academic tasks are at risk for attrition and failure

  b. Organizational staff

   (1) Immediate relevance to area of practice

   (2) Relevance to one's profession or occupation/career

   (3) Publicized relevance to future career goals

   (4) Relevance to professional standards

   (5) Relevance to accreditation guidelines

   (6) Survey background information of learners

   (7) Integrate variety of strategies to match diverse learning styles

  c. Patients

   (1) Immediate relevance to health problem/issue

   (2) Immediate relevance to extrinsic motivators

    (a) Improved health will enhance quality of family life

    (b) Improved health will conserve financial resources

  d. Communities

   (1) Partnerships with key leaders

   (2) Partnerships or role models within group

   (3) Selection of community-based or neighborhood settings

III. Barriers to CC Education in Academic and Clinical Settings (Jeffreys, 2006)

 A. Few faculty and advanced practice nurses formally prepared in

  1. Transcultural nursing

  2. Teaching, curriculum, program development, staff education, evaluation

 B. Even fewer faculty and advanced practice nurses formally prepared in

  1. Theoretical and empirical basis for CC education

  2. Teaching, integrating, and evaluating CC education throughout the curriculum or organizational environment

 C. Even fewer faculty and advanced practice nurses formally prepared in

  1. Teaching, integrating, and evaluating innovative teaching-learning strategies with academically and CD learners

  2. Teaching, integrating, and evaluating innovative, well-sequenced CC teaching-learning strategies with academically and CD learners who must care for many different groups of CD patients

 D. Nursing shortage and nursing faculty shortage

 E. Varying levels of commitment for CC education

  1. Individual

  2. Colleagues and coworkers

  3. Administrators

  4. Organization

IV. Strategies and Modalities for Enhancing CC Education (Jeffreys, 2006)

 A. Educator self-assessment

  1. Values and beliefs about CC in own professional life

  2. Routinely updates knowledge, skills, and attitudes about CC

   a. CD clients, families, communities

   b. CD coworkers and administrators

   c. CD students

  3. Perceived role of faculty in CC education

   a. Active involvement with curriculum integration

      b. Active involvement with course integration

      c. Creates incentives to involve students in events and organizations focused on CC

      d. Publicizes CC continually (ongoing)

   4. Active involvement in professional events related to CC

   5. Active involvement in professional organizations related to CC

B. Academic settings

   1. Curriculum (CC is an integral component)

      a. Program philosophy

      b. Mission statement

      c. Conceptual framework

      d. Program objectives

      e. Program outcomes

      f. Horizontal threads

      g. Vertical threads

      h. Administrator, full-time, part-time faculty input and action

      i. Ongoing curricular evaluation and evidenced-based modification

      j. Outside expert evaluation and consultation for CC and CD

   2. Course

      a. Textbooks and reading assignments

         (1) Textbooks adopted based on CC and CD criteria

         (2) Required additional reading supplement CC and CD gaps

         (3) Class discussion incorporating CC and CD issues

      b. Films, movies, videos

         (1) Clinical and professional topics evaluated in CC and CD

         (2) Assignments further guide students to address CC and CD

         (3) Incorporate non-nursing films related to culture

      c. CAI

         (1) Programs evaluated for CC and CD

         (2) Create cultural scenarios to parallel CAI components

         (3) Focus questions guide students to examine CC and CD

      d. Internet resources

         (1) Scholarly Web sites for CC disseminated with some assignments requiring use

         (2) Reputable ethnic and health Web sites disseminated with some assignments requiring use

      e. Course Web page

         (1) General environment (photos, topics) embraces CD

         (2) Calendar of ethnic and religious holidays

         (3) Links to reputable and scholarly Internet resources on culture and health

         (4) Full-text links to relevant articles on CC and CD

         (5) Discussion questions prompt students to address CC

      f. Nursing skills laboratory (e.g., simulator laboratory)

         (1) General environment embraces cultural diversity

         (2) Bulletin boards contain topics related to CC

         (3) Mannequins/scenarios/charts represent diverse cultural groups

            (a) Physical appearance

            (b) Clothing

            (c) Names

            (d) Religions

            (e) Economic status

            (f) Lifestyles

            (g) Genders

            (h) Ethnicities

            (i) Races

            (j) Insurance coverage

            (k) Immigration status

            (l) Educational backgrounds

        (4) Patient charts and scenarios integrate cultural needs
        (5) Simulated situations incorporate cultural components
        (6) Staff members represent diverse cultural groups

    g. Clinical settings
        (1) Exposure to and interaction with CD clients
        (2) Exposure to and interaction with CD health care personnel
        (3) Clinical objectives include and emphasize CC
        (4) Pre- and postconference discussions address CD and CC
        (5) Planned and unplanned clinical experiences related to CC
        (6) Cultural assessment is part of initial assessment
        (7) Care plans and actual care address cultural needs, such as
            (a) Diet
            (b) Drugs (ethnopharmacology, beliefs about)
            (c) Religious and/or spiritual needs (prayer routines)
            (d) Language needs (interpreter, written materials)
            (e) Referral to cultural or spiritual leaders
            (f) Referral to traditional healers
            (g) Collaboration with cultural expert
            (h) Hygiene and clothing needs
            (i) Others specific to clinical setting or medical issue
            (j) Complementary and alternative medicine
        (8) Alternate culture case scenarios to compare and contrast

    h. Written assignments
        (1) Low stakes (Elbow, 1997; e.g., reflection without grading)
        (2) High stakes (graded; e.g., papers)
        (3) All papers include cultural topics and clinical decision making as a major or minor component
        (4) Visible and equitable point allocation for CC sections
        (5) Select papers focus exclusively on CC topics
        (6) Students must complete all components of the paper to achieve a passing grade

    i. Presentations (PowerPoint, poster, storytelling, etc.)
        (1) All presentations include cultural topics as a major or minor component
        (2) Visible and equitable point allocation for CC sections
        (3) Select presentations focus exclusively on CC topics
        (4) Students must address cultural issue(s) in presentation to achieve a passing grade
        (5) Enhance presentation setting (environment) with culturally linked foods, beverages, music, clothing, scents, traditions
        (6) Several presentations on same culture but different topic or same topic but different cultures for compare and contrast discussion at the end of class

    j. Paired group activity—address and consider
        (1) Group vs. individual orientation
        (2) Noncompetitive vs. competitive approach
        (3) Verbal contextual vs. verbal metaphorical
        (4) Gender roles
        (5) Indirect vs. direct communication patterns
        (6) Perceived value of strategy as teaching-learning activity

    k. Small group activity—consider and address
        (1) Group vs. individual orientation
        (2) Noncompetitive vs. competitive approach
        (3) Verbal contextual vs. verbal metaphorical
        (4) Gender roles
        (5) Indirect vs. direct communication patterns
        (6) Perceived value of strategy as teaching-learning activity

    l. Gaming—consider and address
        (1) Group vs. individual orientation
        (2) Noncompetitive vs. competitive approach

       (3) Verbal contextual vs. verbal metaphorical
       (4) Gender roles
       (5) Indirect vs. direct communication patterns
       (6) Perceived value of strategy as teaching-learning activity

  m. Debate—consider and address
       (1) Group vs. individual orientation
       (2) Noncompetitive vs. competitive approach
       (3) Verbal contextual vs. verbal metaphorical
       (4) Gender roles
       (5) Indirect vs. direct communication patterns
       (6) Perceived value of strategy as teaching-learning activity

  n. Role play—consider and address
       (1) Group vs. individual orientation
       (2) Noncompetitive vs. competitive approach
       (3) Verbal contextual vs. verbal metaphorical
       (4) Gender roles
       (5) Indirect vs. direct communication patterns
       (6) Perceived value of strategy as teaching-learning activity

  o. Immersion experiences
       (1) Sufficient preparation in general transcultural nursing
       (2) Sufficient preparation in cultural values, beliefs, behaviors of host culture
       (3) Sufficient language preparation in host language
       (4) Partnerships/mentors from academic setting sufficiently prepared in transcultural nursing, host culture, and clinical expertise
       (5) Partnerships/mentors in host setting to assist students
       (6) Clear objectives, expectations, and learning outcomes
       (7) Sufficient time frame for immersion
       (8) Reflection journals and other assignments
       (9) Debriefing session

  p. Innovative Field Trip Experience (Jeffreys, Bertone, Douglas, Li, & Newman, 2007)
       (1) Prerequisite components
          (a) Background reading
          (b) Classroom seminar and films
          (c) Literature review
          (d) Written review of literature paper (cultural)
       (2) General required components
          (a) Student-initiated field trip selection
          (b) Cultural purpose and objectives
          (c) Instructor guidance
          (d) Field trip implementation (1–2 days)
          (e) Written paper
       (3) Information-sharing/dissemination components
          (a) Storytelling in class
          (b) Cultural food buffet (foods related to culture)

  q. Cultural discovery integrated learning activity (Jeffreys & O'Donnell, 1997)
       (1) Background reading
       (2) Classroom activity components (lecture, discussion, movie, small group case scenarios)
       (3) Clinical postconference discussions
       (4) Collaborative library introductory program (Xiao, 2005)
          (a) Cultural resources
          (b) Field trip to library
          (c) Hands-on practice session
          (d) Discussion board with library staff
       (5) Videotape program (cultural assessment)
       (6) Interview of culturally different person

   (7) Cultural assessment

   (8) Literature review on interviewee's culture

   (9) Written paper

   (10) Written reflection about cultural interaction, research, etc.

  r. Exams

   (1) Free of cultural bias

   (2) Include cultural topics and clinical decision making

   (3) Equal point allocation for CC questions

   (4) Format and expectations reviewed prior to exam

    (a) Strategies for test taking acknowledge diverse experiences of students educated and tested in other countries and/or at-risk schools

    (b) Academic integrity

3. *Supplementary resources (outwardly and substantively address cultural issues)*

 a. Library

 b. Nursing student resource center/nursing neighborhood

 c. Nursing student lounge

 d. Nursing student club

 e. Sigma Theta Tau chapter

 f. Specialty organizations

 g. Bulletin boards

 h. Web page, blog, discussion board

 i. Guest speakers

 j. Cultural events (e.g., dance, music, drama, food festivals)

C. Health care organizations (outwardly and substantively address cultural issues)

1. *Institutional level*

 a. Philosophy and mission

 b. New employee orientation

 c. In-service education

 d. Newsletter and publications

 e. Library

 f. Web site

 g. Bulletin boards

 h. Committees

  (1) CC in patient care

  (2) Multicultural workplace harmony

  (3) Advisory boards with community leaders

  (4) Recruitment and retention of CD personnel

 i. Special events

  (1) Guest presenters

  (2) Conferences

  (3) Cultural food day (weekly or monthly)

  (4) Cultural holiday recognition and celebration

 j. Employee recognition for CC

  (1) Awards

  (2) Featured spotlight in newsletter or Web site

  (3) Promotional criteria

 k. Employee reimbursement and accommodating work schedule

  (1) College credit courses on CC

  (2) Continuing education courses on CC

  (3) Conferences focused on CC

 l. Policy addressing cultural diverse patient and personnel needs

 m. Cultural community leaders network and advisory board

 n. Advertisements target CD community groups in area

2. *Unit (site) level* (routinely address cultural issues)

 a. In-service education

      b.   Staff meetings
      c.   Patient care conferences
      d.   Walking rounds and report
      e.   Unit-specific cultural assessment forms and care plans

   3. ***Supplementary resources***
      a.   Organizations (local, national, international)
      b.   Local colleges
      c.   Continuing education
      d.   Guest speakers
      e.   Interpreter services
      f.   Written health documents in various languages

D. **Professional associations (outwardly and substantively address cultural issues)**
   1. ***Interpersonal level***
      a.   Board of directors or elected officers
      b.   Members
      c.   Nonmembers or guests

   2. ***Parent association or chapter level***
      a.   Philosophy and mission reflect CC and CD
      b.   Bylaws
         (1) Appropriate to wide range of cultural groups
         (2) Aim to recruit and retain CD members
         (3) Incorporate issues/aims related to CC and CD
      c.   Membership criteria
      d.   Newsletter and publications
      e.   Web site
      f.   Meetings (dates, times, places, accommodate variety of cultures)
      g.   Workshops (dates, times, places, topics, cost, accommodate variety of cultures)
      h.   Conferences (dates, times, places, topics, cost, accommodate variety of cultures)
      i.   Special events
      j.   Cosponsored events with other associations, colleges, or community groups
      k.   Networking
      l.   Mentoring

   3. ***Supplementary resources***
      a.   Other professional associations
      b.   Local colleges
      c.   Health care institutions
      d.   Invited guest speakers

V. Patient and Community Education Program Development (Jeffreys, 2006)
  A. **Determining priorities and goals for teaching programs**
   1. ***Cultural groups*** present in geographic region
      a.   Use health care services
      b.   Do not use health care services
      c.   Underutilize health care services
      d.   Significant health problem(s)
      e.   Largest group
      f.   Newest group
      g.   Victims of discrimination and bias
      h.   Marginalized group
      i.   Poorly understood by health care personnel

   2. ***Learner characteristics***
      a.   Cultural background, identity, values, and beliefs (see Section II)
      b.   Strengths
      c.   Weaknesses

        d.   Gaps in learning

        e.   Biases

        f.   Prior formalized learning related to culture

    3.   ***Educational resources***

        a.   Opportunities for formalized transcultural learning

        b.   Currently available

        c.   Necessary to achieve goals of developing CC

        d.   Most easily attainable

        e.   Qualified personnel to design, implement, and evaluate programs

B. **Selecting culturally appropriate venues for teaching**

    1. Timing

    2. Setting

VI. **Evaluation of Learning Outcomes: Students and Organizational Staff**

    A. **Transcultural Self-Efficacy Tool**—designed to measure and evaluate students (or nurses) confidence for performing general transcultural nursing skills among diverse client populations (Jeffreys, 1994, 2000, 2006; Jeffreys & Smodlaka, 1996, 1998, 1999a, 1999b). Associated model: CCC model (Jeffreys, 2006)

        1. ***Major components and description***—83 items

           a.   Subscales (based on taxonomy of learning and self-efficacy)

              (1) Cognitive (25 items)—respondents rate their confidence about their knowledge concerning the ways cultural factors may influence nursing care

              (2) Practical (28 items)—respondents rate their confidence for interviewing clients of different cultural backgrounds to learn about their values and beliefs

              (3) Affective (30 items)—respondents rate their confidence for their attitudes, values, and beliefs

                  (a) Self-awareness

                  (b) Awareness

                  (c) Acceptance

                  (d) Appreciation

                  (e) Recognition

                  (f) Advocacy

           b.   General item content

              (1) Specific to cultural care issues or transcultural nursing

              (2) Appropriate for entry-level nursing students or nurses

              (3) Focuses on the general transcultural skills needed to care for many different groups of CD patients

           c.   Specific item content

              (1) Addresses only one issue

              (2) Clear and succinct

              (3) Avoids redundancy between items

           d.   Item structure

              (1) Close ended

              (2) Positively phrased

           e.   Rating scale

              (1) 10-point scale from 1 (*not confident*) to 10 (*totally confident*)

              (2) Based on Bandura's use of 10-point scale

              (3) More discriminating than piloted 6-point rating scale

           f.   Item sequence

              (1) Clustering sequentially by content (e.g., pregnancy, birth)

              (2) Least stressful to more stressful or complex

           g.   Emphasis on individual efficacy appraisal

              (1) Personalized items and directions using second pronoun

              (2) Highlighting and underlining important words

           h.   Completion time—approximately 15–20 minutes

           i.   Scoring

              (1) Self-Efficacy Strength—average strength of self-efficacy perceptions within a subscale

              (2) Self-Efficacy Level—number of items perceived at a specified minimum level of confidence (per subscale)

              (3) Grouping (low, medium, high) per subscale

2. **Instrument design process**
    a. Item development following review of literature
    b. Item sequence
    c. Subscale sequence
    d. Expert content review
    e. Expert psychometric review
    f. Revised draft
    g. Pretest
    h. Minor revisions
    i. Second pretest
3. **Validity**
    a. Content validity—6 doctoral-prepared experts certified in transcultural nursing
    b. Construct validity
        (1) Contrasted group approach (longitudinal and cross-sectional)
            (a) Statistically significant differences within groups
            (b) Statistically significant differences between groups
            (c) Novice learners have lower self-efficacy generally
            (d) Advanced learners have higher self-efficacy
            (e) Supremely efficacious (overly confident) learners had decreased self-efficacy (medium range) posttest
            (f) Greatest change in TSE perceptions detected in low self-efficacious learners who are then exposed to formalized transcultural learning
            (g) Learners most confident about attitudes (affective)
            (h) Learners least confident about knowledge (cognitive)
        (2) Factor analysis ($N = 1,260$), accounted for 62% of variance
            (a) Items clustered exclusively under one of three subscales
            (b) Interitem correlation matrix range = .30–.70
                i. Items contribute significantly to TSE construct
                ii. No item redundancy occurred
            (c) 70 items loaded on nine factors
                i. Recognition
                ii. Kinship and social factors
                iii. Professional nursing care
                iv. Cultural background and identity
                v. Lifecycle transitional phenomena
                vi. Awareness of cultural gap
                vii. Communication
                viii. Self-awareness
                ix. Appreciation
            (d) Statistically significant changes in subscale and factor scores in expected direction
                i. Novice learners have lower self-efficacy
                ii. Advanced learners have higher self-efficacy
            (e) Statistically significant subscale intercorrelations
            (f) Learners most confident about attitudes (affective)
            (g) Learners least confident about knowledge (cognitive)
        (3) Reported consistency with underlying conceptual model
    c. Criterion-related validity (predictive validity)
        (1) Statistically significant changes in TSE between first and fourth
        (2) Semester students following integrated CC education
        (3) Demographic variables (age, gender, ethnicity, race) did not influence TSE perceptions or types of changes in TSE
4. **Reliability**
    a. Stability (test–retest = .63–.75)
    b. Internal consistency

          (1) Item-to-total correlations = .30–.70

          (2) Split-half = .76–.92

          (3) Cronbach's alpha = .92–.98

    5. *Reported uses*

      a. Undergraduate and graduate nursing and medical students

      b. Faculty

      c. Nurses and other health professionals in clinical settings

      d. Curricular evaluation and revision: nursing, medicine, dentistry

      e. Adapted versions—Cultural Competence Clinical Evaluation Tool—Teacher Version, Student Version—Content Validity Index (CVI) = .91 for each version; validity testing currently being conducted

B. Cultural Self-Efficacy Scale (CSES)—designed to measure nurses' perceived sense of self-efficacy in caring for African American, Hispanic, Asian, and White patients (Bernal, 1993; Bernal & Froman, 1987; Coffman, Shellman, & Bernal, 2004). Associated model: Culturally relevant community practice model (Bernal, 1993)

    1. *Major components and description*—26 items

      a. Sections

          (1) Knowledge of cultural concepts

          (2) Cultural patterns

          (3) Skills in performing transcultural nursing functions

      b. Subscales

          (1) African American

          (2) Hispanic

          (3) Asian

          (4) White

      c. Rating scale—5-point scale from 1 (*very little confidence*) to 5 (*quite a lot of confidence*) for each of 4 ethnic groups

      d. Scoring

          (1) Item means

          (2) Subscale means

    2. *Validity*

      a. Construct validity

          (1) Contrasted group approach (groups with more cultural exposure had positive effect on CSES score

          (2) Factor analysis—accounted for 90% of variance

      b. Criterion-related validity—significant positive relationships between ethnicity, interaction with diverse clients, work experience, and levels of general self-efficacy

    3. *Reliability—Cronbach's alpha = .86–.98*

    4. *Reported uses*

      a. Nurses in a variety of settings (hospital, community)

      b. Nursing students

      c. Adapted to other ethnic groups (e.g., Native American)

      d. Translated into Spanish language (CSES-S; Jiminez, Contreras, Shellman, Gonzalez, & Bernal, 2006)

C. Eldercare Cultural Self-Efficacy Scale (Shellman, 2006)—designed to determine levels of elder care cultural self-efficacy among nursing students for care of African American, Hispanic, Asian, and White elders

    1. *Major components and description*—28 items

      a. Sections

          (1) Knowledge of cultural concepts

          (2) Cultural patterns

          (3) Skills in performing transcultural nursing functions

      b. Subscales

          (1) Assessing for Lifestyle and Social Patterns

          (2) Determining Cultural Health Practices

          (3) Determining Cultural Beliefs

          (4) Dealing With Grief and Losses Associated With Aging

      c. Rating scale

          (1) Very little confidence

          (2) Little confidence

          (3) Neutral

          (4) Moderate confidence

          (5) Quite a lot of confidence

    d. Scoring

          (1) Item means

          (2) Subscale means

2. ***Instrument design process***
   a. Item development following review of literature
   b. Expert content review
   c. Revised draft
   d. Pretest
   e. Minor revisions
   f. Second pretest

3. ***Validity***
   a. Content validity—five-member expert panel (four knowledgeable about self-efficacy and one gerontological nurse practitioner). CVI = .94
   b. Construct validity
      (1) Contrasted group approach—the more experience with an ethnic group, the higher levels of self-efficacy
      (2) Factor analysis ($N = 248$)
         (a) Accounted for 61% of variance
         (b) Item-total correlations = .30–.70
         (c) Four factors
            i. Assessing for Lifestyle and Social Patterns
            ii. Determining Cultural Health Practices
            iii. Determining Cultural Beliefs
            iv. Dealing with Grief and losses Associated with Aging
      (3) Criterion-related validity (predictive)—the more experience with an ethnic group, the higher levels of self-efficacy

4. ***Reliability—internal consistency***
   a. Cronbach's alpha for total instrument = .97
   b. Cronbach's alpha for subscales = .94–.97
   c. Item-total correlations = .30–.70

5. ***Reported uses—nursing students***

D. **Inventory for Assessing the Process of Cultural Competence Among Healthcare Professionals–Revised (IAPCC-R)**—(Campinha-Bacote, 2003; http://www.transculturalcare.net, retrieved September 23, 2008)—designed to measure the level of CC among health care professionals. Associated model: process of cultural competence in the delivery of health care services (Campinha-Bacote, 2003).

1. ***Major components and description***
   a. Subscales—five items for each proposed construct
      (1) Cultural desire
      (2) Cultural awareness
      (3) Cultural knowledge
      (4) Cultural skill
      (5) Cultural encounters
   b. General item content
      (1) Designed to measure level of CC
      (2) Appropriate for multidisciplinary health professionals
   c. Specific item content
      (1) Specific to constructs in the process of cultural competence in the delivery of health care services model (Campinha-Bacote, 2003)
   d. Item structure
      (1) Close ended
      (2) Positively and negatively phrased

  e. Rating scale (4-point scale)

   (1) Strongly agree, agree, disagree, strongly disagree

   (2) Very knowledgeable, knowledgeable, somewhat knowledgeable, not knowledgeable

   (3) Very aware, aware, somewhat aware, not aware

   (4) Very comfortable, comfortable, somewhat comfortable, not comfortable

   (5) Very involved, involved, somewhat involved, not involved

  f. Completion time—approximately 10–15 minutes

  g. Scoring

   (1) Range = 25–100

   (2) Category ranges based on scoring key for level of CC

 2. *Validity*

  a. Content validity—"was established by national experts in the field of transcultural health care" (Campinha-Bacote, 2003, p. 112)

  b. Construct validity—"was addressed by linking the IAPCC-R with Campinha-Bacote's 1998 conceptual model of cultural competence" (Campinha-Bacote, 2003, p. 112)

 3. *Reliability (English)—Internal consistency*

  a. Split-half = .77

  b. Cronbach's alpha = .73–.90

 4. *Reported uses*

  a. Undergraduate and graduate nursing and other health professions students

  b. Nurses and health care professionals in clinical settings

  c. Translated into other languages

E. Inventory for Assessing the Process of Cultural Competence—Student Version (IAPCC-SV)—(Campinha-Bacote, 2008b; http://www.transculturalcare.net/iapcc-sv.htm, retrieved September 23, 2008)—designed to measure the level of CC among students in the health professions. Associated model: process of cultural competence in the delivery of health care services (Campinha-Bacote, 2003).

 1. *Major components and description*—(20 items total)

  a. Subscales—several items for each proposed construct

   (1) Cultural Desire

   (2) Cultural Awareness

   (3) Cultural Knowledge

   (4) Cultural Skill

   (5) Cultural Encounters

  b. General item content

   (1) Designed to measure level of CC

   (2) Appropriate for multidisciplinary health professions students

  c. Specific item content

   (1) Specific to constructs in the process of cultural competence in the delivery of health care services model (Campinha-Bacote, 2003)

  d. Item structure

   (1) Close ended

   (2) Positively and negatively phrased

  e. Rating scale (4-point scale)—strongly agree, agree, disagree, strongly disagree

  f. Completion time—approximately 10–15 minutes

  g. Scoring

   (1) Range = 20–80

   (2) Category ranges based on scoring key for level of CC

 2. *Validity*

  a. Content validity "was established by reviews of national experts in the field of transcultural health care"; http://www.transculturalcare.net/iapcc-sv.htm, retrieved September 23, 2008)

  b. Construct validity "was addressed in that the items on the IAPCC-SV clearly reflect the review of the literature of cultural competence in healthcare delivery that identifies awareness/attitudes, skill and knowledge as domains of cultural competence" (http://www.transculturalcare.net/iapcc-sv.htm, retrieved September 23, 2008)

3. *Reliability (English)—Internal consistency—Cronbach's alpha = (.78)*
4. *Reported uses* (Campinha-Bacote, 2003)—undergraduate nursing students

F. **Cultural Assessment Scale** (Rew, Becker, Cookston, Khosropour, & Martinez, 2003)—designed to measure multicultural awareness among nursing faculty and students. Associated model: Rew's pathway model (Rew, 1996)

1. *Major components and description*—36 items
    (a) Subscales
        (1) General Educational Experience (14 items)
        (2) Cognitive Awareness (7 items)
        (3) Research Issues (4 items)
        (4) Behaviors/Comfort with Interactions (6 items)
        (5) Patient Care/Clinical Issues (5 items)
    b. General item content: positively phrased
    c. Rating scale: 7-point Likert-type scale, 1 (*strongly disagree*) to 7 (*strongly agree*)
    d. Scoring: mean, standard deviation, subscales

2. *Instrument design process*
    a. Item development following review of literature
    b. Pretest
    c. Expert content review
    d. Revised draft
    e. Second pretest

3. *Validity*
    a. Content validity—10 nursing faculty with a variety of ethnic and racial backgrounds with expertise in culture. CVI = .88
    b. Construct validity
        (1) Contrasted group approach—difference in Research Issues between first and fourth semester students
        (2) Factor analysis ($N = 159$), accounted for 51% variance
            (a) Five factors
                i.   General Educational Experience
                ii. Cognitive Awareness
                iii. Research Issues
                iv. Behaviors/Comfort with Interactions
                v.   Patient Care/Clinical Issues
            (b) Cronbach's alpha = .71–.94
        (3) Reported consistency with underlying conceptual model
            (a) Criterion-related validity—difference in Research Issues between first and fourth semester students

4. *Reliability—internal consistency*
    a. Cronbach's alpha for faculty = .82
    b. Cronbach's alpha for students = .91
    c. Cronbach's alpha for factors = .71–.94

5. *Reported uses*
    a. Nursing students
    b. Nursing faculty

G. **Cultural Competence Assessment** (CCA; Schim, Doorenbos, Miller, & Benkert, 2003)—designed to provide evidence of CC among health care providers and staff. Associated model: Schim and Miller cultural competence model (SMCCM; Schim & Miller, 1999)

1. *Major components and description*—25 items
    a. Subscales
        (1) Awareness and Sensitivity (8 items)
        (2) Competence Behaviors (17 items)
    b. General item content—derived from SMCCM and literature review
    c. Specific item content
        (1) Revised for clarity and conciseness
        (2) Approximately fifth grade reading level

     d. Completion time: 30 minutes

     e. Rating scale: Likert-type scale, where 5 = *always*, 4 = *often*, 3 = *not sure*, 2 = *at times*, 1 = *never*

     f. Scoring—overall score obtained by summing items, ranging from 25 to 125, with high scores suggesting greater CC

2. Instrument design process

     a. Item development following literature review

     b. Expert review for content and face validity

     c. Field test

     d. Pilot test for psychometric evaluation

     e. Revised tool

3. Validity

     a. Content validity—10 hospice experts and 10 end-of-life experts

     b. Construct validity

       (1) Contrasted groups approach

         (a) Recipients of diversity training had statistically significant higher scores than those who had none

         (b) Respondents with high school education had lower scores than baccalaureate graduates

       (2) Factor analysis ($N = 93$), 46% variance, two factors

         (a) Awareness and Sensitivity

         (b) Competence Behaviors

       (3) Criterion-related validity

         (a) Predictive: Recipients of diversity training had statistically significant higher scores than those without

         (b) Concurrent: Moderately correlated ($r = .66$) with scores on the IAPCC

4. Reliability—internal consistency

     a. Total CCA = .92

     b. Cultural Competence subscale = .93

     c. Awareness and Sensitivity subscale = .75

5. Reported uses: hospice workers

H. Cultural Fitness Survey (Rooda, 1993)—designed to examine the knowledge and attitudes of nurses toward patients from culturally different backgrounds

1. Major components and description

     a. Sections

       (1) Section 1—knowledge of cultural diversity related to three minority groups (Black Americans, Hispanics, and Asian Americans)—22 items

       (2) Section 2—Cultural Attitude Scale—developed by Bonaparte (1979)—34 items and four scales

         (a) Hispanic

         (b) Black American

         (c) Asian American

         (d) Anglo-American

       (3) Section 3—Demographic information (eight questions)

     b. General item content

       (1) Knowledge about culturally specific diseases, symptoms, values, family, and issues related to three minority groups (Section 1)

       (2) Vignettes describing four ethnic individuals (Black American, Anglo-American, Asian American, Hispanic (Section 2)

     c. Rating scale

       (1) Section 1—correct answer

       (2) Section 2—5-point Likert-type scale from *strongly disagree* to *strongly agree*

     d. Scoring

       (1) Section 1

         (a) Total correct answer score

         (b) Individual subscores for each of the three minority groups

       (2) Section 2

         (a) Total correct answer score

         (b) Three cultural bias scores calculated by subtracting the respective different race attitude score from the Anglo-American attitude score, with zero indicating no bias

    2.   *Instrument design process—Section 1*
        a.   Item development following literature review
        b.   Content validity review
        c.   Pilot test
        d.   Revisions
        e.   Second test
    3.   *Validity*
        a.   Content validity (Section 1)—three nurse educators with expertise in multicultural nursing education
        b.   Construct validity—predictive validity—cultural attitudes and cultural biases were positively correlated
    4.   *Reliability—internal consistency*
        a.   Section 1—KR-20 = .71
        b.   Section 2—coefficient alpha
            (1) Anglo-American = .88
            (2) Asian American = .87
            (3) Black American = .92
            (4) Hispanic = .92
    5.   *Reported uses—nurses*

VII. Evaluation of Learning Outcomes: Patients and Community

    A. Cognitive outcomes
        1. Pretest knowledge before educational strategy
        2. Posttest knowledge after educational strategy
        3. Comparison of pretest and posttest scores
        4. Focus groups before and after educational strategy

    B. Psychomotor (practical) outcomes
        1. Pretest baseline psychomotor skill and ability
        2. Posttest psychomotor skill and ability after educational strategy

    C. Affective outcomes
        1. Preassessment of attitudes, values, and beliefs concerning health topic
        2. Postassessment of attitudes, values, and beliefs concerning health topic after educational strategy
        3. Focus groups before and after educational strategy
        4. Targeted behavior change implemented independently after educational strategy (evidence that patient/community values new behavior)

VIII. Advancing the Scholarship of Education

    A. Research
        1. Targets CC
           a.   Practice setting (patients)
           b.   Academic setting (students), CD students
           c.   Workplace
        2. Incorporates model to understand the process of CC education
        3. Incorporates valid, reliable measurement tools and plan to measure baseline (before educational strategy) and poststrategy outcomes

    B. Dissemination of findings
        1. Refereed publication (book, journal article)
        2. Professional conference
        3. Internet
        4. Open-review electronic journal
        5. Listserv
        6. Workshop, Webinar
        7. Professional meetings
        8. Professional newsletter, newspaper, Web site
        9. Community agencies
        10. Television and radio
        11. Video

NOTE: All references, additional resources, and important Internet sites relevant to this chapter can be found at the following website: http://tcn.sagepub.com/supplemental

Chapter 9
Organizational Cultural Competency

Journal of Transcultural Nursing
21(Supplement 1) 357S–372S
© The Author(s) 2010
Reprints and permission:
sagepub.com/journalsPermissions.nav
DOI: 10.1177/1043659610374323
http://tcn.sagepub.com
⑤SAGE

Stephen R. Marrone, EdD, RN-BC, CTN-A[1]
Sunita Mutha, MD, FACP[2]
Gayle Tang, MSN, RN[3]

I. INTRODUCTION

A. Globalization, ethnic violence, and wars have increased geographical migrations so that there are scarcely a handful of countries that can claim a single ethnic population.

B. Consequently, health care organizations in most countries are challenged with serving multiple ethnic populations, each with varying health care beliefs and practices.

C. In the late 1980s, the concept of cultural safety was first introduced in New Zealand with the Treaty of Waitangi, in which the cultural health care priorities of the Maori were recognized. It was adopted by the New Zealand Nursing Council in 1992 (Warren, 2002)

D. The need for organizational cultural competency in the U.S. is evidenced by statistics that indicate more than 30% of the total population is composed of ethnic minorities (U.S. Department of Commerce, 2000), more than 47 million people speak a language other than English at home (Greenbaum & Flores, 2004), 28 million Americans are foreign born, and more than 300 different languages are spoken across the country (Joint Commission, 2004 U.S. Department of Commerce, 2000).

E. In order to adequately serve this diverse population, U.S. health care organizations in the mid-1990s were mandated to provide education to health care practitioners to ensure they would be culturally sensitive in the 21st century (Institute of Medicine [IOM], 1994; National Advisory Council on Nurse Education and Practice (US), 1996; Pew Health Professions Commission, 1995, Joint Commission on Accreditation of Healthcare Organizations, 1996).

II. ORGANIZATIONAL STRATEGIES TO ADDRESS WORKPLACE DISCRIMINATION

A. Definition of discrimination

1. Unequal treatment and denial of fundamental rights of individuals or groups based on prejudice related to characteristics such as age, ethnicity, disability, gender, language, marital status, national origin, race, religion, sexual orientation, social class, citizenship, and veteran status, among others (AACN, 2008; Spector, 2004).

B. Discrimination is a behavior

1. Results in disrespect, marginalization, disregard of rights and privileges.
2. There are unique issues relating to discrimination against disabled.
   a. There is no clear, objective dividing line between disabled persons and nondisabled persons; disability relates to perception.
   b. Anyone can become disabled at any time.

C. Types of discrimination

1. *Direct discrimination*—individuals or groups are treated differently based on one or more of the above characteristics. Selected examples are:
   a. Employer treats an African American employee differently due to fear of client disapproval or outside pressure.
   b. Gender differences in pay for equal position and work (Purnell & Paulanka, 2008)

Funding: The California Endowment (grant number 20082226) and Health Resources and Services Administration (grant number D11 HPO9759).
[1]State University of New York, SUNY Downstate Medical Center, Brooklyn, NY, USA (Performance Evaluation and Outcomes Evaluation for Culturally Competent Organizations; Resources for Organizational Cultural Competence; Organizational Resources for Refugees)
[2]University of California, San Francisco, CA, USA (Organizational Strategies to Address Discrimination; Workforce Diversity in Healthcare Organizations)
[3]Kaiser Permanente, Oakland, CA, USA (Language Services for Healthcare Organizations)

Corresponding Author: Stephen R. Marrone, Email: stephen.marrone@downstate.edu

Suggested Citation: Douglas, M. K. & Pacquiao, D. F. (Eds.). (2010). Core curriculum in transcultural nursing and health care [Supplement]. *Journal of Transcultural Nursing, 21*(Suppl. 1).

2. *Indirect discrimination*—certain requirements, conditions, policies or practices imposed by an organization that may appear fair because they apply to everyone equally, but a closer look shows that some people are being treated unfairly. This is because some people or groups of people are unable or less able to comply with the rule or are disadvantaged because of it. If this policy or practice is "not reasonable," it may be indirect discrimination. Selected examples are:
    a. Maternity leave policies may result in preferential hiring of men over women (British Broadcasting Company, 2008).
    b. Policy that no staff can work part-time; employees with children or family responsibilities could be disadvantaged.
    c. All information about workplace health and safety is printed in English. Those whose first language is not English may be disadvantaged.

D. Factors that contribute to discrimination (Dipboye & Colella, 2005)
1. *Prejudice*—usually negative, unjustified attitude toward members of a group.
2. *Stereotyping*—having an attitude, conception, opinion or belief about members of a group (Giger & Davidhizar, 2008; Smedley, Smith, & Nelson, 2003).
3. *Stigma*—a person is identified by a label that sets the person apart and links the person to undesirable stereotypes that result in unfair treatment and discrimination (Link & Phelan, 2001).
4. Ignorance or lack of knowledge
5. Paternalism
6. Policies (see indirect discrimination)

E. Documented impact of workplace discrimination
1. Strong association with mental health disorders (Bhui et al., 2005; Rospenda, Richman, & Shannon, 2008).
2. Associated with work stress (Wadsworth et al., 2007), alcohol consumption (Rospenda et al., 2008; Yen, Ragland, Greiner & Fisher, 1999), and increased likelihood of hypertension (Din-Dzietham, Nembhard, Collins, & Davis, 2004).
3. Also associated with poor health (de Castro, Gee, & Takeuchi, 2008) and morbidity (Asakura, Gee, Nakayama, & Niwa, 2008).
4. Affects subsequent health of women (Pavalko, Mossakowski, & Hamilton, 2003).

F. U.S. federal laws relating to workplace discrimination (U.S. Equal Employment Opportunity Commission, 2008).
1. *Equal Pay Act of 1963*—equal pay for equal work, for both men and women
2. *Title VII of the Civil Rights Act of 1964*—protects individuals against employment discrimination on the bases of race and color, as well as national origin, sex, and religion.
3. *Age Discrimination in Employment Act of 1967*—protects individuals who are 40 years or older from employment discrimination based on age.
4. *Sections 501 and 505 of the Rehabilitation Act of 1973*—prohibit discrimination against qualified individuals with disabilities who work in the federal government.
5. *Title I and Title V of the Americans with Disabilities Act of 1990*—prohibits employment discrimination against qualified individuals with disabilities in private businesses and in state and local governments.
6. *Civil Rights Act of 1991*—series of amendments to Title VII of the Civil Rights Act of 1964 enacted in part to reverse several Supreme Court decisions that limited the rights of persons protected by these laws.

G. Strategies for reducing workplace discrimination
1. *Educational strategies* targeted to all staff in order to:
    a. Increase awareness among staff
        1) Awareness of bias, attitudes, and emotions (e.g., what words/images/feelings spring to mind on hearing the word *disability*)
        2) Awareness of how communication can differ among different groups (e.g., cultural body language, generational differences)
    b. Increase knowledge
        1) Knowledge of history or experiences (e.g., lifestyles/perceptions/priorities) of groups.
        2) Knowledge of health impact of workplace discrimination (see above)
        3) Knowledge of federal laws relating to workplace discrimination
    c. Improve communication skills
        1) Strategies for effectively communicating with diverse individuals
        2) Cross-cultural conflict management skills
        3) Advocacy skills to challenge discrimination through policy and practice

   2. ***Organizational strategies***
      a. Establish an environment committed to respect for diversity through:
         1) Written and widely communicated organizational goals for workforce diversity and nondiscrimination policies
         2) Inclusion of information about diversity, nondiscrimination, policies, and procedures in employee orientation trainings
         3) Similar information in ongoing staff training
         4) Modeling of nondiscriminatory behavior by organizational managers and leaders
      b. Organizational practices and policies
         1) Establish nondiscrimination policy and communicate to all staff
         2) Establish written, objective criteria for hiring and promoting candidates and apply policies consistently to all candidates
         3) Review policies for requirements, conditions, or practices that may disproportionally have an adverse impact on one or more groups (Thornicroft, Brohan, Kassam, & Lewis-Holmes, 2008)
         4) Revise job standards for job performance to reasonably accommodate individuals with disabilities (Tartaglia, McMahon, West, Belongia, & Shier Beach, 2007)
         5) Tie rewards and compensation to success in diversifying the organization's workforce
         6) Establish and communicate formal process for reporting and handling discrimination claims

III. WORKFORCE DIVERSITY IN HEALTH CARE
A. Definitions
   1. ***Diversity***—all-inclusive concept; includes differences in race, ethnicity, national origin, immigration status, religion, age, gender, sexual orientation, education, ability/disability, spirituality, urban versus rural residence, and other attributes of groups of people (Purnell & Paulanka, 2008; Giger & Davidhizer, 2008)
   2. ***Cultural competence***—multiple definitions, among the most useful are:
      a. "Attitudes, knowledge and skills necessary for providing quality care to diverse populations" (Gilbert, 2008)
      b. "An ongoing process that involves accepting and respecting differences and not letting one's personal beliefs have an undue influence on those whose worldview is different from one's own. Cultural competence includes having general cultural as well as cultural-specific information so that the health care provider knows what questions to ask" (Giger & Davidhizer, 2008, p. 197).
      c. Cultural competence is a dynamic, ongoing, developmental process that requires a long-term commitment and is achieved over time (Davidhizer, Bechtal & McEwan, 1999).
B. Background about issues related to workforce diversity in health care (Grumbach et al., 2008; Society for Human Resource Management, 2007)
   1. U.S. health professions workforce does not reflect diversity of the nation's population
   2. Current investments in programs to increase workforce diversity are enhancing numbers of underrepresented minorities in health professions
   3. Lack of rigorous evaluation research makes it difficult to determine effectiveness of such programs and to identify specific interventions that most effectively promote diversity in health professions
   4. Underrepresentation of many minority groups in heath professions is due to profound disparities in educational opportunities and support, starting with the earliest stages of education.
   5. Emphasis is on ethnicity, race and gender.
   6. Focus is generally on compliance.
   7. Efforts focus on awareness rather than actions.
C. How to promote multicultural harmony and teamwork
   1. ***Strategies for increasing staff awareness and knowledge***
      a. Discuss common definitions (e.g., diversity, stereotyping)
      b. Provide activities to raise awareness about diversity
      c. Present data about organization's workforce characteristics and compare to populations served
   2. ***Strategies for improving staff communication skills***
      a. Provide timely feedback (written and verbal) to staff regarding issues related to workforce diversity
      b. Provide instruction in cross-cultural conflict management skills
   3. ***Strategies for changing organizational environment***
      a. Demonstrate visible leadership commitment to workplace diversity through establishment of goals for workforce diversity that align with key business strategies

    b. Establish and maintain a "Diversity Council" to coordinate and oversee cultural activities and issues (Ward, 2008)

    c. Establish and maintain employee cultural network groups (MDB Group, 2008)

    d. Hire, promote, and develop employees committed to diversity vision of organization

D. Resources for staff development (Workforce Diversity Network, 2008)

  1. Cross-cultural communication

    a. American Association of Critical Care Nurses (2008)

    b. Tools for teaching cross-cultural communication and conflict management: UCSF Center for the Health Professions' toolbox for teaching communication strategies (Mutha, Allen, & Welch, 2002)

    c. Kaiser Permanente's National Linguistic and Cultural Programs, National Diversity (National Center for Cultural Competence [NCCC], 2008)

    d. National Center for Cultural Competence (NCCC, 2008)

    e. Health Resources and Services Administration (HRSA, 2008)

    f. Maternal and Child Health Bureau (2008)

  2. Client advocacy—National Center for Cultural Competence (NCCC, 2008)

  3. Leadership for cultural competence

    a. MGH Disparities Solution Center (Disparities Solution Center, 2008)

    b. National Center for Cultural Competence (NCCC, 2008)

IV. LANGUAGE SERVICES FOR HEALTH CARE ORGANIZATIONS

A. Effective Communication With Limited-English-Proficient (or nondominant language) Patients

1. According to the Health Research and Educational Trust Report on hospital languages services (HRET, 2006):

    a. In the United States, 80% of hospitals provide care for patients with limited English proficiency, yet only 3% reported receiving reimbursement for providing those services.

    b. Patients speaking 15 or more different languages are encountered in more than 20% of hospitals in the United States.

    c. Fifty-two million people, 19% of the population of the United States, speak a language other than English at home.

2. In the European Union, 8% to 12% of patients admitted to hospitals annually suffer harm from care received resultant from language discordance (Europa, 2010).

3. The 2000 U.S. Census shows that 33 million people speak a language other than English at home (U.S. Department of Commerce, 2000).

4. Racial and ethnic groups other than Whites are expected to reach 40% of the U.S. population by 2030 (U.S. Census, 2000).

5. Language discordance can lead to decreased access to care, decreased quality of care, increased cost of care, decreased patient satisfaction, recidivism, discrimination, and poor health outcomes (AACN, 2008, 2003; Cary, 2001; Europa, 2010; HRET, 2006; IOM, 2002).

6. Patients who speak little or no English (or nondominant language) are at greater risk of medical errors or misdiagnosis if they are not provided with an interpreter, are less likely to use preventive care services, and more likely to use emergency rooms than English (or dominant language) speakers (Cornelio, 2004).

7. There are no established health care industry standards for ensuring quality translations (Tang, Lanza, Rodriguez, & Chang, 2006).

8. Title VI of the United States Civil Rights Act of 1964 and health care accrediting agencies such as the Joint Commission and the National Committee for Quality Assurance have cultural and linguistic requirements.

9. The U.S. National Standards for Culturally and Linguistically Appropriate Services (CLAS) in Health Care (Office of Minority Health [OMH], 2008) delineate that:

    a. Consumers receive care compatible with their preferred language

    b. Health care organizations:

      1) provide language assistance services in a timely manner

      2) provide consumers in their preferred language verbal and written notices of their right to receive language assistance services

      3) ensure competence of persons providing language assistance

      4) provide patient-related materials and post signage in the languages of the represented in the service area

      5) maintain current language profiles of the community service area

B. Interpretation Services
1. *Language interpretation is* defined as "facilitating oral or sign-language, either simultaneously or consecutively, between users of different languages" (HRET, 2006).
2. *An interpreter* "is a person who converts a thought or expression in *real time* from one language into the expression with a comparable meaning in another language" (HRET, 2006).
3. Studies have shown that improper or inappropriate interpreter usage can increase patient confusion, jeopardize safety, inflict emotional distress, and be costly to an organization (Tang, 2004a, 2004b).
4. Effective interpretation services should be available at the point of care for all client encounters, 24 hours a day, 7 days a week (HRET, 2006)
5. Effective interpretation services include the following (Gilbert, J. 2003a, 2003b, 2003c).
   a. Trained Medical Interpreters who have been evaluated to be competent in a specific language(s).
   b. Clinical Bilingual Staff who have been trained and evaluated to be competent in a specific language(s)
   c. Bilingual Nonclinical Staff (may be used to assist with activities of daily living but not for clinical information)
   d. Interpretation Agencies
   e. Community Language Banks
   f. Telephonic Services at the point of care
   g. Video/Interactive Computer-Based Services for the Deaf/Hearing Impaired
6. In the United States, interpretation by family members and minors is prohibited except in the case of an emergency or if the patient refuses the interpretation services offered by the organization. Use of family members to interpret can violate patient privacy and compromise quality and accuracy of communication (Tang, 2007).
7. Use of interpretation services or patient refusal of interpretation services must be documented in the medical record.

C. Translation Services
1. *Translation is* defined as "the comprehension of the meaning of a text and the subsequent production of an equivalent text that communicates the same message in another language" (HRET, 2006).
2. The original text is referred to as the *source text* and the translated version is referred to as the *target text* (HRET, 2006).
3. When written information is translated from one language to another, it must be confirmed that the translation provides the same (intended) message as the source document.
4. Accuracy of translated documents can be verified by:
   a. Translating the target text back to the source language to verify that the intended meaning has remained consistent with the source document (sometimes referred to as *"back-translation"*). This back-translation must be performed by a native speaker of the target language and who is "blinded" to the original source text.
   b. Engaging native speakers to review target texts and provide suggestions for idiomatic revisions to ensure that the text and pictures or diagrams are culturally sensitive
5. Since errors in translation can have grave consequences, translated documents should be reviewed and approved by the organization's legal and risk management departments in addition to clinical experts and native language speakers.
6. Critical documents to be translated in the major languages spoken among the consumers and within the service area include the following:
   a. patient admission packets, information guides, and admission processes that describe the care environment, services provided, and verbal and written notices of patients' rights to receive language assistance services
   b. Patient's Bill of Rights (United States)
   c. consent forms for treatments (general and procedure specific)
   d. internal and external signage and directions
   e. patient education materials (written and computer-based) particularly related to the patient's disease process(es), aspects of care, including self-care, and medications
   f. pharmaceutical labels and contraindications
7. Use of translation services or patient refusal of translated materials must be documented in the medical record.

D. Health Literacy
1. Health literacy is defined as the degree to which an individual is able to read, understand, and use information to make health care decisions (Rudd, Moeykens, & Colton, 1999).

2. There is mounting evidence that shows that at least half of patients cannot comprehend basic healthcare information. Low health literacy negatively impacts on the health outcomes of the patient and increases the risk of medical errors. The use of simple information and pictorials, avoiding medical jargons, return demonstration techniques, and encouraging patients questions have shown to improve health behaviors in persons with low health literacy (Rudd et al., 1999).

3. Not all speakers of the same language interpret words in the same way. Interpretation and translation services must be followed up by health care providers' evaluation in order to determine if the consumer has understood the information provided.

4. Selection and ongoing evaluation of the effectiveness of interpretation and translational services, including the preparation of patient education materials, should be monitored through formal quality and performance improvement processes.

5. A dedicated, interdisciplinary patient education team of clinical experts, community stakeholders, trained medical interpreters and translators, and legal and quality experts should provide oversight

6. Written policies and procedures for the development and/or purchase of patient education materials in the dominant and nondominant languages should be evaluated by a patient education team and/or diversity council. (See below.)

E. Organizational Infrastructure to Support Interpretation and Translation Services (Language Services)

1. In 2005, Kaiser Permanente's National Linguistic and Cultural Programs staff implemented a survey to examine how providers and staff accessed translated materials at the department and facility levels (Tang et al., 2006). The findings of the survey indicated the following:
   a. Lack of knowledge on how to access translated materials
   b. Lack of departmental and/or facility-wide budgets to translate materials
   c. Lack of organizational structure in general to facilitate the sharing and accessing of materials.
   d. Significant delays in getting translations completed.

2. Organizational preparation for Language Services
   a. Collect demographic and descriptive data of the prevalent cultural, ethnic, linguistic, and spiritual groups represented among patients, families, visitors, the community, and staff in service area (Andrews, 1998).
      (1) Describe the effectiveness of current systems and processes in meeting diverse needs (Andrews, 1998).
      (2) Frequently used techniques to identify the languages spoken within the community and service areas, as well as the need for sign language, include the following (HRET, 2006):
         (a) information from the local community
         (b) community organizations
         (c) directly from patients
         (d) census data
         (e) community needs assessment
   b. Assess the organization's strengths and limitations by examining the institution's ethos toward cultural diversity and the presence or absence of a corporate culture that promotes accord among its constituents (Andrews, 1998)
   c. Determine organizational need and readiness for change through dialogue with key stakeholders aimed at discovering foci of anticipated support and recognizing areas of potential resistance (Andrews, 1998)

3. Organizational Policies and Procedures
   a. Develop a strategic plan of goals, policies, operational plans, and management accountability to provide culturally and linguistically appropriate services (OMH, 2008)
   b. Write a plan for the development, implementation, and evaluation of translated documents and the purchase of patient education materials.
   c. Establish a quality process for health care interpretation and translation services (Tang et al., 2006).
   d. Develop standardized health care terminology in languages other than dominant language (Tang et al., 2006).
   e. Implement strategic plan, policies, and procedures that include measurable benchmarks of success and an ongoing process to ensure that change is maintained (Andrews, 1998).
   f. Evaluate actual outcomes against established benchmarks utilizing performance improvement, quality, and customer satisfaction data (Andrews, 1998).

g. Quantitative and qualitative data should be aggregated to establish a diversity database used to track and trend issues related to demographic indicators, cultural and generational diversity, recruitment and retention patterns, cost, and employee and patient satisfaction, thereby providing a feedback mechanism for continued improvement (Frusti, Niesen, & Campion, 2003).

F. Evaluation Criteria for Organizational Interpretation and Translation Services (Tang, 2007)

1. Written policy on the provision of language services (interpretation and translation).
2. Current list of languages spoken by providers and staff.
3. Systematic, efficient way of connecting persons in need of language services with persons who can provide those services.
4. A system to ensure that nondominant language patients are cared for without delays, at all points of care, 24 hours a day, 7 days a week. (See Section B, No. 5.)
5. Quality management of language services.
6. Patients who do not speak the dominant language have a means to make their needs and complaints known to the unit and/or organizational level.
7. Individuals used for providing language services are qualified, including bilingual staff, interpreter staff, and subcontractors.
8. Patient-informing documents and health education materials available in the patient's preferred language.
9. Language-appropriate signage or maps available in the languages represented in the service area.
10. Signage and pamphlets that inform patients and their families of their rights to interpreter services at no cost, 24 hours a day, 7 days a week, in all patient care areas.

G. Model Case for Using Staff as Interpreters in Health Care Organizations (Tang, 2007)

1. Founded in 1945, Kaiser Permanente is the largest not-for-profit health plan, serving more than 8.6 million members in several regions of the United States. Headquartered in Oakland, California, Kaiser Permanente includes Kaiser Foundation Health Plan, Kaiser Foundation Hospitals and subsidiaries, and the Permanente Medical Groups (Kaiser Permanente, 2010).
2. The National Coalition for Quality Translation in Health Care (Cornelio, 2004), funded by the California Endowment as part of a larger research study, was convened by Kaiser Permanente to evaluate the impact of linguistic services on the health outcomes of limited-English-proficient patients.
3. The Coalition provides guidelines that serve to facilitate the production of high-quality, consistent, easy-to-read, and cost-effective translations throughout the health care industry.
4. The Coalition is the first large-scale U.S. program for the translation of documents in the health care industry, and which puts linguists and translators at the center of the process.
5. *Quick Reference Cards* are used for language service resources and tips.
   a. Series of cards to provide straightforward, insightful guidance in encounters involving language services (Tang, 2004a, 2004b).
   b. Tips for Successful Interpretation
   c. Tips to Share with Untrained Interpreters
   d. Resource Guide for Health Care Interpreters
   e. Guidebook for Language Lab Coaching
   f. Developed to supplement other, more detailed training materials rather than serve as sole training content
6. *Utilization of existing staff*
   a. Bilingual employees use their language skills within two distinct roles (Tang, 2004a, 2004b)
      (1) to perform their regular duties in another language
      (2) to serve as interpreter for individuals who do not share the same language as the health care providers.
   b. Qualified Bilingual Staff (QBS) Model (Tang, 2004a, 2004b)
      (1) Employees who are proficient in at least one language in addition to English, and who serve in a dual-role capacity by providing interpreting services as well as using their language skills as part of their primary position
      (2) QBS employees have completed the KP-QBS Training Program (one of three levels): through assessment of skills, training, evaluation, and monitoring, individuals are certified to perform language assistance according to level of proficiency

     c. Key actions as a model for change
       (1) Building infrastructure and initiatives around the use of existing bilingual or multilingual staff as resources
       (2) Conducting appropriate training that acknowledges a range of abilities in target languages
       (3) Encouraging staff to work within the scope prescribed by their role and by their level of confidence in their abilities
  7. *Health Care Interpreter Certificate Program* (HCICP): Requires five key resources:
     a. Personnel: coordinators/instructors from each partnering academic and health care institution, language lab coaches, and volunteer lecturers such as physicians and nurses
     b. Financial: organization pays for the initial instructor training and provides class materials and space; grants or other sources of funding help support training and education program
     c. Training: the HCI Instructor Training Institute trains faculty at partnering academic institutions and improves skills of existing faculty
     d. Support: Continuous technical support is provided to academic institutions and partner health care institutions
     e. Technology: A dedicated website for HCICP was developed and continues to be maintained
  8. Key actions as a model for change
     a. Creating new and utilizing existing community partnerships in a mutually beneficial manner
     b. Taking advantage of a professional population (interpreters) and honing their skills to be appropriate to and applicable in a health care setting

H. Outcomes of Linguistically Appropriate Health Care Services
  1. Improved patient clinical and health outcomes
  2. Improved client acceptance and satisfaction with care
  3. Improved provider satisfaction and retention
  4. Organizational financial stability
  5. Decreased malpractice suits
  6. See Sections VI (Performance Evaluation) and VII (Outcomes Evaluation)

I. Summary: Key elements of providing quality language services include:
  1. Initial and ongoing organizational self-assessment to ensure that consumers receive care in their preferred language.
  2. Language profiles of the community are kept current and services are implemented that reflect to the health care needs of the service area.
  3. Continued community language profiles of the service area to meet the needs of the changing population.
  4. Trained medical interpreters and translators to provide language assistance services at all points of care across the continuum of care at no cost to the consumers.
  5. Recruitment and retention of a diverse clinical staff and leadership that represents the demographics of the service area.
  6. Signage in the main languages of the health care consumers.
  7. Verbal and written notices of patient's rights to receive language assistance services.
  8. Community partnerships with key community leaders.
  9. Interpretation and translation services that are efficient and accessible at the point of care.
  10. Use of subject matter experts to provide insight in language product development.
  11. Transcultural nurses are in a key position to be able to target areas for improvement or development in language services (Tang, 2007).

V. RESOURCES FOR REFUGEE AND ASYLUM SEEKER SERVICES

  A. A foremost challenge for transcultural nurses caring for refugees and asylum seekers is locating resources. Major resources may be accessed at http://tcn.sagepub.com/supplement.
  B. Refugees are a facet of globalization. Although refugees arriving in the Western world receive the highest profile, most refugees live in developing countries (One World, 2009).
  C. Refugees and asylum seekers are not a homogeneous population. They arrive with diverse experiences and health and nutritional states, often live in poverty, and lack a social support network (Burnett & Peel, 2001).
  D. Racial discrimination and marginalization often result in health care disparities with resultant decrease in quality of life (Bacon, Bourne, Oakley, & Humphreys, 2010).

E. Culturally competent health care organizations maintain the following services and resources for caring for refugees, detainees, and asylum seekers (Bacon et al., 2010; Burnett & Peel, 2001; Gushulak & MacPherson, 2004; One World, 2009):
   1. An organizational infrastructure and strategic plan that includes allocating resources to meet the care needs of sojourners and marginalized populations.
   2. Language assistance programs that represent the dominant languages spoken among refugees, detainees, and asylum seekers.
   3. Community outreach to leaders that represent the demographics of refugees, detainees, and asylum seekers.
   4. Nursing, medical, mental health, social work, and case management professionals that are skilled in the care of oppressed and marginalized individuals and groups and victims of trauma, abuse, and/or disaster.
   5. Infectious diseases specialists who:
      a. are knowledgeable of the impact of globalization on epidemiology
      b. develop management guidelines for nonendemic diseases and access to diagnostic and therapeutic modalities for rare clinical presentations
      c. monitor health outcomes of both the migrant and local populations
   6. Pharmacists knowledgeable of the pharmacologic nuances of marginalized and transient populations.
   7. Registered dieticians/nutritionists that can provide the usual food preferences of oppressed and displaced clients.
   8. Support groups that assist refugees and asylum seekers with integration, cohesion, and activities of daily living.

VI. **PERFORMANCE EVALUATION FOR A CULTURALLY COMPETENT HEALTH CARE ORGANIZATION**
   A. Minority patients are frequently treated and cared for by health care professionals from different cultural backgrounds in what is often referred to as culturally discordant relationships.
   B. Culturally and linguistically discordant patient experiences related to health care processes and outcomes (Cooper & Powe, 2004).
      1. Ethnic minorities were more satisfied with care processes and outcomes when engaged in culturally and linguistically concordant client-provider relationships;
      2. Patients in race-concordant relationships rated their physicians as more participatory;
      3. Minorities were less likely than Whites to have racial or cultural concordance with their regular physicians or nurses;
      4. Patients in race-concordant relationships reported having longer visits with their primary care providers;
      5. Patients who needed an interpreter reported less understanding of their disease and treatment;
      6. Patients receiving interpreter services reported increased use of preventive services; and
      7. Language concordance with health care providers were associated with increased patient satisfaction
   C. Culturally competent health care systems are those that provide culturally and linguistically appropriate services that have the potential to reduce racial and ethnic health disparities (Anderson, 2003; Leininger, 1996).
   D. Organizational interventions to improve cultural competence in health care organizations (Anderson, 2003; Leininger, 1996)
      1. Programs to recruit and retain staff members who reflect the cultural diversity of the community served
      2. Use of interpreter services or bilingual providers for clients with limited language proficiency (language depends on region/country)
      3. Cultural competency training for health care providers
      4. Use of linguistically and culturally appropriate health education materials
      5. Culturally specific health care settings
   E. Performance evaluation of a culturally competent health care organization
      1. must be assessed at least annually
      2. must remain dynamic and responsive to the changing demographics of the service area
      3. organizational outcomes are described in Section VII
   F. Requisite competencies and performance criteria for staff working in a culturally competent health care organization are evidence-based, introduced during orientation, validated upon completion of orientation, and evaluated annually thereafter.
   G. Competencies and performance criteria should include cognitive, psychomotor, and affective domains of learning.

H. Core competencies include the following (AACN, 2002, 2003; Anderson, 2003; Carey, 2001; Cooper & Powe, 2004; IOM, 2002; Marrone, 1999a, 1999b, 2008):
   1. provides safe, meaningful, beneficial, and satisfying care by completing a cultural health assessment for all clients
   2. integrates assessment findings and client health beliefs and values into plans of care across the continuum, including death, dying, and palliative care
   3. initiates appropriate referrals for interpretation/translation services, nutritional support and diet planning, pastoral care, and discharge planning
   4. provides care in the client's preferred language
   5. demonstrates effective cross-cultural communication with clients and families
   6. recognizes diverse learning styles in the delivery of patient education and adjusts education plan to reflect individual client needs and preferences
   7. assesses health literacy as part of patient teaching and evaluation
   8. maintains client dignity and respect throughout the provider-client encounter
   9. documents plans of care and patient responses to facilitate communication among caregivers

VII. OUTCOMES EVALUATION OF A CULTURALLY COMPETENT HEALTH CARE ORGANIZATION
A. Outcome Criteria (Anderson, 2003; Joint Commission, 2008; Marrone, 1999a, 1999b, 2008)
   1. Client satisfaction with care
   2. Improvements in health status of underserved populations
   3. Improvements in inappropriate racial or ethnic differences in use of health services or in received and recommended treatment
   4. Cultural competency with measureable performance criteria integrated into performance appraisals for all job descriptions
   5. Development of documentation systems that include cultural health assessment, integration of assessment data into the plan of care, and evaluation of client satisfaction
   6. Documented use of trained interpreters/use of language telephones for patients who do not understand the primary language of care
   7. Documented use of patient education materials that are culturally sensitive and reflect the health literacy level of the patient
   8. Decreased medical errors related to informed consent
   9. Articulated continuing education learning outcomes that reflect cultural relevant nursing interventions, plans of care, and clinical evaluation strategies
B. Indices of client, provider, and organizational outcomes
   1. Care effective in terms of clinical outcomes
   2. Client acceptance/satisfaction
   3. Provider satisfaction and retention
   4. Financial stability
   5. Few malpractice suits
C. Organizational outcomes of culturally and linguistically competent care with clients (AACN, 2002, 2003; Cary, 2001; IOM, 2002):
   1. Access
      a. Increased access to services by ethnic and vulnerable populations
   2. Quality
      a. Increased consumer satisfaction
      b. Improved public safety
      c. Increased compliance with treatment plan
      d. Increased use of preventive services
      e. Practitioners rated as more participatory
      f. Longer visits with primary care providers
   3. Health Outcomes
      a. Improved patient health outcomes
      b. Decreased recidivism
      c. Decrease in racial and ethnic disparities in health outcomes

4. *Financial*
   a. Decreased health care costs
   b. Increased revenue for the health care organization
   c. Increased use of services by satisfied clients
   d. Decreased emergency department visits and hospital re-admissions
   e. Decreased litigation/malpractice

VIII. RESOURCES FOR ORGANIZATIONAL CULTURAL COMPETENCE

A. ***Governmental and/or regulatory agencies*** that provide the framework for health care organizational cultural competency; selected examples include:
   1. World Health Organization (WHO)
   2. Office of Minority Health (OMH)
   3. The Joint Commission (JC)
   4. The Joint Commission International (JCI)
   5. Institute of Medicine (IOM)

B. ***Professional agencies*** that provide the framework for health care organizational cultural competency; selected examples include:
   1. Transcultural Nursing Society (TCNS) (http://www.tcns.org)
   2. International Council of Nurses (ICN) (http://www.icn.ch/)
   3. Canadian Nurses Association (http://www.cna-nurses.ca/cna/)
   4. Royal College of Nursing, Australia (http://www.rcna.org.au/site/)
   5. Royal College of Nursing, United Kingdom (http://www.rcna.org.uk)
   6. European Council of Nursing Regulators (FEPI) (http://www.fepi.org)

C. **World Health Organization (WHO)** (http://www.who.int)
   1. The mission statement of the World Health Organization (WHO) is specific to each regional project and program.
   2. The objective of WHO is the attainment by all people of the highest possible level of health to include complete physical, mental, and social well-being, not only the complete absence of disease or infirmity (WHO, 2008)
   3. WHO is an agency of the United Nations
   4. The headquarters of WHO are in Geneva, Switzerland, and it maintains six regional offices
   5. WHO provides technical support to assist countries and regions in addressing priority health issues.
   6. WHO engages in partnerships to establish health and care norms and standards, policy, program, and human resource development and the prevention and control of major communicable diseases (WHO, 2008)

D. **U.S. Office of Minority Health** (http://www.omhrc.gov)
   1. The mission of the Office of Minority Health (OMH) is to improve and protect the health of racial and ethnic minority populations through the development of health policies and programs that will eliminate health disparities among the following vulnerable populations in the United States:
      a. American Indians and Alaska Natives
      b. Asian Americans
      c. Blacks/African Americans
      d. Hispanics/Latinos
      e. Native Hawaiians and other Pacific Islanders (OMH, 2008)
   2. Developed National Standards for Culturally and Linguistically Appropriate Services **(CLAS)** in Health Care in order to guide heath care delivery models in meeting clients' culture care needs.
   3. ***CLAS Standards***
      a. Consumers receive effective, understandable, and respectful care compatible with their cultural health beliefs and practices and preferred language;
      b. Recruit, retain, and promote a diverse staff and leadership that represent the demographics of the service area;
      c. Staff receive ongoing education in culturally and linguistically appropriate service delivery;
      d. Provide no-cost language assistance services, including bilingual staff and interpreter services, in a timely manner;
      e. Provide to patients/consumers in their preferred language verbal and written notices of their right to receive language assistance services;

    f. Competence of persons providing language assistance;

    g. Make available easily understood patient-related materials and post signage in the languages of the represented in the service area;

    h. A written strategic plan of goals, policies, operational plans, and management accountability to provide culturally and linguistically appropriate services;

    i. Conduct initial and ongoing self-assessments of CLAS-related activities and integrate CLAS measures into internal audits, performance improvement, patient satisfaction, and outcomes evaluations;

    j. Data on individual patients'/consumers' race, ethnicity, and spoken/written language are collected in health records, integrated into management information systems;

    k. Maintain current demographic, cultural, and epidemiological profiles of the community and implement services that respond to the profiles of the Service Area;

    l. Develop participatory, collaborative partnerships with communities and utilize formal and informal mechanisms to facilitate community and patient/ consumer involvement:

    m. Conflict and grievance resolution processes are culturally and linguistically sensitive; and,

    n. Regularly make available to the public information about innovations in implementing the CLAS Standards (OMH, 2008).

E. **The Joint Commission** (http://www.jointcommission.org/)

    1. "The mission of The Joint Commission (JC) is to continuously improve the safety and quality of care provided to the public through the provision of health care accreditation and related services that support performance improvement in health care organizations" (Joint Commission, 2008).

    2. The mission of The Joint Commission International (JCI) is "to continuously improve the safety and quality of care in the international community through the provision of education and consultation services and international accreditation and certification" (Joint Commission, 2008).

    3. Views the delivery of culturally and linguistically appropriate health care services as an important safety and quality issue.

    4. Joint Commission strategies for enhancing cultural competence in health care delivery:

        a. *Leadership Strategies*

            1) Devote resources to cultural training and educational efforts and integrate initiatives into all levels of the organization

            2) Assess the cultural composition of the staff and make diversity a priority in hiring practices

        b. *Communication Strategies*

            1) Use appropriately trained medical interpreters and translators

            2) Use ad hoc translators with extreme caution

            3) Listen carefully and respectfully to patients' beliefs about illness and traditional cures

        c. *Care Provision Strategies*

            1) Treat others as they expect to be treated

            2) Clarify patient and family instructions through demonstration and visual aides

            3) Avoid stereotyping

        d. *Educational Strategies*

            1) Conduct a cultural audit

            2) Integrate cultural sensitivity into continuing education courses

            3) Make staff aware of diversity information resources

        e. *Evaluation Strategies*

            1) Evidence that the leadership team has:

                (a) devoted resources to initial and ongoing team building and cultural training and educational programs for students and staff, such as such as the development of an interdisciplinary cultural diversity committee and outreach programs to minority nursing and medical organizations.

                (b) integrated cultural diversity initiatives into and cited cultural competency standards within all levels of the organization, such as vision and mission statements, strategic objectives, learning outcomes, clinical performance criteria, policies and procedures, documentation systems, and research.

                (c) assessed the cultural composition of the staff as compared to the demographics of the community of patients served.

                (d) developed hiring practices, promotion strategies within the organization, and outreach programs that support diversity as a priority.

           (e) assessed and integrated patient satisfaction, staff satisfaction, quality improvement, and health outcomes data related to cultural, spiritual, and linguistic diversity into all levels of the organizational infrastructure.

           (f) improved access and quality of care, and reduced cost, for minority patients and families.

           (g) minimized health disparities among minority clients

      2) Evidence that communication strategies within the organization include:

           (a) the use of trained medical interpreters and translators

           (b) the integration of patients' health and illness values and traditions into written plans of care and progress notes

           (c) patient/family understanding of teaching and discharge instructions

      3) Evidence that care provision strategies include:

           (a) attention to respectful care practices based on evidence derived from transcultural research

           (b) clarification of patient and family instructions through demonstration and the use of culturally and linguistically appropriate visual aides and teaching materials

      4) Evidence that educational strategies have:

           (a) conducted a cultural audit of patients, students, staff, faculty, and external community, as applicable

           (b) integrated cultural sensitivity into continuing education, certification, and recertification programs

           (c) informed students, faculty, and staff of the availability and access to diversity information resources

F. **Institute of Medicine** (http://www.iom.edu)

  1. The purpose of the Institute of Medicine (IOM) "is to provide national advice on issues relating to biomedical science, medicine, and health, and its mission is to serve as advisor to the nation to improve health" (IOM, 2008)

  2. The IOM is an independent, nongovernmental, nonprofit organization that is the health arm of the National Academies of Science (U.S.).

  3. The IOM provides independent guidance, analysis, and advice concerning health and science policy development.

  4. Core Competencies for Health Care Professionals

    a. *Provide Patient-Centered Care*

      1) identify, respect, and care about patients' differences, values, preferences, and expressed needs

      2) listen to, clearly inform, communicate with, and educate patients; share decision making and management; and continuously advocate disease prevention, wellness, and promotion of healthy lifestyles, including a focus on population health

    b. *Work as Interdisciplinary Teams*: Cooperate, collaborate, communicate, and integrate care in teams to ensure that care is continuous and reliable

    c. *Employ Evidence-Based Practice*: Integrate best research with clinical expertise and patient values for optimum care, and participate in learning and research activities to the extent feasible

    d. *Apply Quality Improvement*: Identify errors and hazards in care; understand and implement basic safety design principles, such as standardization and simplification; continually understand and measure quality of care in terms of structure, process, and outcomes in relation to patient and community needs; and design and test interventions to change processes and systems of care, with the objective of improving quality

    e. *Utilize Informatics*: Communicate, manage, knowledge, mitigate error, and support decision making using information technology

G. **National Center for Cultural Competence** (http://www11.georgetown.edu/research/gucchd/nccc/)

  1. "The mission of the National Center for Cultural Competence (NCCC) is to increase the capacity of health and mental health programs to design, implement, and evaluate culturally and linguistically competent service delivery systems" (NCCC, 2008).

  2. Guiding Principles

    a. *Organizational Principles* (NCCC, 2008)

      1) Cultural competence includes equal access and nondiscriminatory practices in service delivery

      2) Systems and organizations must integrate cultural knowledge into policy making, infrastructure, and practice

      3) Policies that detail culturally and linguistically competent care provide the infrastructure

         (a) to support the organization's mission and vision

(b) to provide practitioners with the requisite resources to implement culturally and linguistically competent care

(c) to measure the success related to patient outcomes, patient satisfaction, and organizational performance

(d) to embed culturally and linguistically competent care into the essence of the work of the organization

  b. ***Practice and Service Design Principles*** (NCCC, 2008)

    1) Cultural competence is achieved by identifying and understanding the needs and help-seeking behaviors of individuals and families within the service area

    2) "Culturally competent organizations design and implement services that are tailored or matched to the unique needs of individuals, children, families, organizations and communities served" (Cross, Bazron, Dennis, & Isaacs, 1989, p. 15).

    3) "Practice is driven in service delivery systems by client-preferred choices, not by culturally-blind or culturally-free interventions" (Cross et al., 1989, p. 17).

    4) "Culturally competent organizations have a service delivery model that recognizes mental health as an integral and inseparable aspect of primary health care" (Cross et al., 1989, p. 21).

    5) Language services for the population in the service area are to include translated written materials for patient education and informed consent and interpreter services that comply with regulatory agency requirements that govern language access

  c. ***Community Engagement*** (NCCC, 2008)

    1) Cultural competence involve working with community support networks

    2) Communities are self-actualizing, dynamic partners that identify their needs and preferences

  d. ***Family and Consumers*** (NCCC, 2008)

    1) The definition of family and the role of family during times of health and illness are culturally defined.

    2) Family members and consumers are the key decision makers for health care services provided to their children or to themselves.

  3. Resources

    a. Cultural Competence Health Practitioner Assessment (CCHPA)

    b. Cultural and Linguistic Competence Policy Assessment (CLCPA)

    c. Promising Practices: "a listing of evidence-based promising policies, structures, and practices that exemplify cultural and linguistic competence in many healthcare and mental health programs" (NCCC, 2008)

H. **Transcultural Nursing Society** (http://www.tcns.org)

  1. "The mission of the Transcultural Nursing Society (TCNS) is to enhance the quality of culturally congruent, competent, and equitable care that results in improved health and well-being for people worldwide" (TCNS, 2008)

  2. TCNS Position Statement on Human Rights: "TCNS is committed to the rights of all people to enjoy their full human potential, including the highest attainable standard of health and was established to safeguard human rights and quality health care through the discovery and implementation of culturally competent care" (TCNS, 2008)

  3. TCNS Strategies for a Human Rights agenda

    a. "Develop a substantive body of knowledge of the discipline of transcultural nursing by means of research.

    b. Provide a sound knowledge base for nurses to use in order to provide culturally competent care.

    c. Use the TCNS mission statement as a guideline to provide a quality of culturally congruent and competent care that results in improved health and well-being for people worldwide.

    d. Establish and disseminate cultural competency standards for health care professionals and institutions to facilitate the promotion of equitable and ethical policies and practices.

    e. Develop and implement a certification process for nurses and other health care professionals that ensures competency in provision of culturally competent care.

    f. Market the certification program to institutions, organizations, clinics, and academic health care programs worldwide to provide a global commitment to culturally competent care.

    g. Emphasize a focused human rights theme to guide education, research, practice and administration.

h. Explore the process of recognition by the United Nations as a human rights organization, working to improve health conditions and culturally competent care worldwide

i. Become active advocates for changes in healthcare delivery and social policies related to equitable access to health care and the delivery of culturally competent care worldwide". (TCNS, 2008)

I. **American Organization of Nurse Executives (AONE)** (http://www.aone.org)

    1. AONE Guiding Principles for Diversity in Health Care Organizations (AONE, 2008) (http://www.aone.org/aone/resource/PDF/AONE_GP_Diversity.pdf)

        a. "Health care organizations will strive to develop internal and external resources to meet the needs of the diverse patient and workforce populations served."

        b. "Health care organizations will aim to establish a healthful practice/work environment that is reflective of the diversity through a commitment to inclusivity, tolerance, and governance structures."

        c. "Health care organizations will partner with universities, schools or nursing, and other organizations, that train health care workers to support development and implementation of policies, procedures, programs, and learning environments that foster recruitment and retention of a student population that reflects the diversity of the United States."

        d. "Health care organizations will collect and disseminate diversity related resources and information."

    2. AONE Diversity for Health Care Organizations Toolkit (AONE, 2008)
(http://www.aone.org/aone/about/AONE_Toolkit_Diversity.pdf)

J. **International Council of Nurses** (http://www.icn.ch)

    1. The mission of the International Council of Nurses (ICN) is to "lead our societies toward better health" (ICN, 2008).

    2. ICN membership includes national nursing associations representing 130 countries.

    3. Goals are to promote healthy lifestyles, healthy workplaces, and healthy communities.

    4. Supports program development strategies that mitigate poverty, pollution, and other underlying causes of illness.

    5. Integrates ethical caring that includes meeting spiritual and emotional needs.

    6. Advocates that prevention, care, and cure be the right of every human being (ICN, 2008).

K. **Community Resources and Partnerships**

    1. Community leaders

        a. cultural and spiritual leaders and healers

        b. political leaders and regulatory leaders

            1) Advocate on behalf of the underserved

            2) Negotiate with managed care organizations for culturally relevant health services across the continuum of care

        c. formal and informal leaders

        d. natural/lay healers

        e. community elders

    2. Knowledge of community resources

        a. demographics

        b. neighborhood, civic and advocacy associations

        c. local/neighborhood merchants and alliance groups

        d. ethnic, social, and religious organizations, and houses of worship

        e. gathering places and procedures for gaining access

        f. academic community

IX. SUMMARY

A. Culturally competent health care organizations support an organizational infrastructure that respects and celebrates diversity as reflected in the vision, mission, values, strategic plan, quality initiatives, education plan, employee competencies, and clinical and operational performance outcomes.

B. Culturally competent health care organizations design, implement, and evaluate a strategic plan that ensures the provision of culturally and linguistically appropriate services.

C. Culturally competent health care organizations attract and retain nurses prepared in transcultural nursing.

D. Culturally competent health care organizations implement strategies that recruit, retain, the promote diversity at all levels of the organization that are representative of the consumer demographics in the service area.

E. Culturally competent health care organizations provide practitioners diversity-related resources at the point of care.

F. Culturally competent health care organizations ensure that the staff receives initial and ongoing education related to the diverse culture care needs of the consumer demographics in the service area.

G. Culturally competent health care organizations achieve and sustain greater performance and outcomes measures: increased access to care, enhanced quality of care, improved health outcomes, greater patient and staff satisfaction, and secure financial sustainability of the organization.

NOTE: All references, additional resources, and important Internet sites relevant to this chapter can be found at the following website: http://tcn.sagepub.com/supplemental

Chapter 10
Research Methodologies for Investigating Cultural Phenomena and Evaluating Interventions

Journal of Transcultural Nursing
21(Supplement 1) 373S–405S
© The Author(s) 2010
Reprints and permission:
sagepub.com/journalsPermissions.nav
DOI: 10.1177/1043659610369679
http://tcn.sagepub.com
⑨SAGE

Marilyn K. Douglas, DNSc, RN, FAAN[1]
Jeanne K. Kemppainen, PhD, RN[2]
Marilyn R. McFarland, PhD, RN, FNP-BC, CTN-A[3]
Irena Papadopoulos, PhD, MA, RN, RM, FHEA[4]
Marilyn A. Ray, PhD, MA, RN, CTN-A[5]
Janice M. Roper, PhD, MS, RN[6]
Melissa Scollan-Koliopoulos, EdD, APRN, CDE[7]
Jill Shapira, PhD, RN, FNP-C[8]
Hsiu-Min Tsai, PhD, RN[9]

I. Introduction

A. This chapter is an overview of the most common research methods used to study cultural phenomena and test interventions that can be used in practice.

B. Most of the research in transcultural nursing has been qualitative in nature, which is appropriate for the phenomena of study.

C. The future of transcultural nursing research is in both evaluating interventions and validating outcomes of culturally appropriate care practices for specific populations.

D. Implementation of scientifically tested, evidence-based strategies and practices that are targeted to the health needs and life ways of specific cultural groups may be one approach to decreasing global racial and ethnic disparities in health outcomes.

II. Specific Considerations In The Conduct Of Transcultural Research

A. Problem Identification

    1. Is the study's purpose or question appropriate for the population and sociocultural context where the study is being conducted?

    2. Does the problem statement/hypothesis reflect the researchers' bias about a cultural group?

B. Theoretical Framework

    1. Is the theoretical framework appropriate to the cultural phenomenon being investigated?

    2. Does the framework fit the methodology selected?

C. Literature Review

    1. Does the literature review provide sufficient information to gain an understanding of the culture and the people being studied?

Funding: The California Endowment (grant number 20082226) and Health Resources and Services Administration (grant number D11 HPO9759).

[1]University of California, San Francisco, Palo Alto, CA, USA (Human Subjects Protection in Research)
[2]University of North Carolina Wilmington, Wilmington, NC, USA (Critical Incident Analysis Research Method)
[3]University of Michigan -Flint, Bay City, MI, USA (Ethnonursing Research Method)
[4]Middlesex University, London, UK (Participatory Action Research [PAR] Method)
[5]Florida Atlantic University, Boca Raton, FL, USA (Phenomenological-Hermeneutical Research Method; Ground Theory Method)
[6]American University of Health Sciences, Santa Monica, CA, USA (Ethnography Research Method, Ethnographic Interviewing Techniques, Participant Observation, Triangulation, Validity and Reliability; Computer Software for Qualitative Analysis)
[7]University of Medicine and Dentistry of New Jersey, Newark, NJ, USA (Quantitative Research Methodologies)
[8]University of California Los Angeles Health Systems, Los Angeles, CA, USA (Ethnography Research Method, Ethnographic Interviewing Techniques, Participant Observation, Triangulation, Validity and Reliability; Computer Software for Qualitative Analysis)
[9]Chang Gung Institute of Technology, Kwei-Shan, Tao-Yuan, Taiwan (Internet Research Method)

Corresponding Author: Marilyn K. Douglas, Email: martydoug@comcast.net

Suggested Citation: Douglas, M. K. & Pacquiao, D. F. (Eds.). (2010). Core curriculum in transcultural nursing and health care [Supplement]. *Journal of Transcultural Nursing, 21*(Suppl. 1).

2. Does the author analyze the research from a transcultural or cross-cultural perspective?

3. Is the literature review comprehensive to include both qualitative and quantitative studies on the variables being studied?

4. If instruments are used, (a) do they have established reliability and validity, and (b) is there evidence of fit to the people and phenomenon being studied?

III. **Qualitative Methodologies For Investigating Questions Related To Culture:** The strengths of qualitative methods are flexibility, giving of insights to the research findings, reliability, and rarely, generalizing (Ryan-Nichols & Will, 2009).

    A. **Ethnography:** Ethnographic research answers questions about why people do what they do by learning about their customs, practices, beliefs, and interpretations of the world.

        1. Overview

            a. Developed within the tradition of anthropology

            b. Usually involves one researcher living for an extended period of time among a group of people with quite different ways of life

            c. The product of this inquiry consists of a holistic description of the social framework of the community, including political, economic, kinship, and religious aspects organizing specific behavioral patterns.

            d. Descriptions of illness episodes and health practices are situated within these social systems and include cultural beliefs about disease, healing rituals, and processes of birth and death. (Chagnon, 1992; Lévi-Strauss, 1963; Turner, 1967).

            e. Most nursing ethnographies focus on a distinct health issue or nursing problem within a specific context among a small group of people.

            f. The researcher hopes to learn *from participants* the salient areas of the topic under study.

        2. Strategies for data collection

            a. *Participant observation*

                1) The primary data collection method of ethnography

                2) All observations—events, behaviors, and relationships—are linked with the meanings held by the group as well as historical influences upon the process.

                3) Usually requires intensive face-to-face contact over an extended period of time (Roper & Shapira, 2000)

                4) Involves active involvement in group activities, studying real-life situations as they occur in their natural settings

                5) Level of engagement moves along a continuum from total involvement (participant only) to no involvement (observer only).

                6) Identify key events by listening to what people talk about and learning their daily routines and where they routinely go (Agar, 1980).

                7) Identify customary behaviors and frequency of significant events (Bernard, 1994; Gross, 1984; Johnson, 1978).

                8) *Emic* perspective: group members' ("insiders'") view of the world, meanings associated with health issues or significant relationships involved with health care issues

                9) *Etic* perspective: the "outsider's" view of the situation, attempt to make sense of what is seen by identifying patterns of behavior

             10) A system of continuous feedback emerges as the researcher watches an event, asks a group member to explain its meaning, and then applies an interpretation based on previous experiences within the community.

            b. *Ethnographic interviewing*

                1) The most important characteristics of the interview are that it has to be descriptive, structured, and includes a contrast among the questions and how the questions are asked (Spradley, 1979).

                2) Relevant human subjects procedures need to be executed prior to the interviews.

                3) *Group interviews* highlight variations in concepts present among the population, used for topics that are reasonably public and not sensitive or embarrassing (Lofland, 1971, p. 88).

                4) *Focused or formal interviews* pose specific questions to individuals after the researcher gains a general understanding of the setting and interactions among participants.

5) Questions are open-ended and semistructured. They start with general questions (i.e., "What is it like to be a healer?") and proceed with using prodding or prompting questions (i.e., "What healing situations have been most difficult for you?").

6) Asking how others in the community act, believe, or feel illuminates shared cultural values and practices (Roper & Shapira, 1999).

7) Group and formal interviews are often audio or video recorded.

8) *Informal interviews* occur when the ethnographer has immediate questions about something in the setting or wants to confirm the accuracy of an interpretation.

9) "Key informants" provide broad knowledge of their culture and have directly experienced relevant issues related the study.

10) "Key informants" often explain things from different perspectives (Fetterman, 1989) and suggest further lines of inquiry.

11) Those selected because of their expertise or specialized knowledge are considered as part of a purposeful, theoretical, or judgmental sample of people (Agar, 1980; Fetterman, 1989; Glaser & Strauss, 1967).

c. ***Review of pertinent documents and objects***

1) Review of relevant documents will supplement data obtained through participant observation activities and interviews.

2) Earlier ethnographies, histories, biographies, newspaper articles, written protocols, photographs, and family letters may provide a historical context for current happenings.

3) It may be appropriate to use inventories, such as a patient's medical history, to collect standardized information from participants.

4) Exercise caution when using supplemental sources, as reliance on information developed from "outsider" assumptions negates discovering the meaning of events from the perspective of group members (Germain, 1993, p. 254).

5) The review of documents includes descriptions of documents used, rationale for their use, and findings that were interpreted from these documents (J. M. Morse & Field, 1995).

d. ***Systematic data collection with field notes***

1) Documenting observations, conversations, feelings, and interpretations in concrete and detailed field notes provides the principal means for understanding what is learned about the people and events in the setting.

2) Observation guidelines, forms, and checklists make data collection easier and serve as reminders of what to observe or ask.

3) Objective and verbatim descriptions of observations and interviews are compared with investigators' personal feelings about these experiences.

4) Explicit accounting of emotional reactions to community members becomes crucial when moving between subjective and objective research modes.

5) This accounting helps identify unrecognized biases and preconceived notions of why events and relationships happen and the meaning they hold for individuals in the group

6) Ethnographers develop their own styles of keeping track of information for analysis, including written descriptions by hand or computer, audiotapes, and video recordings, but all share a commitment to structured and organized methods of collecting data.

3. Data analysis

a. Analysis of ethnographic data actually begins *while* data are collected.

b. The investigator makes decisions about what avenues are most promising and deserve more intensive scrutiny.

c. Spending extended periods of time in the research setting allows the opportunity to further validate initial thoughts about potential meanings and patterns of the information with further observations and questions.

d. More formal analysis occurs once leaving the research site.

e. The process of ethnographic data analysis involves breaking up raw data from field notes and interviews, reassembling these segments into patterns (Jorgensen, 1989).

f. Next, constructs or theories are formulated to explain the experiences learned from the people and events of the setting.

    g. Specific procedures help with this process, including coding data into descriptive labels and then sorting or grouping the labels into categories or patterns (Roper & Shapira, 2000).

    h. General themes discovered from these patterns provide a more global understanding of why things happen as they do in the community and explain recurring relationships between individuals and events.

    i. Finally, connections made between the emic meanings of study participants and the investigator's etic interpretation of those meanings encourage the development of explanatory theories.

4. **Triangulation:** a method to enhance the rigor of the ethnographic study by increasing its *reliability* and *validity*

    a. ***Reliability***

       1) Reliability means that the test procedures, questionnaires are measuring what they are supposed to measure.

       2) Reliability is generally not questioned in ethnographic studies as long as the subject matter and research question are <u>obviously</u> threaded into the collection of data and the analysis.

       3) Reliability or trustworthiness is measured by the repeatability of the study or of the measures used.

       4) Use of an independent researcher to review the outcomes from study is one strategy to enhance reliability.

       5) Keeping detailed notes of observations and diaries of the decisions made throughout collection of data and analysis will also increase the ability for others to repeat the research.

       6) The use of codes in sorting the data during analysis will make the process more transparent.

       7) Computer software may be used to assist in the data sorting, but the investigator must complete the analysis in a transparent manner (Brink & Wood, 2004; Miles & Huberman, 1994).

       8) The process of transcribing the interviews is crucial to maintaining reliability.

       9) The interviews must be transcribed word for word and also must indicate pauses, interviewee questions, and concerns over and above the interview questions.

      10) Keeping notes about observations, feelings and thoughts about observations, and what else is happening besides the verbal interaction will help support conclusions.

      11) A qualitative study, especially ethnographic research, does not have a specific test or procedure to guide rigor, such as the Cronbach's alpha for quantitative studies.

    b. ***Validity***

       1) Validity is determining that the proposed measures results in information about the true or real variable being studied (Brink & Wood, 1994; Macnee & McCabe, 2008).

       2) Validity in the qualitative (ethnographic) study may be influenced by interview questions that may not ask the right questions, believing that verbal information from participants connects with behavior, and that observations may not reflect the research question or the overreaction of the investigator towards the observed situations (Begley, 2003).

       3) It is vital to maintaining the validity of the study that investigators keep awareness of themselves and their feelings in the process of data collection.

       4) To increase validity, ensure that the data reflects the research question/problem (Burns & Grove, 2001).

       5) Make contrasts and comparisons when analyzing the data.

       6) Asking the informants to give feedback about the findings and the conclusions will increase validity.

    c. Triangulation means to apply more than one method of data collection and/or analysis to strengthen validity for qualitative research.

    d. Two types of triangulation (Casey & Murphy, 2009)

       1) Across-methods triangulation: use both qualitative and quantitative methods

       2) Within-methods triangulation: more than one qualitative method for data collection

    e. Issues related to application of more than one method include the following:

       1) Checking for representativeness of the research topic

       2) How do the measurements compare?

       3) How are comparisons, contrasts, and outliers handled in each method?

       4) Assuring that the quantitative measure has established validity and reliability (Jones & Bugge, 2006)

    f. Some researchers combine ethnography with other qualitative strategies, such as phenomenology (Maggs-Rapport, 2000).

    g. Other researchers combine one of the three strategies of ethnography with quantitative methods, such as measurement tools or questionnaires (Barton, 2008).

Table 10.1. Strategies in Triangulation: Advantages and Disadvantages

Strategies	Advantages	Disadvantages
Use of the three methods of ethnography: 1) interview 2) participant observation 3) review of documents, photos, and artifacts	• These three methods are already a part of an ethnography as identified by anthropologists and nurses. • The three processes work together to validate and establish reliability in collection, analysis and findings	
Combined use of ethnography with other qualitative methods, such as phenomenology or grounded theory, etc.	• May increase the amount of information collected and subsequent findings by asking the same qualitative question but by using different methods of interviews, observation, analysis of findings. • Enhances the research skills of nurses because they learn other qualitative methods.	• Potential risk of not staying focused on the original ethnographic research question. • May increase the length of the study, which is already time-consuming, in order to get data needed to answer question(s)
Combined use of ethnography with the use of quantitative methods	• May enhance amount of data/findings if the disadvantages are able to be mastered in order to accomplish the increase in knowledge	• Potentially violates the principle of the ethnography focus, which is usually having little or no knowledge about the subject prior to the study. • Finding the right quantitative tool that supports the focus of the ethnography may be difficult. Quantitative and qualitative research serves two different purposes: a) Qualitative is to find the information from the voices of the subjects and thus is inductive in analysis. b) Quantitative is deductive in that the researcher already has information about the research question/problem. • They are two very different approaches.

  h. In ethnography, observation, interview, and reviewing pertinent documents are a natural triangulation; therefore, triangulation may or may not increase the rigor of the ethnographic study (Roper & Shapira, 2000).

  i. There is no consensus about the correct use of triangulation in the nursing literature; researchers are adapting the ethnographic methods and including other qualitative measures in a triangulation effort. See Table 10.1.

 5. Computer software programs for qualitative data analysis

  a. The use of computers in the last decade has been limited to sorting data after the investigator has identified the sorting topics.

  b. Following the completion of the computer sorting, the investigator(s) finish the analysis by identifying categories and themes as part of the findings, which is often a time-consuming process.

  c. These programs are particularly important where there is a large volume of data that might take months or years to sort manually.

  d. Having the computer conduct the preliminary steps of sorting saves the investigator time as well as reduces human error.

  e. The software programs used in studies during this last decade are Atlas.ti (http://www.atlasti.com), Ethnograph (Green, Meaux, Huett, & Ainley, 2009), NUD*IST (Harper, Ersser, & Gobbi, 2007) and QRR N 6th (Kelly & Patterson 2006).

  f. NVivo (formerly NUD*IST): permits management of data tracking and assists researcher in development of categories and themes (www.qsrinternational.com/products_nvivo.aspx)

  g. Ethnograph: permits management of interview transcripts, field notes, survey responses, and collections of documents (letters, newspaper articles, diaries, essays, etc.); analysis tools; compatible with Windows XP and Vista (www.qualisresearch.com)

    h. The advantages of the software is in saving time, decreasing human errors, and standardizing the initial step in content analysis.

    i. The disadvantages are the potential lack of the human review process or missing sorting topics.

B. **Ethnonursing:** a research method designed to facilitate discovery of data focused on Leininger's Theory of Culture Care Diversity and Universality (Leininger, 2002a, p. 85).

  1. *Ethnonursing* refers to a qualitative research method focused on naturalistic, open discovery and largely inductive (emic) modes to document, describe, explain, and interpret informants' worldview, meanings, symbols, and life experiences as they bear on actual or potential nursing care phenomena.

  2. Principles (Leininger, 2006b, pp. 71-72)

    a. Maintain an open discovery, active listening, and genuine learning attitude in working with informants; show a willingness to learn from the people.

    b. Maintain an active and curious posture about the "why" of whatever is seen, heard, or experienced and appreciation of whatever informants share.

    c. Record what is shared by informants in a careful and conscientious way with full meanings, explanations, or interpretations in order to preserve informant ideas.

    d. Seek a mentor who has experience with the ethnonursing method.

    e. Clarify the purposes of additional qualitative research methods if combined with the ethnonursing method, such as combining life histories, ethnography, phenomenology, or ethnoscience.

  3. Purposes

    a. To discover largely unknown or vaguely known complex nursing phenomena bearing on care, well-being, health, and related cultural knowledge;

    b. To facilitate the researcher to enter the people's emic (insider's) cultural world and learn from them first-hand of their beliefs, values, experiences, and life world about human care and health;

    c. To gain in-depth knowledge about care meanings, expressions, symbols, metaphors, and daily factors influencing health and well-being as depicted by the Sunrise Model;

    d. To use standard and new Enablers to tease out covert or embedded care and nursing knowledge related to the Culture Care Theory with both emic and etic data;

    e. To use a rigorous, detailed, and systematic method of qualitative data analysis that would preserve naturalistic, cultural, and contextual data related to the theory;

    f. To use qualitative criteria for accurate, meaningful, and credible analysis of findings; and

    g. To identify strengths and limitations of the ethnonursing method.

  4. Process/Steps (Leininger, 2002a, p. 93)

    a. Fully review the literature directly or closely related to domain of inquiry (DOI), including both qualitative and quantitative studies.

    b. State researcher's theoretical interests and assumptive premises about the DOI in relation to the Culture Care Theory.

    c. State the orientational definitions (not operational ones), purpose(s), goal(s), and significance of study.

    d. Select the site and obtain appropriate approvals.

    e. Submit proposal to Institutional Review Board for approval prior to initiation of study.

    f. Select key and general informants thoughtfully and purposefully.

    g. Use Stranger to Friend Enabler, Observation-Participation-Reflection (OPR) Enabler, and Sunrise Model Enabler.

      1) Researcher should frequently assess own attitude, verbal and nonverbal communication modes, gender, and any other factors that may influence informant responses

      2) Confer with experienced transcultural nursing mentor who may provide insights

  5. Strategies for ensuring qualitative rigor (Leininger, 2002a)

    a. *Credibility:* direct sources of evidence or information from the people within their environmental contexts of their "truths" held firmly as accurate or believable to them

    b. *Confirmability:* repeated direct, documented verbatim statements and direct observational evidence from informants, situations, and other people who firmly and knowingly affirm and substantiate the data for findings upon repeated explanations to the researcher

    c. *Meaning-in-Context:* understandable and meaningful referents, meanings, or findings in situations, instances, settings, or life events, experiences, communications, symbols, or other human activities that are known and held relevant to the people within their familiar and natural living environmental contexts and the culture

    d. ***Recurrent Patterning:*** documented evidence of repeated instances, sequences of events, activities, experiences, expressions, lifeways, patterns, themes, and acts over time reflecting consistency in lifeways or patterned behaviors

    e. ***Saturation:*** very full, comprehensive, exhaustive, in-depth "taking in" of information of all that is or can be known or understood by the informants about phenomena related to a domain of inquiry under study with no further data or insights forthcoming

    f. ***Transferability:*** refers to whether the findings from a completed study have similar (but not necessarily identical) meanings and relevance to be transferred to another similar situation, context, or culture while still preserving the particularized meanings, interpretations, and inferences of the culture under study

6. Selection of appropriate instruments (Leininger, 2006b)
   a. Sunrise Model as Enabler. Inquiry Guide for Use with the Sunrise Model to Assess Culture Care and Health, which includes Culture Care Values and Meanings Enabler; Audio-Visual Guide; and Generic and Professional Care Enabler Guide (Leininger, 1995; McFarland, 1995)
   b. OPR Enabler
   c. DOI Enabler
   d. Stranger to Trusted Friend Enabler
   e. Ethnodemographic Enabler (Leininger, 2006a; McFarland, 1995)
   f. Acculturation Healthcare Assessment Enabler (McFarland, 1995)

7. Sampling methods to include sufficient representation (Leininger, 2002a, 2006b)
   a. Study size
      1) Mini: 6-8 key informants and 12-16 general informants
      2) Maxi or Macro: 12-15 key informants, or approximately twice as many key as general informants.
   b. Informants: Ratio of 1:2 regardless of study size is advised.
      1) **Key:** thoughtfully and purposefully selected (often by persons in the culture or subculture) to provide in-depth data about the domain of inquiry; are held to reflect the norms, values, beliefs, and general lifeways of the culture; and are usually interested and willing to participate
      2) **General:** selected to provide reflection and for representation of the wider community; not as fully knowledgeable about the DOI, but do have general ideas that they are willing to share
   c. Sampling issues (Leininger, 2006b)
      1) Large numbers of informants alone are not the rule.
      2) Focus is on obtaining *in-depth* knowledge to understand fully the phenomena under study.

8. Data collection procedures: field notes (Leininger, 2006b, p. 75)

9. Interpretation of the data: identifying cultural themes and patterns
   a. Phases of Ethnonursing Data Analysis (Leininger, 1991, 2006b)
      1) Fourth (last) Phase: major themes, theoretical formulations, and recommendations
      2) Third Phase: patterns and contextual analysis
      3) Second Phase: identification and categorization of descriptors and components
      4) First Phase: collecting, describing, and documenting raw data; use of field journal and computer
   b. Coding Scheme: Partial overview of approach used in ethnonursing research study is provided in McFarland (1995).
      1) Categories and Domains of Information: includes observations, interviews, interpretative material, and nonmaterial data
         a) Category I: General Cultural DOIs (worldview; cultural and social lifeways; ethnohistorical and environmental contexts; linguistic terms; cultural foods; material and nonmaterial culture; ethnodemographics; racism, prejudice, and race)
         b) Category II: Domain of Cultural and Social Structure Data (includes normative values, patterns, functions, and conflicts)
         c) Category III: Care, Cure, and Health (Well-Being) and Illness of Folk and Professional Lifeways
         d) Category IV: Health and Social Service Institutions (includes administrative norms, beliefs, and practices with meanings-in-context)
         e) Category V: Lifecycle and Intergenerational Patterns (includes ceremonies and rituals)
         f) Category VI: Methodological and Other Research Features of the Study

   2) Themes using example of African American (AA) residents in retirement home (McFarland, 1995)

      a) Generic Care Theme: AA residents viewed, expressed, and lived generic care to maintain their preadmission generic lifeways and to maintain beneficial and healthy lifeways in the retirement home. Generic Care Patterns supporting this theme were care as doing physical tasks, activities, or special things for others; care as family help or assistance; care as religious or spiritual helping; care as watchfulness or surveillance; and care as presence.

      b) Professional Care Theme: Anglo and AA professional nurses, licensed practical nurses, and nursing assistants provided aspects of professional care to support beneficial and satisfying lifeways to residents in the retirement home.

      c) Environmental Context Theme: Retirement home care patterns and expressions were expressed and viewed within the daily and nightly environmental context as a continuing life experience but with major differences between the apartment section and nursing home units.

      d) Generic Health Theme: The Anglo and AA residents shared a view of good health that included being mobile and have a clear mind, which was supported by the nursing home staff.

      e) Institutional Culture Theme: The institutional culture of the retirement home reflected some unique lifeways and shared care and health expressions, patterns, and practices for elderly residents, which were embedded in their worldview.

10. Acculturation as a mitigating factor on outcomes (Leininger, 2006b)

   a. Acculturation Enabler Guide was developed

      1) to assess the extent of acculturation of an individual or group with respect to a particular culture or subculture,

      2) to assess the extent to which the group or individual are more traditionally or nontraditionally oriented, and

      3) to identify cultural variability or universality features.

   b. The Acculturation Enabler Guide was developed to assess cultural variabilities of individuals and groups of a particular culture along major lines of differentiating cultural experience.

   c. With Enabler,

      1) A profile can be obtained with respect to traditional and nontraditional orientations;

      2) Data can be analyzed and findings reported in different creative ways, such as pictorial graphs, bar graphs, narratives, or informant/group profiles; and

      3) Percentages or simple numerical data may also be used to show direction or degree of acculturation.

C. Phenomenology

1. Description

   a. *Phenomenology* is a qualitative human science research approach used to study the meaning of lived experience.

   b. *Human science* relates to the human world characterized as mind, thoughts, consciousness, values, feeling, emotions, actions, culture, and purposes, which are discovered in languages, beliefs, arts, and institutions.

   c. Human science is different from natural sciences, which are characterized by objects of nature, things, or natural events.

2. Purpose

   a. ***Phenomenological hermeneutics*** studies persons or beings that have consciousness and act purposefully by creating intentional meanings that are expressions of how human beings exist in the world. *Hermeneutics* relates to interpretation.

   b. Phenomenological hermeneutics offers insight into and understanding of the world itself. It addresses what we want to know, that which is most essential to being (van Manen, 1992).

   c. Study the world as we immediately experience it, pre-reflectively rather than as we conceptualize or categorize it, and as it is interpreted by both research participants and the researcher.

   d. Capture both the description and interpretation of human phenomena—the mind, thoughts, values, feelings, emotions, culture, and actions of human beings.

   e. From a transcultural nursing perspective, phenomenology explicates the meaning of transcultural human caring phenomena by describing and seeking understanding of the life world phenomena in the narrative texts to illuminate the meaning of culturally oriented themes, metathemes, or even a phenomenological theory generated in a culturally dynamic universe.

f. Overall, phenomenological hermeneutic research meets human beings where they are. For transcultural nursing, this research meets people in the transcultural context for the purposes of description, interpretation, and analysis of the caring relationship and the meanings embedded in the sociocultural nursing situation.

g. Van Manen (1992, pp. 8-13), a noted phenomenologist, described *phenomenological hermeneutic* human science research as follows:
   1) Phenomenology is the study of lived experience. Central questions:
      a) What is the nature or essence of the experience, for example, what is the nature of transcultural caring for a person of a different culture than one's own?
      b) What is it like to experience something?
      c) What does it mean?
   2) Phenomenology is the explication of phenomena as they present themselves to consciousness, which is the only access to how human beings are related to the world. It is reflection on experience that is already passed or lived through.
   3) Phenomenological hermeneutics is the study of lived or existential meanings and endeavors to describe and interpret these meanings deeply and richly.
   4) Phenomenological research is the study of essences.
      a) It is interested in what makes something what it is, without which it could not be what it is.
      b) It attempts to uncover and describe the internal meaning structures and significance of lived experience.
      c) It is the description of the experiential meanings we live as we live them.
      d) It is the attentive practice of thoughtfulness, described as a minding, heeding, and caring attunement about life, of living, or what it means to live a life.
   5) Phenomenological research is the human scientific study of phenomena.
      a) Its research is systematic and focused, using specific modes of questioning, such as what is it like to experience something in life; what does it mean.
      b) Uses reflection and intuition
      c) It is an explicit attempt to communicate, through the narrative content of the text, the structures of meaning of the lived experience.
   6) Phenomenological research is a search for what it means to be human.
      a) Explores and describes one's identity, culture, and sociocultural world
      b) The researcher has a moral obligation to take an active responsibility for becoming more fully who he/she is as the researcher and facilitate that process for research participants.
   7) Phenomenological research is a poetizing activity.
      a) There is an active link between the interview process and the results.
      b) The link is a process of communicating that is both an inspired and expressive illumination of the world.
      c) Phenomenology aims at making explicit and seeking universal meaning where poetry and literature remain "implicit and particular" (van Manen, 1990, p. 19).

3. ***The Phenomenological Hermeneutic Research Process*** (Ray, 1991, 1994; van Manen, 1990)
   a. The *intentionality of the inner being* of the researcher imagines the vision of transcultural caring in nursing, past and future, within the present and listening to the voice within embodied consciousness for caring-directed research.
   b. Turning to the *nature of lived experience* means that the researcher turns to things themselves and embraces a human experience, a project of someone or people who live in the context of particular individual, sociocultural, and historical life circumstances in order to make sense (meaning) of a certain aspect of human existence.
   c. The researcher brackets existing presuppositions for the purposes of validly turning to the "things" themselves.
   d. Investigating *experience as we live it* focuses on a renewed contact with the original experience.
      1) Engaging with and exploring the basic experience of the world and human relationships in diverse situations through caring dialogue to penetrate the meaning of experience
      2) Transcribed texts are created from the interview process.
   e. Reflecting on *essential themes* is a reflective grasp of the essence of the lived experience expressed in the text by first feeling the presencing of the participants' state of being, followed by describing and interpreting the meaning of aspects of their life world.

1) According to Gadamer, researchers are interpreting an interpretation of the participant's recollective understanding of their life world experience (van Manen, 1990, p. 26).
2) These essences are communicated as *themes* (direct experiences framed linguistically), and *meta-themes* (linguistic abstractions of the descriptive themes).
3) Essences can be intuited as a direct apprehension of the whole of the experience and can be expressed as metaphors or a unity of meaning (universal or a phenomenological hermeneutic theory).

   f. Maintaining a *strong and oriented relation with the text* in the process of interpretation (theorizing) about the essence of experience.
   1) A theory of meaning may be generated that captures the universal.
   2) It does not relate to generalizability as in the positivist tradition; rather, it is an integral understanding and way of communicating the aesthetic act (harmony) or the universal meaning of the whole experience.

   g. The *art of writing and rewriting* refers to the "bringing to speech" of something by writing (van Manen, 1990, p. 32).
   h. Phenomenological hermeneutics is the application of language and thoughtfulness to illuminate its essence.
   i. *Dialoguing with the written texts* allows for considering the parts and the whole of the text—the individual phrases, sentences, paragraphs, and the whole of the text—to examine differences and similarities.
   j. The form or structure of the *meanings* (themes, metathemes, metaphors, and theory) gives rise to its value and further examination in relation to existing literature to advance implications or recommendations for (transcultural) nursing education, practice, administration, and research.

4. ***Credibility and Significance of the Process of Phenomenological Hermeneutics***
   a. Illuminates the processes of recognizing, believing, and acknowledging the dynamics of the credibility of the research. Did the study illuminate the caring attunement of the researcher and the research participant (reality-as-meant)?
   b. Did the study properly ground the questions: What is it like to experience the phenomenon? What does the experience mean in the context of a life and sociocultural environment?
   c. Phenomenology should enlarge human awareness directly and expand the range of human perception, the possibilities of being—the quality of making humans more human, humane, and spiritual (whole) rather than mechanistic.

5. ***Affirming and confirming meanings of the lived experience*** are the dynamics of the significance of the research.
   a. The universal meaning is deep; it is a sympathetic relationship through which the researcher and the textual knowledge are transposed into the interior lives of others.
   b. It resonates with the lived life of others. Buytendijk referred to this experience as "*the phenomenological nod . . .* indicating that a good phenomenological description [and interpretation] is something that we can nod to, recognizing it as an experience that we have had, or could have had . . . the validating circle of inquiry"(van Manen, 1990, p. 27).

D. Grounded Theory

1. Description
   a. ***Grounded theory method*** is a qualitative research approach that uses the constant comparative method of analysis and is associated with qualitative data collection in the field, open coding, theoretical sampling, and memo writing of specific sociocultural phenomena in order to generate both substantive and formal theories.
   b. Theory in this method relates to induction, discovery, and emergence from experiential, systematic, or procedural thematic inquiry and analysis.

2. **Origins of Grounded Theory**
   a. Grounded theory originated in sociology and in the philosophy and sociology of symbolic interaction described mainly by Mead and Blumer (Glaser & Strauss, 1967).
   b. Glaser and Strauss (1967; Glaser, 1978, 1992; Strauss & Corbin, 2008) were the first sociologists to present the perspective of grounded theory research, that is, the generation of a substantive and formal theory emerging from the social world.
   c. Glaser was more committed to a creative process and outlined the notion of discovery and emergence in theory generation. Glaser (1992) reported that the importance of theory grounded in reality is its evolution from the nature and active roles of the subjects and the researcher in shaping the worlds

they live in through the processes of *symbolic interaction* (patterns of relationship and sociocultural meaning).

    d. Corbin, Quint Benoliel, Ray, Stern, and Swanson are a few of the nurse scholars credited with some of the first contributions to the evolution of the Grounded Theory Method in nursing.

3. **Use of Grounded Theory in Transcultural Nursing**

    a. Grounded theory is very applicable to transcultural nursing and the study of transcultural interactions.

    b. Highlights the holistic nature of nursing, the transcultural context, and the procedural analysis of sociocultural or transcultural categories, subcategories, and core variables in the transcultural nursing situation.

    c. Integration of descriptors of sociocultural processes facilitate the discovery of a basic social process (*substantive theory* grounded in reality) and the assimilation of conceptual data with general patterns of culture and transcultural nursing knowledge (*formal theory*).

    d. There is emphasis on change, social and cultural processes, and the variability (diversity) of and complexity of life.

    e. The research experience is the constant comparative analysis by the researcher of data collection, coding of data (variables, categories, subcategories, discovery of the basic social process), memo writing, theoretical sampling, and emergence of substantive and formal theories.

    f. Transcultural nurses can use grounded theory methodology to study transcultural interaction and patterns of culture that illuminate the meaning of relationships, holism (body, mind, and spirit), health, and healing in the transcultural context.

    g. Generating theory in the transcultural nursing situation facilitates and increases understanding and meaning of cultural diversity, universality, and competence in the sociocultural world of nursing.

    h. The theories that are generated respect and reveal perspectives of subjects in the substantive area under study.

    i. The theories emerge from:

        1) First, an in-depth comparative approach that focuses on the discovery of action and interaction associated with the social world (*substantive theory*)

        2) Second, the analytic process of assimilation of the substantive theory with knowledge that has been generated in the primary or related disciplinary fields, such as nursing, sociology, or anthropology (*formal theory*)

    j. Substantive theory is often compared with middle range theory.

        1) Generally, middle range theories are considered narrower in scope than grand theories but not as broad as the formal theory in the Grounded Theory tradition.

        2) In nursing, middle range theories are intermediate in scope, are testable, are grounded in research, are focused on limited aspects of reality, are less concrete than practice theory, have a limited number of variables, and can be built on the work of other middle range theories (Liehr & Smith, 1999). On the other hand, substantive theory in Grounded Theory is focused on the discovery and emergence of theory grounded systematically in the field data or concepts of reality.

4. **Procedures for the Use of the Grounded Theory Method in Transcultural Nursing**

    a. Data generation and analysis

        1) The researcher is the principal instrument of the generation and analysis of data through the process of interviewing to describe and compare and contrast the social and cultural processes of the life world as it is lived in the reality of the nursing situation.

        2) The researcher not only participates with subjects but also observes and engenders memos (written notes) of the social transcultural nursing process.

    b. Constant Comparative Analysis provides for the investigation and analysis of data in which each part of the interview and written data (transcribed lines, sentences, phrases, paragraphs) is compared with other parts and then coded into categories and subcategories (Glaser, 1978).

    c. Categories and subcategories and their properties are identified and compared for similarities and differences in patterns of culture.

    d. Theoretical coding proceeds simultaneously and demonstrates how categories relate to each other.

    e. Saturation of data occurs when no new data are generated.

    f. When all data are compared and contrasted, a *basic social process* emerges, which allows for the discovery and emergence of *substantive theory*.

      1) The conceptual level of substantive theory illuminates the integration of the data of the study, what the integrative data indicate, and what is revealed in the study of the social process (Glaser, 1978).

      2) Many studies conclude with the discovery of substantive theory only.

    g. The generation of formal theory provides another level of power in the challenge of Grounded Theory research.

    h. Formal theory is then generated from an analysis of the substantive theory in relationship to the meaning of the social unit (Glaser, 1978), which can be linked to a discipline, such as nursing; an organization, such as a hospital; a community, such as a pattern of social governance; or a global unit, such as the concept of globalization itself.

5. **Evaluation of Grounded Theory method** requires that the credibility of a theory or theories meet specific criteria.

    a. *Fit* means that the theory must fit the substantive area from which the application was made and must correspond to the data generated in the social (nursing) situation.

    b. *Understanding* means that the theory must make sense and be understandable to subjects and professionals familiar with the subject matter.

    c. *Generality* means that the theory must be applicable to any diverse life world situation within the substantive area.

    d. *Control* means that the theory allows the user control over the structure and processes that describe social interaction in a given group or the nursing situation (Hutchison & Skodol-Wilson, 2001).

E. Participatory Action Research (PAR)

1. Definition and description of method

    a. Research that involves all relevant parties in actively examining together current action (which they experience as problematic) in order to change and improve it (Wadsworth, 1998).

    b. PAR is sometimes referred to as "participatory research," "collaborative inquiry," or "participative inquiry."

    c. Papadopoulos (2006a, 2006b) uses the term *culturally competent research* to describe her version of PAR that is specifically applied to investigate cross-cultural/transcultural health-related questions.

    d. Further, Papadopoulos (2005) defined culturally competent research as research that both utilizes and develops knowledge and skills that promote the delivery of health care that is sensitive and appropriate to individuals' needs, whatever their cultural backgrounds.

2. **Distinguishing characteristics**

    a. Wadsworth (1998) identifies PAR's characteristics as

      1) more conscious of "problematizing" an existing action or practice and by whom,

      2) more explicit about "naming" the problem,

      3) more planned and deliberate about involving others who should or could be involved,

      4) more systematic and rigorous in the effort to get answers,

      5) more carefully documenting and recording action,

      6) more self-skeptical, and

      7) changing actions as part of the research process and then researching these changed actions.

    b. Finn (1994) provides three key elements that distinguish participatory research from traditional approaches to research: people, power, and praxis.

      1) People: PAR is people centered, as the research is informed by and responds to their experiences and needs.

      2) Power: PAR gives power/empowerment to ordinary people to construct knowledge based on their reality, language, and rituals of truth.

      3) Praxis: PAR recognizes the inseparability of theory and practice and the personal—a political dialectic.

    c. In her specific version of PAR—that of culturally competent research—Papadopoulos states that culturally competent research is

      1) Reflexive,

      2) Inclusive,

      3) Relevant,

      4) Nonessentializing,

      5) Rigorous,

6) Ethical, and

7) Liberating.

3. **Philosophical and disciplinary underpinnings**

   a. The Colombian sociologist Orlando Fals-Borda gave PAR its worldwide recognition by organizing the first PAR conference in 1975.

   b. PAR has many of its roots in social psychology.

   c. PAR builds on critical pedagogy put forward by Paulo Freire (1970/1990).

   d. It also builds on Action Research and Group Dynamics models developed by psychologist Kurt Lewin in the early to mid-1900s.

   e. PAR's philosophical underpinnings are based on the democratic principles of participation, social justice, collaborative decision making, and redistribution of power.

4. **Phenomena and types of questions** that can best be investigated using this method

   a. Any issue that needs to be explored from patients'/clients' perspective

   b. Investigations about ordinary people's health-related interests and problems

   c. Questions that prioritize working with the oppressed or people whose issues include inaccessibility, marginalization, exploitation, racism, and cultural isolation

   d. Inquiries about ordinary people's construction of illness and how it impacts on their lives

   e. Inquiries during which people are empowered to appropriate knowledge about their health and unveil the power monopoly of the experts and professional researchers

   f. Examples of research questions:

      1) What are the health and social care needs of Ethiopian refugees and asylum seekers in the United Kingdom and how can these inform the voluntary and statutory service providers? (Papadopoulos & Gebrehiwot, 2002)

      2) What are the risks of sexual maltreatment of Ethiopian unaccompanied asylum-seeking minors in England and how can these be prevented? (Lay, Papadopoulos, & Gebrehiwot, 2007)

      3) What are the meanings and experiences of cancer of the Chinese community in London, and how can these inform the future development of culturally appropriate cancer information for Chinese people in the United Kingdom? (Lees, Papadopoulos, & Ridge, 2004)

5. **Ethical issues** that need to be addressed specific to this method are many, but here are some examples:

   a. True participation, not manipulation: Is there real power sharing in the partnership or are lay participants being exploited by the powerful "experts" who simulate power sharing by involving people who do not have the necessary skills to be truly influential?

   b. The consensual processes of participation can be a form of manipulation by the powerful members to gain "powerful" agreements, as these are believed to be consensual.

   c. Relativism of those who participate: Is it possible for the few people to be representative of all views? Or are they representing their own views and interests? How are they recruited or get involved?

   d. Whose research is it anyway? Was it initiated by the people and/or have they been involved from the start and at every stage? Or is this the result of an "expert" to promote knowledge (whatever the motive) without a real commitment to promoting change and the right action?

   e. How is the confidentiality and anonymity of the lay members of the research team being protected from the members of the communities/groups they "represent"? Should this be a concern and could this result in harm?

   f. Participating in a research study takes time and effort. Should lay members be paid, and if so, how?

   g. Participating in a research study can be daunting. How are lay members prepared/trained/empowered to become equal members of the team and not remain "junior partners"? Can training institutionalize them, thus removing the edge of their perspective?

   h. Who owns the research outputs? Whose names go on the research report and published papers? Who presents the findings at conferences?

   i. If PAR is about people actively examining together problems they are experiencing in order to change and improve their situation, do they need professional researchers? If they conduct PAR in ways that suit them and by using "unconventional" methods of research, can they gain research funding, and will politicians, policy makers, academics, and other politically powerful take their findings and recommendations seriously?

6. **Potential for use with other methods,** that is, combined methodologies: Although most PAR frequently uses qualitative research methods, it does not exclude the use of relevant quantitative methods and instruments.

7. **Strategies for ensuring validity and reliability**
   a. If a mixed methodology is used, the validity and reliability of the data collected through quantitative methods is the same as for all quantitative studies (see segment on quantitative methodologies).
   b. For qualitative methods, the terms *verification, applicability, trustworthiness, credibility, transferability,* and *confirmability* are more appropriate than *validity* and *reliability.*

8. **Recruitment and retention of research participants**
   a. Sampling issues: Since PAR is driven by people's need to know in order to solve their problems and bring about desired change, the size and type of sample is entirely guided by this agenda.
   b. However, PAR also sets out to produce deeper understandings and more useful and more powerful theory; frequently, qualitative methodologies and thus qualitative sampling considerations need to be observed.
   c. Whether the PAR project is originated and sponsored by the people concerned or it is done in partnership with experts and professional researchers, it is imperative that members of the target community or communities are involved in the recruitment of participants.
   d. Successful retention of research participants depends on the cultural competence of the research team, which is manifested in
      1) spending time to understand their cultural context and backgrounds;
      2) spending time within the community to develop collaborations;
      3) acknowledging the participants' experiences and contributions;
      4) acknowledging the effort and time given by them to the project and providing them with desired rewards, such as paying for their expenses, providing training and accreditation opportunities; and
      5) showing genuine interest in them and commitment to sustainable change.

9. **Setting selection**
   a. Selecting the setting is always a matter of negotiation with the participating community/group.
   b. Entry is gained through discussions with gatekeepers.
   c. The role of the professional researcher in culturally competent PAR varies. This may depend on
      1) the funder's conditions,
      2) the available and/or accessible resources,
      3) the type of project,
      4) the research skills within the project team,
      5) the participating community's/group's wishes, and/or
      6) what will bring the best outcome.
   d. The range of researcher roles in PAR projects can be thought of as on a continuum:
      1) taking the lead,
      2) being a coinvestigator,
      3) providing advice on research design and procedures,
      4) training and empowering members of the participating community to be effective investigators,
      5) being a learner (particularly if he or she is an "outsider"),
      6) or any combination of the above.

10. **Authenticity of context** is one of the main strengths of PAR, since the investigation and the main actors of it originate from and are part of the context.

11. **Instruments**
    a. Culturally sensitive and appropriate instruments must be selected. If existing validated instruments are used, these may have to be modified and/or translated (and back-translated to achieve conceptual and semantic equivalence) from the source language to the target language.
    b. As PAR is frequently aimed at specific problems and contexts, specific culturally and linguistically sensitive instruments need to be developed. These could range from self-administered questionnaire surveys to individual interviews, focus groups, participant observations, and so on.
    c. Questions in these instruments must not offend; what is acceptable in one culture may not be so in another. The strength of PAR is that through the participation of members of the target group—ideally in all stages of the research process—such issues will not arise.

12. **Data collection procedures**
    a. Ensuring authenticity of data: Culturally competent PAR researchers aim to observe and participate in authentic experiences that can be described and explained with the purpose of achieving a deeper understanding of a particular phenomenon.
    b. All participants—professional researchers, service providers, service users, patients' health advocates, and so on—should, according to Guba and Lincoln (1989), experience the following:
       1) catalytic authenticity, because the research would change their practice or lifeways;
       2) tactical authenticity that would lead all participants feeling empowered to act;
       3) ontological authenticity, since to ensure fairness, all participants should be involved in constructions and interpretations of data; and
       4) educative authenticity, since through the research, participants develop an awareness of, and empathy for, others' constructions.
    c. Minimizing researcher's bias through cultural self-awareness, reflexivity, establishing explicit criteria of authenticity, and trustworthiness.
    d. Use of emerging questions: These are explored through the continuous PAR cycles of question-fieldwork-analysis-reflection-action.
    e. Primary and secondary informants/sources are used depending on the research question.
    f. Ensuring saturation (thick) of data: Thick description and deep understanding is the purpose of PAR. Personal narratives and community testimonies are some of the methods used.
13. **Data analysis procedures**
    a. Verbatim transcriptions of all interviews. Issues of translation are of paramount importance (see above).
    b. Contextual and concept analysis as per qualitative methodology's good practice: Coding, identifying categories/domains, determining recurrent patterns, and identifying emerging themes. c. Context, such as ethnohistory, is always provided in some detail.
    d. Criteria for assuring valid interpretation of findings:
       1) data analysis and interpretation involves members of participating communities/groups
       2) findings verified with the broader participating community/group through a process of discussion and consensus
       3) care is taken not to promote or establish essentialisms through privileging homogenous personal experiences
       4) care is taken not to impose a single interpretation that denies the cultural, psychosocial, environmental, and economic complexities of personal experiences
14. **Generating conclusions**
    a. If cultural bias was not minimized, results will reflect these biases.
    b. Overgeneralization to communities and cultural groups should be avoided, as PAR is not concerned with generalizable findings, but these could function as exemplars that can have applicability and transferability to other cultural groups. Thus PAR research generates useful knowledge for cross-cultural studies.
    c. Although PAR privileges firsthand personal experiences and uses these to generate the desired useful and powerful theory, the philosophical basis underpinning PAR and the explosion in PAR research in many disciplines enable culturally competent PAR in health to link and be linked with theories generated by such studies as well as other non-PAR resultant theories. This promotes comparison and help to generate further conclusions.
15. **Reporting the study findings**
    a. User-friendly reports with low to medium readability difficulty and available in variety of formats. Summary, in a variety of languages, if needed.
    b. Professional researcher–participating member coauthorship of report.

F. Critical Incident Analysis as a Research Method
   1. This practical and efficient qualitative research methodology offers a wide application for nursing research.
   2. It is unique and different from other qualitative research methods that describe phenomena in naturalistic settings.
   3. Critical incident studies are more highly focused and are aimed at pinpointing facts and producing data to solve practical problems.

    a. Developed by John Flanagan during World War II (Flanagan, 1954).

        1) Urgently needed understanding of behaviors associated with being a successful pilot and of doing the job well.

        2) More traditional research methods were cumbersome and time-consuming.

        3) A highly reliable method of intensive interviewing identified critical behaviors of pilots and other key military positions.

        4) Technique proved useful for solving other practical problems.

        5) Since World War II, this method has been used for a variety of purposes by business, industry, and organizational psychology.

    b. Research applications in health services research.

        1) Developing faculty appraisal instruments in medical and nursing schools

        2) Assessing patient and spouses' experiences in health care settings

          a) Patients perceptions regarding quality of care (Cheek, O'Brian, Ballantyne, & Pincombe, 1997; Grant, Reimer, & Bannatyne, 1996; Kemppainen et al., 2000)

          b) Spouses' decision making in chronic illness (Martinsson, Dracup, & Frilund, 2001)

        3) Determining patient responses to illness and treatment

          a) Self-care strategies for symptom management in HIV/AIDS (Eller et al., 2005; Kemppainen, Levine, Mistal, & Schmidgall, 2003; Nicholas et al., 2002)

          b) Compliance with treatment or medication regimens (Kemppainen et al., 2001, 2004)

        4) Identifying essential components for staff and patient education programs

        5) Identifying best practices within a health care discipline (Nadine et al., 2009; Prochaska et al., 2009)

        6) Integration within a randomized controlled trial to expand quantitative results (Bormann et al., 2006)

4. **Basic rationale and advantages of the critical incident approach**

    a. Critical incident studies are typically conducted to identify effective or ineffective behaviors causally linked with specific outcomes.

    b. They are highly focused on finding solutions to practical problems and finding out "why people do something."

    c. Critical incident studies offer many advantages.

        1) Can be used in a wide variety of situations to study a wide variety of behaviors.

        2) Data can be collected by a variety of means (face-to-face interviews, phone interviews, group settings, Internet).

        3) Persons have the opportunity to generate detailed descriptions of incidents as they see them.

        4) Since only simple types of judgments and responses are required from study participants, the research method is highly effective for interviewing persons who are acutely ill or have limited attention spans (Flanagan, 1954).

        5) Critical incident interviews may be as brief as 10 to 15 min. They are designed to pinpoint facts and eliminate personal opinion or generalization.

        6) This method is considered highly reliable and valid. When a large number of participants offer the same description of a behavior, it becomes fact (Flanagan, 1954).

5. **Process for conducting a critical incident study**

    a. The critical incident technique provides an organized structure for data collection that focuses on identifying specific behaviors that persons perform or fail to perform (Flanagan, 1954).

    b. Key terms/concepts

        1) An *incident* is a report of an observable, specific behavior.

        2) *Critical* means that the behavior was crucial to the outcome of concern (Flanagan, 1954).

        3) The emphasis is on obtaining behavioral descriptions as opposed to opinions or generalizations.

        4) When many incidents are collected and analyzed, a comprehensive picture is developed.

    c. Three essential elements are required for a useful critical incident (Kemppainen, 2000):

        1) A description of the situation that led up the incident

        2) A description of the actions or behaviors of the person in the incident

        3) A description of the outcomes of those actions

    d. Essential study prerequisites for maintaining reliability and validity

        1) Respondent sample is representative of the population being studied.

2) Respondents are knowledgeable and can accurately determine the critical nature of the behavior being studied.

3) They can provide an accurate description of an incident related to the outcome of the behavior.

e. Steps in developing a critical incident study

1) Clearly define the general *Aim* of the study.

2) Develop a clear, simple statement of behaviors to be studied.

3) Carefully consider sample selection and size.

   a) Must be diverse so incidents provide a complete picture

   b) Nonrandom sample is acceptable

   c) Sample size should be based on number of critical incidents, not the number of subjects (the critical incident is the unit of analysis)

      (1) For simple topics, 50 to 100 incidents may be adequate

      (2) For complex issues, may need several thousand

   d) Important considerations for questionnaire development

      (1) Write an introductory statement of the problem.

      (2) Ask about specific events related to the study *Aim*.

4) Following essential steps in collecting critical incident data

   a) Ask participants to be as specific as possible in describing an incident and include all relevant details.

   b) The accuracy of this technique depends on the researcher's ability to help participants be as specific as possible in providing concise descriptions of behavior in a given circumstance (Flanagan, 1954).

   c) The persons collecting the data should be very familiar with the task or issue being studied.

5) Reviewing an example of a typical critical incident questionnaire format

   a) What led up the situation?

   b) What happened? What did you do?

   c) How did your behavior lead to a successful/unsuccessful outcome?

6) Auditing and processing data for analysis

   a) Use notes from the critical incident interview to prepare a succinct summary of each incident.

   b) Enter each incident onto an index card or into an electronic database for easy sorting.

   c) Read through each incident to determine which ones include all three essential key elements.

   d) Essential criteria for usable incidents

      (1) The behavior of only a single person is included

      (2) The behavioral description is critical to the outcome of the situation

      (3) Discard incidents that are vague or lack sufficient detail

7) Adhering to Flanagan's essential steps in sorting and analyzing the critical incidents

   a) Have at least two teams of experts classify the incidents independently into major categories.

   b) Sort incidents into highly specific minor subcategories.

   c) Calculate statistical measures of agreement between the teams for both major and minor subcategories.

   d) Refine and modify both major and minor categories based on team discussions.

   e) Conduct a second and third sort and continue to modify categories as needed.

   f) Independent judges are essential for providing reliability checks.

   g) Classification scheme for the categories should relate to the *Aim* of the study.

8) Interpret and report the findings

IV. Quantitative Methodologies: for testing hypotheses, interventions, and instruments.

A. Observational or Descriptive Designs

1. Also known as correlational studies that typically utilize survey procedures.

2. Include cross-sectional, retrospective, or prospective sampling methods.

   a. *Cross-sectional* means the data are collected at only one time.

   b. *Retrospective* means the data are based on past or current perspectives or events.

   c. *Prospective* designs are planned to measure future behaviors, perspectives, or events through tracking and at specific time points. Data collection occurs on more than one occasion.

3. **Description of method**
   a. Used to establish the function of relationships among variables, such as moderation and mediation, but are unable to establish causality.
      1) *Moderators* are third variables that influence the effect of independent variables on the outcome or dependent variable. When a moderator is present, the value of the independent variable will change. An example is a descriptive characteristic such as gender, age, race, education, and income level.
      2) *Mediators* are third variables that are the "go-between" between an independent and dependent variable. The independent variable works through the mediator to influence the dependent variable. Without the mediator variable, the independent variable has little (partial mediation) or no (complete mediation) effect on the dependent (outcome) variable.
   b. The strength of the relationship between an independent (or combination of an independent variable and third variable or predictor variables) and dependent (outcome) variable is called an *effect size.*
      1) Effect size can be small, medium, or large
      2) Is interpreted for validity and clinical significance in relation to the sample size
   c. The direction of the relationship between the variables is either positive or negative (inverse).
      1) In a *positive relationship*, the participants' scores on both the independent and dependent variable are either high or low. The scores move in the same direction for both variables.
      2) In a *negative or inverse relationship*, the participants' scores on one variable will be high while the value of the other will be low. The scores move in opposite directions for the variables.
4. **Philosophical and disciplinary underpinnings**
   a. The use of quantitative methods in health care delivery from a deductive worldview is based on the belief that the statistical effect size of a research-tested intervention (efficacy) is what will predict future outcomes.
   b. The evidence-based practice paradigm is deductive by nature and conservatively relies on findings of randomized controlled trials (RCTs).
5. **Phenomena and types of questions** that can best be investigated using this method (hypothesis testing). Examples of hypotheses about cultural phenomena include the following:
   a. There will be a change in intention to obtain a dilated eye exam pre- and postreceipt of tailored health threat messages about eye disease based on their Afrocentric cultural scores. Useful statistical analysis: regression analysis.
   b. Those self-reporting race as Black or ethnicity as African American will be more likely than those who report White ethnicity to also report suboptimal quality of life. Useful statistics analysis: regression analysis, chi-square, or analysis of variance.
   c. Spirituality (third variable) will mediate the relationship between perceived risk (independent variable) of developing cardiovascular disease and dietary fiber intake (dependent or outcome variable). Useful statistical analysis: regression analysis.
6. **Potential for use with other methods, that is, combined methodologies**
   a. Use of a focus group to obtain themes or patterns of beliefs among group members initially, naming the themes (variables) and then selecting existing validated surveys to estimate a statistical effect and direction of relationships between the variables.
   b. Beginning with a survey procedure can sometimes be useful in determining which probing questions may be relevant for future focus groups.
   c. Having a sample of survey participants "speak aloud" about their reactions to questions, called *protocol analysis*, can provide insight about cultural variations in survey responses.
   d. Postintervention study evaluation focus groups about patient satisfaction, preference, and cultural sensitivity of intervention procedures or study staff.
7. **Instruments: Selection and cultural appropriateness**
   a. Measures are content validated by field experts or a clinical population to ensure question appropriateness and applicability to target group characteristics.
   b. Survey questions need to be linguistically appropriate to reading level, common language, and dialects. Surveys are translated and back-translated for content validity.
   c. Psychometric analysis is the principal component analysis used to validate surveys by assessing whether or not respondents are answering the questions as they were constructed. Reliability analyses are calculated

(i.e., internal consistency reliability seeking a Cronbach's alpha over .70 per subscale of questions) based on how the questions cluster together in the factor analyses.

   d. An additional factor analyses and internal consistency reliability is indicated whenever the survey is used on a new population for the first time.

   e. Additional analyses include assessing likelihood of responses according to cultural characteristics when a diverse sample is used (i.e., chi-square and odds ratio).

8. **Data collection procedures**

   a. Self-report using paper-and-pencil surveys, computer-based testing, such as ecologic momentary assessment (data assessed in real time).

   b. Behaviorally framed questions minimize respondent bias.

   c. Bias includes overestimating one's ability in comparison to others, impression management, wanting to please the researcher, selection of extreme scores, and various other tactics.

   d. Computer-based testing using handheld devices will feed questions based on the response to particular antecedent questions. This avoids responder fatigue.

   e. Objective assessment includes various methods used to minimize self-report bias. Examples include home glucose monitor downloads, pill counts, and pharmacy refill records.

9. **Data analysis procedures**

   a. Parametric data are continuous data with a wide range of scores. An example is data obtained from a Likert-type scale (i.e., *strongly agree*, *agree*, *no opinion*, *disagree*, and *strongly disagree*).

     1) Statistical analyses include Pearson's correlation and multiple regression analyses used to estimate the effect of independent variables on dependent variables.

     2) *T* tests and analysis of variance are used to estimate differences among subjects in the sample or between groups on scores on a dependent variable. This is usually used in experimental designs.

   b. Nonparametric data are categorical and have a range restriction. An example is gender (i.e., one is either male or female) or a 2-point scale (agree or disagree).

     1) Analyses include chi-square analyses to estimate the likelihood of an association between the independent and dependent variable.

     2) Logistic regression can be used to estimate the effect of an independent variable on a categorical dependent variable.

   c. *Effect size* estimation estimates the magnitude of the relationships based on the standardized mean difference. It is, for example, the actual correlation, described as small, medium, or large.

     1) A perfect correlation of 1.0 would be a strong effect.

     2) Effect size differs from significance level. Significance level is the probability that the effect size is due to chance (represented as p level or less, which is determined by the alpha level set by the researcher).

   d. Confidence intervals are usually set at a lower and upper bound of 95% to reduce the chance of a Type II error. This prevents the researcher from missing an effect.

   e. Levels of alpha error. Type I error is controlled using an appropriate alpha coefficient, typically <.05 for psychological constructs and <.01 for clinical response to pharmaceutical intervention. This prevents the researcher from finding an effect that may not be replicable in future studies.

10. **Generating conclusions**

   a) If cultural bias has been built into the research, results will reflect these biases.

   b) Avoid overgeneralization to ethnic groups.

     1) Data should be collected using assessments that are culturally appropriate and can measure degrees to which the respondent identifies with cultural characteristics to avoid making assumptions that a finding applies to all of a self-described ethnicity.

     2) Not all individuals of a particular ethnicity will fully identify with all cultural characteristics to the same degree due to different levels of acculturation and assimilation.

     3) Ethnicity and race are self-described by the respondents and not determined by the researcher.

11. **Strengths and weaknesses of this method**

   a. Inability to confirm causal relationships

   b. Strengths include the ability to estimate the effect size of relationships between variables, determine mediators, and the role of third variables that may be important to consider in health intervention trials

B. Ex Post Facto Design
1. Retrospective studies without a pretest but group comparisons are included. Examples include case-control designs used to determine a single effect, for example, a characteristic linked with a rare diagnosis.
2. If population-based samples are not used, incidence rate calculations cannot be estimated.
3. Designs typically include comparison of a group with a particular characteristic (e.g., rare disease) with those who do not have the characteristic. Medical record reviews are typically conducted.
4. Controls are randomly selected under ideal circumstances but more typically are matched based on shared characteristics.
5. Multiple controls are needed to ensure that variables are cause and not confounding variables.
6. Phenomena and types of questions that can best be investigated using this method (hypothesis testing):
   a. Do elevated insulin levels lead to diabetes?
   b. Is secondhand smoke linked to ear infections?
   c. Are Hispanic teenage girls more likely to have a preterm birth than White teenage girls?
7. Ethical issues specific to this method: Informed consent is not always possible (e.g., deceased subjects).
8. Threats to validity may include the following:
   a. Adequacy of knowledge of the field
   b. Specification and selection of the study population
   c. Executing the exposure
   d. Measuring the exposure or outcome variable
   e. Data analyses
   f. Interpretation of findings of data analysis
9. Data analyses
   a. Estimation of relative outcome frequency in a sample or maximum likelihood estimation
   b. Odds ratio, chi-square analysis, and logistic regression when estimating more than one predictor variable contributing to the effect on the outcome variable
10. Generating conclusions are limited by:
    a. If cultural bias has been built into the research, results will reflect these biases
    b. Overgeneralization to ethnic groups
    c. Lack of sufficient data to draw conclusions
    d. Sufficient "power" to make conclusions based on power analyses
       1) Typically the sample size is determined in advance of the study or a priori and is a function of the statistical tests planned to test the hypotheses.
       2) Parametric methods (regression) typically require a smaller sample size than nonparametric methods (chi-square tests) for detecting an effect.
11. Strengths and weaknesses of this method include the inability to make predictions or confirm causality.

C. Experimental and Quasi-Experimental Designs
1. Are similar by all accounts except that *quasiexperimental designs* lack random assignment and unlike experimental designs use self-selection, self-assignment, or investigator assignments for comparison among groups.
2. *Examples* include randomized controlled trial, cluster randomized design (where providers or care sites and patients are both randomized), and intention-to-treat designs (where participants are treated as if they are receiving the treatment for the group to which they were assigned).
3. *Phenomena and types of questions that* can best be investigated using this method (hypothesis testing):
   a. Is quality of life improved in those who receive telephone calls about health promotion versus in those who do not?
   b. Does tailoring talking points based on scores on a cultural assessment about lifestyle promote dietary fiber intake in those diagnosed with heart disease compared to those who receive information the routine way?
   c. Does assignment to a culturally similar peer group result in more disclosure about health-related fears than assigning peers based on gender?
4. *Ethical issues*
   a. Individuals volunteer for research trials and need to be aware that they can drop out at any time without any repercussion.

    b. Volunteers of research trials provide informed consent and are fully educated in the risks and benefits of the trial, including risks to privacy and the purposes for which the data are being collected and how these will be utilized, destroyed, and who has access to the data.

    c. Ethnic minorities and the uninsured may be especially vulnerable to feeling obligated to join a trial to prevent compromise in routine care (e.g., resulting from oppression).

    d. Excessive incentives and payment may result in unintentional coercion.

5. ***Strategies for ensuring rigor***

    a. ***Construct validity:*** How valid are the inferences about the hierarchy of the constructs under study?

        1) Concerns whether or not the appropriate variables are being addressed in the study to meet the study aims and the tools are valid and reliable means of measuring the variables under study.

        2) Avoid treatment diffusion. Did the subjects receive the treatment they were assigned and not other treatments?

        3) Reacting to the experimental situation or questions on the measures, experimenter expectations, novelty effects, compensatory rivalry (control group subjects show they can do as well as the intervention group), equalization (study staff compensate by offering control group subjects services or goods to compensate), and resentful demoralization (control subjects respond more negatively than expected because they did not get the desirable study intervention).

    b. ***Internal validity:*** Does the relationship between constructs (covariation) represent a causal relationship as measured or intervened on?

        1) Concerns elements such as treatment fidelity, which questions whether the treatment was carried out consistently in a way that prevents crossover between a control group and intervention group.

        2) Systematic bias occurs when respondent characteristics cause the effect more than the intervention (e.g., motivated participants).

        3) Study attrition as a result of the study conditions.

        4) Mere exposure to a test can affect the scores on repeat tests. Additionally the nature of the instruments may change over time.

        5) Failure to consider interaction effects of multiple threats to validity in advance of the study.

        6) Naturally occurring changes over time known as *maturation* (i.e., natural improvement) or events occurring concurrently known as *history* (i.e., treatment for a different condition affects the condition under study).

        7) Were subjects selected for extreme scores on particular measures? If so, *regression* can occur whereby the individuals do not score as high on other measures, making it difficult to infer whether or not effects were due to the intervention. Is the investigator certain that the cause preceded the effect as hypothesized, known as *ambiguous temporal precedence*?

        8) High concordance with ensuring internal validity as a means for ensuring efficacy of the intervention under study can be demonstrated.

    c. ***Statistical conclusion validity:*** Validity of inferences about the correlation between the independent and dependent variable.

        1) Assumes the correct statistical tests and procedures are followed and that the assumptions of the statistical tests are not violated.

        2) Was there adequate power to detect effects? Was the sample size calculated before the study was conducted based on the researcher's risk for a Type I error (alpha level)?

        3) Fishing and experiment-wise error avoided by not conducting excessive statistical tests seeking significance (leads to a Type I error).

        4) Use of unreliable measures, a restriction in the range of the measurement response options (e.g., categorical versus continuous data) can make it difficult to detect effects (leads to a Type II error).

        5) Heterogeneity of subjects leads to increased variability in responses on dependent variables and increases error making it difficult to detect effects (leads to a Type II error).

        6) Awareness that certain statistics will overestimate effect sizes.

    d. ***External validity/generalizability*** is the most difficult element of rigor to achieve.

        1) Inferences of the extent to which relationships will hold over various settings and people.

        2) There is a constant compromise between internal validity and external validity. A similar (homogenous) sample increases internal validity yet jeopardizes external validity; a heterogenous sample is needed for true generalizability to the general population. Typically, findings can only be generalized to a population similar to the research sample characteristics.

  3) External validity is concerned with translatability and effectiveness. Will the same intervention work on a real-world population?
  e. Recruitment and retention of research participants
  1) Power analysis is calculated statistically (eta squared) based on a set level by the researcher and what is common in the discipline (i.e., 80% power) to detect effects of an independent variable on a dependent variable.
  2) Power works like a microscope. It is calculated based on the desired confidence interval or alpha level or the degree of risk the researcher is willing to take that he or she may make a Type I error (finding an effect that cannot be replicated).
  3) The appropriate sample size is determined by the power calculation, and each calculation is specific to the proposed statistical tests to be used to test the hypotheses in advance of the study.
  f. Simple random sampling (SRS) is the technique used to ensure that selection bias does not creep in.
  1) SRS allows for every possible sample to have an equal chance of being selected up to the desired sample size.
  2) Tossing a coin, random number tables, and computer generation of random numbers assigned to the sample members is often used in SRS.
  g. Investigator observations can bias the interpretation of findings. Many experiments use blinding or masking so the group assignment (control or treatment) is concealed from the interventionist, subject, or both ("double-blind").
  h. Equal opportunity can change as the study progresses.
  1) Although equal at randomization, attrition by dropping out of the study or switching groups can unequalize the characteristics of the sample.
  2) Intention-to-treat analyses analyze data as if the sample remained intact and received the treatment they were allocated, even if they did not get it. Many translational or real-world studies use this design.
  i. Instruments
  1) Selection of instruments with established validity and reliability
  2) Intervention studies usually have physiologic and quality-of-life measures as outcome variables
  j. Estimation of relative outcome frequency in a sample or maximum likelihood estimation
  1) Odds ratio, chi-square analysis, and logistic regression when estimating more than one predictor variable contributing to the effect on the outcome variable.
  2) Effect size estimation depends upon whether nonparametric tests are used or multiple regression analysis.
  3) Confidence intervals are set at a lower and upper bound of 95% to reduce the chance of a Type II error. This prevents the researcher from missing an effect.
  4) Type I error is controlled using an appropriate alpha coefficient, typically <.05 for psychological constructs and <.01 for clinical response to pharmaceutical intervention. This prevents the researcher from finding an effect that may not be replicable in future studies.
6. ***Generating conclusions*** are limited similar to the descriptive quantitative designs previously described.
7. ***Strengths and weaknesses*** of this method include the inability to make predictions or establish causality.
  a. Strengths of the method include the ability to establish the efficacy of clinical interventions in a randomized controlled trial and effectiveness in an intention-to-treat real-world trial.
  b. Strengths of cluster-randomized designs include the ability to account for provider effects as well as the target subjects.

D. Use of the Internet for Research

1. Description
  a. The *Internet* is a research resource and tool for generation of knowledge and the exploration of different human experiences and behaviors.
  b. *Internet or online research* offers an interdisciplinary and transdisciplinary collaborative approach (James & Busher, 2007). Facilitates wider involvement of research teams and other experts, such as computer technologists, Internet methodologists, Web programmers, social scientists, and health and nursing educators.
  c. Provides a globally accessible platform independent infrastructure (Dix, 1997) using synchronous and asynchronous communication channels between researchers and the researched (Im & Chee, 2004).

      d. Facilitates communication with diverse participants across racial-ethnic groups, social class, and educational levels with less expensive cost. Gives opportunity to test a large, heterogeneous population (Reimers, 2007; Yu & Yu, 2007).

2. ***Characteristics of Internet research***

      a. A special kind of "cyberspace" with structural features that provides a unified means of delivering a vast range of online information (Dix, 1997)

      b. Provides a social and cognitive space for the activation of interpersonal and psychosocial relationships between users (Riva, 2001)

3. ***Phenomena that can be examined by Internet research:*** Several studies have used the Internet approach.

      a. Study of women's experiences (Beck, 2005; Bunting & Campbell, 1990; Huntington, 2009; Im, 2001; Im & Melies, 2001; Taylor, 2000)

      b. Health behavior change in vulnerable groups (Graham et al., 2006) and managing symptoms of chronic illness (Whitehead, 2007)

      c. Comparison of psychometric properties of Internet-based instruments and traditional paper versions (Aluja et al., 2007; Henning, 2004; IJmker et al., 2007; Zlomke, 2009)

4. ***Advantages of Internet research***

      a. Although all proposals for Internet research need approval by the Institutional Review Board, generally, an Internet study is granted an I "exempt" status (Im & Chee, 2003).

      b. An Internet study poses minimal risk to participants' anonymity and confidentiality (Reimers, 2007).

         1) In general, e-mail addresses are requested from participants, and a user name may be created to log onto the study Web site. No personal identities are requested.

         2) All participants in an Internet study are volunteers.

         3) Without participants' login names and passwords, they are not allowed admittance to the questionnaire site.

         4) Collected electronic data can be saved and stored on a personal computer that only the investigator can access. Firewalls and secure socket layers could be used to protect confidentiality of data reported by participants (O. L. Strickland, et al., 2003).

      c. An electronic informed consent is provided to participants via e-mail or on the study Web page (see Table 10.2).

         1) Potential participants visiting the study Web site are able to review the electronic informed consent.

         2) To enter the study Web page, potential participants must first give their consent by clicking "I agree to participate in this study."

      d. Participants have greater freedom and comfort to withdraw from the study because the researcher is not physically present (Nosek, Banaji, & Greenwald, 2002).

      e. Participants from different cultural backgrounds may be more willing to divulge their insights and experiences when the researchers are physically absent.

         1) Reimers (2007) found a higher rate of nonheterosexuality reported by college students in an Internet study.

         2) Participants were more comfortable in reporting symptoms of depression of smoking cessation (Graham et al., 2006).

         3) An Internet approach tends to protect research participants against unwanted interference and observation from researchers (Kralik, Warren, Price, Koch, & Pignone, 2005).

         4) May decrease participants' feelings of shyness, embarrassment, and fear (Whitehead, 2007)

         5) Participants were more likely to speak honestly rather than report socially "correct" views (Szabo & Frenkl, 1996).

         6) May be an effective medium for collecting comprehensive, in-depth information and experiences without fear of reprisal

5. ***Potential for use with other methods***

      a. A triangulation method can be used in Internet research.

      b. Triangulation, using both Internet qualitative and quantitative approaches, allows the researcher to observe both objective and subjective research data, increases the validity and completeness of the research findings, enriches the quality of data, obtains a more realistic interpretation of findings, and ultimately achieves a holistic view of a single phenomenon (Kimchi, Ploivka, & Stevenson, 1991).

Table 10.2. Example of an Informed Consent Form for an Internet Study

Informed Consent

Thank you so much for visiting the study website. You are being invited to participate in a study of the physical activity in Taiwanese women with menstruation symptoms. This form provides you with information about the study. The Principal Investigator (the person in charge of this research), XXXXXXXX and XXXXXX or their representative will also describe this study to you and answer all of your questions. You are one of 160 Taiwanese women with menstrual symptoms being asked to participate in this research and to give your ideas about your physical activity and menstruation experience. Please read the information below and ask questions about anything you don't understand before deciding whether or not to take part. Your participation is entirely voluntary and you can refuse to participate without penalty or loss of benefits to which you are otherwise entitled.

Title of the Research Study:
Physical Activity among Taiwanese Women with Menstrual Symptoms

Principle Investigator (include faculty sponsor), UT affiliation, and Telephone Number(s):
XXXXXX Doctoral Candidate, School of Nursing, Tel: (512) 000-0000 (PI)
XXXXXX Associate Professor, School of Nursing, (512) 000-0000 (Faculty Sponsor)
Funding Source: None

What is the purpose of this study?
The purpose of the study is to explore physical activity involvement among Taiwanese women with menstrual symptoms using a national approach through the Internet. The focus of the study is given on gender and cultural issues within the psycho-socio-cultural contexts of the women experiences.

What will be done if you take part in this research study?
This study includes two sections: (a) an Internet survey and (b) an e-mail group discussion.
If you agree to participate in the Internet survey,

1) You will be invited to visit the study website at least twice.
2) You will be asked to review the informed consent sheet on the study website at least once.
3) You will be asked to click "I agree to participate in the study" in order to give your content to participate in the study.
4) You will be asked to provide your email address.
5) You will be asked to answer the Internet survey questions on demographic characteristics, physical activity, and menstrual experience. It will take about 20 minutes to complete the Internet survey.

If you agree to participate in additional e-mail group discussion,

1) You will receive an invitation e-mail that asks you to participate in e-mail group discussion.
2) Within one week after receiving an invitation e-mail, you will be asked to join the e-mail group discussion. The investigator of this study will start an e-mail group discussion with one topic per week.
3) At your convenience, you can join the e-mail discussion and share your experience of menstruation, meaning of being a woman, and physical activity experience.
4) In a three-week period during e-mail group discussions, you may receive many e-mails from other women participants who share their experience of menstruation, meaning of being a woman, and physical activity experience.
5) The e-mail group discussion in this study will take 3 weeks. No personal identity (such as name, mailing address, and phone number) will be requested. You may be free to join the discussion and share your experience, thought, and words at your convenience.

What are the possible discomforts and risks?
Some questions in the Internet survey or some discussion in e-mail group discussion may make you feel uncomfortable. You are free to not answer any question or share any experience that makes you uncomfortable. You are free to withdraw from the study at any time. There is no more risk than 'everyday life' from participation.

(continued)

Table 10.2 (continued)

What are the possible benefits to you or to others?
There is no direct benefit for you from participation. However, you may gain some awareness about your experience of physical activity and menstruation after you complete the Internet survey or e-mail group discussion. Information gained from this study may help other women in the future.

If you choose to take part in this study, will it cost you anything?
If you choose to take part in this study, there is no cost to you.

Will you receive compensation for your participation in this study?
You will not be paid for your participation in this study. You may receive the results of the study when they become available, upon request.

What if you are injured because of the study?
No physical risk will be involved in this study.

If you do not want to take part in this study, what other options are available to you?
If you decide to participate, you do not have to answer any question and share any experience that makes you feel uncomfortable and you can withdraw from this study at any time without any explanation and without fear of penalty. Your decision whether or not to participate will not prejudice your present or future relations with The University of *XXXXXX* in any way.

How can you withdraw from this research study and who should I call if I have questions?
If you want to stop your participation or you have any question about the study at any time, you may call me, XXXXX, at (512) 0000000, or by e-mail: 00000@0000.0000.edu, or by mail: XXXXXXXXXXXXXXX. Or you may contact my faculty sponsor, XXXXXXXX by telephone 0021-512-000-0000, or by e-mail: 0000000@000000000.edu. In addition, if you have questions about your rights as a research participant, please contact XXXXXX Chair, The University XXXXXXX Institutional Review Board for the Protection of Human Subjects, at 0021-512-000-0000.

How will your privacy and the confidentiality of your research records be protected?
Authorized persons from XXXXXXXXXXX and the Institutional Review Board have the legal right to review your research records and will protect the confidentiality of those records to the extent permitted by law. Also, the faculty sponsors have the legal right to review your research records. Otherwise, your research records will not be released without your consent unless required by law or a court order. All your responses will be kept confidential in only one personal computer. Only the principal investigator of the study has access to reach your responses. Only authorized persons and the investigator can review your responses. Names will not be used in any way and only group response will be reported. Your e-mail address will be used only for this study and eliminated from the database after the data collection of the study.

Will the researchers benefit from your participation in this study (beyond publishing or presenting the results)? No
You have been informed about the title of the study, information of principal investigator, the purposes of the study, inclusion criteria of participants, possible discomforts and inconvenience, potential benefits and risks, confidentiality, anonymity, their contribution to the study, and their right to withdraw from the study at any time. You also have reviewed a computerized format of this informed consent form. Please print out this page for your record or we can send you a hard copy of this informed consent sheet, upon request (please email XXXXXXXXXX at 00000000@00000.edu). You have been given the opportunity to ask any question before you sign, and you have been told that you are free to ask any other questions at any time. You voluntarily agree to participate in the study. Clicking the bottom "I agree to participate in study" indicates that you are at least 20 years of age, you understand the information provided above, and you are giving your informed consent to be a participant in the study.

☐ YES, I AGREE TO PARTICIPATE IN THIS STUDY

☐ NO, I DO NOT AGREE TO PARTICIPATE IN THIS STUDY

By clicking "yes, I agree to participate in this study", you are not waiving any of your legal rights.

6. ***Strategies for ensuring validity and reliability***
   a. Strategies for quantitative research using the Internet
      1) Use of *probability sampling* (random selection of study participants from a population) ensures validity and generalizability. Yu and Yu (2007) used random sampling to examine the psychometric properties of an Internet-based questionnaire on a population from the Taiwan Ministry of Education Web site. Eight teachers from each sampled school were randomly selected and invited to participate.
      2) Pilot testing of instruments
         a) There is lack of Internet-based instruments.
         b) Adapted paper-and-pencil instruments should be pilot-tested, as the Internet is a different format (Napolitano et al., 2003).
      3) Adding pictures to the questionnaire can enhance its validity. Im and colleagues (2008) constructed a Web-based questionnaire with added pictures to provide visual guidance to participants.
      4) Criteria for Internet-based qualitative research
         a. *Credibility*: Categories and themes extracted from the narrative text should be shared and validated with participants through e-mail or online group discussion.
         b. *Dependability* is enhanced by accounting for changes in context during the research, which should be described and integrated in the analysis.
         c. *Confirmability* is the degree to which the results could be confirmed or corroborated by others in terms of their relevance and meanings.
         d. Using an independent auditor or external reviewer to examine the research process and validate that findings are supported by the data enhances both *dependability* and *confirmability*.
         e. *Transferability* is the degree to which the results can be generalized to other settings, groups, or contexts. Thick description allows for a comprehensive description of participants' responses, including research contexts and data collection process, to make evident for readers the process of decision making (Polit & Hungler, 1999).
7. ***Recruitment and retention of sufficient participants***
   a. Randomized sampling is not possible because the total population in the World Wide Web is immense (Bar-Ilan & Peritz, 2002; Reimer, 2007).
   b. Researchers recruit Internet participants via an open accessibility method that is open to whoever is able to find the study Web site and voluntarily choose to participate (Nosek et al., 2002). Voluntary samples recruited through the Web are not considered random samples (Yu & Yu, 2007).
   c. Individual e-mails might be sent to members of the Internet communities to recruit potential study participants. Samples of an Internet study tend to be extremely diverse.
   d. Snowball Internet sampling works better than convenient Internet sampling in recruiting specific ethnic groups. For example, H. M. Tsai (2005) failed to recruit aboriginal Taiwanese women using convenience sampling. Using snowball sampling, more than 50 aboriginal Taiwanese women participated in the research.
   e. Quota sampling (nonrandom sampling using identified strata of the population followed by a determination of the composition of a population to target) is more likely to ensure that diverse segments are represented in the sample.
   f. Quota sampling works better than convenience sampling for ensuring recruitment and retention of sufficient ethnic participants. Im and associates (Im, Liu, Dormire, & Chee, 2008) used quota sampling to ensure adequate numbers of early perimenopausal, late perimenopausal, and postmenopausal participants from diverse social and cultural groups.
   g. A potential concern is that participants are more likely to be younger, better educated, and more affluent (Lenert et al., 2002; Im & Chee, 2003), excluding ethnic groups who are impoverished, poorly educated, and with little or no access to a computer.
      1) Strategies for recruitment and retention of culturally diverse participants include reducing the reading level of instruments to fifth grade or lower; placing study announcements in public Web sites, such as those of schools, public libraries, and community centers; and distributing flyers in community laundry rooms.
      2) Targeting Internet support groups, Bender and associates (Bender, Clark, Guevara, Chee, & Im, 2006) successfully recruited African Americans with cancer.
      3) H. M. Tsai (2005) used several recruitment strategies to obtain aboriginal women participants through the general Internet communities, Internet support groups, and nationwide warehouses, and using an aboriginal woman as informal recruiter.
   h. Four major search engines are generally used for recruitment (AOL, MSN, Yahoo, and Google).

7. ***Data collection***
   a. There is no specific research setting in an Internet study; hence, there is no limitation in localities for recruitment of participants.
   b. A researcher can undertake an Internet study to reach diverse groups in national and international locations simultaneously.
   c. The research Web site is developed and maintained following the guidelines and policies of Health Insurance Portability and Accountability Act (HIPAA) regulations and the Systems Administration, Audit, Network, Security (SANS)/ Federal Bureau of investigation (FBI) recommendations (Im et al., 2005) to protect personal privacy and information.
   d. When potential participants visit the study Web site, they are asked to review the informed consent and give their consent to participate by clicking "I agree to participate."
   e. Once they agree to participate, they are checked for eligibility. If they are eligible, they are directed to the study Web page and asked to fill out the questionnaire (Im et al., 2005).
   f. Qualitative data can be collected by using e-mail, group discussion, e-mail interview, online forum, and online support group. Im et al. (2009) used an online forum to collect qualitative data from four ethnic groups in the United States.
   g. The main procedure for data collection in an Internet quantitative study includes e-mail surveys and online questionnaires. Rabius, Pike, Wiatrek, and McAlister (2008) conducted experimental research using Internet surveys of daily smokers. Etter (2004) conducted a comparative study of smokers in four countries using online surveys.
   h. Data entry is rapid, as all the data are already in file format, which can be easily converted to any file format for data analysis.

8. ***Role of the researcher***
   a. Develop advanced computer competence to have the knowledge and skill in computer technology and software to be able to apply an Internet method in research.
   b. Minimize researcher bias by bracketing own perceptions and assumptions so interpretations are derived from the data. Researchers should be aware of the social, cultural, and political contexts that impact on participants. Researchers should have integrity to honor and respect the personal and group experiences of participants, particularly, racial and ethnic minorities.
   c. Ensure authenticity of Internet research participants.
      1) It is not possible to verify statements of participants who may incorrectly self-identify as eligible participants. Several approaches were used by researchers to prevent this error: using preselection questions to verify eligible participants, preestablished inclusion criteria for participation, and two or three screening questions to verify eligibility.
      2) Another possibility is for participants to submit information multiple times to the survey. A password and account number can be provided to each participant.
      3) Reaching a meaningful online interaction with participants enhances authenticity of their response. Building rapport with participants requires sensitivity to their culture, language, and communication.
   d. Selecting appropriate instruments and design
      1) Know the psychometric properties of the instrument and conduct pilot-testing of the Internet version.
      2) Pay attention to the cultural relevance and appropriateness of language used.
      3) Use culturally sensitive measures that are relevant to the target population and reflect the authentic lifeways of participants. For example, martial arts and gardening may be common physical activities among Taiwanese but not relevant to other groups.
      4) Design the Web page to be user friendly and inviting for visitors.
   e. Ensuring saturation of data
      1) Low response rate is a threat to obtaining data saturation.
         a) According to Dillman and colleagues (2008), the response rates varied greatly, from 13% for the Internet, to 28% for interactive voice response (IVR), 44% by telephone, and 75% for mail.
         b) Strategies to promote increased response include using different modalities for contacting participants, innovative invitations and greetings, e-mail addresses of participants, and providing incentives.
      2) Early withdrawal is another threat to data saturation. Measures to sustain continued participation include providing supportive contact to help participants with technology and address their concerns. Technological failure results in involuntary withdrawal, which can be prevented. Maintaining

Table 10.3. Description of Types of Inferential Statistics and Their Use for Specific Research Questions

Inferential statistics	Definition (Vogt, 1993)	Examples of research questions/ hypothesis
Chi-square tests	To test statistically significant difference between the observed (or actual) frequencies and expected (or hypothesized) frequencies	Whether the females' Internet usage differs significantly from males
Correlation analyses	To test two or more variables (measured at interval or ratio level) that are related but not mean one variable causes the other	What is the relationship between the severity of menstrual symptoms and physical activity involvement among Asian women?
T tests	To test differences between two group means	Are there differences in the cancer pain symptoms of African American compared with Asians?
ANOVA tests	To test the differences among two or more group means	Are there differences in response rates of online semistructured questionnaire among Hispanics, Asians, and African Americans?
Regression	Methods of predicting the variability of a dependent variable based on the variability of one or more independent variables	What are the significant physio-psycho-socio-cultural predictors of physical activity involvement among aboriginal and nonaboriginal women?

consistent dialogue through e-mails and offering emergency technical support can alleviate these problems. It is important that e-mail addresses should be obtained from each informant early.

9. ***Quantitative data analysis***
   a. Quantitative data collected through the Internet survey can be saved in ASC II (American Standard Code for Information Exchange) format that conforms to the SPSS data format and are later imported to an SPSS data file.
   b. Descriptive statistics include frequency, percentage, mean, standard deviation, and range for continuous data and proportions and frequencies for nominal data.
   c. Descriptive statistics are generated to describe social and cultural demographic characteristics of the participants.
   d. In general, inferential statistics include correlation analyses, chi-square tests, *t* tests, bivariate correlation, ANOVA tests, and regression. Table 10.3 provides examples of inferential statistics.

10. ***Qualitative research analysis***
    a. In general, content and thematic analysis is applied for contextual analysis of qualitative data to interpret psycho-social-cultural contexts among Internet participant groups.
    b. The major procedures of narrative analysis consist of line-by-line coding, member and peer checking, and examining relationships among the categories and themes. The researcher reads and systematically codes the narrative text line by line. Coded words, phrases, or other text units that have similar meanings are placed into one category. The extracted categories are constructed by analyzing contents and contexts (Im et al., 2008). Ultimately, categories that emerge reveal the main themes of the texts.
    c. To enhance credibility of contextual analysis, revealed themes of the texts should be shared with and validated by the participants (Campbell & Bunting, 1999). With member validation, researchers can be much more confident that their interpretation of research finding accurately reflects the phenomena being explored.

11. ***Generating conclusions***
    a. The conclusions of an Internet study have limited generalizability due to issues with recruitment and use of convenience sampling.
    b. To increase the generalizability of the findings, sociodemographic background of participants can be carefully considered.
       1) In the study of physical activity among Taiwanese women with menstrual symptoms, H. M. Tsai (2005) included five target sociodemographic compositions of the sample: (a) 50% women ages 20 to 30 years and 50% women ages 31 to 40 years, (b) 30% aboriginal women and 70% nonaboriginal women, (c) 50% women who were college graduates or higher and 50% women with associate degrees or less, (d) 60% employed women and 40% unemployed women, and (e) 60% unmarried women and 40% married women.
       2) Im and colleagues (2008) used quota sampling method to recruit four socioeconomic groups of midlife women. By recruiting participants with numerous sociodemographic compositions, the results of an Internet research are likely to gather sufficient data to draw conclusions.

3) Multiple strategies can be employed to reach potential participants from diverse socioeconomic and ethnic backgrounds, such as use of e-mail and Web-based communication. E-mails can be sent to members of organizations or online support groups, discussion groups (moderated or unmoderated), or in commercial surveys. Web-based communication can be used for newsgroups (moderated or unmoderated) and linking with other Web sites or chat rooms (Lenert & Skoczen, 2002).

12. *Strengths and limitations*
   a. Major strengths of an Internet method
      1) It has no time zone or geographic limitations for recruitment of participants or communication between the researcher and participants.
      2) Facilitates immediate and reciprocal communication. Online forums are ideal for this purpose. Timely communication can clarify ambiguities immediately.
      3) Improves data completeness and saturation through automatic notification of beginning and end of participation, acknowledgement of participation, and sending follow-up and frequent reminders. Kongsved and associates (2007) reported that the completeness rate of Internet questionnaires without missing any data was approximately 98%, compared to 63.4% in the paper-and-pencil questionnaire.
      4) Increases accuracy of data entry through direct downloading of data into a secured computer data file system for each participant. Upon completion, respondents' data can be automatically transferred to an Excel file and then imported into SPSS for further data analysis (O.L. Strickland et al., 2003).
      5) Offers convenience in time, place, and pace
   b. Major limitations of an Internet method
      1) Recall bias has been described as a serious problematic issue in self-reported Internet surveys.
      2) Sample bias
         a) Internet participants are more likely to be younger, better educated, more affluent, and White (Im & Chee, 2004; Reimers, 2007; Yu & Yu, 2007).
         b) A second concern with sampling bias is incorrect self-identification as eligible participants (Lenert et al., 2002; Riva & Galimberti, 2001).
         c) The third concern relates to convenience sampling. Convenience sampling is frequently used in Internet research to recruit potential participants who are able to find the study Web site and voluntarily choose to participate in the study (Nosek et al., 2002).
      3) Indirect measurement: Using a self-reported Internet method is an indirect and non-face-to-face measurement, and researchers have very limited ability to verify accuracy of self-reported data.
      4) Cost of an Internet study may include equipment, software, programming, and training.
      5) Literacy and linguistic competence: Culturally diverse participants with low literacy may encounter informational obstacles on the Internet because study Web sites require at least a high school reading proficiency for optimal access (Mehret et al., 2006).

V. Ethical Issues
A. The Ethical Mandate to Protect Human Subjects in Research
   1. *The Nuremberg Code*: Addressed the necessity of requiring the voluntary consent of the human subject and that any individual "who initiates, directs, or engages in the experiment" must bear personal responsibility for ensuring the quality of consent (www.citiprogram.org)
   2. *The Declaration of Helsinki*: Calls for prior approval and ongoing monitoring of research by independent ethical review committees
   3. *The Belmont Report*: Defines the ethical principles and guidelines for protecting human subjects
      a. Respect for persons (applied by obtaining informed consent, consideration of privacy, confidentiality, and additional protections for vulnerable populations),
      b. Beneficence (applied by weighing risks and benefits), and
      c. Justice (applied by the equitable selection of subjects and avoidance of exploitation of vulnerable populations)
B. Risks to Human Subjects in Social and Behavioral Research (SBR)
   1. The risks in SBR may be routinely underestimated and not perceived to have severe outcomes because the risks are subtle and often pertain to interpersonal relationship.

2. The types of risks of harm that may result from SBR include the following:
   a. **Psychological**
      1) It is important to consider the participant's reaction to the subject matter.
      2) Some interview questions or questionnaires may induce significant psychological discomfort. For example, people interviewed about domestic violence may experience anxiety, insomnia, and/or clinical depression when asked about these experiences.
      3) Researchers must have a management plan to deal with these possibilities.
   b. **Social**
      1) Social harm may result when sensitive and personal information is inappropriately disclosed.
      2) Explicit security precautions with data management must be planned and submitted to the ethics committee for approval.
   c. **Economic**
      1) Inappropriate disclosure of study data about participants' beliefs, values, behaviors, and health may result in damage to their economic status.
      2) These harms include loss of employment, health insurance, housing, or life insurance. For example, disclosing HIV status could cause an individual to lose health insurance.
      3) Rigorous coding of data may reduce this risk.
   d. **Physical**
      1) Unlikely but possible with inadvertent disclosure of confidential information, especially with HIV status information.
      2) Researchers must be aware that maintaining the confidentiality of the *participant* may be as important as securing the confidentiality of the research data.
   e. **Legal**
      1) On rare occasions, researchers may be subpoenaed to release study data about participant's illegal behavior.
      2) For example, a disclosure of illicit drug use could have legal consequences.
      3) In the United States, a researcher may obtain a *Certificate of Confidentiality*, which protects against compulsory legal demands, such as court orders and subpoenas, for identifying information about a research participant.

C. **Institutional Review Boards**
   1. Definition: An Institutional Review Board (IRB) is a board, committee, or other group formally designated by an institution to review, approve, require modification, disapprove, and conduct continuing oversight of human subject research. Its purpose is to protect the rights and welfare of human research subjects.
   2. Institutions may vary in how they name their IRB, for example, Committee for Protection of Human Subjects, Research Ethics Committee, and so on.
   3. In the United States, federal regulations require IRB review and approval for research involving human subjects (Department of Health and Human Services [DHHS], 2009).
   4. Most research institutions, professional organizations, and scholarly journals apply the same requirements to all human subjects.
   5. Definition of terms relevant to a required IRB review:
      a. Research: "A systematic investigation designed to develop or contribute to generalizable knowledge" (DHHS, 2009, 45 CFR 46.102[d]). If an investigator is unclear about whether a planned activity is research, the investigator should contact his/her IRB office.
      b. Human Subjects: "a living individual about whom an investigator (whether professional or student) conducting research obtains:
         1) Data through intervention or interaction with an individual, OR
         2) Identifiable private information" (DHHS, 2009, 45 CFR 46.102).
   6. Minimal IRB requirements for Human Subjects: An application must be submitted and approved by the IRB prior to initiation of research. The application must include the following:
      a. Analysis of anticipated benefits and risks
      b. Informed Consent process and documentation, including Consent Form
      c. Selection of subjects
         1) Equitable selection in terms of gender, race, and ethnicity, depending on topic

2) Benefits are distributed fairly among the community's populations.

3) Safeguards are provided for vulnerable populations susceptible to pressure to participate.

d. Protection of participants' privacy: Procedures to assure *confidentiality* of information collected during the research

e. Security of data: Research plan for collection, locked storage, and analysis of data. For example, the recruitment log with names linked with code numbers must be locked with separate key in a separate location.

f. Description of research methodology: Research design and methods must be appropriate, scientifically valid.

g. Approval letters from sites where research will be conducted

h. Copies of all questionnaires, surveys, instruments, data collection tools

7. Types of IRB reviews

   a. **Full committee review**

     1) The standard review, requiring all elements of the application

     2) The review must be conducted at a convened meeting with a quorum of members present.

     3) A majority of the members must approve the research.

     4) The IRB must inform the researcher in writing of its decisions to approve, modify, or disapprove the research.

     5) Detailed notes of the discussion of the application must be made.

   b. **Expedited review**

     1) A review of a study that involves no more than minimal risk and fits within certain categories

     2) Describes only the process; the information to be reviewed by the committee is the same as for a full review.

     3) The chair of the IRB or an experienced member may review the application, using same criteria for approval.

   c. **Review for exempt status**

     1) NOT applicable for studies involving pregnant women, most children, or prisoners

     2) The decision to apply exempt status is made by the IRB; the investigators *cannot* make this determination for themselves.

     3) Categories eligible for exempt status (DHHS, 2009, 45 CFR 46.101[b]):

       a) Research conducted in established educational setting, involving normal educational practices

       b) Research involving the use of educational tests, survey or interview procedures, or observation of public behavior

       c) NOTE: Some observational studies, specifically, participant observation, do *not* qualify for exemption.

       d) Research involving the collection or study of freely available deidentified existing data, documents, records, specimens

       e) Research conducted by heads of governments or agencies that are designed to evaluate public programs

       f) Food quality evaluations and consumer acceptance studies

D. Informed Consent Process

1. Informed consent is a process, not just a form.

2. Information must be presented to enable persons to voluntarily decide whether or not to participate as a research subject.

3. The procedures used in obtaining informed consent should be designed to educate the subject population in terms that they can understand.

4. Informed consent language and its documentation must be written in "lay language" (i.e., understandable to the people being asked to participate).

5. The written presentation of information is used to document the basis for consent and for the subjects' future reference.

6. *Elements of a Consent Form* for Social and Behavioral Research studies (see Table 10.2 for an example)

   a. Name of research protocol

   b. Name of Principal Investigator with address and phone number

   c. Statement that the study involves research

    d. Explanation of the purpose of the study

    e. Description of the procedures involved

    f. Expected duration of the participant's involvement; for example, if a number of surveys or questionnaires are to be completed, state the approximate time involved to complete them.

    g. Description of any foreseeable risks

    h. Description of any benefits to the participants or others that may reasonably be expected from the research

    i. Description of measures taken to ensure confidentiality of records that identify the participant

    j. If payment is given, state the amount.

    k. An explanation of whom to contact for answers about the subject's rights and to lodge complaints about the study (this cannot be the investigator, but rather the contact is usually the approving IRB)

    l. A statement that participation is voluntary

    m. A statement that the participant may discontinue participation at any time, or may decline to answer any question, without penalty or loss of benefits

    n. If applicable: I give consent to be audiotaped/videotaped during this study: __Yes __No

    o. If applicable: I give consent for tapes resulting from this study to be (describe proposed use): __Yes __No

    p. A line for signature and date of participant

    q. A line for signature and date for person obtaining consent

    r. A statement that one copy of the consent form is theirs to keep

    s. Each page of the Consent Form should be initialed by the participant.

7. When conducting research in a number of countries around the world, or in certain communities in the United States, it may be inappropriate to consent potential participants by using the standard written and signed consent form that is used in most research studies.

    a. If written and/or signed consent form is not culturally appropriate in the communities of proposed research, an application for a waiver of signature requirement or alteration of consent procedures may be an option.

    b. Examples when a waiver or alternation of the consent process may be acceptable:

        1) Research is proposed to be carried out in a location where no written and/or signed contracts are used.

        2) The presentation of a written consent form that requires the signature of the prospective subject would introduce an element of fear and distrust towards the researcher.

        3) The research presents no more than minimal risk.

        4) The waiver or alteration of consent will not adversely affect the rights and welfare of the subjects.

        5) The research could not practicably be carried out without the waiver or alteration.

    c. When a consent form is not used, an information sheet should be provided for the potential participant to read or have read to them. It should contain the following:

        1) A statement that the study involves research

        2) A description of any foreseeable risks; if there are none, state as such.

        3) A description of any benefits; if none, state as such (not including payment).

        4) A statement describing confidentiality of records

        5) A statement of whom to contact about research questions (bilingual card)

        6) A statement of whom to contact about subjects' rights (bilingual card)

        7) A statement that participation is voluntary

        8) A statement that subjects may discontinue participation at any time without penalty

        9) A statement that subjects can decline to answer specific questions

E. Research Involving Vulnerable Populations

1. Within the context of research, vulnerability refers to a limitation on the ability of the human subject to exercise his or her autonomy.

2. Those who are vulnerable are more likely to have their rights abused because of a potential for control, coercion, undue influence, or manipulation.

3. Specific classes of vulnerable subjects include the following (International Conference on Harmonization, 1996; Guideline 1.61):

    a. Children

    b. Mentally disabled individuals

    c. Marginalized social groups may lack influence in society as a result of age, race, ethnicity, gender, and disability. These groups often do not have full access to social institutions such as the legal system.

      d. Hierarchical social structures create situations where voluntariness can be compromised, such as in the case of students, some ethnic groups, prisoners, hospitalized patients, and prisoners.

      d. Educationally disadvantaged subjects may have limitations in reading the consent form and understanding the study in which they will participate.

      f. Economically disadvantaged subjects may be vulnerable due to limitations to voluntariness. They may enroll in a study because of being unduly influenced by the monetary compensation and not fully weigh the risks.

   4. Special precautions need to be included in the research protocol to safeguard persons in these vulnerable groups.

VI. Summary

  A. Qualitative research methodologies are valuable for describing cultural phenomena relevant to nursing, caring, and health care.

  B. However, as members of a practice profession, health care researchers need to move beyond solely describing the phenomena and advance toward examining how the integration of this knowledge into care practices contributes to improved health outcomes for the clients.

  C. In order to expand the scope of transcultural health research and to achieve a balance between the descriptions of phenomena and their relationship to care practices and outcomes, health care researchers might address the strengths of triangulation, which uses multiple research methods to study phenomena.

  D. Finally, culture is dynamic, is complex, and exists within a multidimensional context. In order to adequately investigate cultural phenomena, researchers need to collaborate with their interdisciplinary colleagues to gain their perspectives, appreciate their research methodologies, and aid in adding new knowledge to the field of transcultural nursing and health care.

NOTE: All references, additional resources, and important Internet sites relevant to this chapter can be found at http://tcn .sagepub.com/supplemental

Journal of Transcultural Nursing
21(Supplement 1) 406S–417S
© The Author(s) 2010
Reprints and permission:
sagepub.com/journalsPermissions.nav
DOI: 10.1177/1043659610370341
http://tcn.sagepub.com

Chapter 11
Professional Roles and Attributes of the Transcultural Nurse

Ani Kalayjian, EdD, RN, DDL, BCETS[1]
Stephen R. Marrone, EdD, RN-BC, CTN-A[2]
Connie Vance, EdD, RN, FAAN[3]

I. Introduction
   A. The scope of practice of transcultural nursing is broad and yet specific (Murphy, 2006). The professional roles of transcultural nurses are as expert clinicians, educators of students, patients, and staff, interdisciplinary consultants and colleagues, researchers, and entrepreneurs (Leininger, 2000).
   B. The transcultural nurse serves as an advocate, leader, mentor, role model, collaborator, and scholar Seisser, 2002.
   C. Certification in transcultural nursing is one means of validating the knowledge, skills, and experience required to provide culturally competent health care.

II. Attributes of a Transcultural Nurse
   A. Advocate
      1. Cultural Brokering on behalf of clients
         a. A cultural broker is one who is familiar with the values, practices, and beliefs of two or more cultures; he or she works to foster understanding between peoples of different cultures, enhancing their interaction with one another by translating, interpreting, and breaking down each culture's own nuances and rich points (Singh, McKay, & Singh, 1999).
         b. For a patient or client, the benefits of positively working with a cultural broker can include a better outlook toward the health care system and practices, a feeling of mutual respect and consideration, a desire from the hospital to provide and maintain linguistic and culturally competent care, and a desire from the patient to continue care as well as an interest in preventative measures and overall general health (National Center for Cultural Competence, 2004).
      2. Negotiation with managed care systems
         a. Managed care programs include "[h]ealth insurance plans intended to reduce unnecessary health care costs through a variety of mechanisms, including: economic incentives for physicians and patients to select less costly forms of care; programs for reviewing the medical necessity of specific services; increased beneficiary cost sharing; controls on inpatient admissions and lengths of stay; the establishment of cost-sharing incentives for outpatient surgery; selective contracting with health care providers; and the intensive management of high-cost health care cases" (National Library of Medicine, 1990).
         b. As cultural brokers and advocates for patients, the nurse can work with managed care systems to provide quality care that is cost effective.
      3. Advocacy for cultural competent/congruent care by other professionals and staff
         a. Community health workers of all kinds, including *promotoras* (health promoters), natural healers, doulas, lay health advisers, and frontline workers also need to be culturally competent.
         b. The role of a community health worker is comprehensive in scope and can include increasing access to care as well as providing health services ranging from health education and immunization to complex clinical procedures (Perez & Martinez, 2008).

Funding: The California Endowment (grant number 20082226) and Health Resources and Services Administration (grant number D11 HPO9759).
[1]Fordham University, Cliffside, NJ USA (Transcultural Nurse as an Advocate, Role Model, Entrepreneur, and in Policy Development)
[2]State University of New York, SUNY Downstate Medical Center, Brooklyn, NY, USA (Leadership Roles: Collaboration, Scholarship, Evidence-based Practice, Credentialing & Certification; The Transcultural Nurse as an Educator and Researcher)
[3]College of New Rochelle, New Rochelle, NY USA (The Mentoring Role of the Transcultural Nurse)

Corresponding Author: Stephen R. Marrone, Email: stephen.marrone@downstate.edu.

Suggested Citation: Douglas, M. K. & Pacquiao, D. F. (Eds.). (2010). Core curriculum in transcultural nursing and health care [Supplement]. *Journal of Transcultural Nursing, 21*(Suppl. 1).

    4. ***Preventing and combating bias, prejudice and stereotypes***

       a. Any comprehensive theory or practice of transcultural nursing must be culture inclusive and holistic in nature.

       b. Transcultural nurses must be able to clearly identify the different scientific and political issues that surround culture so that they can provide unbiased care and accurately articulate policy decisions regarding prevention of prejudice and stereotyping.

       c. Transcultural training is necessary to embrace the knowledge and practice in transforming others and the organization toward respect for cultural differences and cultural competence.

    5. ***Cultural competent/congruent care for vulnerable populations***

       a. Refugees, asylum seekers, the underrepresented, the uninsured, and those with limited economic means are also examples of client groups that need to be respected, included, and understood.

       b. Caution is needed when attempting to revise policies to accommodate one cultural group as it may result in the exclusion of another.

    6. ***Legal implications of culturally based practices***

       a. Legal restrictions may limit accommodation of culturally based practices, such as female circumcision or coin rubbing of a sick newborn. However, an attitude of cultural imposition needs to be avoided.

       b. Cultural imposition refers to the tendency to impose one's own values, beliefs, and practices on another culture because they are believed to be superior to or better than those of another group or individual.

    7. ***Ethical Practice***

       a. Ethics can be defined as a set of moral principles concerning how individuals and/or groups should behave.

       b. Common ethical dilemmas encountered in practice are usually negotiated based on the dominant culture's legal and ethical protocols. Advanced directives, informed consent, and Health Insurance Portability and Accountability Act directives are examples of protocols that are largely based on individual autonomy that is valued in individualistic cultures but are contrary to the collective ethos of other cultural groups.

       c. An ethical practice entails one that is sensitive to cultural differences in health beliefs and incorporates the patient's wishes and cultural perspectives into the plan of care (Maier-Lorentz, 2008).

B. Leadership

    1. ***Mentoring***

       a. The mentor connection is a developmental, empowering, and nurturing relationship among colleagues, extending over time in which mutual sharing, learning, and growth occur in an atmosphere of respect, collegiality, and affirmation (Vance & Olson, 1998).

       b. Mentors influence the profession by serving as teachers, professional guides, professional and transcultural role models, and advocates to students, peers, and colleagues throughout the nursing career.

       c. Mentoring is an essential leadership role and activity (Kosininen & Tossavainen, 2003).

         (1) The leader-mentor plays a crucial developmental role in the professional-cultural socialization of students and colleagues.

         (2) The leader-mentor is actively involved in the personal and career growth and development of their protégés.

         (3) The leader-mentor influences the principles and practice of transcultural nursing in academe, the workplace, and associations in local and global communities.

       d. Mentors have a professional privilege and obligation to develop and promote transcultural awareness, education, and competency of the nurse, the profession, the organizational workplace, and communities. This should occur locally and globally and through the preparation of culturally competent nurses in every specialty area of the profession.

       e. Importance of mentoring for the nurse, profession, and workplace.

         (1) Professional nurse

           (a) Career success and satisfaction

           (b) Professional and personal confidence

           (c) Cultural/transcultural awareness in profession, organizational workplace, and community

           (d) Career and leadership role socialization and preparation

         (2) Nursing profession

           (a) Knowledge development, research, and innovation

      (b) Excellence in nursing education, practice, and research
      (c) Leadership development and succession
      (d) Commitment and bonding to the profession
      (e) Establishment of networks, mentor connections, and associations (e.g., transcultural)
    (3) Organizational workplace
      (a) Culture of learning and development
      (b) Exemplary professional and transcultural nursing practice
      (c) Empowerment of professional potential and talent
      (d) Legacy of organizational leadership and nursing practice
  f. Components of the mentor connection
    (1) Relationship. Mentors and protégés share a relationship of trust and reciprocal growth and development. Mentor-leaders influence and transmit the cultural values, beliefs, attitudes, and behaviors of the profession and the organizational workplace through personal and professional relationships.
    (2) Partnership. Mentors and protégés are professional partners and colleagues who engage in mutual teaching and learning to improve cultural competence in nursing practice; strengthen professional values, ethics, and standards; and enhance cultural awareness and competence in the profession and the workplace on behalf of patients and colleagues.
    (3) Networking. Mentors and protégés establish and share networks that promote access and connections to persons and associations, and expand sociocultural-based information, education, and practice.
    (4) Advocacy. Mentor-leaders support and protect colleagues and protégés by establishing cultural environments that promote empowerment and autonomy and excellence in nursing practice.
  g. Mentor-leader as culture guide in:
    (1) The profession
      (a) Embodies the cultural values, beliefs, and attitudes of the profession
      (b) Serves as an exemplar of excellence and cultural competence in professional practice and service
    (2) Students, professional nurses, and other colleagues
      (a) Transmits the culture of the profession to students and colleagues through role modeling, guidance, and teaching
      (b) Employs personal and professional networks to expand connections among nurses for information sharing, career development, and change activity
    (3) The organizational workplace
      (a) Promotes cultural competence in nursing practice, research, and patient care policies and service
      (b) Establishes a culture of mentorship and transcultural nursing and health care throughout the organization
    (4) The community
      (a) Establishes partnerships with community organizations, community leaders, and policy makers to support and build healthy communities (Davis, 1997)
      (b) Develops culturally competent community-based educational, health care delivery, and research initiatives (Andrews & Boyle, 2008)
  h. The culture of mentorship
    (1) Local contexts
      (a) Mentoring occurs in individual (dyadic) and collective relationships in academic, workplace, professional association, and community settings.
      (b) Local mentoring is based on the models of novice to expert and peer-to-peer relationships or a blend of both.
    (2) Global contexts
      (a) Transcultural global mentoring is characterized by a diversity of partnerships and collaborative linkages across many types of boundaries.
      (b) Global mentoring relationships are challenged by communication, distance, social, cultural and language differences, politics, and economics.

(c) Personal, professional, and social change occur through cross-cultural mentoring that provides transformation in perspectives, knowledge, skills, and attitudes (Morales-Mann & Higuchi, 1995)

    i. Education for mentoring and transcultural nursing cultures

        (1) Theoretical

            (a) Use of descriptive, anecdotal, and research-based literature

            (b) Offering academic and staff education courses and programs in mentoring

        (2) Experiential

            (a) Fostering traditional mentor relationships and formal mentoring programs in academic and workplace settings

            (b) Linking with professional associations offering mentor programs to their constituent members and in partnership with other associations

            (c) Mentoring at every career stage necessary for every student and nurse

        (3) Research

            (a) Extensive body of anecdotal and research data in mentorship and transcultural nursing cultures

            (b) Collaborative mentorship model supports scholarship and research activities

2. Role Modeling

    a. Role modeling theory encompasses five different components:

        (1) building trust

        (2) promoting positive orientation

        (3) promoting perceived control

        (4) promoting strengths

        (5) setting health-directed mutual goals

    b. Role modeling theory can be actualized using Maslow's Hierarchy of Needs

        (1) physiological

        (2) safety

        (3) love and belonging

        (4) esteem

        (5) self-actualization

3. Collaboration

    a. Collaboration refers to a recursive process in which two or more people, groups, or organizations work together toward achieving mutually agreed on common goals for the purposes of

        (1) an intellectual endeavor

        (2) sharing knowledge

        (3) learning

        (4) building consensus

        (5) sharing resources

    b. Internal and external partnerships with key stakeholders are critical elements to collaboration.

    c. Internal partnerships are accomplished by conducting a five-step Cultural Assessment Process (Andrews, 1998) to:

        (1) "Gather demographic and descriptive data by identifying the prevalent cultural, ethnic, linguistic, and spiritual groups represented among patients, families, visitors, the community, and staff and describing the effectiveness of current systems and processes in meeting diverse needs;

        (2) Assess the organization's strengths and limitations by examining the institution's ethos toward cultural diversity and the presence or absence of a corporate culture that promotes accord among its constituents;

        (3) Determine organizational need and readiness for change through dialogue with key stakeholders aimed at discovering foci of anticipated support and recognizing areas of potential resistance;

        (4) Implement the change by developing a strategic plan that includes measurable benchmarks of success and an ongoing process to ensure that change is maintained; and

        (5) Evaluate the change by measuring actual outcomes against established benchmarks utilizing performance improvement and satisfaction data" (Andrews, 1998, pp. 62–66.).

    d. External partnerships include drivers, linkages, cultures, and measurements (Frusti, Niesen, & Campion, 2003).

      (1) Drivers

        (a) Key drivers include the integration of multiculturalism into the organizational infrastructure and collaboration among the nursing diversity committee, nursing recruitment and retention committee, and transcultural patient care committee.

        (b) Committee memberships should reflect a conscious effort to enlist nurses from minority cultures and subcultures.

      (2) Linkages

        (a) Linkages "examine how the organization integrates diversity throughout all levels of the workplace" (Frusti et al., 2003, p. 33).

        (b) Interdepartmental and intradepartmental linkages must establish an internal network for cooperative decision making and collective understanding of diversity issues throughout the organization.

        (c) External linkages are achieved by collaborating with minority nursing organizations and advertising in nursing journals reflective of the diversity within the internal and external communities.

      (3) Cultures

        (a) Culture "describes how the organization creates a work environment that reinforces behaviors" (Frusti et al., 2003, p. 33).

        (b) Respect for diversity must be integrated into all aspects of corporate culture.

      (4) Measurements

        (a) Measurements "examine how the organization evaluates and improves toward continuous progress and business results" (Frusti et al., 2003, p. 33).

        (b) Quantitative and qualitative data must be aggregated to establish a diversity database used to track and trend issues related to demographic indicators, cultural and generational diversity, recruitment and retention patterns, cost, and employee and patient satisfaction, thereby providing a feedback mechanism for continued improvement (Frusti et al., 2003).

    e. International partnerships expand the scope of influence of transcultural nurses through joint ventures in grassroots projects, policy development, and humanitarian efforts. Notable international agencies include:

      (1) International Council of Nurses (ICN; http://www.icn.ch/)

      (2) Sigma Theta Tau International (STTI; http://www.nursingsociety.org)

      (3) European Transcultural Nurses Association (ETNA; http://etna.middlesex.wikispaces.net/)

      (4) United Nations (http://www.un.org/)

      (5) Direct Relief International (http://www.directrelief.org)

      (6) Hope for a Healthier Humanity (http://www.hopeforahealthierhumanity.org/)

      (7) Transcultural Nursing Society (TCNS) (http://www.tcns.org)

    f. Community partnerships with community, cultural, and spiritual leaders and natural/lay healers, application of knowledge of community resources, and advocacy with managed care agencies enable transcultural nurses to reduce health disparities, improve access to care, and enhance client self-advocacy and self-efficacy.

4. *Scholarship*

    a. Scholars seek knowledge.

    b. Scholarship in nursing combines theory, research, philosophy, and practice (Meleis, 2007).

    c. Scholarship is the foundation of the discipline of transcultural nursing.

    d. The four components of scholarship include discovery, integration, application, and teaching (Boyer, 2008).

      (1) Transcultural nurses seek new knowledge and evidence for practice through original research and scientific inquiry using qualitative, quantitative ethnonursing, and triangulation research methodologies.

      (2) Transcultural nurses integrate the findings of original research (evidence), combined with clinical judgment and client preferences, through formal and informal channels by influencing organizations to adopt innovations in culture care practice(s) and translate practice changes into sustainable systems.

        (3) Transcultural nurses apply research findings (evidence-based practice [EBP]) as they fit with the culture care needs of patients, families, and communities and evaluate the impact of the evidence on health outcomes, provider and client satisfaction, efficacy, efficiency, cost, and health status impact.

        (4) Transcultural nurses teach patients, families, communities, organizations, and staff in formal and informal settings using best culture care practices derived from the process of scholarly inquiry.

  e. Evidence-based practice

        (1) EBP includes the application and integration of research evidence with clinical expertise and patient values (Sackett, Straus, & Richardson, 2000).

        (2) Nursing practice based on evidence is more likely to result in desired outcomes across various care settings and geographic locations (Youngblut & Brooten, 2001).

        (3) EBP requires changes in education of students and practitioners, more practice relevant research, and collaborative partnerships between clinicians and researchers.

        (4) EBP provides opportunities for individualized nursing care that is effective, streamlined, and dynamic that maximizes clinical judgment and critical thinking (Youngblut & Brooten, 2001).

5. *Policy Development*: Developing and implementing effective culturally competent policies depends on adequately trained, empowered, and proactive nurses who promote collaboration between health institutions and local communities.

  a. Local level

        (1) Proper training in culturally competent care and business and policy planning are necessary

        (2) Strengthening community-based initiatives

  b. Regional and national levels

        (1) Cross-cultural partnerships and collaboration are key to successful policy development

        (2) Policy development should focus on strengthening community support services and locally developed implementation models.

  c. International levels

        (1) Collaborations and strategic partnerships between different international organizations and communities necessary in international policy should be a global initiative.

        (2) Continued reinforcement of nurse empowerment and leadership for effective policy development and its implementation on the ground.

6. *Credentialing and Certification*

  a. Credentialing refers to the official recognition by a professional discipline or an organization of a practitioner's professional or technical competence as validated through registration, certification, licensure, admission as a member into a professional or clinical specialty association, and/or the award of an academic degree or diploma.

        (1) Registration and licensure ensure the legal right to practice a professional discipline.

        (2) Registration and licensure requirements for practice vary depending on the country, state, province, or jurisdiction.

  b. Certification refers to the formal recognition of the specialized knowledge, skills, and experience by the achievement of standards identified by a nursing specialty to promote optimal outcomes for patients, families, communities, and/or populations (American Board of Nursing Specialties [ABNS], 2008; National Organization for Competency Assurance [NOCA], 2008).

  c. Recertification ensures health care consumers that certified nurses have maintained a level of knowledge and competency in the nursing specialty by meeting rigorous practice and continuing education requirements (ABNS, 2008).

  d. Transcultural nursing certification "aims to validate the ability to provide culturally competent and congruent care to clients, families, communities, and organizations" (Transcultural Nursing Certification Commission [TCNCC], in press).

  e. The purposes of transcultural nursing certification and recertification are to:

        (1) promote and maintain safe and culturally meaningful care with the aim of protecting individuals, groups and communities;

        (2) recognize the expertise of transcultural nurses prepared to care for clients of diverse and similar cultures; and

        (3) provide quality-based standards of transcultural nursing practices (TCNCC, in press).

f. Benefits of transcultural nursing certification
   (1) Improved public safety
   (2) Improved patient outcomes (American Association of Critical Care Nurses, 2002, 2003; Cary, 2001; Institute of Medicine [IOM], 2002)
      (a) Increased compliance with treatment plans
      (b) Decreased recidivism
      (c) Decreased emergency department visits and hospital readmissions
      (d) Decreased health care costs
   (3) Improved patient satisfaction (IOM, 2002)
      (a) Cultural and linguistic concordance between patients and practitioners
      (b) Culturally sensitive care
      (c) Increased access to care
      (d) Increased quality of care
   (4) Culture care needs of diverse patients, families, communities, and populations are met.
   (5) Diverse learning needs of students are met.
   (6) Evidence of competence and clinical expertise based on the Domains of Transcultural Nursing Practice (TCNCC, in press)
   (7) Recognition and validation of transcultural nurses' contributions in the provision of culturally competent care to consumers
   (8) Recognition and acceptance by governing boards, accrediting agencies, insurers, and the military (American Nurses Credentialing Center [ANCC], 2008)
   (9) Certified nurses are in greater demand and command higher salaries (ANCC, 2008).
  (10) Nurse empowerment, pride, and accomplishment from mastering specialized practice knowledge and skills

g. Nursing Specialty Certification
   (1) Eligibility criteria for certification and recertification vary as they reflect the knowledge and competency requirements specific to each nursing specialty practice.
   (2) Criteria typically include:
      (a) unrestricted license or registration as a registered nurse (RN; as per country of origin)
      (b) minimum hours of clinical practice in the specialty within 2 to 3 years prior to certification
         i. hours of clinical practice frequently vary and are in relation to level of academic preparation in nursing
      (c) minimum level of academic preparation in nursing
      (d) specified number of continuing education or contact hours in specialty within 2 to 3 years prior to certification/recertification
   (3) Certification in advanced transcultural nursing is achieved by (TCNCC, in press):
      (a) Meeting all eligibility criteria
         i. Current, active, unrestricted RN license in a state or territory of the United States or the professional, legally recognized equivalent in another country
         ii. Master's, postmaster's, or doctorate in nursing, education, philosophy, or related field from an accredited nursing program or legally recognized equivalent in another country
         iii. Employed in nursing
         iv. Completed one 3-credit course (contact hour equivalent) in cultural diversity or cultural competency
         v. Completed 2400 hours of transcultural nursing practice as a RN prior to submitting application
         vi. Refer to www.tcns.org for most current information
      (b) Completion of the application packet
      (c) Submission of required application fee
      (d) Submission of a professional portfolio that includes evidence of
         i. Professional growth in transcultural nursing
         ii. Creative and innovative ways to promote and maintain transcultural nursing practice
         iii. Transcultural nursing research
         iv. Substantive or unique contributions made to advance transcultural nursing
         v. Leadership in teaching, research, or consultation to improve care in diverse cultures

(e) Successful completion of a written examination

(f) Credential awarded (CTN-A)

  i. Length of initial certification: 5 years

  ii. Length of recertification: 5 years

(g) Credential awarded by the TCNCC

(4) Certification in basic transcultural nursing is achieved by (TCNCC, in press):

(a) Meeting all eligibility criteria

  i. Current, active, unrestricted RN license in a state or territory of the United States or the professional, legally recognized equivalent in another country

  ii. Diploma, associate, or baccalaureate degree in nursing or legally recognized equivalent in another country

  iii. Employed in nursing

  iv. Completed one 3-credit course (contact hour equivalent) in cultural diversity or cultural competency

  v. Completed 2,400 hours of transcultural nursing practice as a RN prior to submitting application

  vi. Refer to www.tcns.org for most current information

(b) Completion of the application packet

(c) Submission of required application fee

(d) Successful completion of a written examination

(e) Credential awarded (CTN-B)

  i. Length of initial certification: 5 years

  ii. Length of recertification: 5 years

(f) Credential awarded by the TCNCC

(5) Notable nurse certifying/accrediting/credentialing agencies

(a) ABNS (http://www.nursingcertification.org)

(b) ANCC (http://www.nursecredentialing.org)

(c) NOCA (http://www.noca.org;USA)

(d) National Commission for Certifying Agencies (http://www.noca.org/Resources/NCCA Accreditation; USA)

(e) Canadian Nurses Association (http://www.cna-nurses.ca/cna/)

(f) Royal College of Nursing, Australia (http://www.rcna.org.au/site/)

(g) Royal College of Nursing, United Kingdom (http://www.rcna.org.uk)

(h) European Council of Nursing Regulators (http://www.fepi.org)

III. ROLES OF TRANSCULTURAL NURSES

A. Educator

1. As a socially responsible discipline, transcultural nursing requires both formal and informal educational processes that are designed to ensure the initial and continuing competency of its practitioners (Jeffreys, 2006).

2. Regardless of their primary roles and responsibilities, all nurses are educators.

3. Transcultural nurses serve as educators to patients, families, communities, staff, and students in both formal and informal settings.

4. A "formal" description of the nurse educator is an RN (or recognized equivalent depending on country) who has advanced academic preparation and experience in a clinical nursing specialty as well as demonstrated mastery of the principles of adult learning, educational design, curriculum development, test design, and evaluation of educational outcomes (National League for Nursing [NLN], 2008).

5. Academic (educational) and experiential requirements for the nurse educator role vary depending on country and setting.

6. Transcultural nurse educators design, implement, and evaluate learning activities that

   a. Enable learners (students and practitioners alike) to meet the culture care needs of diverse patients, families, communities, and populations

   b. Facilitate engagement of learners who are culturally, spiritually, linguistically, and generationally diverse

   c. Ensure that staff and patient learning materials are culturally appropriate

   d. Ensure that patient education materials reflect an awareness of linguistic and health literacy levels

7. Global influences that affect nursing education and the educator role include
   a. "Specialization in nursing cultural backgrounds, changes in educational levels, and other demographic characteristics of nursing adult learners;
   b. Changes in demographic characteristics of health care consumer populations; and
   c. Political, social, economic, legislative, and regulatory requirements" (American Nurses Association [ANA], 2000).
8. Nurse educators serve in a variety of formal roles and settings:
   a. Academic and/or clinical faculty in college of nursing
      (1) Dean/administrator/chairperson
      (2) Professorial role (professor, associate professor, assistant professor)
      (3) Adjunct
      (4) Lecturer
      (5) Clinical instructor
   b. Health care organizations
      (1) Director of nursing education
      (2) Nurse educator/education specialist
      (3) Staff development educator
      (4) Continuing education specialist
9. Roles and responsibilities
   a. Nurse educators in the academic setting (NLN, 2008)
      (1) Facilitate, teach, and guide undergraduate and graduate student learning
      (2) Facilitate student learner development and socialization
      (3) Advise students
      (4) Assist students to identify their own learning needs and learning opportunities to meet those needs
      (5) Use assessment and evaluation strategies
      (6) Participate in curriculum design, course and program development, and evaluation of program outcomes
      (7) Pursue continuous quality improvement in the academic nurse educator role
      (8) Engage in scholarship, service, and leadership
   b. Nurse educators in health care organizations (ANA, 2000)
      (1) Educator role (staff education and patient education)
         (a) Provide an appropriate learning environment and facilitate adult learning that respects learners as practicing clinicians (also applies to the teaching of graduate nursing students in the academic setting)
         (b) Ensure learners are actively engaged in the assessment of learning needs and outcomes by establishing the *need to know*
         (c) Evaluate the effectiveness of the learning outcomes in clinical practice
      (2) Facilitator role: facilitate learner identification of learning needs and effective learning strategies to meet those needs
      (3) Change agent role: leadership and participation in nursing and health care associations and facilitating evidence-based sustained practice, policy, and legislative changes at the local, regional, national, and international levels
      (4) Consultant role (formal or informal)
         (a) Assist with the integration of new learning and best practice into the practice environment
         (b) Serve on unit-based, departmental, and/or organizational committees, councils, and task forces
      (5) Researcher role
         (a) Integrate relevant evidence into the design of educational programs and clinical practice requirements
         (b) Facilitate the development of staff knowledge and skills in the research process
         (c) Serve as principal or coinvestigator in the research process
      (6) Leader role: serve as role models in the achievement of departmental and organizational goals
   c. Informal educator roles
      (1) Informal learning typically occurs outside of the classroom and includes bedside teaching, *just-in-time* teaching, mentoring, and self-directed learning.

   (2) Informal educator roles and activities include
    (a) Preceptorship
    (b) Mentorship
    (c) Participation in committees that affect clinical practice and affect the health of clients
    (d) Attendance at community groups and organizations such as schools, houses of worship, local cultural
  d. Educators in academic settings and organizational settings frequently partner for the purposes of student clinical practice and research projects and initiatives.

B. Researcher
 1. The goal of transcultural nursing research is to gain in-depth and substantive transcultural nursing knowledge and to evaluate effective, culturally competent nursing care practices.
 2. Research dissemination and utilization must be planned.
 3. Transcultural nurses test research methodologies associated with underserved, vulnerable, and/or misunderstood populations.
 4. Research utilization refers to the purpose of the research and to the intended impact on the end user.
 5. Research dissemination refers to the process of knowledge transfer from the knowledge source to the intended recipient of the knowledge.
 6. Search engines that are useful for transcultural nurses to locate culturally relevant knowledge sources include
  a. CINAHL (Cumulative Index of Nursing and Allied Health Literature; http://www.ebscohost.com/cinahl/)
  b. PubMed (http://www.ncbi.nlm.nih.gov/pubmed/)
  c. Medline (http://medlineplus.gov/)
  d. Embase (http://www.embase.com/)
  e. Cochrane Database of Systematic Reviews (http://www.cochrane.org/)
  f. U.S. Veterans Administration/Department of Defense National Guideline Clearinghouse (http://www.guideline.gov/summary/summary.aspx?doc_id=9907)
  g. Joanne Briggs Institute (Australia; http://www.joannabriggs.edu.au/about/home.php)
  h. Social science database
 7. Utilization of research
  a. Transcultural nurses utilize research through the implementation of evidence-based best practices for the care of patients, families, communities, and populations and for the education of staff and students
  b. Research utilization is evidenced by
   (1) Educational and clinical practice policies, procedures, care practices, performance criteria, and learning outcomes based on evidence derived from
    (a) systematic reviews and meta analyses
    (b) research that generates substantive culture care knowledge regarding a particular culture or subculture
    (c) systematic evaluation of culture-based interventions
    (d) expert opinion
   (2) Integration of best evidence into educational program curricula for the initial education of students and continuing competency of practitioners
   (3) Improved health outcomes of vulnerable and underserved populations
 8. Dissemination: Research dissemination is evidenced by
  a. Publication(s) in refereed nursing research journals, such as *Journal of Transcultural Nursing*
  b. Publication of findings in nursing texts
  c. Presentation (oral/poster) at local, regional, national, and international professional nursing conferences, workshops, and professional meetings
 9. Research priorities
  a. Transcultural nursing research priorities are derived from the culture care needs that are affected by global changes in health, migration, emigration/immigration, pandemics, and human rights.
  b. Research priorities, as identified by governmental agencies and private foundations. A few examples of these priorities are:

(1) Minority and vulnerable populations
  (a) women
  (b) children
  (c) indigenous populations
  (d) people affected/displaced by war or disaster
  (e) gay/lesbian, transgender, transsexual
  (f) uneducated/illiterate, low health literacy
(2) Eliminating health disparities
  (a) improved access
  (b) improved quality
  (c) improved outcomes
(3) Culture care needs of subcultures, such as racial minorities
(4) Cultural and linguistic concordance/discordance
  (a) the influence of provider–client concordance on health care processes and outcomes
  (b) the influence of provider–client concordance on access to health care and compliance with medical regimens
  (c) the influence of linguistic discordance on health care processes and outcomes
  (d) the relationship between provider and client attitudes toward each other in both concordant and discordant relationships
  (e) the influence of cost on access to care, satisfaction with health care provided, and health outcomes among minority clients as compared to the Whites (or the majority population)

10. Proposals and Projects (Polit & Hungler, 1999)
  a. Research Proposal format
    (1) Introduction
    (2) Statement of the problem
    (3) Significance of the problem
    (4) Review of the literature—including gaps
    (5) Purpose of the study (addressing gaps in knowledge)
    (6) Research hypotheses or questions
    (7) Methods
      (a) Design
      (b) Sampling
        i.   Selection of site
        ii. Procure access of participants
        iii. Inclusion criteria
        iv. Exclusion criteria
      (c) Data collection procedures
      (d) Protection of human research subjects/participants
      (e) Data analysis
    (8) Findings
    (9) Discussion and conclusions
    (10) Implications for future research
    (11) Implication for practice
  b. Projects (Gilbert, 2003a, 2003b, 2003c)
    (1) U.S. Department of Health and Human Resources Health Resources and Services Administration (HRSA)
      (a) increase nursing workforce diversity
      (b) increase cultural competency of nursing workforce
      (c) benefit rural and underserved populations
      (d) HRSA and TCNS grant Cultural Competency Train-the-Trainer (www.tcns.org)
      (e) For grant opportunities (www.grants.gov)
    (2) U.S. National Institute for Nursing Research
      (a) eliminate health disparities
      (b) for grant opportunities see (http://www.ninr.nih.gov/)

(3) Additional sources of grant funding to initiate and sustain transcultural nursing research and organizational cultural competency programs
    (a) The California Endowment (www.calendow.org)
    (b) U.S. National Institute of Health (http://www.nih.gov/)
    (c) STTI (www.nursingsociety.org)
    (d) http://www.nursingsociety.org/Research/Small Grants/
    (e) NLN (http://www.nln.org/research/index.htm)
    (f) Specialty nursing organization seed grants
(4) Association for Common European Nursing Diagnoses, Interventions, and Outcomes (http://www.acendio.net/education/html)

C. Entrepreneur

1. A common definition of a nurse entrepreneur is a nurse who chooses to work independently and directly with patients in a private practice (Elango, Phil, & Hunter, 2006; Faugier, 2005; Sankelo & Akerblad, 2008). However, this overlooks the entrepreneur's ability to be innovative within the field (Drucker, 1985; Faugier, 2005).

2. According to Drucker (1985), "Entrepreneurs create something new—something different—[they] change values" (p. 21).

3. Nurse entrepreneurs, then, reimagine nursing practices, ethics, and culture, always improving their methods to individual patients and/or issues.

4. Employee innovation behavior and leadership abilities are precursors to successful nurse entrepreneurship.

5. New venture creation

6. Advancement through entrepreneurship. If nurses can broaden their scope of "spheres of influence" to include all facets of the health care industry, they simultaneously can facilitate better policy development and collaboration while improving their own professional status and demands.

IV. SUMMARY

A. Transcultural nurses are specialists, generalists, and consultants, educators, and researchers who practice in diverse clinical, academic, community, and organizational settings.

B. By means of their diverse roles, transcultural nurses influence nursing education, practice and health care policy development by improving health outcomes and minimizing health disparities among vulnerable and diverse patients, families, communities, populations, and staff.

NOTE: All references, additional resources, and important Internet sites relevant to this chapter can be found at the following website: http://tcn.sagepub.com/supplemental